HANDBOOK OF

Geriatric
Assessment

FIFTH EDITION

The John A. Hartford Foundation
Dedicated to Improving the Care of Older Adults

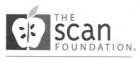

Transforming Care for Older Adults

EDITED BY

Terry Fulmer, PhD, RN, FAAN
President, The John A. Hartford Foundation

Bruce Chernof, MD, FACP
President, The Scan Foundation

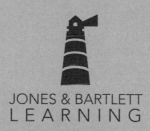

JONES & BARTLETT
LEARNING

World Headquarters
Jones & Bartlett Learning
5 Wall Street
Burlington, MA 01803
978-443-5000
info@jblearning.com
www.jblearning.com

Jones & Bartlett Learning books and products are available through most bookstores and online booksellers. To contact Jones & Bartlett Learning directly, call 800-832-0034, fax 978-443-8000, or visit our website, www.jblearning.com.

Substantial discounts on bulk quantities of Jones & Bartlett Learning publications are available to corporations, professional associations, and other qualified organizations. For details and specific discount information, contact the special sales department at Jones & Bartlett Learning via the above contact information or send an email to specialsales@jblearning.com.

Production Credits

VP, Product Management: David D. Cella
Director of Product Management: Amanda Martin
Product Manager: Teresa Reilly
Product Assistant: Anna-Maria Forger
Production Manager: Carolyn Rogers Pershouse
Production Editor: Kelly Sylvester
Director of Marketing: Andrea DeFronzo
Marketing Communications Manager: Katie Hennessy
Production Services Manager: Colleen Lamy

Product Fulfillment Manager: Wendy Kilborn
Composition: S4Carlisle Publishing Services
Cover Design: Kristin E. Parker
Director of Rights & Media: Joanna Gallant
Rights & Media Specialist: Wes DeShano
Rights & Media Specialist: John Rusk
Media Development Editor: Troy Liston
Printing and Binding: Edwards Brothers Malloy
Cover Printing: Edwards Brothers Malloy

Library of Congress Cataloging-in-Publication Data

Names: Fulmer, Terry T., editor. | Chernof, Bruce, editor.
Title: Handbook of geriatric assessment / [edited] by Terry Fulmer, Bruce Chernof.
Description: Fifth edition. | Burlington, Massachusetts : Jones & Bartlett
  Learning, [2019] | Includes bibliographical references and index.
Identifiers: LCCN 2018007485 | ISBN 9781284144307 (paperback)
Subjects: | MESH: Geriatric Assessment
Classification: LCC RC953 | NLM WT 30 | DDC 618.97/075--dc23
LC record available at https://lccn.loc.gov/2018007485

6048

Printed in the United States of America
22 21 20 19 18   10 9 8 7 6 5 4 3 2 1

*Dedicated in loving memory to
my Aunt Mary, 1921–2015.*

–TF

Brief Contents

Preface   xiv

Contributors   xvi

Acknowledgments   xxiii

Chapter 1   Through the Older Person's Eyes: What Matters 1

Chapter 2   The Context and Future of Geriatric Care 9

Chapter 3   Demographic Trends: A Success Story 19

Chapter 4   Age-Friendly Health Systems 31

Chapter 5   Payment Reform, Health System Transformation, and the Impact on Older Adults .41

Chapter 6   The VA Health System for Older Adults 49

Chapter 7   Following the Assessment Data—Whose Data Is It: Open Notes in Real Time 55

Chapter 8   Assessment and Care Plans That Support Goals That Matter to the Person 65

Chapter 9   Self-Care Self-Management 73

Chapter 10   The Family Context 81

Chapter 11   The Social Determinants of Health 89

Chapter 12   Multiculturalism and Geriatric Assessment 103

Chapter 13   Vulnerable Populations 115

Chapter 14   Targeting Older Persons for Optimal Team Care Outcomes 125

Chapter 15   Developing and Managing a High-Functioning Interprofessional Team 133

Chapter 16   Building on Geriatric Interdisciplinary Team Training (GITT) 141

Chapter 17   Community Team-Based Geriatric Care 149

Chapter 18   Effects of Team Care on Quality and Outcomes...... 157

Chapter 19   Evidence-Based Models in Action That Work 165

Chapter 20   Advance Care Planning 179

Chapter 21   Cognitive Assessment 185

Chapter 22   Depression Assessment and Other Mental Illnesses 197

Chapter 23   Recognizing Mistreatment in Older Adults 215

Chapter 24   Functional Assessment of Older Adults 231

Chapter 25   Physical Assessment 241

Chapter 26   Pain Assessment.............................. 265

Chapter 27   Caregiver Assessment 275

Chapter 28   Spiritual Assessment as a Key Component of Comprehensive Geriatric Care.................... 281

Chapter 29   Substance Use Assessment 291

Chapter 30   Medication Assessment in Older Adults 305

Chapter 31   Mobility Assessment 313

Chapter 32   Nutritional Assessment as a Key Component of Comprehensive Geriatric Care.................... 323

Chapter 33   Transitions of Care 331

Chapter 34   Assessment of Older Adults in Their Home 349

Chapter 35   Aging in Place: Transitional Housing and Supported Housing Models...................... 365

Chapter 36   Thriving in Community 373

Chapter 37   Geriatric Assessment in Nursing Homes 383

Chapter 38   Emergency Department Assessment at the Time
of Hospitalization 401

Chapter 39   The Older Adult Driver 417

Chapter 40   Advance Care Planning Through the Incorporation
of Values History Discussions 431

Chapter 41   Clinical Assessment of Older Persons with
Developmental Disabilities 447

Chapter 42   Assessing Disaster Preparedness and Response 461

Index   **473**

Contents

Preface . . . . **xiv**

Contributors . . . . **xvi**

Acknowledgments . . . . **xxiii**

Chapter 1 Through the Older Person's Eyes: What Matters **1**

Introduction 1

The Importance of Soliciting and Acting on
What Matters 3

Patient-Centered Versus Person-Centered:
Sources of Variation Are More Than
Just Medical 6

Summary 7

References 7

Chapter 2 The Context and Future of Geriatric Care **9**

Introduction 9

Historical Perspectives 14

Future Directions 15

Summary 17

References 17

Chapter 3 Demographic Trends: A Success Story **19**

Introduction 19

What Constitutes Healthy Aging? 20

Current and Projected Aging Population
Growth in the United States 20

Social and Economic Capital .21

Disparities in Health and Life Expectancy 22

Age-Friendly Cities and Communities:
A Movement to Maximize Participation,
Reduce Disparities, and Improve
Quality of Life 25

Conclusion 26

References 27

Chapter 4 Age-Friendly Health Systems **31**

Introduction 31

Defining Age-Friendly Health Systems 32

The Challenge 33

Aim, Purpose, and Expected Benefits 33

Methods 34

Scale-Up Design and Social Movement 36

Expected Next Steps 38

Summary 39

References 39

Chapter 5 Payment Reform, Health System Transformation, and the Impact on Older Adults . . . **41**

Introduction 41

Bigger Bundles
Are Better 42

Total Joints: Yesterday, Today, and Tomorrow 43

Summary 47

Acknowledgments 47

References 47

Chapter 6   The VA Health System for Older Adults 49

Introduction 49
Present State of Geriatric Evaluation in VA 52
Summary 54
References 54

Chapter 7   Following the Assessment Data—Whose Data Is It: Open Notes in Real Time 55

Introduction 55
Trends in Geriatric Access to Electronic
    Patient Portals 56
Current Best Practices 57
Future Possibilities 58
Challenges 59
Practical Application 61
Summary 61
References 62

Chapter 8   Assessment and Care Plans That Support Goals That Matter to the Person 65

Introduction 66
Contextual Frame of Older Adults with Complex
    Health and Social Care Needs 67
What Is Person-Centered Care and How Does
    It Relate to Assessment and Care Planning? 68
Timing and Nuance of Ascertaining Goals
    in the Assessment Process 69
Using Assessment Information for Care Planning . . .70
Summary 72
References 72

Chapter 9   Self-Care Self-Management . . . 73

Introduction 73
Self-Management and Older Adults 74
Self-Management Best Practices 75
Practice Challenges 77
Summary 77
References 78

Chapter 10   The Family Context 81

Introduction 81
Who Are the Family Caregivers of Older
    Adults and What Do They Do? 82
Value-Based Purchasing and Implications for
    Family Caregivers 84
Hospital Readmissions and the Family
    Caregiver 85
The CARE Act Brings Policy into Practice 85
Family Caregivers and Healthcare Professionals:
    Practice Challenges and Resources 86
Summary 87
References 87

Chapter 11   The Social Determinants of Health 89

Introduction 89
Access to Comprehensive Health Services 90
Poverty and Economic Stability 91
Food Insecurity 92
Housing and Neighborhood Settings 92
Discrimination Based on Race and Ethnicity 93
Social Isolation 94
Addressing the Social Determinants of Health . . .94
Summary 96
References 98

Chapter 12   Multiculturalism and Geriatric Assessment 103

Introduction 103
Heterogeneity Within Older Ethnic Minority
    Groups 104
Reliability, Validity, and Use of Instruments
    for Ethnic Minorities 105
Enhancing Communication with Ethnically
    Diverse Older Adults 106
Eliciting Beliefs and Attitudes About Illness 107
Selected Domains of Geriatric Assessment 107
Depression Assessment 109
Social and Economic Issues in Assessment 110
Summary 111
References 111

Chapter 13 Vulnerable Populations 115

Introduction. 115

Defining Vulnerability. 116

Understanding How Vulnerable Older Adults
    Get Their Care. 118

Using Assessment Data for Policymaking and
    Program Planning. 120

Programmatic Issues and Practice Challenges . . . 121

Summary. 122

References 122

**Chapter 14 Targeting Older Persons for
               Optimal Team Care
               Outcomes 125**

Introduction. 125

Epidemiological Challenges of Demographic
    Changes 126

The Changing Healthcare System
    and Practice Model 128

Older Adults Most Likely to Benefit
    from Team Care 129

Summary. 130

References 130

**Chapter 15 Developing and Managing
               a High-Functioning
               Interprofessional Team 133**

Introduction. 133

What Are Teams? 134

Evidence for the Effectiveness of Teams 134

Team Training 137

Summary. 139

References 139

**Chapter 16 Building on Geriatric
               Interdisciplinary Team
               Training (GITT) 141**

Introduction. 141

Why GITT-PC? 142

Implementation of GITT-PC. 145

Summary. 147

References 147

**Chapter 17 Community Team-Based
               Geriatric Care 149**

Introduction. 149

Targeting and Assessment 151

Models of Effective Community Team-Based
    Care for Older Adults 153

Summary. 153

References 154

**Chapter 18 Effects of Team Care on
               Quality and Outcomes 157**

Introduction. 157

Best Practices. 158

Practice Challenges. 161

Summary. 162

References 162

**Chapter 19 Evidence-Based Models in
               Action That Work. 165**

Introduction. 165

Geriatrics Models of Care 166

Strategies to Implement, Sustain, and
    Disseminate Geriatrics Models of Care. 175

Summary. 176

References 176

Chapter 20 Advance Care Planning. 179

Introduction. 179

Advance Directives 180

Why Is Advance Care Planning Important? 180

Best Practices in Advance Care Planning 182

Practice Challenges. 183

Summary. 184

References 184

Chapter 21 Cognitive Assessment. 185

Introduction. 185

Defining Dementia and Cognitive Impairment . . . 186

Differential Diagnosis 186

Pre-assessment Process. 187

Test Selection. 188

The Mental Status Examination 188
Standardized Brief Assessments. 192
Practical Considerations 193
Summary. 194
References 194

**Chapter 22   Depression Assessment and
Other Mental Illnesses 197**

Introduction. 197
Depression 198
Assessment of Late-Life Depressive
   Disorders 198
Challenges and Best Practices in Assessment. . . 205
Suicide 207
Differential Diagnosis 209
Recommendations for Practice 210
Summary. 211
References 212

**Chapter 23   Recognizing Mistreatment
in Older Adults. 215**

Introduction. 215
Scope and Consequences of EM. 216
EM Risk and Vulnerability 217
EM Assessment. 217
Documentation 221
Reporting to the Authorities 221
Tools for Formal Screening. 222
Practice Challenges. 226
Approach for Readers. 227
Summary. 227
References 227

**Chapter 24   Functional Assessment of
Older Adults 231**

Introduction. 231
Assessment and Best Practices. 232
Assessment Tools. 233
Functional Assessment: Case Exemplar. 237
Summary. 238
References 238

Chapter 25   Physical Assessment. 241

Introduction. 241
Approach to the Geriatric Patient 242
History Taking 243
Sexual Health Assessment 244
Physical Assessment. 247
Components of the Examination. 247
Practice Challenges. 261
Summary. 261
References 261

Chapter 26   Pain Assessment 265

Introduction. 265
Importance of Pain Assessment. 266
Best Assessment Practices 267
Practice Challenges: Barriers and Facilitators. . . . 270
Summary. 272
References 272

Chapter 27   Caregiver Assessment. 275

Introduction. 275
Why Caregiver Assessment Is Important:
   Demographics and Prevalence 276
Best Practices. 276
Where to Start. 277
Practice Challenges. 278
Summary. 278
References 279

**Chapter 28   Spiritual Assessment as a Key
Component of Comprehensive
Geriatric Care. 281**

Introduction. 281
Spirituality and Health Outcomes 282
Spiritual Assessment. 282
Spiritual Screening Tools 283
Practice Challenges in Performing a Spiritual
   Assessment 285
Which Tool to Use? 286
Summary. 287
References 288

Chapter 29 Substance Use Assessment 291

Introduction. 291
Screening, Brief Intervention, and Referral
   for Treatment: A Best Practice. 294
Screening 294
A Brief Discussion of Brief Intervention 298
Practice Challenges. 300
Summary. 300
References 300

Chapter 30 Medication Assessment in Older Adults. 305

Introduction. 305
Importance of Polypharmacy 306
Medication Assessment Tools. 306
Challenges 310
Summary. 311
References 311

Chapter 31 Mobility Assessment. 313

Introduction. 313
Mobility: Definition and Epidemiology 314
Measures of Mobility. 314
Clinical Characteristics 317
Intent of the Measure. 317
Challenges 319
Summary. 320
References 320

Chapter 32 Nutritional Assessment as a Key Component of Comprehensive Geriatric Care. 323

Introduction. 323
Why Under-nutrition Is Common in
   Older Adults 324
Health Outcomes from Under-nutrition 326
Nutritional Assessment and Assessment
   Tools. 327

Summary. 329
References 329

Chapter 33 Transitions of Care 331

Introduction. 331
Key Factors That Contribute to Poor Care
   Transitions 332
Models of Care Transitions in the Era of
   Value-Based Care. 332
Patient Assessment in the Context of
   Transitional Care Models. 336
Patient Assessments 336
Summary. 345
Additional Resources for Healthcare
   Professionals 346
References 346

Chapter 34 Assessment of Older Adults in Their Home 349

Introduction. 349
Why Is In-Home Assessment Important? 350
Best Practices. 351
Assessment Domains: Priorities for the
   Home Visit 352
Practice Challenges. 355
Sample Assessment Tool or Approach 357
Assessing the Geriatric Population Living
   with Homelessness 362
Summary. 363
References 364

Chapter 35 Aging in Place: Transitional Housing and Supported Housing Models 365

Introduction. 365
Aging in Place 367
Importance of Aging in Place 368
Practice Challenges. 370
Summary. 370
References 371

Chapter 36 Thriving in Community.....373

Introduction.....................................373
Models of Aging in Community................374
Practice Challenges...........................380
Summary.......................................381
References 381

Chapter 37 Geriatric Assessment in Nursing Homes 383

Introduction.....................................383
Goals of Assessment in the Nursing Home 384
Roles of Interprofessional Team Members in
    Assessment..................................385
Standardized Assessments and Components...387
Challenges and Opportunities 398
Summary.......................................400
References 400

Chapter 38 Emergency Department Assessment at the Time of Hospitalization 401

Introduction.....................................402
Epidemiology 402
Challenges to Geriatric Care in the ED.........402
ED Crowding and Boarding....................403
Variability of the ED Admission Decision 404
The Future of Geriatric ED Care: Geriatric
    Emergency Department Guidelines 412
Summary.......................................413
References 413

Chapter 39 The Older Adult Driver 417

Introduction.....................................417
Older Drivers 418
Behaviors and Characteristics of
    Older Drivers................................418
Older Drivers at Risk for a Motor
    Vehicle Crash 419
Normal Aging, Preclinical Alzheimer's Disease,
    Mild Cognitive Impairment, and Dementia...421
Assessing Driving Skills 422

Driving Retirement 423
Ethical, Legal, and Policy Issues................424
Future Trends in Older Adult Mobility 424
Summary.......................................425
References 425
Appendix 39A..................................430

Chapter 40 Advance Care Planning Through the Incorporation of Values History Discussions...............431

Introduction.....................................432
The Living Will..................................433
The Durable Power of Attorney for
    Health Care 434
The Family Covenant 434
The Values History 435
POLST/MOLST Forms 437
Barriers to Using Advance Directives 439
Legal Considerations 440
Summary.......................................440
References 440
Appendix 40A 442

Chapter 41 Clinical Assessment of Older Persons with Developmental Disabilities...............447

Introduction.....................................447
Developmental Disabilities Are Important
    to Geriatric Clinical Assessment 448
Disparities in Care and Health Are
    Substantial..................................449
Geriatric Care for People with DD Should Be
    Tailored Based on Their Conditions 449
Challenges to Providing High-Quality Care
    for Older Adults with DD 451
Clinical Assessment............................451
Preventive Health..............................454
Summary.......................................457
References 457

Chapter 42 Assessing Disaster Preparedness and Response 461

Introduction................................ 461

Why Community-Dwelling Older People and Nursing Home Residents Are More Vulnerable to the Effects of Disasters 462

Types of Disasters............................ 464

Best Practices in Disaster Management 465

Psychiatric, Ethical, and Social Needs of Elderly Victims of Disasters 467

Summary..................................... 470

References 471

Index.......................................473

Preface

The Handbook for Geriatric Assessment, Fifth Edition is an exceptional compilation of over three decades of extraordinary interdisciplinary research and practice experience from leaders in the field of aging who have established the gold standard for assessing older adults. We are proud of the role our respective foundations have played in supporting the individuals who have advanced our understanding of geriatric assessment, many of whom are authors here. What has changed over five editions? The fields of geriatrics and gerontology have grown dramatically. We have more tools to help people live longer and we know a great deal more about what works well and what doesn't, particularly when it comes to older adults. Maybe the most important change over the five editions is the growing realization that what matters to older people needs to play a much larger role in how we assess needs and plan care.

It goes without saying that in the absence of excellent assessment, there can be no effective care planning, care management, or understanding of appropriate measurement, of outcomes stemming from that assessment. As healthcare professionals we all worry about errors of omission: Did I forget to do the right thing? Excellent assessment helps us make sure not only that we remember to do the right thing but maybe even more importantly, protects us from errors of commission–actually doing something that doesn't improve clinical outcomes or even worse, goes against the functional or personal goals that older people have for themselves. When clinicians start with the right data that can illuminate strengths and weaknesses of those older persons being assessed, the plan of care is created appropriately with an appreciation for the unique individuality of every older adult.

As we set out to build on the strong work of previous editions, we had a strong sense that a more extensive discussion of the context of care along with external forces that shape geriatric assessment would be useful to our reading audience. There has been a strong and positive shift over the past several years to focus on what matters most to the older person who is being assessed in order to ensure that his or her goals are met and that the subsequent care plan is co-developed between the older adult and the care team with those goals very intentionally stated and recorded. We are pleased that all the authors here have made a concerted effort to align their assessment recommendations with this in mind.

We have organized the *Fifth Edition* very purposefully, leading with the context and future of geriatric care along with a salute to the success story of our aging demographics over the past century. We believe that the greatest success story of the past century is longevity and our assessment skills have needed to be continually honed to address the "longevity dividend." Chapters 4 through 6 discuss system issues as related to geriatric care and take us from current innovations to goals and aspirations for the future. Chapters 9 through 13 underscore the importance of person-centered goals with an emphasis on self-care in the family context within the framework of vulnerability and risk. We're especially pleased that we are at an inflection point in health care where this emphasis on goal-directed, person-centered care is evolving rapidly.

Chapters 14 through 18 underscore the essential value of excellent interdisciplinary teams in geriatric care and the way in which high-functioning teams lead to quality outcomes, value, and allow each team member to contribute unique knowledge that can be brought to bear on this work. Chapter 19 is rich with examples of models of care that are effective once assessment data lead to plans that require such models and Chapter 20 provides essential information related to advance care planning.

Chapters 21 through 26 take a deeper look at key aspects of the of geriatric assessment that focus on well-being, dignity, and interdependence and underpin the quality of life of older adults, including cognitive assessment, recognizing elder mistreatment assessment, function physical assessment, and pain assessment. We believe this cluster of chapters recognizes the inherent interactions of pain, cognition, mistreatment, and function.

An area of growing research, enhanced policy focus, and increased visibility among the general public is the profoundly important role that family caregivers play in the lives of older adults and the risks that caregivers' themselves face. There are over 40 million family caregivers in our country, with over 18 million providing care for frail older adults. Caregivers may be spouses, adult children, extended family, or friends. Mounting evidence demonstrates that caregivers may face worsening health status, increased likelihood of depression, and, for working-age adults, a substantial loss of income and productivity. As a result, we believe that inclusion of caregiver assessment is absolutely mandatory for contemporary best practice. As our population ages, both care recipients and caregivers must be thought of as a continuous dyad with attention to both for successful outcomes.

Another area of growing understanding is the special risk that transitions represent in the lives of older adults. For older adults, particularly those with chronic medical problems and functional limitations, continuity and stability are the key to preserving health and function. Evidence shows that even when completely clinically appropriate—a hospitalization for pneumonia for example—an older person may well be discharged at a lower functional status and that this functional loss may never be regained. Assessment of transitions (such as hospital to home or skilled nursing facility), home assessment, and a strong understanding of the community setting assessment parameters are paramount to understanding the lived experience of the older adult. Furthermore, assessing safety for older adults is a critical aspect of care planning whether it's in the context of driving or in the context of a natural or man-made disaster scenario. Unfortunately, assessment of specific settings of care including nursing homes and emergency rooms, and the entire continuum of care has traditionally been extremely fragmented. In response to this expanded and more holistic need, in this *Fifth Edition* we have intentionally brought increased focus to proactively planning for and managing transitions as part of the assessment and care planning.

This *Fifth Edition* documents the important advances that geriatrics and gerontology have made over past decade. We have endeavored to bring together absolutely the best thinking about how to put these learnings to work to improve direct clinical care to improve both the quality of life and quality of health of older adults. Strong, evidence-based, holistic, and person-centered assessment provides the basis to achieve these important goals. We wish to acknowledge all of the previous editors and authors of *Handbook of Geriatric Assessment*; because of their excellent work, we've had a solid roadmap for this fifth edition.

Contributors

▶ Contributors

Gretchen Alkema, PhD, LCSW
The SCAN Foundation
Long Beach, CA

Richard M. Allman, MD
Department of Veterans Affairs
Washington, DC

Alicia Arbaje, MD, MPH, PhD
John Hopkins University
Baltimore, MD

Patricia A. Areán, PhD
University of Washington
Seattle, WA

Garima Arora, MS, MD
Univeristy of Texas Health Science Center at
    Houston
Houston, TX

Sandy Atkins, MPA
Partners in Care Foundation
San Fernando, CA

John Auerbach, MD
Trust for America's Health
Washington, DC

Stephen J. Bartels, MD, MS
Dartmouth College
Geisel School of Medicine at Dartmouth
Hanover, NH

Amy Berman, RN, LDH, FAAN
The John A. Hartford Foundation
New York, NY

Staja Q. Booker, PhD, RN
The University of Iowa
College of Nursing
Iowa Cita, IA

Carla Bouwmeester, PharmD, BCPS, BCGP, FASCP
Northeastern University
School of Pharmacy
Boston, MA

Jennifer Brach, PhD, PT
University of Pittsburgh
Department of Physical Therapy
Pittsburgh, PA

Megan Burke, MD
John Hopkins University
Baltimore, MD

David B. Carr, MD
Washington University School of Medicine
The Rehabilitatin Institute of St. Louis
St. Louis, MO
Parc Provence
Creve Coeur, MO

Bruce Chernof, MD
President, The SCAN Foundation
Long Beach, CA

Anna C. Davis, PhD, MPH
Kaiser Permanente
Pasadena, CA

Karen Desalvo, MD, MPH, MSc
University of Texas at Austin
Deli Medical School
Jefferson, LA

John W. Devlin, PharmD
Northeastern University
School of Pharmacy
Boston, MA

David Doukas, MD
James A. Knight Chair of Humanities and
    Ethics in Medicine
Tulane University
New Orleans, LA

Carmel Bitondo Dyer, MD
UTHealth Consortium on Aging
McGovern Medical School
Houston, TX

Thomas Edes, MD, MS
U.S. Department of Veterans Affairs (10NC4)
Washington, DC

Alyssa Elman, LMSW
Weill Cornell Medicine
New York, NY

Betty Ferrell, PhD, RN, MA FAAN, FPCN, CHPN
City of Hope, Beckman Research Institute
Duarte, CA

Ellen Flaherty, PhD, APRN, AGSF
Geisel School of Medicine at Dartmouth
Dartmouth-Hitchcock Medical Center
Lebanon, NH

Renee Flores, MD
McGovern Medical School
University of Texas Health Science Center
Houston, TX

Terry Fulmer, PhD, RN, FAAN
President, The John A. Hartford Foundation
New York, NY

Colleen Galambos, PhD, ACSW, LCSW, LCSW-C FGSA
School of Social Work
University of Missouri
Columbia, MO

Lynn M. Garofalo-Wright, DPPD, MHA
Kaiser Permanente
Pasadena, CA

Sarah Givens, PhD, RN-BC
Case Western Reserve University
Cleveland, OH

Lindsay Goldman, LMSW
The New York Academy of Medicine
New York, NY

Sherry A. Greenberg, PhD, RN, GNP-BC
Senior Training Specialist; Adjunct Clinical
    Associate Professor of Nursing
Hartford Institute for Geriatric Nursing
    and Nurses Improving Care for Health
    System Elders
New York University Rory Meyers College
    of Nursing
New York, NY

Aaron Hagedorn, PhD
Assistant Clinical Professor of
    Gerontology
University of Southern California
Andrus School of Gerontology
Los Angeles, CA

Stephen Hanson, PhD
Department of Philosophy
University of Louisville
Louisville, KY

Annie C. Harmon, PhD, MS
Washington University School
    of Medicine
St. Louis, MO

Maureen Henry, JD, PhD
National Committee for Quality
    Assurance (NCQA)
Washington, DC

Keela Herr, PhD, RN, AGSF, FGSA, FAAN
The University of Iowa
College of Nursing
Iowa Cita, IA

Nancy A. Hodgson, PhD, RN, FAAN
Biobehavioral Health Sciences
Florida Atlantic University
Boca Raton, FL

Teresita M. Hogan, MD, FACEP
Associate Professor of Medicine
University of Chicago
Medicine & Biological Sciences
Chicago, IL

Victoria Hornyak, DPT, GCS
University of Pittsburgh
Department of Physical Therapy
Pittsburgh, PA

Kathryn Hyer, PhD, MPP
University of South Florida
Tampa, FL

Paul Andrew Jones, AGPCNP-BC, MS, RN-BC
New York Presbyterian Hospital
Weill Cornell
New York, NY

Vanya C. Jones, PhD, MPH
Johns Hopkins Bloomberg School
    of Public Health
Baltimore, MD

Kate E. Koplan, MD, MPH
The Southeast Permanente
    Medical Group
Kaiser Permanente Georgia
Atlanta, GA

Mary Jane Koren, MD, MPH
The John A. Hartford Foundation
New York, NY

Alexandra Kruse, MSG, MHA
Senior Program Officer, Center for Health
    Care Strategies
Hamilton, NJ

Kari Lane, PhD, RN
University of Missouri
Sinclair School of Nursing
Columbia, MO

Bruce Leff, MD
John Hopkins University
School of Medicine
Baltimore, MD

Rosanne M. Leipzig, PhD, MD
Icahn School of Medicine at Mount Sinai
New York, NY

Stacie Levine, MD, FAAHPM
Professor of Medicine
Section of Geriatrics and Palliative
    Medicine
Univeristy of Chicago
Medicine & Biological Sciences
Chicago, IL

Nanxing Li, MSW Candidate
The John A. Hartford Foundation
New York, NY

C.T. Lin, MD
University of Colorado
School of Medicine
Aurora, CO

Jonny Macias, MD
Aurora Health Care
Milwaukee, WI

Michael L. Malone, MD
Aurora HealthCare
Milwaukee, WI

Amy Pacos Martinez, PsyD
University of Rochester Medical Center
Rochester, NY

Kedar S. Mate, MD
Weill Cornell Medical College
Department of Medicine
Boston, MA

Donna McCabe, DNP, APRN-BC, GNP
Clinical Assistant Professor of Nursing
New York University Rory Meyers College
    of Nursing
New York, NY

Christine McDonough, PT, PhD, MS, CEEAA
University of Pittsburgh School of
    Rehabilitation Sciences
Department of Physical Therapy
University of Pittsburgh School of Medicine
Department of Orthopaedic Surgery
Pittsburgh, PA

Rhonda J. V. Montgomery, PhD, MA, BS
University of Wisconsin
Milwaukee, WI
Tailored Care Enterprises LLC
Sun Prairie, WI

Shirley M. Moore, PhD, RN, FAHA, FAAN
Grances Payne Bolton School of Nursing
Case Western Reserve University
Cleveland, OH

Charles Mouton, MD, MS
University of Texas Medical Branch
Galveston, TX

Carol M. Musil, PhD, RN, FAAN
Case Western Reserve University
Cleveland, Ohio

Ronald A. Navarro, MD
Regional Coordinating Chief of
Orthopedic Surgery
Southern California Permanente Medical
Group
Harbor City, CA

Jennifer Ouellet, MD
Yale University School of Medicine
New Haven, CT

Joseph G. Ouslander, MD
Florida Atlantic University
Charles E Schmidt College of Medicine
Boca Raton, FL

Neha Pawar, MD
Department of Psuchiatry
University of Rochester School of Medicine
and Dentistry
Rochester, NY

Leslie Pelton, MPA
Institute for Healthcare Improvement
Boston, MA

Kara Peterik, BA
Boson University School of Public Health
Department of Health Law, Policy and
Management
Boston, MA

Cheryl Phillips, MD, AGSF
Leading Age
Washington, DC

Lorraine Phillips, PhD, RN, FAAN
University of Missouri
Sinclair School of Nursing
Columbia, MO

Lori Popejoy, PhD, APRN, GCNS-BC
University of Missouri
Sinclair School of Nursing
Columbia, MO

Diane Powers, MA, MBA
University of Washington
School of Medicine
Department of Psychiatry and Behaviorial
Sciences
Seattle, WA

Marilyn Rantz, PhD, RN, FAAN
University of Missouri
Sinclair School of Nursing
Columbia, MO

Anne Reb, PhD, NP
City of Hope, Beckman Research Institute
Duarte, CA

George W. Rebok, PhD, MA
John Hopkins Bloomberg School of Public
Health
Baltimore, MD

Susan C. Reinhard, RN, PhD, FAAN
AARP Public Policy Institute
Washington, DC

Brenna N. Renn, PhD
University of Washington
Seattle, WA

David B. Reuben, MD
David Geffen School of Medicine at UCLA
Los Angelas, CA

Bernardo Reyes, MD
Florida Atlantic University
Boca Raton, FL

Vanessa M. Rodriguez, MD
Icahn School of Medicine at Mount Sinai
  Hospital
New York, NY

Anthony Rosen, MD, MPH
Weill Cornell Medical College
New York, NY

Paul Sacco, PhD, MSW
University of Maryland—Baltimore
Baltimore, MD

Judith Salerno, MD, MS
The New York Academy of Medicine
New York, NY

Mandi Sehgal, MD
Florida Atlantic University
Charles E. Schmidt College of Medicine
Boca Raton, FL

Nirav R. Shah, MD, MPH
Pasadena, CA

Kenneth Shay, DDS, MS
Department of Veteran Affairs
Washington, DC

Eugenia L. Siegler, MD
Division of Geriatrics and Palliative Medicine
Weill Cornell Medical College
New York, NY

W. June Simmons, MSW
Partners in Care Foundation
San Fernando, CA

Stephen A. Somers, PhD
President and CEO
Center for Health Care Strategies
Hamilton, NJ

Sarah L. Szanton, PhD, ANP
John Hopkins University
Baltimore, MD

Sheena Thakkar, BS
The John A. Hartford Foundation
NYU College of Global Public Health
New York, NY

Kali S. Thomas, PhD, MA
U.S. Department of Veterans Affairs
  Medical Center
Center for Gerontology and Health Care
  Research, Brown University
Providence, RI

Mary Tinetti, MD
Yale School of Medicine
Section of Geriatrics
New Haven, CT

Jürgen Unützer, MD, MPH, MA
University of Washington
Seattle, WA

David Wert, PhD, MPT
University of Pittsburgh
Department of Physical Therapy
Pittsburgh, PA

Jan Busby-Whitehead, MD, CMD, AGSF
Center for Aging and Health
University of North Carolina at Chapel Hill
Chapel Hill, NC

Marsha N. Wittink
Department of Psychiatry and Family
  Medicine
University of Rochester School of Medicine
  and Dentistry
Rochester, NY

Amber M. Zulfiqar, MD
UT Houston
Family and Community Medicine
Houston, TX

▶ Reviewers

**Elizabeth R. Barker, PhD, FNP, FAANP, FACHE,
  FNAP, FAAN**
Faculty Emerita, The Ohio State University
  College of Nursing [Mount Carmel College
  of Nursing]
Columbus, OH

Gloria Brandburg, PhD, RN, GNP-BC
Associate Professor, University of Texas
  Medical Branch
Galveston, TX

Bonnie Brown, BS Pharm, PharmD
Professor of Pharmacy Practice, Butler
  University College of Pharmacy and Health
  Sciences
Indianapolis, IN

Maria Claver, PhD, MSW, CPG
Program Director and Associate Professor,
  California State University Gerontology
  Program
Long Beach, CA

Jacqueline DeBrew, PhD, MSN, RN, CNE
Clinical Professor, UNC Greensboro
Greensboro, NC

Evelyn G. Duffy DNP, AGPCNP-BC, FAANP
Associate Professor, Case Western Reserve
  University, Frances Payne Bolton School of
  Nursing
Cleveland, OH

Julie Fisher, PhD, RN
Professor, Wesley College
Dover, DE

Mellisa Hall, DNP, AGPCNP-BC, FNP-BC
Graduate Nursing Program Chair, University
  of Southern Indiana
Evansville, IN

Kathleen A. Hill-O'Neill, DNP, CRNP, NHA
Lecturer/Clinical Site Coordinator
Family Nurse Practitioner Program
Adult-Gerontology Primary Care
  Nurse Practitioner Program
University of Pennsylvania School of Nursing
Philadelphia, PA

Bonita L. Huiskes, RN, FNP-BC, PhD
Assistant Professor, Azusa Pacific University
Azusa, CA

Linda J. Keilman, DNP, GNP-BC, FAANP
Associate Professor, Michigan State
  University, College of Nursing
East Lansing, MI

Joanne Kern, PHD, DNP
Assistant Professor, Maryville University
St. Louis, MO

Laura Kneale, MS
PhD Candidate, University of Washington
Seattle, WA

Donna Konradi, PhD, RN, CNE
Associate Professor, Graduate Nursing,
  University of Indianapolis
Indianapolis, IN

Cheryl Kruschke, EdD, MS, RN, CNE
Associate Professor, Regis University
Denver, CO

Cindy Manjounes, MS, EdD, PhD
Professor and Dean, School of Accelerated
  Degree Programs, Lindenwood University
St. Charles, MO

Patti A. Parker, PhD, RN, ANP, GNP, BC
Assistant Clinical Professor, University of
  Texas at Arlington College of Nursing and
  Health Innovation
Arlington, TX

Rebekah Penton, DNP, RN, AGPCNP-BC
Clinical Instructor The University of Texas
  Medical Branch–Galveston
Galveston, TX

Sue Polito, MSN, APN,C, GNP,C
Specialist Professor, Monmouth University
West Long Branch, NJ

Maria Scott, DNP, RN
Associate Professor & Chair ASN Program,
  Miss. University for Women
Columbus, MS

Amy L. Silva-Smith, PhD, APN
Professor, Associate Dean for Academic
   Affairs and Operations
Helen and Arthur E. Johnson Beth-El College
   of Nursing and Health Sciences
University of Colorado Colorado Springs
Colorado Springs, CO

Wendy Swope, DNP
Professor, Maryville University
St. Louis, MO

Meica Valen, DNP, FNP-BC
Professor at Winona State University
Winona, MN

Tracy Van Oss, DHSc, MPH, OTR/L FAOTA
Clinical Professor of Occupational Therapy,
   Quinnipiac University
Hamden, CT

Pamela Becker Weilitz, DNP, ANP-BC
Adjunct Faculty, Maryville University
St. Louis, MO

Lynn Wimett, EdD, AORN-C
Full Professor, Regis University
Denver, CO

Ann Marie Zvorsky, MSN,RN,CNE
Medical-Surgical Nursing Instructor, Joseph
   F. McCloskey School of Nursing
Pottsville, PA

Acknowledgments

We wish to thank the wonderful staff of our foundations, especially Jennifer Phillips, Executive Administrative Assistant to the President at The John A. Hartford Foundation, and Gina Alferez, Executive Administrative Assistant to the President at The SCAN Foundation, for their constant support and coordinating efforts throughout this project. Added thanks to Kevin De La Cruz, Administrative Assistant at JAHF for his support as well! We further wish to recognize the exceptional JAHF student intern support of Ocean Le (Northeastern University), JiHo Chang (University of Utah), Nanxing (Clare) Li (Columbia University), Maya Zamek (Northeastern University), Sheena Thakkar (New York University), and Carrie Lehman (University of Missouri). Without them, this project would not have been possible. Their energy and commitment to getting us across the finish line has been inspiring! Finally, we would both like to recognize the boards of our respective foundations; it is their longstanding passion and commitment to improving the lives of older adults that drives this work. Please know how grateful we are to all of you.

CHAPTER 1

Through the Older Person's Eyes: What Matters

Terry Fulmer and Bruce Chernof

CHAPTER OBJECTIVES

1. Recognize the history and trajectory of older persons' participation in their own health care.
2. Understand the role of healthcare providers in changing the paradigm to person-directed care.

KEY TERMS

Patient-directed

Person-centered

Person- and family-centered

Shared decision-making

▶ Introduction

The greatest success story of the 20th century has been the story of longevity. As illustrated in **FIGURE 1-1**, at the beginning of that century, the human lifespan was approximately 46 years; today, it is nearly 80 years. With added years to life, there has been a paradigm shift away from acute medical management and disease management and toward chronic disease management, with the average person older than the age

of 65 having 3 to 5 chronic conditions and taking 5 to 10 medications. With this complexity in the healthcare regime for older people comes multiple decisions and an important and deeply personal need for older persons to feel that their clinicians are truly in sync with their personal preferences and wishes for care.

The future of health care for older adults—particularly those who have complex chronic needs, functional limitations, or cognitive impairment—will be founded on strong care

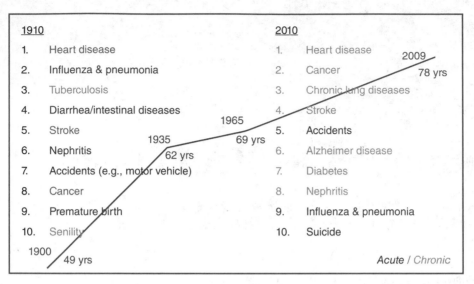

FIGURE 1-1 Life expectancy improvements in the 20th century, Washington.

Data from Arias, E., Heron, M., & Xu, J. Q. (2016). *United States life tables, 2012.*
National Vital Statistics Reports, 65(8), 1-64. Hyattsville, MD: National Center for Health Statistics.

planning and coordination that encompass not just medical problems, but an older person's full range of needs. Next generation care planning for older adults will have to balance their personal goals and desires alongside their medical needs. This care planning can be both complicated and nuanced when personal goals and perceptions about best medical care don't entirely align. It is human nature to want autonomy for ourselves and safety for others—sometimes what healthcare providers might recommend as the safest course or the possibility that there might be one more medical intervention that could be attempted—may not be what the older person wants.

The key to care planning in this more complicated and nuanced environment is multifaceted assessment. There are a wide range of general and specific assessment strategies and tools that can help clinicians screen for needs and assess treatments and interventions as well as deeply explore an older adult's personal goals. This multi-faceted approach, using a set of assessment tools tailored to the specific needs of an older adult, provides the foundation by creating the database that underpins **person-centered** care.

The evolution of the person-centered care imperative and the language that describes it really tell the story. In 1973, Woody and Mallison addressed the issue of the problem-oriented system for patient-centered care, drawing on Weed's work in 1969 at Case Western Reserve University. Weed (1969, cited in Woody & Mallison, 1973) was quoted as saying, "the medical record is such a tangle of illogically assembled bits of information that one cannot reliably discern from it how or whether the physician defined and logically pursued each problem." In those early years, as intensive care units were beginning to flourish and technology was developing at an exponential pace, documentation of the person's health, let alone the individual's thoughts or preferences, was extremely limited in the face of this gain in complexity. Rothman's powerful book, *Strangers at the Bedside: A History of How Law and Bioethics Transformed Medical Decision Making* (1991), traces the history of medical decision making from the mid-1960s to today, describing why the doctor–patient relationship has been so dramatically changed by lawyers judges, legislators, and academics. A review of the literature shows

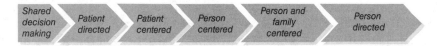

FIGURE 1-2 Evolution of person-centered decision-making in healthcare.

a clear longing by the public and by a vast majority of clinicians to get back to relational care and care planning. Interestingly, the **shared decision-making**, **patient-directed**, patient-centered, person-centered, **person-and family-centered**, person-directed narrative has been evolving in a strong and positive way, and this trend continues today (**FIGURE 1-2**). As the baby boomers have come of age—more than 10,000 Americans turn 65 every day—a new type of care, with the person driving that care, is the expectation.

Early on, Charles, Gafni, and Whelan (1997) reminded us that shared decision making in a medical encounter requires at least two people—a patient and a physician. One might argue today that this process now requires the person seeking care and the appropriate clinician—whether that be the social worker, the nurse, the pharmacist, the rabbi, or any other appropriate member of the healthcare team. The notion of patient empowerment and self-efficacy have been another important part of the medical decision-making narrative over many decades (Anderson et al., 1995; Eskildsen et al., 2017; Sak, Rothenfluh, & Schulz, 2017).

▶ The Importance of Soliciting and Acting on What Matters

In this new era of value- and quality-based payment, what matters to the older person receiving care is now even more important. The tectonic shift that took place in 2001 with the publication of *Crossing the Quality Chasm: A New Health System for the 21st Century* (Berwick, 2002) changed the way healthcare professionals think about the patient voice. Recommendation

4 of that report proposed eight rules for ensuring the patient voice (Berwick, 2002):

1. *Care based on continuous healing relationships.* Patients should receive care whenever they need it and in many forms, not just face-to-face visits. This rule implies that the healthcare system should be responsive at all times (24 hours a day, every day) and that access to care should be provided over the Internet, by telephone, and by other means in addition to face-to-face visits.

2. *Customization based on patient needs and values.* The system of care should be designed to meet the most common types of needs, but have the capability to respond to individual patient choices and preferences.

3. *The patient as the source of control.* Patients should be given the necessary information and the opportunity to exercise the degree of control they choose over healthcare decisions that affect them. The health system should be able to accommodate differences in patient preferences and encourage shared decision making.

4. *Shared knowledge and the free flow of information.* Patients should have unfettered access to their own medical information and to clinical knowledge. Clinicians and patients should communicate effectively and share information.

5. *Evidence-based decision making.* Patients should receive care based on the best available scientific knowledge. Care should not vary illogically from clinician to clinician or from place to place.

6. *Safety as a system property.* Patients should be safe from injury caused by the care system. Reducing risk and ensuring safety require greater attention to systems that help prevent and mitigate errors.

7. *The need for transparency.* The healthcare system should make information available to patients and their families that allows them to make informed decisions when selecting a health plan, hospital, or clinical practice, or when choosing among alternative treatments. This should include information describing the system's performance on safety, evidence-based practice, and patient satisfaction.

8. *Anticipation of needs.* The health system should anticipate patient needs, rather than simply reacting to events.

All clinicians long for faster progress in the march toward this paradigm shift so that we can better hear the voice of the person in the direction of their care. Indeed, 16 years after the publication of *Crossing the Quality Chasm*, we still struggle to put its recommended concepts into practice. The Institute for Healthcare Improvement has done more than any other organization in the country to keep our feet to the fire on this issue, but much remains to be done to make real changes in the system.

The Lown Institute has helped practitioners in the aging field understand how value, resource utilization, and patient satisfaction are inextricably bound together (Brownlee & Berman, 2016). The monograph by Brownlee and Berman (2016) posits that several barriers to achieving value-based (person-centered) care exist, including a public appetite for the "more is better" concept, our inherent dislike as consumers for understanding healthcare value and costs, a lack of appreciation for the harm that can ensue from overtreatment, and lack of discussion related to price, value, and trade-offs. The following vignette illustrates these points.

CLINICAL VIGNETTE

Mr. T was 98—almost 99—when he died. He was physically small but had a great wide smile, piercing blue eyes, and a shock of white hair. It seemed he spent more time in the hospital than home with his wife owing to his end-stage dilated cardiomyopathy, chronic poorly compensated congestive heart failure, and a host of different arrhythmias. In the same month, Mr. T was admitted to my service three times. During that third admission, I sat down with Mr. T and his wife and said, "I know you understand we can't cure these things, but we can try and manage them so that you can do what is really important to you. Tell me your goals, and let's see if can get there together."

What became clear immediately was that Mr. T wanted to be home with his wife as much as possible and not in the hospital unless it was really necessary. What also became clear was that his biggest goal was to be alive and as healthy as possible so he could attend his daughter's wedding, which was some six months away. With this brief but clear discussion, we had the outlines of a plan. Every medical decision needed to be made with the plan in mind—that is, would *X* treatment or *Y* medication help Mr. T stay at home and increase his chances of getting to his daughter's wedding?

This "plan" mystified most of the hospital staff at first because Mr. T and his wife guarded it jealously. The couple asked lots of questions when new providers appeared with one more new treatment option that could be tried. They said no even when doctors and nurses stood in front of them, perplexed by their refusal. And most challenging of all, the couple would often say, "We won't say yes or no until you talk to my personal doctor." Ultimately, though, the plan worked really well. When arrhythmias became more frequent and complex, worsening Mr. T's heart failure, a big family conference resulted in a change in medications but no pacemaker. The risk of the procedure just wasn't worth it with wedding drawing closer.

Unfortunately, Mr. T spent his 98th birthday in the hospital. When our ward team rounded on him that morning, we asked him what he wanted for his birthday. His reply: "Honestly, just a plate of piping hot spaghetti with lots and lots of red sauce." So, we sent a medical student out to the Italian restaurant around the corner to arrange a birthday lunch. As you might imagine, that plate of spaghetti didn't quite meet the low salt dietary restrictions imposed by the cardiologist.

When the wedding arrived, Mr. T was able to attend and had a marvelous time. The pictures from the day shared by his wife with all the hospital staff were a revelation for everyone. Mr. T died in sleep at home, two days after his daughter's wedding. In retrospect, he had spent less time in the hospital over the past six months compared to similar time periods over the last several years. Also, he felt better than he had in a long time even though his medical problems never went away and were actually getting progressively worse. At the end of his life, Mr. T's care shifted from volume to value, quality of life and quality health were both considered, and ultimately both the providers and the patients were more satisfied.

BEST PRACTICES AND PRACTICE CHALLENGES

This brief synopsis of the genesis and trajectory of patient inclusion is presented here very intentionally in a handbook of geriatric assessment. It highlights the intersection between the goals of the healthcare system (quality of health: to improve health outcomes and prolong life) and the goals of the individual (quality of life: to live with dignity, agency, and a high level of function). In that overlap lies value for healthcare payers, providers, and the older adults who are the recipients of care. Key questions in finding that sweet spot include the following: Are we practicing prudent geriatric assessment? What is the time spent and value of the assessment? To which end, for whom, and with which type of systematic evidence and evidence-based follow-up is the assessment taking place?

Older people have unique needs that are often overlooked. Notably, the traditional public health prevention framework of primary, secondary, and tertiary prevention applies as much to older people as it does to other populations.

Primary prevention focuses on universal opportunities to help people prepare for their needs as they age (such as disease prevention in younger adulthood), as well as the strategies that can help older persons remain successfully in the homes and communities of their choice. These strategies address issues ranging from the physical fabric of the communities in which those individuals live (e.g., are there curb cuts at all crosswalks?), to proactive modifications in the home setting, thinking through transportation options, and explicitly expressing their desires as they age to both family and healthcare providers.

Secondary prevention expressly targets those at risk, providing additional supports and/or services to help mitigate these risks. The traditional acute-care-oriented U.S. healthcare system tends to view secondary prevention as the aggressive treatment of disease (think about a cancer diagnosis or diabetes), with the explicit goal of cure or disease complication mitigation and the prolongation of life. In older adults, however, secondary prevention might include interventions such a robust falls prevention program for an older person whose vision is limited by diabetic complications or a community engagement strategy to stave off social isolation and depression.

Tertiary prevention in older adults seeks to mitigate the impact of serious chronic, life-impacting conditions and preserve or enhance functional status. Cure is not generally an option in tertiary prevention. Thus, the focus of the healthcare system needs to remain squarely on quality of life and simply the technical quality of health or healthcare delivery.

▶ Patient-Centered Versus Person-Centered: Sources of Variation Are More Than Just Medical

In the 1980s, frustration with an increasingly fragmented healthcare delivery system caused the Picker Commonwealth Institute (Picker Foundation) to define patient-centered care as healthcare delivery that explicitly incorporates the experience and desires of the patient (Gerteis, Edgman-Levitan, Daley, & Delbanco, 1993). The definition of patient-centered care represented an important step forward, ushering in the goal of shared decision making as a critical tenet of the provider–patient relationship. The principles that define effective shared decision making are the backbone the *Crossing the Quality Chasm* report's recommendations outlined earlier.

As population longevity has increased, however, more and more older adults are living with chronic illnesses and functional limitations for many years of their lives and not simply when they are very sick or toward the end of life. They live with these impacts every day, not just when they are formally "patients" lying in a hospital bed waiting for a procedure or sitting in the doctor's office exam room. Research demonstrates that these social determinants of health are important drivers of the variability in medical expenditures (**FIGURE 1-3**).

For older adults, four important sources of variation drive direct healthcare spending: their medical care, health behaviors, social support network, and physical environment (including their home and surrounding community). Patient-centered care largely (but not entirely) focuses on the medical sources of variation and measures quality mostly through the paradigm of "quality of health" measures. As we age, quality of life may be just as important as—and possibly more important than—quality of health alone. Work by Fried and colleagues (2011) has given us a roadmap for helping older persons achieve healthcare decision making that is centered

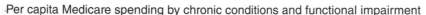

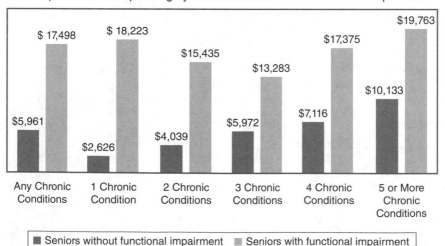

FIGURE 1-3 Per capita Medicare spending by chronic condition and functional impairment.

Rodriguez, S., Munevar, D., Delaney, C., Yang, L., & Tumlinson, A. (2014). *Effective management of high-risk Medicare populations.* Washington, DC: Avalere Health LLC.

on dignity and independence. Addressing the needs of older adults from a whole-person perspective, rather from the narrower perspective of just a patient, is the key to providing better care at lower costs.

To provide a gold standard to guide future program development, the American Geriatrics Society (2016) convened a national expert panel to create a consensus definition for person-centered care:

> Person-centered care means that individuals' values and preferences are elicited and, once expressed, guide all aspects of their healthcare, supporting their realistic health and life goals. Person-centered care is achieved through a dynamic relationship among individuals, others who are important to them, and all relevant providers. This collaboration informs decision-making to the extent that the individual desires.

The principles of sound person-centered care include the following:

- An individualized, goal-oriented care plan based on the person's preferences
- Ongoing review of the person's goals and care plan
- Care supported by an interprofessional team in which the person is an integral team member
- One primary or lead point of contact on the healthcare team
- Active coordination among all healthcare and supportive service providers
- Continual information sharing and integrated communication
- Education and training for providers and, when appropriate, the person and those important to the person
- Performance measurement and quality improvement using feedback from the person and caregivers

Each of these principles requires some form of assessment, whether it be of the elder persons themselves, their caregivers, their healthcare system, or their homes or the community where they live. The chapters that follow capture the best available evidence and practical tools to help healthcare practitioners and systems leaders implement geriatric assessment that improves both quality of health and life—thereby leading to better care at lower costs. In the future, a new generation of quality measures, such as person-reported outcomes and goal attainment, will help drive the balance between quality of health and quality of life.

▶ Summary

Geriatric assessment plays a critical role in helping meet the specific needs of older adults, supporting their caregivers, improving the quality of their health care, and increasing the efficiency of the enormous resources we dedicate to healthcare delivery in the United States. The ultimate goal should be to improve the quality of life and health for the older persons themselves. The assessment at every level provides critical insight but not definitive answers. It is important to listen to older persons and honor their desires, and to recognize that their right to agency (choices that they alone control) trumps the healthcare system's overarching expectation of safety and longevity at the expense of all else. Judgment and empathy, rather than just medical expertise, are what healthcare professionals bring to the table in the provider–patient relationship. Geriatric assessment provides an important mapping function to guide shared decision making and inform a plan of care.

References

American Geriatrics Society. (2016). Person-centered Care: A definition and essential elements. *Journal of the American Geriatrics Society, 64,* 15–18.

Anderson, R. M., Funnell, M. M., Butler, P. M., Arnold, M. S., Fitzgerald, J. T., & Feste, C. C. (1995). Patient empowerment: Results of a randomized controlled trial. *Diabetes Care, 18*(7), 943–949.

Berwick, D. M. (2002). A user's manual for the IOM's "Quality Chasm" report. *Health Affairs, 21*(3), 80–90.

Brownlee, S., & Berman, A. (2016). *Defining value in healthcare resource utilization: Articulating the role of the patient.* Washington, DC: Academy Health.

Charles, C., Gafni, A., & Whelan, T. (1997). Shared decision-making in the medical encounter: What does it mean? (Or it takes at least two to tango). *Social Science & Medicine, 44*(5), 681–692.

Eskildsen, N. B., Joergensen, C. R., Thomsen, T. G., Ross, L., Dietz, S. M., Groenvold, M., & Johnsen, A. T. (2017). Patient empowerment: A systematic review of questionnaires measuring empowerment in cancer patients. *Acta Oncologica (Stockholm, Sweden), 56*(2), 156.

Fried, T. R., Tinetti, M. E., Iannone, L., O'Leary, J. R., Towle, V., & Van Ness, P. H. (2011). Health outcome prioritization as a tool for decision making among older persons with multiple chronic conditions. *Archives of Internal Medicine, 171*(20), 1856–1858.

Gerteis, M., Edgman-Levitan, S., Daley, J., & Delbanco, T. (1993). *Through the patient's eyes.* San Francisco, CA: Jossey-Bass.

Rothman, D. J. (1991). *Strangers at the bedside: A history of how law and bioethics transformed medical decision making.* New York, NY: Basic Books.

Sak, G., Rothenfluh, F., & Schulz, P. J. (2017). Assessing the predictive power of psychological empowerment and health literacy for older patients' participation in healthcare: A cross-sectional population-based study. *BMC Geriatrics, 17*(1), 59.

Woody, M., & Mallison, M. (1973). The problem-oriented system for patient-centered care. *American Journal of Nursing,* 1168–1175.

CHAPTER 2

The Context and Future of Geriatric Care

Jennifer Ouellet and Mary Tinetti

CHAPTER OBJECTIVES

1. Illustrate differences between the geriatric approach to patient care and the traditional disease-based approach.
2. Describe how geriatric assessment enables patient-centered, goal-aligned clinical care for older adults.
3. Discuss strategies for dissemination of geriatric principles among the full range of healthcare providers and health systems.

KEY TERMS

Functional limitations   Geriatrics   Person-centeredness

▶ Introduction

The rapid growth of the 65-years-and-older age group mandates a healthcare workforce that is trained and prepared to address unique clinical and psychosocial needs. Older adults may experience multiple chronic conditions, functional disability, and multifactorial geriatric syndromes (e.g., falls, delirium) that affect their ability to live independently and enjoy a good quality of life. Both health and function become more heterogeneous with increasing age. Furthermore, older adults vary in their health and healthcare priorities. The heterogeneity of healthcare needs and variability in health priorities necessitate that healthcare services be tailored to patient-specific goals and preferences. Tailoring care to each individual's needs, goals, and preferences is the guiding premise of geriatric care.

The geriatric approach to clinical care is a departure from the traditional disease-based diagnosis and treatment paradigm that has dominated healthcare professionals' education and medical care for at least the last century. The concept of multifactorial geriatric syndromes provides the opportunity to identify modifiable contributions to those syndromes' development that can be addressed via multipronged intervention strategies. The **geriatrics** approach allows for nuance and does not force-fit "one size fits all" solutions to every patient as are encouraged by many clinical guidelines. Tailoring care to the individual is essential, as the potential benefits and harms of guideline-based care are uncertain for older adults given their many different potential vulnerabilities, including frailty,

multiple chronic conditions, and functional disability (Fried, Tinetti, & Iannone, 2011). Furthermore, these patients may differ in the outcomes that they most hope to achieve from their health care. Preservation of function and relief of symptoms may be higher priorities for older patients than mortality, the "hard outcome" on which many guidelines were built (Fried, Tinetti, Iannone, O'Leary, et al., 2011).

In this context, the use of the geriatric assessment allows implementation of a structured yet tailored approach to the identification of potential patient needs and priorities. Identification of these needs and priorities then guides development of a personalized healthcare plan and supports shared decision making between health professionals and older adults. In this chapter, we explore the historical context of geriatric principles and propose future directions in improving the care of older adults. Several key geriatric principles are highlighted in **TABLE 2-1**.

TABLE 2-1 Geriatric Principles with Examples of Their Current State and Proposed Future Directions		
Principle	**Examples of the Current State**	**Examples of Future Directions**
Older adults are physically, functionally, and cognitively heterogeneous, requiring clinicians to adapt individualized treatment plans within the context of each patient's unique combination of biological, psychological, and social needs.	Older adults with multiple conditions and functional limitations either receive the same disease guideline-based care as persons with single conditions, ignoring the uncertainty of benefits or harms, treatment burden, and variability in patient goals and preferences, OR they are assumed not to benefit from some treatment, so that they are denied access to potentially beneficial treatments.	*Training/Education and Clinical Care* Individualized treatment plans with focus on what matters to patients, in the context of their health conditions and health trajectory. *Health Policy* Quality metrics and payment that reflect individualized treatment plans.

Principle	Examples of the Current State	Examples of Future Directions
Older adults often experience decreased function, quality of life, and increased mortality due to multiple chronic conditions.	Patients interact with multiple siloed providers, often resulting in conflicting and burdensome recommendations. There is minimal communication among providers. Multiple health record systems, with minimal ability to cross-talk.	*Training/Education* Incorporation of education regarding management of multiple chronic conditions into a nationwide curriculum for health professionals and trainees, including discussion of trade-offs and uncertainty. *Clinical Care* Geriatrics-trained professionals are recognized by health systems and the public as specialists in multiple chronic conditions. *Technology* Through use of existing electronic records, development of strategies for improved communication and easier dissemination of health records among providers. Creation and transmission of an integrated care plan based on the patient's specific goals and preferences.
Functional status and quality of life are key outcomes in older adults.	Clinical care and research usually focus on therapies and interventions that extend life, or improve only discrete disease-specific outcomes, which may not be what all patients value (Fried, Tinetti, & Iannone, 2011).	*Training/Education* Incorporation of geriatric principles early and throughout all health professionals' training. *Clinical Care* Assessment and management (and accompanying documentation) focus on patients' goals and preferences, function, and quality of life. *Health Policy* Development and implementation of quality metrics that drive payment that reflect patients' goals and preferences, function, and quality of life, rather than disease-specific measures.

(continues)

TABLE 2-1 Geriatric Principles with Examples of Their Current State and Proposed Future Directions *(continued)*		
Principle	**Examples of the Current State**	**Examples of Future Directions**
Older adults should receive care that is aligned with each patient's goals and preferences.	Much current clinical care focuses on guidelines-based therapy, which is not necessarily generalizable to older adults with multiple conditions and limited life expectancy and is not always focused on what matters most to the individual.	*Training/Education* Training modules for current health professionals and trainees on goals and preferences ascertainment, and a framework for incorporating these considerations into individualized patient care plans. Development of training for public dissemination encouraging patients to communicate with their health professionals about their goals and preferences. *Clinical Care* Development of a unified, integrated plan of care that is consistent with patient goals and preferences. Changes to documentation to include prioritization of patient goals and preferences instead of individual diseases. *Health Policy* Reimbursements tied to meeting patient goals and preferences. Alignment of financial incentives to promote care that is consistent with patient goals and not tied to procedures and management that do not result in achievement of what matters to patients.
Geriatric care is interprofessional.	Geriatric models of care often include interprofessional teams. Evidence for the benefit of interprofessional clinical care and education is growing.	*Training/Education* Incorporation of interprofessional education sessions in national curricula. *Clinical Care* Development of integrated models of care maximizing benefits of interprofessional teams.

Principle	Examples of the Current State	Examples of Future Directions
Iatrogenic illnesses are common and many are preventable.	Older adults are especially vulnerable to iatrogenic illnesses, including infection, delirium, and falls in healthcare settings. Polypharmacy is common and has been shown to have adverse events including falls, hospitalizations, increased costs, reductions in function and cognition, and mortality (Budnitz, Lovegrove, Shehab, & Richards, 2012; Fried et al., 2014).	*Training/Education* Increased education regarding the benefits and harms of interventions embedded (such as medication management) into a national curriculum for health professions trainees (Kostas et al., 2014). *Clinical Care* Growth of geriatric services across healthcare settings; geriatric expertise available in all health systems. *Technology* Reminders regarding potentially harmful medications in the medical chart; incorporation of decision algorithms based on individual patient characteristics, goals, and preferences into electronic health records to identify best treatment options (Stevens et al., 2015).
Geriatric syndromes are abnormal clinical signs and symptoms that are often the result of vulnerabilities in multiple domains in older adults.	There has been increased recognition in mainstream health care of many geriatric conditions, including falls, delirium, and dementia. Many geriatric syndromes continue to be under-recognized and under-treated. Ongoing research is seeking to define new potential geriatric syndromes.	*Training/Education* Development of educational sessions designed to change the way that providers seek a unifying "one size fits all" approach to diagnosis and treatment. *Clinical Care* Incorporation of core elements of geriatric models across healthcare settings to improve recognition of conditions early in patient encounters. Inclusion of interprofessional treatment plans with opportunities to develop multimodal and stepwise approaches to patient care.

(continues)

TABLE 2-1 Geriatric Principles with Examples of Their Current State and Proposed Future Directions *(continued)*

Principle	Examples of the Current State	Examples of Future Directions
Development of models of care utilizing geriatric expertise leads to improvements in quality care to older adults.	Geriatric "co-management" is gaining popularity in many fields, including orthopedic surgery, based on clear evidence showing its benefits (Friedman, Mendelson, Bingham, & Kates, 2009; Schnell, Friedman, Mendelson, Bingham, & Kates, 2010). Many other fields continue to practice without adequate input from geriatric specialists, leading to fractured clinical care and poor outcomes.	*Training/Education* All health professionals who care for older adults must master understanding of geriatric principles and skills. *Clinical Care* Build consensus regarding core elements of successful geriatric models of care to allow broad dissemination. All health professionals who care for older adults have training in geriatric principles and care. Continued collaboration between geriatric and specialty services to result in improved clinical care for older adults. *Health Policy* Development and implementation of reimbursements that support evidence-based geriatric models of care.

▶ Historical Perspectives

While older adults have always been significant users of the healthcare delivery system, geriatrics as a field is relatively new. Its emergence partly reflects the changing demography in the United States in the last hundred years. For example, in 1910, average life expectancy was 49 years and the top 10 causes of death were almost entirely acute illnesses. By comparison, in 2015, life expectancy was almost 79 years and a majority of the top 10 causes of death were related to chronic conditions. During this roughly 100-year period, the U.S. healthcare system has added many years of life through new treatments and technologies. As a consequence, older adults today

live with far more chronic conditions (which cannot be cured but need to be managed) and **functional limitations** that can impact their quality of health and life. Geriatrics as a field for all health professionals grew in response to the substantial new needs of this population.

Over the last 30 years, the field of geriatrics has built an impressive research base and has begun to contribute its unique knowledge to the broader healthcare community. Better understanding of the multifactorial nature of many geriatric health conditions has resulted in development of effective, targeted interventions for those conditions. Furthermore, principles that were once championed by few health professionals other than geriatricians and nursing professionals have entered the clinical mainstream. For example, function—which has always played a large role in the geriatric assessment—is now understood as an important outcome in clinical research and quality measurement. The field of geriatrics has also widely disseminated ground-breaking healthcare delivery models that demonstrate the value of interprofessional team-based care as well as care planning that focuses on quality of life, not just quality of health—for example, Acute Care of the Elderly units (Landefeld, Palmer, Kresevic, Fortinsky, & Kowal, 1995), Geriatric Resources for Assessment and Care of Elders (Counsell et al., 2007), Program of All-inclusive Care for the Elderly (Eng, Pedulla, Eleazer, McCann, & Fox, 1997), Hospital Elder Life Program (Inouye et al., 1999), Nurses Improving Care for Health System Elders (Fulmer et al., 2002), and Interprofessional Approach to Fall Prevention (Eckstrom et al., 2016).

More recently, geriatrics has played a larger role in shaping the operations of healthcare organizations that either include a larger number of older adults among their patient populations or specifically target these older populations. Examples include co-management interventions such as ortho-geriatric services (Friedman et al., 2009; Schnell et al., 2010.), dementia care (Jennings et al., 2016), and age-friendly emergency rooms.

The United States spends more money on health care on a per capita basis than any other country in the world, yet has worse health outcomes than many other industrialized countries. There is an increasing recognition that continued growth in healthcare costs is not sustainable and, moreover, that we ought to be able to deliver better efficiency and effectiveness for the dollars we spend. Policymakers seeking to inject value into the system have begun to appreciate the importance of geriatric principles. For example, hospital readmissions of persons with multiple chronic conditions is now a quality measure, as are assessment and management of several geriatric syndromes (Centers for Medicare and Medicaid Services [CMS], 2015, 2016b;

RTI International, 2015a, 2015b). The Medicare program has recently introduced a number of new tools to support this broader role for geriatric principles, including modest payments for home visits, transitional care, and care coordination and payment for advance care planning discussions (CMS, 2015, 2016a).

▶ Future Directions

There is growing recognition that the field of geriatrics does not fit the classic model of a medical specialty. As a result, its role in the future, while exciting, remains incompletely defined. What is clear is that geriatrics, unlike the traditional medical specialties such as oncology or neurosurgery, is not defined by a specific disease, organ, or set of medical procedures. So what roles will geriatrics play in the future?

As the population continues to age and healthcare delivery becomes more complicated, the core concepts of geriatrics will need to be infused across the various delivery system, the training of all types of healthcare professionals, and the development of healthcare policy. Table 2-1 details several key geriatric principles, examples of the current management approach to address them, and future directions within the areas of clinical training/education, clinical care, health policy, and technology.

Because we will never have a sufficient number of geriatric specialists to meet the needs of all older people, the training of all types of healthcare professionals will need to embrace geriatric principles and competencies. One way to accomplish this goal could be to develop a national geriatrics curriculum intended for all health professional trainees, so that the core principles of geriatrics can be widely disseminated to providers in all healthcare settings. A national geriatric curriculum would have components designed to reach multiple audiences, including patients and caregivers, trainees, and the full spectrum of health professions and practicing providers. Its dissemination would ensure that these principles reach broad audiences and would provide necessary expertise to providers facing the unique challenges of treating older adults with complex needs. Such a national curriculum would facilitate the exposure of trainees from varied health professions, such as nursing, medicine, pharmacy, and rehabilitative therapies, to a common knowledge and skill base, further ensuring a well-trained, integrated, interprofessional workforce. The core of this curriculum would be the geriatric principles outlined in Table 2-1, with the mode of delivery tailored to the target audience.

In the direct clinical care environment, there will be an ongoing and increasing need for discipline-specific individuals who have specialized training in geriatrics. These professionals could play a variety of roles, including direct providers to the highest-need, most-complicated older adults; expert consultants to other healthcare providers who have only basic geriatric training; leaders of interprofessional care teams; and developers of tailored geriatrics programs and services within their institutions that are responsive to the needs of their communities.

Geriatrics as a field must continue to stress the importance of **person-centeredness** and interprofessional teams to improve patient care. In the last several years, the patient-centered care movement has gained a wide audience, whose members are seeking to improve the value of delivered clinical care. By its very nature, the geriatric approach to patient care has necessarily been patient-centered in its broad assessment of patient needs and tailored treatment plans. Moving forward, geriatrics can help the wider healthcare audience define value in clinical care. One truly patient-centered approach would be to transition from value as measured by lab values and disease-specific outcomes and events, to metrics based on providing care appropriate to the priorities of each individual older adult (Tinetti, Esterson, Ferris, Posner, & Blaum, 2016; Tinetti, Naik, & Dodson, 2016).

To achieve these improvements, health systems and clinical leaders will need to develop electronic medical records that can capture more than older individuals' medical problems—that is, records that can capture their functional limitations, the composition and strength of their social support networks, and, most importantly, their goals and preferences, both medical and personal. The current focus of clinical assessment and management documentation, which in turn drives decision making and care, is on traditional disease-based lists of conditions and their corresponding siloed management strategies. What is needed in the future is targeted assessment of patient goals and preferences as well as assessment and management of function, which tends to be the outcome of greatest importance to most older adults and persons of all ages with multiple conditions. Focus should be on interpreting results and findings in the context of each patient's unique goals and health preferences, health conditions, and healthcare trajectory.

Healthcare systems will also increasingly rely on technology to facilitate day-to-day tasks and to form networks of geriatrically trained professionals and patients across the globe to improve patient care. The advent of telemedicine has resulted in improved access to care, allowing wide dissemination of care to rural, isolated, and vulnerable communities. Within the field of geriatrics, telemedicine has shown the ability reduce both emergency room visits (Shah et al., 2015) and hospitalizations (Catic et al., 2014).

Finally, there will substantial need for geriatrically trained professionals to provide leadership in shaping public policy around programs that serve vulnerable adults. For older adults with complex histories, care in the current system is often fragmented among many siloed providers and geared toward achieving outcomes that may not be relevant to patients. In the face of the growing consensus about the need to improve the value of clinical care, the Institute for Healthcare Improvement introduced the ambitious Triple Aim (Berwick, Nolan, & Whittington, 2008), which focuses on improving population health, improving patient experience, and reducing costs. At this juncture, however, policymakers continue to argue about relevant outcomes.

Certainly geriatric principles have informed some progress in this area, as evidenced by Medicare's coverage of advance care planning and transitional care models. However, many quality metrics are still tied to mortality or to disease-specific outcomes or laboratory measures that may not be relevant to medically complex older adults. As such, there is significant opportunity for geriatrics to contribute to a much wider sphere of influence through national health policy.

▶ Summary

The population of patients age 65 years and older is expanding rapidly throughout the world. These patients have heterogeneous healthcare and psychosocial needs, as well as variable health goals, preferences, and priorities. These characteristics demand an evolution of the healthcare system from the traditional disease-based evaluation and intervention care, to a system tailored to each patient's unique set of goals, preferences, conditions, and needs. Through use of the geriatric assessment, individual patient needs can be identified in a thorough and structured fashion, allowing for individualized and tailored treatment plans. Geriatric principles are increasingly defining quality patient care, and advances in geriatrics will continue to guide the future directions of healthcare delivery.

References

Berwick, D. M., Nolan, T. W., & Whittington, J. (2008). The Triple Aim: Care, health, and cost. *Health Affairs, 27*(3), 759–769.

Budnitz, D. S., Lovegrove, M. C., Shehab, N., & Richards, C. L. (2012). Emergency hospitalization for adverse drug events in older Americans. *Survey of Anesthesiology, 56*(2), 65–66.

Catic, A. G., Mattison, M. L., Bakaev, I., Morgan, M., Monti, S. M., & Lipsitz, L. (2014). ECHO-AGE: An innovative model of geriatric care for long-term care residents with dementia and behavioral issues. *Journal of the American Medical Directors Association, 15*(12), 938–942. doi: 10.1016/j.jamda.2014.08.014

Centers for Medicare and Medicaid Services (CMS). (2015). *2015 physician quality reporting system (PQRS): Implementation guide.* Retrieved from https://www.cms.gov/Medicare/Quality-Initiatives-Patient-Assessment-Instruments/PQRS/Downloads/2015_PQRS_ImplementationGuide.pdf

Centers for Medicare and Medicaid Services (CMS). (2016a). *Chronic care management services.* Retrieved from https://www.cms.gov/Outreach-and-Education/Medicare-Learning-Network-MLN/MLNProducts/Downloads/ChronicCareManagement.pdf

Centers for Medicare and Medicaid Services (CMS). (2016b). *Proposed policy, payment, and quality provisions changes to the Medicare physician fee schedule for the calendar year (BY) 2017.* Retrieved from https://www.cms.gov/Newsroom/MediaReleaseDatabase/Fact-sheets/2016-Fact-sheets-items/2016-07-07-2.html

Counsell, S. R., Callahan, C. M., Clark, D. O., Tu, W., Buttar, A. B., Stump, T. E., & Ricketts, G. D. (2007). Geriatric care management for low-income seniors: A randomized controlled trial. *Journal of the American Medical Association, 298*(22), 2623–2633.

Eckstrom, E., Neal, M. B., Cotrell, V., Casey, C. M., McKenzie, G., Morgove, M. W., . . . Lasater, K. (2016). An interprofessional approach to reducing the risk of falls through enhanced collaborative practice. *Journal of the American Geriatrics Society, 64*(8), 1701–1707. doi: 10.1111/jgs.14178

Eng, C., Pedulla, J., Eleazer, G. P., McCann, R., & Fox, N. (1997). Program of All-inclusive Care for the Elderly (PACE): An innovative model of integrated geriatric care and financing. *Journal of the American Geriatrics Society, 45*(2), 223–232.

Fried, T. R., O'Leary, J., Towle, V., Goldstein, M. K., Trentalange, M., & Martin, D. K. (2014). Health outcomes associated with polypharmacy in community-dwelling older adults: A systematic review. *Journal of the American Geriatrics Society, 62*(12), 2261–2272.

Fried, T. R., Tinetti, M. E., & Iannone, L. (2011). Primary care clinicians' experiences with treatment decision making for older persons with multiple conditions. *Archives of Internal Medicine, 171*(1), 75–80.

Fried, T. R., Tinetti, M. E., Iannone, L., O'Leary, J. R., Towle, V., & Van Ness, P. H. (2011). Health outcome prioritization as a tool for decision making among older persons with multiple chronic conditions. *Archives of Internal Medicine, 171*(20), 1854–1856. doi: 10.1001/archinternmed.2011.424

Friedman, S. M., Mendelson, D. A., Bingham, K. W., & Kates, S. L. (2009). Impact of a comanaged geriatric fracture center on short-term hip fracture outcomes. *Archives of Internal Medicine, 169*(18), 1712–1717. doi: 10.1001/archinternmed.2009.321

Fulmer, T., Mezey, M., Bottrell, M., Abraham, I., Sazant, J., Grossman, S., & Grisham, E. (2002). Nurses Improving

Care for Healthsystem Elders (NICHE): Using outcomes and benchmarks for evidenced-based practice. *Geriatric Nursing, 23*(3), 121–127.

Inouye, S. K., Bogardus, S. T. Jr., Charpentier, P. A., Leo-Summers, L., Acampora, D., Holford, T. R., & Cooney, L. M. Jr. (1999). A multicomponent intervention to prevent delirium in hospitalized older patients. *New England Journal of Medicine, 340*(9), 669–676.

Jennings, L. A., Tan, Z., Wenger, N. S., Cook, E. A., Han, W., McCreath, H. E., . . . Reuben, D. B. (2016). Quality of care provided by a comprehensive dementia care comanagement program. *Journal of the American Geriatrics Society, 64*(8), 1724–1730. doi: 10.1111/jgs.14251

Kostas, T., Zimmerman, K., Salow, M., Simone, M., Whitmire, N., Rudolph, J. L., & McMahon, G. T. (2014). Improving medication management competency of clinical trainees in geriatrics. *Journal of the American Geriatrics Society, 62*(8), 1568–1574. doi: 10.1111/jgs.12933

Landefeld, C. S., Palmer, R. M., Kresevic, D. M., Fortinsky, R. H., & Kowal, J. (1995). A randomized trial of care in a hospital medical unit especially designed to improve the functional outcomes of acutely ill older patients. *New England Journal of Medicine, 332*(20), 1338–1344.

RTI International. (2015a). *Accountable care organization 2015 program analysis quality performance standards narrative measure specifications.* Retrieved from https://www .cms.gov/Medicare/Medicare-Fee-for-Service-Payment /sharedsavingsprogram/Downloads/RY2015-Narrative -Specifications.pdf

RTI International. (2015b). *Skilled nursing facility quality reporting program: Specifications for the quality measures adopted through the fiscal year 2016 final rule.* Retrieved from https://www.cms.gov/Medicare /Quality-Initiatives-Patient-Assessment-Instruments /NursingHomeQualityInits/Downloads/SNF-specs.pdf

Schnell, S., Friedman, S. M., Mendelson, D. A., Bingham, K. W., & Kates, S. L. (2010). The 1-year mortality of patients treated in a hip fracture program for elders. *Geriatric Orthopaedic Surgery & Rehabilitation, 1*(1), 6–14.

Shah, M. N., Wasserman, E. B., Gillespie, S. M., Wood, N. E., Wang, H., Noyes, K., . . . McConnochie, K. M. (2015). High-intensity telemedicine decreases emergency department use for ambulatory care sensitive conditions by older adult senior living community residents. *Journal of the American Medical Directors Association, 16*(12), 1077–1081. doi: 10.1016/j.jamda.2015.07.009

Stevens, M. B., Hastings, S. N., Powers, J., Vandenberg, A. E., Echt, K. V., Bryan, W. E., 3rd, . . . Vaughan, C. P. (2015). Enhancing the Quality of Prescribing Practices for Older Veterans Discharged from the Emergency Department (EQUiPPED): Preliminary results from Enhancing Quality of Prescribing Practices for Older Veterans Discharged from the Emergency Department, a novel multicomponent interdisciplinary quality improvement initiative. *Journal of the American Geriatrics Society, 63*(5), 1025–1029. doi: 10.1111/jgs.13404

Tinetti, M. E., Esterson, J., Ferris, R., Posner, P., & Blaum, C. S. (2016). Patient priority-directed decision making and care for older adults with multiple chronic conditions. *Clinics in Geriatric Medicine, 32*(2), 261–275. doi: 10.1016/j.cger.2016.01.012

Tinetti, M. E., Naik, A. D., & Dodson, J. A. (2016). Moving from disease-centered to patient goals-directed care for patients with multiple chronic conditions: Patient value-based care. *JAMA Cardiology, 1*(1), 9–10. doi: 10.1001/jamacardio.2015.0248

CHAPTER 3

Demographic Trends: A Success Story

Lindsay Goldman and Judith Salerno

CHAPTER OBJECTIVES

1. Define healthy aging.
2. Identify major sociodemographic trends associated with aging of the U.S. population.
3. Describe potential social and economic benefits associated with an aging population.
4. Discuss Age-Friendly Cities and Communities as one model to advance healthy aging.

KEY TERMS

Age-Friendly Cities and Communities

Health disparities
Healthy aging

Longevity dividend

▶ Introduction

Advances in medicine and technology, coupled with reductions in fertility and infant and childhood mortality rates, have led to significant gains in life expectancy around the world, with the global average life expectancy at birth now being 69 years for men and 73 years for women (United Nations, 2017). As a result, the proportion of people age 60 and older is increasing in both developed and developing countries. The United Nations estimates that 13% of the world population is currently 60 and older, representing 962 million people, and projects growth of this population to proceed at a rate of 3% per year, to total 1.4 billion people in 2030 and 2.1 billion in 2050. Within this cohort, the subpopulation of persons age 80 and older is projected to grow the fastest, tripling from 137 million in 2017 to 425 million in 2050.

This demographic shift has the potential to produce a **"longevity dividend,"** in the form of "social, economic, and health benefits for current and future generations" (Olshansky, Perry, Miller, & Butler, 2007), if older people are able to remain actively involved in public life. However, social systems and institutions, which were generally designed when life expectancy was much shorter, require adaptation and improvement to sustain engagement in later life (Rowe & Kahn, 2015). To reap the possible rewards associated with population aging, all sectors must prioritize maximizing the health, well-being, and full participation of older adults (Sadana, Blas, Budhwani, Koller, & Paraje, 2016).

This chapter illustrates the larger theoretical, environmental, and sociodemographic context within which geriatric care is delivered in the United States. We first define the concept of **healthy aging**. We then present an overview of current and projected population trends, the social and economic effects associated with changing demographics, and disparities in health and life expectancy experienced by marginalized populations. Finally, we suggest **Age-Friendly Cities and Communities** as a global model that can mobilize stakeholders across the public and private sectors to promote healthy aging.

▶ What Constitutes Healthy Aging?

The World Health Organization (WHO) defines healthy aging as the "process of developing and maintaining the functional ability that enables well-being in older age . . . [which] reflects the ongoing interaction between individuals and the environments they inhabit" (Beard et al., 2016). This person–environment relationship begins in the prenatal period and continues throughout the lifespan (Stein & Moritz, 1999). For example, evidence shows that fetal under-nutrition is associated with negative health outcomes in adulthood, such as diabetes, coronary heart disease, and chronic lung and kidney disease (Fall, 2013). At every stage of life, personal, interpersonal, behavioral, and socioeconomic factors can mitigate or exacerbate both normative and pathological age-related changes (Rowe & Kahn, 2015).

The Centers for Disease Control and Prevention (CDC, 2017) has identified 15 key health status indicators of older people, including perceived physical and mental health status, loss of teeth, disability, consumption of fruits and vegetables, obesity, current smoking, physical inactivity, and receipt of preventive services. Analyzing 2015 data from the Behavioral Risk Factor Surveillance System (BRFSS), the CDC found that among those respondents age 65 and older in the United States, 74% reported their health as good, very good, or excellent; 25.5% reported their health as fair or poor; and 36.3% reported having a disability. This cohort also reported an average of a little more than 5 physically unhealthy days and 6 days with activity limitations in the past month. Successful interventions to support healthy aging can improve perceptions of well-being, quality of life, and autonomy; maximize functional ability; and minimize activity limitations. These interventions require a multipronged approach that includes modifying the built environment, providing social and technological supports, and changing public policies to facilitate ongoing participation of people as they age, even in the presence of chronic conditions and disability (Tesch-Römer & Wahl, 2017).

▶ Current and Projected Aging Population Growth in the United States

The United States experienced significant gains in life expectancy at birth from 1975 to 2015 for both men (from 68.8 to 76.3 years) and women (from 76.6 to 81.2 years) (National Center for

Health Statistics, 2017). In 2015, approximately 15% of the U.S. population was age 65 and older (nearly 48 million people), with this proportion projected to increase to 22% by 2050 (He, Goodkind, & Kowal, 2016). The largest increase, consisting of an additional 18 million people, is expected to occur between 2020 and 2030 (Colby & Ortman, 2015). The United States is not, however, among the world's oldest countries, ranking 34th of 160 countries on this basis in 2015, and anticipated to decline to 56th by 2050 (He et al., 2016). In Japan, the world's oldest country, more than 26% of the population was age 65 and older in 2015, with this proportion projected to increase to 40% by 2050 (He et al., 2016).

According to the Federal Interagency Forum on Aging-Related Statistics (2016), by 2060 the older population will be more racially and ethnically diverse than previous generations. Within the 65 and older population, the proportion accounted for by those persons identifying as non-Hispanic white is expected to decrease from 78% to 55%, while the proportion accounted for by those persons identifying as Hispanic or Latino (any race) is expected to increase from 8% to 22%, representing 21.5 million people. Projections also indicate that the proportion accounted for by those persons identifying as non-Hispanic black will increase from 9% to 12%, and the proportion accounted for by those persons identifying as non-Hispanic Asian will increase from 4% to 9%. Within this same time frame, the population age 65 and older born outside of the United States is projected to increase by 300% (Colby & Ortman, 2015). These demographic changes have implications for the prevalence of certain conditions and the human and financial resources that will be required to care for this older population.

In 2014, the state with the largest proportion of residents age 65 and older was Florida (more than 19%), followed by Maine, West Virginia, Vermont, Montana, Pennsylvania, Delaware, Hawaii, and Oregon (16% or more) (Federal Interagency Forum on Aging-Related Statistics, 2016). While most older people live in metropolitan or micropolitan areas, people age 65 and older also represent larger proportions of rural populations (Werner, 2011). Of the 2013 Medicare-insured population age 65 and older, 93% lived in traditional community settings without services or supports, 3% lived in community settings that provided services and supports,[1] and 4% lived in long-term care facilities. Members of the age 85 and older population were more likely to reside in community settings with services (8%) and long-term care facilities (15%), reflecting the increased challenges associated with activities of daily living that can accompany advanced age (Federal Interagency Forum on Aging-Related Statistics, 2016).

▶ Social and Economic Capital

Spending and Working

A large older population can stimulate economic growth and bring added social capital to communities and institutions. Holding 83% of household wealth in the United States, the population age 50 and older was responsible for $5.6 trillion in spending in 2015, representing a $7.6 trillion contribution to the U.S. gross domestic product (GDP) (AARP & Oxford Economics, 2016). This amount includes

---

1 A community setting with services and supports includes people who reported living in retirement communities or apartments, senior citizen housing, continuing care retirement facilities, assisted living facilities, staged living communities, board and care facilities/homes, and similar situations *and* who reported they had access to one or more of the following services through their place of residence: meal preparation, cleaning or housekeeping services, laundry services, or help with medications.

$1.8 trillion in federal, state, and local tax revenues and $4.7 trillion in labor income that supported 61% of American jobs.

According to a 2017 report from the U.S. Bureau of Labor Statistics, approximately 40% of people age 55 and older participated in the U.S. labor force in 2014, and between 2012 and 2024, the fastest annual labor force growth is projected to be among those age 65 to 74 (4.5% increase) and age 75 and older (6.4% increase) (Toossi & Torpey, 2017). Older workers have been found to be more engaged in their work than their younger counterparts, and higher levels of employee engagement are associated with greater revenue growth (Aon Hewitt for AARP, 2015).[2] Studies have also shown that an age-diverse workforce may be more creative, productive, and better at solving problems (Paullin, 2014; Pitt-Catsouphes, Mirvis, & Berzin, 2013). Older people have higher rates of self-employment than younger people (Toossi & Torpey, 2017), with people age 55 to 64 making up nearly 26% of all new entrepreneurs in the United States in 2015 (Fairlie, Morelix, Reedy, & Russell, 2015). A 2008 survey found that even in the technology field, there were twice as many company founders older than age 50 than younger than age 25 (Wadhwa, Freeman, & Rissing, 2008).

Civic Engagement, Volunteerism, and Charitable Giving

Older people are often among the most long-term, civically engaged community members. People older than age 65 typically have the highest rates of voting in general elections (File, 2017), as well as high rates of volunteerism and philanthropy. A study by Merrill Lynch and Age Wave projects that as more baby boomers (those born between 1946 and 1964) retire, they will generate an additional $8 trillion in charitable giving and in-kind volunteering (Bank of America Corporation, 2016). Evidence suggests that volunteering among older people is associated with reduced mortality (Musick, Herzog, & House, 1999), improved perceptions of well-being (Morrow-Howell, Hinterlong, Rozario, & Tang, 2003), and increased physical, cognitive, and social activity (Fried et al., 2004). Research on Experience Corps—an intergenerational program that places older volunteers in inner-city public elementary schools—demonstrated improved mobility and ability to accomplish instrumental activities of daily living (IADLs) among older volunteers and improved reading and classroom behavior among children in participating schools (Fried et al., 2013).

▶ Disparities in Health and Life Expectancy

Age

Longer lives can mean more years in both good and poor health. In the United States, as in other parts of the world, increases in life expectancy are associated with increases in years with disability (Tesch-Römer & Wahl, 2017). Increased age is associated with a higher prevalence of chronic conditions and related physical and cognitive challenges. Based on data from the 2006 and 2010 Medical Expenditure Panel Survey, the Agency for Healthcare Research and Quality (AHRQ) reported that more than 30% of all non-institutionalized Americans have multiple chronic conditions, as compared to 80% of those age 65 and older (Gerteis et al., 2014). People with multiple chronic conditions account for 71% of all healthcare spending (Gerteis et al., 2014).[3]

---

2 Engagement is defined as the emotional and intellectual involvement that motivates employees to do their best work and contribute to an organization's success.

3 Chronic conditions are defined as those lasting or expecting to last 12 or more months and resulting in functional limitations and/or the need for ongoing medical care.

The most common chronic conditions experienced by people age 65 and older include hypertension, high cholesterol levels, arthritis, ischemic heart disease, and diabetes (Centers for Medicare and Medicaid Services [CMS], 2012). The evidence suggests that today's older Americans are experiencing more chronic conditions than their counterparts in previous generations; for example, an analysis of data from the Health and Retirement Study indicated that the prevalence of diabetes increased by 37% and arthritis by 41% between 2004 and 2010 (Beltrán-Sánchez, Jiménez, & Subramanian, 2016). The higher prevalence of certain conditions may be related to risk factors such as poor nutritional habits, tobacco use, obesity, and physical inactivity (University of Michigan Institute for Social Research, 2017).

Gender and Sexual Orientation

Women have longer life expectancy than men and account for 56% of the population age 65 and older and two-thirds of the population age 85 and older (Federal Interagency Forum on Aging-Related Statistics, 2016). However, women experience certain conditions at higher rates than men, including arthritis, osteoporosis, and hypertension, resulting in higher rates of reported physical and cognitive disabilities (Henry J. Kaiser Family Foundation, 2013). For women, increased disease burden may be related to and exacerbated by higher levels of poverty, more out-of-pocket medical expenses, and limited access to resources (Henry J. Kaiser Family Foundation, 2013).

Projections indicate that by 2060, the population older than age 50 self-identifying as lesbian, gay, bisexual, or transgender (LGBT) will increase from 2.7 million to more than 5 million (Fredriksen-Goldsen, 2016). This population has a higher risk of disability, poor physical and mental health, and substance abuse compared to their non-LGBT peers (Fredriksen-Goldsen, Kim, Shui, & Bryan, 2017). LGBT older people are also more likely to live in poverty, experience social isolation, and face discrimination when accessing supportive services in both residential and community-based settings (Hughes, Harold, & Boyer, 2011; National Senior Citizens Law Center et al., 2011).

Race and Ethnicity

While life expectancy at birth has increased among all racial and ethnic groups, non-Hispanic black males and females live 4.5 and 3 fewer years, respectively, than their white counterparts (National Center for Health Statistics, 2017). This gap declines with age, yet significant **health disparities** persist in later life. In 2013, the CDC reported that at age 65, on average, whites could expect to live an additional 14.3 healthy years, while blacks could expect to live only 11.1 more healthy years.

Illustrating these health discrepancies, blacks have higher death rates than whites for all types of cancers combined (24% higher for males and 14% higher for females) as well as for heart disease (26% higher) (American Cancer Society, 2016). Black males are more likely to experience and die from cancer of the prostate, lung, colon or rectum, kidney, and pancreas (American Cancer Society, 2016). Black females have a 2% lower incidence rate of breast cancer than white females but have a 42% higher death rate from this cause (DeSantis, Ma, Goding Sauer, Newman, & Jemal, 2017). Similarly, while black females are slightly less likely to experience uterine cancer, they have a 92% higher death rate from this cause compared to white females (American Cancer Society, 2016). Blacks also have higher rates of multiple chronic conditions and disabilities (CMS, 2012) and are twice as likely to develop dementia compared to whites (Alzheimer's Association, 2015).

Hispanics and Latinos have the highest life expectancy at birth (National Center for Health Statistics, 2017), but they also have high rates of multiple chronic conditions and disabilities in advanced age (CMS, 2012). Although 35% less likely to experience heart disease and 49% less likely to experience cancer than whites, Hispanics and Latinos are 24% more likely to suffer from poorly controlled high blood pressure, are 23% more likely to be obese, and have a 50% higher rate of death from diabetes (CDC, 2015).

Disparities in health and life expectancy may be attributable to a complex interplay of social, environmental, behavioral, and genetic factors. Differences in socioeconomic status, stress, perceived discrimination, and neighborhood conditions have been found to influence higher levels of functional limitations among black men (Brown, Hargrove, & Griffith, 2015). Lack of access to high-quality health services can contribute to poor health outcomes; for example, blacks are less likely to be screened for colorectal cancer and more likely to die of this disease than whites (CDC, 2015; Williams et al., 2016). Finally, while evidence remains inconclusive at present, future genomic research has the potential to identify increased risks for certain conditions among different racial and ethnic groups (Peprah, Xu, Tekola-Ayele, & Royal, 2015).

Income and Education

Independent of, but often aligned with, patterns of race and ethnicity, lower levels of income and education have been found to be associated with poorer health and lower life expectancy (Braveman, Cubbin, Egerter, Williams, & Pamuk, 2010). A 2016 study published in the *Journal of the American Medical Association* found that men and women in the poorest 1% of the population could expect to live 14.6 and 10.1 fewer years, respectively, than men and women in the wealthiest 1% at age 40; this inequality increased over time (Chetty et al., 2016). Blacks and Hispanics and Latinos with higher levels of education (16 or more years) have been shown to live significantly longer than whites with lower levels of education (less than 12 years) (Olshansky et al., 2012).

Other studies have focused on the effects of neighborhood socioeconomic conditions over the life course. Living in economically disadvantaged communities, which are often characterized by lower-quality housing, high levels of crime and pollution, and fewer resources, is associated with more chronic health conditions, mobility challenges, high levels of stress, and earlier death among older residents (Population Reference Bureau, 2017). Wight et al. (2006) found that regardless of individual educational attainment, older people in low-education urban communities demonstrated lower cognitive functioning than those in communities with higher levels of education. Neighborhood characteristics can facilitate or limit access to health-promoting assets and influence behavior. For example, economically disadvantaged neighborhoods may be associated with reduced physical activity among older people who perceive their surroundings as unsafe, and who lack access to green space, well-lighted and well-maintained streets and sidewalks, and age-inclusive exercise programs (Population Reference Bureau, 2017; Tucker-Seeley, Subramanian, Li, & Sorensen, 2009).

Social Network

Evidence suggests that social isolation contributes to morbidity and mortality from cancer and cardiovascular disease (Hawkley, 2003), rehospitalization (Mistry, 2001), and depression and cognitive impairment (Cacioppo & Hawkley, 2009). Social isolation is also a risk factor for elder abuse (Mysyuk, Westendorp, & Lindenberg, 2015), as well as negative health outcomes, including death, following emergency events (Goldman, Finkelstein, Schafer, & Pugh, 2014; Klinenberg, 2002). Older people at higher risk of social isolation include those who are divorced, separated, or widowed; have disabilities; live alone; earn less than 100% of the federal poverty level; and have limited English proficiency (AARP Foundation, 2012). Inadequate intergenerational contact has also been shown to perpetuate stereotyping and exclusion that contribute to the social isolation of older people (Hagestad & Uhlenberg, 2005).

▶ Age-Friendly Cities and Communities: A Movement to Maximize Participation, Reduce Disparities, and Improve Quality of Life

Background and Framework

In 2006, WHO launched the Global Age-Friendly Cities and Communities project to address the converging trends of urbanization and population aging using the Active Aging Framework.[4] Grounded in evidence, the Active Aging Framework posits that a person's disability trajectory can be slowed or reversed through increased engagement in the community, which is associated with better physical and mental health (World Health Organization [WHO], 2007). The WHO Age-Friendly Cities and Communities model was created to identify and address barriers to engagement faced by older people throughout the course of daily life within eight domains (WHO, 2007):

1. Outdoor spaces and buildings
2. Transportation
3. Housing
4. Social participation
5. Respect and social inclusion
6. Civic participation and employment
7. Communication and information
8. Community support and health services

Through qualitative and quantitative data collection methods, feedback from older people is solicited across the eight domains and used by policymakers, community leaders, and residents to make local resources, institutions, services, and amenities more inclusive. When viewed through the Active Aging Framework, an aging population presents an opportunity to make communities more livable for people of all ages and abilities. Notably, the provision of health care, where most aging-related attention and investment are directed, is but one of eight domains within this framework, which suggests that aging must also become a focal point for government, architecture and design, urban and regional planning, arts and culture, education, and business.

Age-Friendly NYC

New York City was one of the first cities to implement the Age-Friendly Cities and Communities model and to join the WHO Global Network, which currently includes 500 cities and communities across 37 countries (WHO, 2017). Age-Friendly NYC was founded in 2007 as a public–private partnership between the New York Academy of Medicine (a private nonprofit organization), the Mayor's Office (administrative branch of city government), and the New York City Council (legislative branch) to maximize the social, physical, and economic participation of older people to improve their health and well-being and strengthen communities. In direct response to concerns expressed by older people across the city, but paying special attention to those in under-resourced neighborhoods, this partnership has catalyzed new programs, legislation, and enhancements to the built environment.

For example, a 2006 survey found that 52% of New York City residents age 75 and older were likely to walk to a destination rather than use another form of transportation (Stowell-Ritter, Bridges, & Sims, 2006); however, older people frequently reported significant barriers to

---

4 While the model initially focused on cities, WHO has since expanded the model to include communities of all sizes and geographic areas.

walking, including inadequate street crossing times, poorly maintained streets and sidewalks, and lack of seating. To address these issues, the Department of Transportation installed thousands of newly designed benches; redesigned bus shelters to include seating and transparent walls; and implemented mitigation measures at the most dangerous intersections, such as extending pedestrian crossing times, constructing pedestrian safety islands, widening curbs and medians, and installing new stop controls and signals. These interventions resulted in a 16% decrease in senior pedestrian fatalities citywide, from an average of 65 deaths per year between 1999 and 2007 to an average of 54 deaths between 2008 and 2016 (New York City Department of Transportation, 2017).

Other age-friendly improvements include new programs at parks, pools, and cultural institutions; legal protections under New York City Human Rights Law for employees with caregiving responsibilities; and a better consumer experience offered by countless local businesses (New York City Department for the Aging, 2017). Many of these solutions are low cost and optimize existing assets that can facilitate connections between the generations and build social cohesion.

Challenges and Areas for Future Growth

While the Age-Friendly model has proved adaptable to diverse populations and localities, it is not without its challenges. Sustaining the interest and commitment of stakeholders across many different sectors through political changes, shifting priorities, and contractionary fiscal policies requires strong organizational commitments, buy-in from local community leaders, and mobilization of consumers. Macro-level social and economic forces often underlie and compound these difficulties. In global cities such as New York, unconstrained development, the privatization of public space, and foreign investment in real estate may make housing and other resources unaffordable

to many older people and threaten the social fabric of neighborhoods (Buffel & Phillipson, 2016). Policies that incentivize affordable housing construction and preservation, promote universal design principles, and require community engagement and participatory planning can help to mitigate some of these dynamics.

Evaluation of Age-Friendly initiatives poses another challenge. Numerous efforts have been made to identify indicators of an Age-Friendly community using existing data tracked over time, including AARP's Livability Index (AARP Public Policy Institute, 2017) and the WHO Kobe Center's Core Indicators (WHO, 2015); however, there have been few studies of the health outcomes, costs, and benefits associated with the Age-Friendly model, which is inherently multifactorial. The fundamental goal of Age-Friendly Cities and Communities is to enable older people to remain actively and meaningfully engaged where they live, but that outcome is very difficult to measure at a population level given the myriad systemic and environmental variables involved. Additional research is needed to demonstrate the short- and long-term impacts of living in an Age-Friendly locality and to evaluate the potential for Age-Friendly interventions to advance health equity.

▶ Conclusion

Significant opportunities are associated with an aging, and particularly with an increasingly diverse population, that can be realized if people can continue to participate in and contribute to public life. All too often, health challenges, socioeconomic conditions, and pervasive ageism can impede working and volunteering, consuming goods and services, socializing, and recreation in life's later years. While most of the chapters in this text focus on assessments of the older individual, this chapter highlights the physical, social, and economic environments of older individuals that can either compromise or enhance their optimal functioning and autonomy. The

Age-Friendly Cities and Communities model is one innovative approach to assessing and improving these environments that can be used by local governments, health systems, faith- and community-based organizations, academic and cultural institutions, business-serving organizations, and grassroots movements to enhance the health and quality of life of current and future aging populations.

References

AARP Foundation. (2012). *Framework for isolation in adults over 50.* Retrieved from https://www.aarp.org/content/dam/aarp/aarp_foundation/2012_PDFs/AARP-Foundation-Isolation-Framework-Report.pdf

AARP Public Policy Institute. (2017). AARP Livability Index: Great neighborhoods for all ages. Retrieved from https://livabilityindex.aarp.org/

AARP & Oxford Economics. (2016). *The longevity economy: How people over 50 are driving economic and social value in the US.* Retrieved from http://www.aarp.org/content/dam/aarp/home-and-family/personal-technology/2016/09/2016-Longevity-Economy-AARPpdf

Alzheimer's Association. (2015). *What is Alzheimer's?* Retrieved from http://www.alz.org/alzheimers_disease_what_is_alzheimers.asp

American Cancer Society. (2016). *Cancer facts & figures for African Americans 2016–2018.* Retrieved from https://www.cancer.org/content/dam/cancer-org/research/cancer-facts-and-statistics/cancer-facts-and-figures-for-african-americans/cancer-facts-and-figures-for-african-americans-2016-2018.pdf

Aon Hewitt for AARP. (2015). *A business case for workers age 50+: A look at the value of experience.* Retrieved from http://states.aarp.org/wp-content/uploads/2015/08/A-Business-Case-for-Older-Workers-Age-50-A-Look-at-the-Value-of-Experience.pdf

Bank of America Corporation. (2016). *Giving in retirement: America's longevity bonus. A Merrill Lynch retirement study conducted in partnership with Age Wave.* Retrieved from https://mlaem.fs.ml.com/content/dam/ML/Articles/pdf/ML_AgeWave_Giving_in_Retirement_Report.pdf

Beard, J. R., Officer, A., de Carvalho, I. A., Sadana, R., Pot, A. M., Michel, J.-P., . . . Chatterji, S. (2016). The world report on ageing and health: A policy framework for healthy ageing. *Lancet, 387*(10033), 2145–2154. http://doi.org/10.1016/S0140-6736(15)00516-4

Beltrán-Sánchez, H., Jiménez, M. P., & Subramanian, S. V. (2016). Assessing morbidity compression in two cohorts from the Health and Retirement Study. *Journal of Epidemiology and Community Health, 70*(10), 1011–1016. http://doi.org/10.1136/jech-2015-206722

Braveman, P. A., Cubbin, C., Egerter, S., Williams, D. R., & Pamuk, E. (2010). Socioeconomic disparities in health in the United States: What the patterns tell us. *American Journal of Public Health, 100*(Suppl. 1), S186–S196. http://doi.org/10.2105/AJPH.2009.166082

Brown, T. H., Hargrove, T. W., & Griffith, D. M. (2015). Racial/ethnic disparities in men's health: Examining psychosocial mechanisms. *Family & Community Health, 38*(4), 307–318. http://doi.org/10.1097/FCH.0000000000000080

Buffel, T., & Phillipson, C. (2016). Can global cities be "age-friendly cities"? Urban development and ageing populations. *Cities, 55*, 94–100. http://doi.org/10.1016/J.CITIES.2016.03.016

Cacioppo, J., & Hawkley, L. (2009). Perceived social isolation and cognition. *Trends in Cognitive Sciences, 13*(10), 447–454. http://doi.org/10.1016/j.tics.2009.06.005

Centers for Disease Control and Prevention (CDC). (2013). State-specific healthy life expectancy at age 65 years—United States, 2007–2009. *Morbidity and Mortality Weekly Report, 62*(28), 561–566. Retrieved from https://www.cdc.gov/mmwr/preview/mmwrhtml/mm6228a1.htm

Centers for Disease Control and Prevention (CDC). (2015). Vital signs: Leading causes of death, prevalence of diseases and risk factors, and use of health services among Hispanics in the United States—2009–2013. *Morbidity and Mortality Weekly Report, 64*(17), 469–478. Retrieved from https://www.cdc.gov/mmwr/preview/mmwrhtml/mm6417a5.htm?s_cid=mm6417a5_w

Centers for Disease Control and Prevention (CDC). (2017). Healthy Aging Data Portal. Retrieved from https://www.cdc.gov/aging/agingdata/index.html

Centers for Medicare and Medicaid Services (CMS). (2012). *Chronic conditions among Medicare beneficiaries, chartbook, 2012 edition.* Retrieved from https://www.cms.gov/research-statistics-data-and-systems/statistics-trends-and-reports/chronic-conditions/downloads/2012chartbook.pdf

Chetty, R., Stepner, M., Abraham, S., Lin, S., Scuderi, B., Turner, N., . . . Cutler, D. (2016). The association between income and life expectancy in the United States, 2001–2014. *Journal of the American Medical Association, 315*(16), 1750. http://doi.org/10.1001/jama.2016.4226

Colby, S. L., & Ortman, J. M. (2015). *Projections of the size and composition of the U.S. population: 2014 to 2060.* Retrieved from https://www.census.gov/content/dam/Census/library/publications/2015/demo/p25-1143.pdf

DeSantis, C. E., Ma, J., Goding Sauer, A., Newman, L. A., & Jemal, A. (2017). Breast cancer statistics, 2017, racial disparity in mortality by state. *CA: A Cancer Journal for Clinicians.* Retrieved from http://onlinelibrary.wiley.com/doi/10.3322/caac.21412/abstract;jsessionid=F3005373B8811B79BE547B0E3A371ABB.f03t01

Fairlie, R., Morelix, A., Reedy, E., & Russell, J. (2015). The Kauffman Index: Startup activity national trends. Retrieved from http://www.kauffman.org/kauffman-index

Fall, C. H. D. (2013). Fetal malnutrition and long-term outcomes. *Nestle Nutrition Institute Workshop Series, 74,* 11–25. http://doi.org/10.1159/000348384

Federal Interagency Forum on Aging-Related Statistics. (2016). *Older Americans 2016: Key indicators of well-being.* Washington, DC: Author. Retrieved from https://agingstats.gov/docs/LatestReport/Older-Americans-2016-Key-Indicators-of-WellBeing.pdf

File, T. (2017). Voting in America: A look at the 2016 presidential election. Retrieved from https://www.census.gov/newsroom/blogs/random-samplings/2017/05/voting_in_america.html

Fredriksen-Goldsen, K. I. (2016). The future of LGBT+ aging: A blueprint for action in services, policies, and research. *Generations, 40*(2), 6–15. Retrieved from http://www.ncbi.nlm.nih.gov/pubmed/28366980

Fredriksen-Goldsen, K. I., Kim, H.-J., Shui, C., & Bryan, A. E. B. (2017). Chronic health conditions and key health indicators among lesbian, gay, and bisexual older US adults, 2013–2014. *American Journal of Public Health, 107*(8), 1332–1338. http://doi.org/10.2105/AJPH.2017.303922

Fried, L. P., Carlson, M. C., Freedman, M., Frick, K. D., Glass, T. A., Hill, J., . . . Zeger, S. (2004). A social model for health promotion for an aging population: Initial evidence on the Experience Corps model. *Journal of Urban Health : Bulletin of the New York Academy of Medicine, 81*(1), 64–78. http://doi.org/10.1093/jurban/jth094

Fried, L. P., Carlson, M. C., McGill, S., Seeman, T., Xue, Q.-L., Frick, K., . . . Rebok, G. W. (2013). Experience Corps: A dual trial to promote the health of older adults and children's academic success. *Contemporary Clinical Trials, 36*(1), 1–13. http://doi.org/10.1016/j.cct.2013.05.003

Gerteis, J., Izrael, D., Deitz, D., LeRoy, L., Ricciardi, R., Miller, T., & Basu, J. (2014). *Multiple chronic conditions chartbook.* AHRQ Publications No, Q14-0038. Rockville, MD: Agency for Healthcare Research and Quality. Retrieved from https://www.ahrq.gov/sites/default/files/wysiwyg/professionals/prevention-chronic-care/decision/mcc/mccchartbook.pdf

Goldman, L., Finkelstein, R., Schafer, P., & Pugh, T. (2014). *Resilient communities: Empowering older adults in disasters and daily life.* Retrieved from https://nyam.org/media/filer_public/64/b2/64b2da62-f4e7-4e04-b5d1-e0e52b2a5614/resilient_communities_report_final.pdf

Hagestad, G. O., & Uhlenberg, P. (2005). The social separation of old and young: A root of ageism. *Journal of Social Issues, 61*(2), 343–360. http://doi.org/10.1111/j.1540-4560.2005.00409.x

Hawkley, L. (2003). Loneliness in everyday life: Cardiovascular activity, psychosocial context, and health behaviors. *Journal of Personality and Social Psychology, 85*(1), 105–120.

He, W., Goodkind, D., & Kowal, P. (2016). *An aging world: 2015.* International Population Reports, P95/16-1. Washington, DC: U.S. Census Bureau. Retrieved from https://www.census.gov/content/dam/Census/library/publications/2016/demo/p95-16-1.pdf

Henry J. Kaiser Family Foundation. (2013). *Medicare's role for older women.* Retrieved from https://www.kff.org/womens-health-policy/fact-sheet/medicares-role-for-older-women/

Hughes, A. K., Harold, R. D., & Boyer, J. M. (2011). Awareness of LGBT aging issues among aging services network providers. *Journal of Gerontological Social Work, 54*(7), 659–677. http://doi.org/10.1080/01634372.2011.585392

Klinenberg, E. (2002). *Heat wave: A social autopsy of disaster in Chicago.* Chicago, IL: University of Chicago Press.

Mistry, R. (2001). Social isolation predicts re-hospitalization in a group of older American veterans enrolled in the UPBEAT Program. *International Journal of Geriatric Psychiatry, 16*(10), 950–959.

Morrow-Howell, N., Hinterlong, J., Rozario, P. A., & Tang, F. (2003). Effects of volunteering on the well-being of older adults. *Journals of Gerontology, Series B: Psychological Sciences and Social Sciences, 58*(3), S137–S145.

Musick, M. A., Herzog, A. R., & House, J. S. (1999). Volunteering and mortality among older adults: Findings from a national sample. *Journals of Gerontology, Series B: Psychological Sciences and Social Sciences, 54*(3), S173–S180.

Mysuyk, Y., Westendorp, R. G. J., & Lindenberg, J. (2015). Perspectives on the etiology of violence in later life. *Journal of Interpersonal Violence.* Retrieved from http://journals.sagepub.com/doi/10.1177/0886260515584338

National Center for Health Statistics. (2017). *Health, United States, 2016: With chartbook on long-term trends in health.* Hyattsville, MD: Author. Retrieved from https://www.cdc.gov/nchs/data/hus/hus16.pdf

National Senior Citizens Law Center, National Gay and Lesbian Task Force, Services & Advocacy for GLBT Elders, National Center for Lesbian Rights, Lambda Legal, & National Center for Transgender Equality. (2011). *LGBT older adults in long-term care facilities: Stories from the field.* Retrieved from http://www.lgbtagingcenter.org/resources/pdfs/NSCLC_LGBT_report.pdf

New York City Department for the Aging. (2017). *Age-Friendly NYC: New commitments for a city for all ages.* Retrieved from http://www.nyc.gov/html/dfta/downloads/pdf/age_friendly/AgeFriendlyNYC2017.pdf

New York City Department of Transportation. (2017). Safe streets for seniors. Retrieved from http://www.nyc.gov/html/dot/html/pedestrians/safeseniors.shtml

Olshansky, S. J., Antonucci, T., Berkman, L., Binstock, R. H., Boersch-Supan, A., Cacioppo, J. T., . . . Rowe, J. (2012). Differences in life expectancy due to race and educational differences are widening, and many may not catch up. *Health Affairs (Project Hope), 31*(8), 1803–1813. http://doi.org/10.1377/hlthaff.2011.0746

Olshansky, S. J., Perry, D., Miller, R. A., & Butler, R. N. (2007). Pursuing the longevity dividend: Scientific goals for an aging world. *Annals of the New York Academy of Sciences, 1114*(1), 11–13. http://doi.org/10.1196/annals.1396.050

Paullin, C. (2014). *The aging workforce: Leveraging the talents of mature employees.* Retrieved from https://

www.shrm.org/hr-today/trends-and-forecasting/special-reports-and-expert-views/Documents/Aging-Workforce-Talents-Mature-Employees.pdf

Peprah, E., Xu, H., Tekola-Ayele, F., & Royal, C. D. (2015). Genome-wide association studies in Africans and African Americans: Expanding the framework of the genomics of human traits and disease. *Public Health Genomics, 18*(1), 40–51. http://doi.org/10.1159/000367962

Pitt-Catsouphes, M., Mirvis, P., & Berzin, S. (2013). Leveraging age diversity for innovation. *Journal of Intergenerational Relationships, 11*(3), 238–254. http://doi.org/10.1080/15350770.2013.810059

Population Reference Bureau. (2017). How neighborhoods affect the health and well-being of older Americans. *Today's Research on Aging, 35.* Retrieved from http://www.prb.org/pdf17/TRA 35.pdf

Rowe, J. W., & Kahn, R. L. (2015). Successful Aging 2.0: Conceptual expansions for the 21st century. *Journals of Gerontology, Series B: Psychological Sciences and Social Sciences, 70*(4), 593–596. http://doi.org/10.1093/geronb/gbv025

Sadana, R., Blas, E., Budhwani, S., Koller, T., & Paraje, G. (2016). Healthy ageing: Raising awareness of inequalities, determinants, and what could be done to improve health equity. *Gerontologist, 56*(suppl 2), S178–S193. http://doi.org/10.1093/geront/gnw034

Stein, C., & Moritz, I. (1999). *A life course perspective of maintaining independence in older age.* Retrieved from http://apps.who.int/iris/bitstream/10665/65576/1/WHO_HSC_AHE_99.2_life.pdf

Stowell-Ritter, A., Bridges, K., & Sims, R. (2006). *Good to go: Assessing the transit needs of New York Metro AARP members.* Retrieved from http://assets.aarp.org/rgcenter/il/ny_transit_06.pdf

Tesch-Römer, C., & Wahl, H.-W. (2017). Toward a more comprehensive concept of successful aging: Disability and care needs. *Journals of Gerontology, Series B: Psychological Sciences and Social Sciences, 72*(2), 310–318. http://doi.org/10.1093/geronb/gbw162

Toossi, M., & Torpey, E. (2017). Older workers: Labor force trends and career options. *Career Outlook.* U.S. Bureau of Labor Statistics. Retrieved from https://www.bls.gov/careeroutlook/2017/article/older-workers.htm

Tucker-Seeley, R. D., Subramanian, S. V., Li, Y., & Sorensen, G. (2009). Neighborhood safety, socioeconomic status, and physical activity in older adults. *American Journal of Preventive Medicine, 37*(3), 207–213. http://doi.org/10.1016/j.amepre.2009.06.005

United Nations. (2017). *World population ageing.* Retrieved from http://www.un.org/en/development/desa/population/publications/pdf/ageing/WPA2017_Highlights.pdf

University of Michigan Institute for Social Research. (2017). *The Health and Retirement Study: Aging in the 21st century: Challenges and opportunities for Americans.* Retrieved from http://hrsonline.isr.umich.edu/sitedocs/databook/inc/pdf/HRS-Aging-in-the-21St-Century.pdf

Wadhwa, V., Freeman, R., & Rissing, B. (2008). *Education and tech entrepreneurship.* Retrieved from http://citeseerx.ist.psu.edu/viewdoc/download?doi=10.1.1.560.1474&rep=rep1&type=pdf

Werner, C. A. (2011). The older population: 2010. *2010 Census Briefs.* Retrieved from https://www.census.gov/prod/cen2010/briefs/c2010br-09.pdf

Wight, R. G., Aneshensel, C. S., Miller-Martinez, D., Botticello, A. L., Cummings, J. R., Karlamangla, A. S., & Seeman, T. E. (2006). Urban neighborhood context, educational attainment, and cognitive function among older adults. *American Journal of Epidemiology, 163*(12), 1071–1078. http://doi.org/10.1093/aje/kwj176

Williams, R., White, P., Nieto, J., Vieira, D., Francois, F., & Hamilton, F. (2016). Colorectal cancer in African Americans: An update. *Clinical and Translational Gastroenterology, 7*(7), e185. http://doi.org/10.1038/ctg.2016.36

World Health Organization (WHO). (2007). *Global age-friendly cities: A guide.* Geneva, Switzerland: Author. Retrieved from http://www.who.int/ageing/publications/Global_age_friendly_cities_Guide_English.pdf

World Health Organization (WHO). (2015). *Measuring the age-friendliness of cities: A guide to using core indicators.* Kobe, Japan: WHO Centre for Health Development. Retrieved from http://apps.who.int/iris/bitstream/10665/203830/1/9789241509695_eng.pdf?ua=1

World Health Organization (WHO). (2017). *Age-friendly world.* Retrieved from https://extranet.who.int/agefriendlyworld/who-network/

CHAPTER 4

Age-Friendly Health Systems

Kedar S. Mate, Leslie Pelton, Amy Berman, and Terry Fulmer

CHAPTER OBJECTIVES

1. Describe the aims, purpose, and expected benefits addressed by Age-Friendly Health Systems.
2. Identify core content principles underlying an Age-Friendly Health System.

KEY TERMS

Geriatric care models Health systems Triple Aim

▶ Introduction

The population of older adults with complex needs in the United States is growing rapidly. The age 65 and older population increased 15.1% between 2000 and 2010, compared with a 9.7% increase for the total U.S. population over the same period (West, Cole, Goodkind, & He, 2014). Individuals age 65 and older now make up 13% of the total U.S. population, compared with 12.4% in 2000 and 4.1% in 1900. Coupled with this increase in the number of older adults is their greater projected needs for health care

and long-term services and supports: The U.S. Department of Health and Human Services estimates that 70% of people older than age 65 will need long-term care at some point in their lives (Chernof & Warshawsky, 2014).

Safe and effective care of older adults (the **Triple Aim**) is actually a pressing need on a global scale, given the rapid growth of the aging population in many countries around the world. Current healthcare delivery systems are not, and have never been, adequately prepared to support these complex needs, and care systems often fall short in this area (Coleman, 2013; Coleman & Boult,

2003; Knight, 2013; Levison, 2010; Pham, O'Malley, Bach, Saiontz-Martinez, & Schrag, 2009). These shortcomings are not for lack of substantial, creditworthy effort. Dozens of models to improve care for older adults have been shown to lead to improved outcomes in different care settings, but the spread and scale of these models have been limited (Fulmer et al., 2002; Hirth, Baskins, & Dever-Bumba, 2009; Malone, Capezuti, & Palmer, 2015; Mezey, Fulmer, & Fletcher, 2002; SteelFisher, Martin, Dowal, & Inouye, 2011). In the United States, the policy and payment environment continues to evolve toward value-based care, which may offer long-sought incentives and opportunities to improve the care of older adults (Institute of Medicine et al., 2010).

This chapter describes the concept design for an Age-Friendly Health System—a model that is long overdue, but just might be possible to implement in today's healthcare environment (Mate, Berman, Laderman, Kabcenell, & Fulmer, 2017). An Age-Friendly Health System is clearly defined, and its aims, purpose, and expected benefits elaborated. The core content principles underlying an Age-Friendly Health System are described, including how they were derived. The chapter concludes with a description of how the concept of an Age-Friendly Health System is being tested today and how it will spread and scale rapidly throughout the United States in the coming years.

▶ Defining Age-Friendly Health Systems

Much is known about what older adults need to be healthy and to improve their health when illness strikes. Evidence-based models to improve care and outcomes for older adults exist across both clinical and nonclinical settings, including the home and community settings (Malone et al., 2015). Every day across the United States, excellent care is delivered to older adults in hospitals, skilled nursing facilities, physician offices, and community-based settings by leveraging these evidence-based models and applying them with empathy and compassion. And yet, every day across the United States, some older adults "fall through the cracks" in hospitals, as they transition from hospital to home, and in their homes and communities. In hospitals, despite our best intentions, some older adults are given medications that are known to cause harm (Field et al., 2005), delirium is disregarded as "understandable confusion," and there is inadequate attention to mobility and home safety (Kosar, Thomas, Inouye, & Mor, 2017; Oh, Fong, Hshieh, & Inouye, 2017). Across all settings, it remains a rare event to invite patients into a dialogue about what truly matters to them as they transit through the health system (Fulmer, Mate, & Berman, 2017).

There is a gap between the evidence-based models of health care for older adults and the care that our **health systems** put into practice at every touch point that older adults experience with those health systems. This is the "know–do" gap: We "know" the right way to care for older adults, yet our practices have not been able to consistently "do" it every day for every patient.

There are two distinguishing characteristics of Age-Friendly Health Systems: They eliminate that knowledge to action gap, and they ensure that the gap is closed for every patient, every day, and at every touch point. Age-Friendly Health Systems "do" what they "know" is best with older adults through implementation of evidence-based interventions that improve the building blocks of Age-Friendly care (defined further in "Methods" section). Further, Age-Friendly Health Systems commit to system-level outcome measures that are stratified by age. They also commit to leadership engagement in issues of aging and align their strategic priorities with Age-Friendly care. These commitments ensure that interdisciplinary teams in all care settings are enabled and expected to deliver Age-Friendly care.

▶ The Challenge

Health care historically has focused on the cure of acute disease, with the hospital seen as the primary entity within the healthcare delivery system. While hospitals remain critical to communities and serve as financial hubs for healthcare delivery, the population of both the United States and the world has aged—a factor that means care today is primarily devoted to the management of chronic disease. The goal of healthcare delivery in the face of this demographic shift and the rise of chronicity is the management of multimorbidity to prevent sentinel hospital admissions, which are largely acute exacerbations of chronic conditions, and subsequent hospital readmissions.

As health care moves from an emphasis on volume to a focus on value, the older adult population offers one of the greatest opportunities to improve care, health outcomes, and costs of care by deploying the existing strong evidence base for geriatric care. Healthcare systems are slowly awakening to the need to address population health. All too often, though, health system leaders have not sufficiently addressed the unique needs of older adults—despite the reality that this is the largest population segment they serve, and a group associated with disproportionately poor cost and quality outcomes. Avoidable harms in older adult patients include medication errors, falls, pressure ulcers, and delirium. A set of equally insidious harms are experienced when healthcare providers and systems either fail to identify and respect the wishes of older adults or do not address the supports and services needed by vulnerable elders to live independently in the community.

The John A. Hartford Foundation, in partnership with the Institute for Healthcare Improvement, established Age-Friendly Health Systems as a way to address two goals: (1) consistently address preventable harms across the continuum of care and (2) fundamentally shift the culture of care by laying a foundation consisting of essential evidence-based elements of care that are known to improve health and cost outcomes while focusing on what matters most to older adults.

▶ Aim, Purpose, and Expected Benefits

The healthcare delivery environment is rapidly changing, offering a new set of opportunities to improve the care of older adults. In this age of concerns about population health and financial risk beyond the hospital stay, hospitals are consolidating into health systems that incorporate a wide but inconsistent array of services—ranging from home health care, hospice, post-acute rehabilitation, primary care, Programs of All-Inclusive Care for the Elderly (PACE), and palliative care, to contracts with social services agencies. This consolidation and integration of disparate services offers health systems an opportunity to better deploy their existing resources and introduce evidence-based strategies that can improve the quality of care for older adults, drawing upon the John A. Hartford Foundation's investment in geriatric experts and models of care.

The Age-Friendly Health Systems initiative aims to ensure that the fundamentals of evidence-based geriatric care are consistently implemented across the continuum of care, from inpatient settings to care in the community. It targets common failures of health systems by focusing on essential elements of care as markers aimed at improving the health of older adults and value for the health system.

The Age-Friendly Health Systems initiative has been co-designed by geriatric care experts, health systems leaders, and experts in improvement science and dissemination. Building on these core strengths, the effort is taking the best of what we know of good geriatric care and coupling it with what is feasible in healthcare delivery systems to build with spread and scale in mind. This co-design effort is testing and validating a health-system-wide approach to care for older adults, measuring the impact on health systems that embrace this perspective as compared with those lacking such an approach. The Age-Friendly Health Systems model is designed to measurably improve the quality of care for older adults and optimize value for health systems.

In November 2015, the John A. Hartford Foundation adopted the bold and important aim of establishing an Age-Friendly Health Systems approach to measurably improve the quality of care for the growing older adult population and optimize value for health systems. The goal is to reach 20% of U.S. hospitals and health systems by December 2020 with the Age-Friendly Health Systems model of care.

▶ Methods

Eliminating the knowledge to action gap in more than 20% of U.S. hospitals requires implementation of a rigorous methodology. In June 2016, the John A. Hartford Foundation engaged with the Institute for Healthcare Improvement (IHI) to apply its expertise in innovation, improvement science, and health-related campaigns to create Age-Friendly Health Systems.

Creating an Age-Friendly Prototype Model for Testing by Early-Adopter Health Systems

Given the breadth and depth of evidence-based models of care with older adults, IHI's first step was to synthesize the knowledge on the "know" side of the gap. The Research & Development team at IHI analyzed 17 evidence-based **geriatric care models** and programs serving older adults for common elements: Which population is served? Which outcomes have been achieved? What are the core features of the intervention? More than 90 core features of these 17 programs were identified, though there was considerable overlap in the features. Ultimately, they were clustered into 13 distinct core features

that served as the design basis for a prototype model of Age-Friendly Health Care.

IHI then engaged health systems in the next step of the prototype development and encouraged them to engage with geriatric research experts. Researchers, clinical geriatric specialists, and health system leaders convened in an expert meeting to further refine the core features and select four or five features that would form the basis for the Age-Friendly model of care. The integration of health systems with the researchers at this step in the development of the prototype was itself a narrowing of the "know–do" gap. The outcome was the set of core features of the Age-Friendly Prototype, known as the "4M's":

1. *What Matters*: Know and act on each patient's specific health outcome goals and care preferences.
2. *Mobility*: Maintain mobility and function and prevent/treat complications of immobility.
3. *Medication*: Optimize use to reduce harm and burden, focusing on medications affecting mobility, mentation, and what matters.
4. *Mentation*: Focus on delirium and dementia and depression.

The next step was to build out the Age-Friendly core features with descriptions of what would be included in each of the 4M's. To further develop the core features, IHI and the John A. Hartford Foundation engaged a group of nine geriatric experts to further map out the high-level interventions that would occur within each of the 4M's. Five health systems were enlisted to serve as a testing community to investigate locally developed implementation ideas to reliably execute each of these high-level interventions (**TABLE 4-1**).

Testing of the Age-Friendly Prototype Model by Innovator Health Systems

Applying Everett Rogers's diffusion of innovations theory, IHI and The John A. Hartford

TABLE 4-1 The 4Ms: Interventions and Actions

		High-Level Interventions
What Matters	1	Know what matters: health outcome goals and care preferences for current and future care, including end-of-life care
	2	Act on what matters for current and future care, including end-of-life care
Mobility	3	Implement an individualized mobility plan
	4	Create an environment that enables mobility
Medication	5	Implement a standard process for Age-Friendly medication reconciliation
	6	De-prescribe and adjust doses to be Age-Friendly
Mentation	7	Ensure adequate nutrition and hydration, sleep, and comfort
	8	Engage and orient to maximize independence and dignity
	9	Identify, treat, and manage dementia, delirium, and depression

Foundation identified five innovator health systems that began testing the specific implementation ideas. The health system teams were able to move forward with creativity and navigate the inevitable ambiguity of a testing phase; they were inspired by starting something new and being in on the ground floor of its development, and were motivated through relationships with other early-adopter health systems and experts and geriatrics (**FIGURE 4-1**).

The prototype health system senior sponsors selected team leaders, microsystems for testing, and front-line teams. The leaders and teams were convened into a learning system for two-way sharing: (1) the teams learned a model for iterative testing and learning from IHI (see the nearby box) and (2) IHI captured the teams' experiences testing the Age-Friendly prototype and plans to illustrate the Age-Friendly model with practical implementation ideas that will be collated into "how-to" guides and other implementation support materials.

THE MODEL FOR IMPROVEMENT

To apply changes in their local settings, Age-Friendly Health Systems participants learn an approach for organizing and carrying out their improvement work, called the Model for Improvement. This model, developed by Associates in Process Improvement, identifies four key elements of successful process improvement: specific and measurable aims, measures of improvement that are tracked over time, key changes that will result in the desired Improvement, and a series of testing "cycles" during which teams learn how to apply key change ideas to their own organizations.

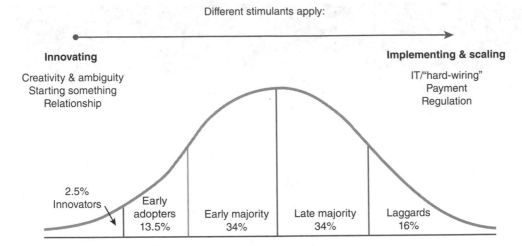

FIGURE 4-1 Rogers' Diffusion of Innovation.

Measurement

Concurrent to the development of the Age-Friendly prototype model, IHI engaged health system leaders, clinical geriatric experts, and its own improvement experts to develop a set of measures at the system level and for each of the 4M's. The approach was consistent with the development of the prototype model, in that it sought to narrow the "know–do" gap. For example, researchers and clinicians "know" that ambulation is critically important to the health of older adults, but there is a gap in what health systems consistently "do" with this knowledge. Health systems measure the number of falls among this population and, therefore, may inadvertently reduce the mobility of older adults to improve the reported measures. IHI applied the same two approaches to narrow the "know–do" gap with measures as it did when building the prototype: (1) bring geriatric experts together with health system leaders and (2) use the Model of Improvement, by testing the measures first on a small scale and then on a larger scale as confidence in the measures increased.

▶ Scale-Up Design and Social Movement

Spreading use of the model from the five innovator health systems to the early adopters and early majority was an intentional part of the work of the Age-Friendly Health Systems initiative. That intentionality included four components:

- Establish an aim for the scale-up by answering the following question: How many care delivery organizations did the Age-Friendly Health Systems initiative want to include?
- Define what will be spread and scaled up by answering the following question: What is an Age-Friendly Health System?
- Create demand and capacity among healthcare delivery organizations for becoming an Age-Friendly Health System.
- Build or utilize distribution channels for healthcare delivery organizations to become Age-Friendly Health Systems.

The goal of 1000 healthcare organizations becoming Age-Friendly by December 2020 was the bold and explicit aim established at the start of the initiative. This goal guided the design of each phase of the work. Following the initial testing phase (described earlier), the five initial health systems participants began a test of scale-up within their systems, with the eventual goal of spreading the Age-Friendly practices to all care sites within these five systems by the end of 2020. Beginning in 2019, new health systems will be recruited to join the initiative. These systems will adapt a well-established set of interventions to their local environments.

Spread of the Age-Friendly Health System model is dependent upon Age-Friendliness being adopted by initially tens, then hundreds, and then a thousand organizations. The design for its distribution is based on Rogers's (2010) diffusion of innovation theory. To be adopted widely, however, becoming an Age-Friendly Health System must convey a relative advantage to the organization, it needs to be compatible with the organizations' priorities, and its design needs to be simple, trial-able, and observable.

Recognizing that creating Age-Friendly Health Systems would require methods beyond the traditional quality improvement effort, Dr. Terry Fulmer, President of The John A. Hartford Foundation, characterized the work as a social movement. Social movement theory and practices, particularly those advocated by Marshall Ganz, senior lecturer in public policy at the Kennedy School of Government at Harvard University, were integrated into the design and development of the Age-Friendly initiative (see the nearby box) (Ganz, 2010). Ganz has written:

> . . . [S]ocial movements emerge from the efforts of purposeful actors, individuals or organizations, to respond to changes, to conditions experienced as unjust—not just inconvenient, but unjust—so as to assert new public values, form new relationships, and mobilize political, economic, and cultural power to translate those values into action. . . . The aim of such movements is not simply to reallocate goods, or "win the game," but instead to change the game's rules. (Roundtable on Population Health Improvement, Roundtable on the Promotion of Health Equity and the Elimination of Health Disparities, Board on Population Health and Public Health Practice, & Institute of Medicine, 2014)

THE MODEL FOR IMPROVEMENT

The Model for Improvement is a simple but powerful tool for accelerating change that has been used successfully by thousands of organizations to improve many different aspects of health care. This model has three components (**FIGURE 4-2**):

- Aim: What are we trying to accomplish? Here, participants determine which specific outcomes they are trying to change through their work.
- Measures: How will we know that a change is an improvement? Here, team members identify appropriate measures to track their success.
- Changes: Which changes can we make that will result in improvement? Here, teams identify key changes that they will actually test.

Once these components are in place, key changes are implemented in a cyclical fashion: Teams thoroughly plan to test the change, taking into account cultural and organizational characteristics; they do the work to make the change in their standard procedures, tracking their progress using quantitative measures; they closely study the results of their work for insights on how to do better; and they act to make the successful changes permanent or to adjust the changes that need more work. This process continues serially over time and refinement is added with each cycle; these are known as "plan–do–study–act" (PDSA) cycles of learning.

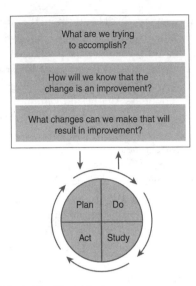

FIGURE 4-2 The Model for Improvement.

The core elements of nurturing and developing a social movement were integrated into each stage of the Age-Friendly Health System. For example, in the first stage, the innovator teams built relationships with one another and articulated first the narrative of *why* this work was important to each individual, *why* it was important to each team, and, finally, *why* it was important to their health systems. In addition to relationship building and narrative development, the Age-Friendly Health Systems initiative has developed strategies for engaging others in specific actions that will improve care for older adults. On this score, the American Hospital Association, with its state chapters and far reach into all or most U.S. hospitals, and the Catholic Health Association, with its well-development membership structure, were engaged early to help disseminate the Age-Friendly efforts. Others are planned to join in subsequent stages of the effort. At all points, the backbone supporting infrastructure of IHI and The John A. Hartford Foundation will be further developed to ensure execution of a well-organized campaign (Roundtable on Population Health Improvement et al., 2014).

▶ Expected Next Steps

At the end of year one of the work on creating Age-Friendly Health Systems, we have a clear operational definition of an Age-Friendly Health System with an attendant set of measures that will guide us, a set of high-leverage principle changes (the 4M's) for the content of what it will take to become Age-Friendly, and a group of initial health systems testing and learning about how to reliably execute those four principles across care settings. The next phase of the work will involve spreading and scaling across the five initial health systems. This will require clear and concise descriptions of the 4M's, how they interact, and how to implement them across various practice environments. Concrete guidance and implementation advice will come from the specific experiments that the participating health systems have led to date. The 4M's will be deployed by the five participating health systems employing various specific strategies. In some settings, the 4M's will be embedded condition by condition (starting with the most common conditions among older adults); in others, they will be embedded as part of strategic initiatives to partner with patients and engage families more routinely.

In all cases, the spread and scale-up of the 4M's and the Age-Friendly Health System will require a complex set of supporting changes that reach well beyond the specific technical changes. **FIGURE 4-3** identifies the primary changes that we now recognize to be essential to getting unstuck—that is, to moving beyond the pilot phase and toward large-scale change. The community of geriatric experts, in conjunction with the health system leaders, have set bold, inspiring aims and sourced a set of evidence-based practice changes. The five prototype testing health systems have developed dozens of practical implementation tactics, and The John A. Hartford/IHI team has begun the work of communicating the concept of an Age-Friendly Health System to key stakeholders.

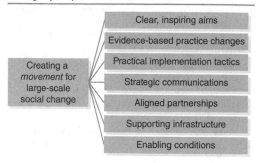

Getting beyond pilot: Let's build a movement

FIGURE 4-3 Creating a movement for large-scale social change.

More remains to be done to develop the partnerships needed to ensure that Age-Friendly Health Systems will thrive. Early partners have included the American Hospital Association, the Catholic Health Association, and The Joint Commission. Other professional societies, membership organizations, and government (federal and state) agencies, including local area Departments of Aging, are beginning to take notice, and the next phase of this work will include considerable effort at building collaborations to create the financial, regulatory, and payment conditions that will allow Age-Friendly Health Systems to thrive.

Finally, the supporting infrastructure for a national campaign to improve care for older adults will need to be cultivated. Distribution "nodes" from hospitals to home care agencies will need to be developed and nurtured. Candidates from the first five health systems and others that voluntarily began the process of transformation into Age-Friendly systems will be actively sought and cultivated as potential change agents that can help with the transformation of others during the efforts to reach national scale.

▶ Summary

Among all patient groups, older adults are at greatest risk for preventable harms and death caused by their healthcare experience. The Age-Friendly Health Systems initiative targets common failures of health systems by focusing on essential elements of care that will lead to better outcomes across the continuum of care. These essential elements of care, known as the 4M's, set the stage for a broader culture shift within healthcare delivery to address the needs of an aging population.

References

Chernof, B. A., & Warshawsky, M. J. (2014). Recommendations from the Federal Commission on Long-Term Care: Blueprint for a bipartisan path forward. *Public Policy & Aging Report, 24*(2), 37–39. doi: 10.1093/ppar/pru008

Coleman, E. (2013). The Care Transitions Program: Healthcare services for improving quality and safety during care hand-offs. Retrieved from https://caretransitions.org/about-the-care-transitions-intervention/

Coleman, E. A., & Boult, C. (2003). Improving the quality of transitional care for persons with complex care needs. *Journal of the American Geriatrics Society, 51*(4), 556–557.

Field, T. S., Gilman, B. H., Subramanian, S., Fuller, J. C., Bates, D. W., & Gurwitz, J. H. (2005). The costs associated with adverse drug events among older adults in the ambulatory setting. *Medical Care, 43*(12), 1171–1176.

Fulmer, T., Mate, K. S., & Berman, A. (2017). The Age-Friendly Health System imperative. *Journal of the American Geriatrics Society*. doi: 10.1111/jgs.15076

Fulmer, T., Mezey, M., Bottrell, M., Abraham, I., Sazant, J., Grossman, S., & Grisham, E. (2002). Nurses Improving Care for Healthsystem Elders (NICHE): Using outcomes and benchmarks for evidenced-based practice. *Geriatric Nursing, 23*(3), 121–127.

Ganz, M. (2010). Leading change: Leadership, organization, and social movements. Handbook of leadership theory and practice, 19.

Hirth, V., Baskins, J., & Dever-Bumba, M. (2009). Program of All-Inclusive Care (PACE): Past, present, and future. *Journal of the American Medical Directors Association, 10*, 155–160. doi: 10.1016/j.jamda.2008.12.002

Institute of Medicine, Roundtable on Value & Science-Driven Health Care, Yong, P. L., Olsen, L., McGinnis, J. M., & National Academies Press. (2010). *Value in health care: Accounting for cost, quality, safety, outcomes, and innovation: Workshop summary*. Washington, DC: National Academies Press.

Knight, S. J. (2013). Bridging the gap at the center of patient centeredness: Individual patient preferences in health care decision making. *JAMA Internal Medicine, 173*(5), 369–370. doi: 10.1001/jamainternmed.2013.3370

Kosar, C. M., Thomas, K. S., Inouye, S. K., & Mor, V. (2017). Delirium during postacute nursing home admission and risk for adverse outcomes. *Journal of the American Geriatrics Society, 65*(7), 1470–1475. doi: 10.1111/jgs.14823

Levison, D. (2010). *Adverse events in hospitals: National incidence among Medicare beneficiaries.* Retrieved from https://oig.hhs.gov/oei/reports/OEI-06-09-00090.pdf

Malone, M. L., Capezuti, E., & Palmer, R. M. (2015). *Geriatric models of care.* Cham, Switzerland: Springer International.

Mate, K. S., Berman, A., Laderman, M., Kabcenell, A., & Fulmer, T. (2017). Creating Age-Friendly Health Systems: A vision for better care of older adults. *Healthcare (Amsterdam).* doi: S2213-0764(17)30012-X

Mezey, M., Fulmer, T., & Fletcher, K. (2002). Nurses Improving Care to Healthsystems Elders (NICHE): Using outcomes and benchmarks for evidenced-based practice. *Geriatric Nursing, 23*(3), 1–7.

Oh, E. S., Fong, T. G., Hshieh, T. T., & Inouye, S. K. (2017). Delirium in older persons: Advances in diagnosis and treatment. *Journal of the American Medical Association, 318*(12), 1161–1174. doi: 10.1001/jama.2017.12067

Pham, H. H., O'Malley, A. S., Bach, P. B., Saiontz-Martinez, C., & Schrag, D. (2009). Primary care physicians' links to other physicians through Medicare patients: The scope of care coordination. *Annals of Internal Medicine, 150*(4), 236–242.

Rogers, E. M. (2010). *Diffusion of innovations 4th Edition.* New York, NY: Simon and Schuster.

Roundtable on Population Health Improvement, Roundtable on the Promotion of Health Equity and the Elimination of Health Disparities, Board on Population Health and Public Health Practice, & Institute of Medicine. (2014). *Supporting a movement for health and health equity: Lessons from social movements: Workshop summary.* Retrieved from https://www.ncbi.nlm.nih.gov/books/NBK268728/

SteelFisher, G. K., Martin, L. A., Dowal, S. L., & Inouye, S. K. (2011). Sustaining clinical programs during difficult economic times: A case series from the Hospital Elder Life Program. *Journal of the American Geriatrics Society, 59*(10), 1873–1882.

West, L. A., Cole, S., Goodkind, D., & He, W. (2014). *65+ in the United States: 2010.* U.S. Census Bureau. Retrieved from https://www.census.gov/content/dam/Census/library/publications/2014/demo/p23-212.pdf

CHAPTER 5

Payment Reform, Health System Transformation, and the Impact on Older Adults

Anna C. Davis, Ronald Navarro, Lynn M. Garofalo-Wright, Kate E. Koplan, and Nirav R. Shah

CHAPTER OBJECTIVES

1. Understand key concepts in payment reform and financial incentives in health care.
2. Describe the rationale for payment reform.
3. Explain how payment reform may impact older adults.

KEY TERMS

Payment reform	Shared savings/shared risk	Triple Aim

▶ Introduction

In 2008, Don Berwick established the vision of the "**Triple Aim**"—that is, better care and improved health at a lower cost (Berwick, Nolan, & Whittingon, 2008). Since that time, the vision of higher-value care for the United States has proliferated, and acceptance of the importance of Triple Aim outcomes has become widespread.

Historically, health care in the United States was financed through a "fee for service" (FFS) mechanism in which providers were paid a fixed price for units of service delivered to patients. Such a "retail" approach is relatively simple to administer, but creates financial incentives for providers to deliver more care and more expensive care—sometimes called a "volume over value" or "heads in beds" mindset. Although academicians have long debated the existence of "induced demand" (i.e., utilization driven by the FFS incentives felt by providers to deliver more care; Evans, 1974), there is little disagreement now that reframing healthcare incentives to align with the Triple Aim goals of care, health, and value is the right path ahead (Porter, 2009).

The field of behavioral economics can shed much light on the incentives experienced by both providers and patients. Thoughtful benefit designs and payment systems can "nudge" both producers and consumers in the economic equation to act in a manner that promotes overall welfare and well-being (Thaler & Sunstein, 2009). Delivery system and **payment reform** initiatives use economic principles to create financial incentives that can be fine-tuned to tap into intrinsic and extrinsic motivators and help people do the right thing, whether that is to get recommended screenings and preventive care, avoid unnecessary or goal-discordant procedures, or attend well-child visits. We believe that these payment and delivery system reforms are the key to achieving the Triple Aim,

and hold the promise of better value in a truly attainable light.

This chapter first reviews concepts in payment and care transformation, and defines risk, savings, and bundling. We then describe the evolution of total joint replacement procedures over the last decade as a teaching example of the powerful effect of payment reform and delivery system transformation. Finally, we discuss how payment reform and system transformation may impact older adults, and conclude by describing barriers on the path to comprehensive payment reform.

▶ Bigger Bundles Are Better

In general, payment reform involves the "bundling" of reimbursement into aggregated groups of (1) services, (2) patients, or (3) time. As illustrated in **FIGURE 5-1**, we can conceptualize a continuum of payment reforms, which move from the fee-for-service system to increasingly aggregated payment models, including bundled payments, partial or full capitation, and global budgets. As bundles get bigger, they wrap in

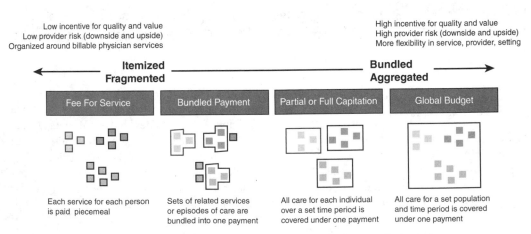

FIGURE 5-1 Payment bundling incentivizes quality, value, and flexibility by introducing risk.

Courtesy of Dana Barnes MPH, Kaiser Permanente.

more services and can be defined to include both upside and downside risk for providers (commonly called **shared savings** and **shared risk**) (Burke, 2013; Delbanco, Anderson, Major, Kiser, & Toner, 2011).

The following basic definitions of payment models are drawn from the work of Davis and Long (2013):

- *Bundled payment:* Grouped reimbursements for all services used by a patient within a single episode of care related to a specific medical treatment or event (e.g., total knee replacement).
- *Partial or full capitation:* Prospective payments for the total cost of care per person across settings and for a defined time period; can be specific to care related to a single condition (e.g., diabetes) or a cluster of conditions.
- *Global budget:* A total fixed budget, prospectively defined for the care of a specific population (e.g., based on geography) or organization (e.g., a hospital) over a defined period of time.

These core payment models can be supplemented by strategies layered on to fine-tune incentives for quality and value:

- *Pay for performance:* Financial rewards or penalties tied to provider or system performance, which are typically based on quality-of-care benchmarks.
- *Shared savings/shared risk:* An arrangement in which providers are offered a portion of savings (or take on a portion of risk) for a population. Agreements can be one-sided or two-sided, and include upside risk, downside risk, or both. In shared risk arrangements, providers are accountable for excess expenditures, so they accept some risk that has traditionally been held by the purchaser or the payer.

In 2015, the Centers for Medicare and Medicaid Services (CMS) set a goal of tying 50% of its reimbursement to quality or value through alternative payment models by 2018 (Burwell,

2015; Ginsburg & Patel, 2017). Waves of payment reform demonstrations have come from CMS over the last decade, including the Bundled Payment for Care Improvements (BPCI) Model (CMS, 2017) and the Comprehensive Care for Joint Replacement (CJR) Model (CMS, 2015). This ongoing shift has already transformed the organization of care, as providers increasingly move from solo practice to larger organizational structures that have the capacity to accept bundled payments and manage the risk that accompanies them (Burke, 2013). The rise in Accountable Care Organizations (ACOs) is one example of an organizational structure that supports value-based payment.

In concert with efforts to bundle an increasing share of payments and shift provider-side incentives, payers can also work to rationalize the incentives faced by consumers (Loewenstein, Asch, & Volpp, 2013). Adjusting copayment and coinsurance algorithms to encourage health maintenance activities is one clear opportunity. The removal of patient cost-sharing for preventive services under the Affordable Care Act was one example of such a policy (Koh & Sebelius, 2010).

▶ Total Joints: Yesterday, Today, and Tomorrow

More than 1 million total hip and knee replacement procedures are done each year in the United States (Kremers et al., 2015). Total joint replacement (TJR) procedures can alter the life-course of patients who receive them, granting continued independence and dignity, easing pain, and enabling mobility even in patients with advanced arthritis. With the aging of the U.S. population, total hip and knee replacements are projected to become the most common elective surgical procedures (Kremers et al., 2015). TJRs are regarded as safe and highly effective, although elderly patients receiving a TJR may experience a higher risk of potential complications (Talmo, Aghazadeh, & Bono, 2012).

Yesterday

Yesterday's TJR might be characterized by fragmentation and just-in-time management. In the fee-for-service paradigm, there are few incentives for providers to coordinate care or minimize inpatient days and days spent in a skilled nursing facility (SNF), and some payment arrangements actually dis-incentivize shortened stays. Despite the promise of improved quality of life for older adults who receive a TJR, the period of recovery can be extended. During the average hip replacement surgery, for example, the patient receives general anesthesia, delaying postoperative mobilization and making recovery time slower. After a three-day stay in the hospital, the patient is discharged to a SNF for rehabilitation prior to recovery at home. Too many patients are readmitted for inadequate pain control or other challenges during the period of recovery. Some frail patients experience cascading decline linked to postoperative events (e.g., delirium, blood clots, pneumonia) that might have been preventable with adequate preoperative planning and postoperative management (Talmo et al., 2012).

In many cases, the patient receives little information about what to expect prior to the surgery. Shared decision making is limited, with patient preferences regarding pursuit of surgery (versus more conservative choices) and preferred location of recovery largely unknown or ignored. Care is organized to optimize efficiency and convenience for surgeons. Taken together, patients receive narrow preoperative and postoperative management, ultimately leading to greater costs and worse outcomes. Fee-for-service reimbursement establishes few incentives for providers to reorganize or reframe TJR processes.

Today

Patients needing a TJR today in many systems have a phenomenally better experience than the traditional FFS-based experience. A growing body of literature recognizes the improvement potential of enhanced recovery interventions (Ibrahim, Alazzawi, Nizam, & Haddad, 2013; Proudfoot, Bennett, Duff, & Palmer, 2017), which are becoming the new standard for TJR in a framework of bundled payments that incentivizes this approach.

In Kaiser Permanente Southern California, orthopedic surgeons perform approximately 3600 elective hip surgeries and 8000 elective knee surgeries each year. Most recently, about 20% of our hip and knee patients recovered at home with no hospital stay. By the end of 2018, we hope to grow that percentage to 50% (Shah, Garofalo-Wright, Navarro, & Kanter, 2017). Orthopedic teams in Kaiser Permanente regions across the country are building and spreading similar programs. This shift respects each patient's preferred pathway through shared decision making, and reflects the recognition that patient preference is frequently for recovery at home.

These patients receive preoperative and postoperative supportive care at home to ensure successful recovery (**FIGURE 5-2**). Patients in this care pathway get what they want: recovery at home where they can sleep better, they have total control over visiting hours, and they can access all the comforts of home. Our data show that the readmission rate for our patients who go home immediately after surgery is as good as or better than the rate for patients who recover in the hospital.

We achieve this ambitious model through a standardized and multidisciplinary workflow that begins four to eight weeks before the procedure. What happens before surgery is foundational and important: the patient and family receive education on what to expect from a total joint care coordinator in a group class or by phone; the correct-sized walkers or canes are delivered; in some cases, a physical therapist visits the patient's home to conduct a safety evaluation and basic accessibility in the home is addressed, such as by moving the patient's bed to the ground floor or setting up sleeping arrangements to accommodate this state. This preparation sets expectations for "normal" during the subsequent home recovery, and introduces important members of the care team to the patient and family.

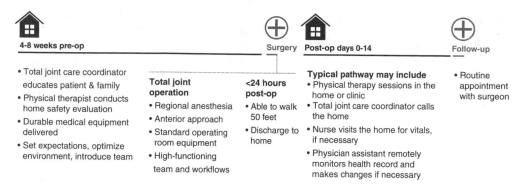

FIGURE 5-2 Total joint replacement at Kaiser Permanente today entails maximum time at home—and minimal time in the intensive, expensive hospital setting.

Courtesy of Dana Barnes MPH, Kaiser Permanente.

On the day of the surgery, the patient receives a regional anesthesia protocol (e.g. periarticular injections, regional block) and the orthopedic surgeon uses an anterior approach in many cases (innovative for a hip replacement). Such an approach reduces the pain of surgery and recovery, and together with the avoidance of general anesthesia, allows the patient to walk almost immediately after the operation. Operating room teams are highly functioning, and use a standard set of implant devices and surgical tools, enabling protocolized workflows and better safety practices for nurses and operating room technicians.

After surgery and recovery, the patient demonstrates walking safely at least 50 feet and goes home within a few hours of leaving the operating room—by lunch time for the first case of the day. The post-discharge pathway varies somewhat, but might typically include the following: On the following morning, a physical therapist arrives at the patient's home to begin the first of several physical therapy sessions. The care coordinator calls to check in and makes certain the patient has the care coordinator's phone number should the patient or family have any questions or concerns. A nurse may arrive to take vital signs if clinically necessary. A physician assistant reviews the electronic

health record and, if necessary, makes changes to the care regimen. Approximately two weeks later, there is an appointment in the orthopedic surgeon's outpatient office, closing the traditional loop.

This is reliably excellent care with multiple safety nets. Every workflow is created for and with patients, to empower caregivers and promote healing at home instead of deconditioning in the hospital. This careful choreography works only if the care team is highly functioning and all parties adhere to the appropriate standards and protocols, but an important part of the work is customization—to the important preferences and expectations of the patient and family, and to the local needs of the surgical and clinical care teams.

In Kaiser Permanente, we continue to work to standardize and optimize this process across our national footprint. Kaiser Permanente is not alone in pursuing this approach. Other systems have radically rethought care processes for TJRs, made possible by the shift to bundled payments and the resulting changes in provider and system incentives (Mouille, Higuer, Woicehovich, & Deadwiler, 2016; Navathe et al., 2017). The bundled payment allows health systems to spend funds on home-based services that might not have been feasible in a FFS framework.

Tomorrow

In a future where payment models support high-value approaches, incentives are aligned, and systems have the necessary supports (e.g., infrastructure, health information technology, workforce), all patients will experience a robust shared decision-making process prior to choosing to receive a TJR. Within a model such as the perioperative surgical home (Chimento & Thomas, 2017), patient preferences alongside necessary safety criteria will guide the place of surgery (ambulatory surgical center or hospital) and recovery pathway, with many being offered the option to recover at home. Regardless of the place of recovery, all patients will mobilize on postoperative day zero to speed the pace of recovery and to minimize the risk of postoperative complications. Providers will plan and conduct these procedures with the goal of same-day mobilization above physician- or facility-oriented productivity goals.

Moreover, this approach to care planning and execution will be translated to other services wherever safe and effective. Care pathways will focus on optimizing patient-centered outcomes. Bundled payments will flow to the providers or systems that can deliver the best quality and value for specific conditions or services (Porter & Lee, 2013). The window of the bundle will grow longer, extending further back in time.

Multidisciplinary "premanagement" will maximize quality of life, and will ensure "right-place and right-time" care for each patient, rather than waiting until the patient presents with a pressing need. Predictive analytics, population segmentation, and early assessment will help identify patients on a trajectory toward an event. Dedicated workflows will maintain optimal functioning for each patient as long as possible. The healthcare workforce will be cross-trained, just as some systems are already testing (Offord, Harriman, & Downes, 2017). In this framework, older adults receive assessment in their homes by a single "geriatric assessor" rather than individual physical therapy, occupational therapy, speech therapy, social needs, and nutrition specialists. These midlevel multispecialists will be equipped to recognize early indicators of vulnerability and risk, and will support the healthcare team in responding to patient needs across the spectrum of total health. Using a shared decision-making framework, they will know the patient and understand what matters most to them, and care will be approached with the patient's goals in the center. For patients undergoing TJR, this approach may prevent months or years of unnecessary pain and other needless suffering.

To support this vision of tomorrow, payment bundles will be expansive, enabling flexibility in services, provider, and setting. Providers and systems will experience incentives that align so as to encourage them to keep people well throughout the context of their life, rather than only when they enter the healthcare system (Westphal, Alkema, Seidel, & Chernof, 2016). Hospital rate setting as established in Maryland (Murray, 2009) and global budgets as tested in the Alternative Quality Contract (Song et al., 2012) are examples of payment arrangements that incentivize such approaches. Their aggregated nature encourages systems to deliver more proactive, preventive, and high-value care.

As we move toward increasing use of bundled payments, providers will require strategies for targeting specialized or customized services to patients with greater needs to realize the promise of shared savings (Kelley et al., 2017). As shown in **FIGURE 5-3**, patient segmentation methods could

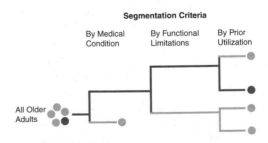

FIGURE 5-3 Mass customization of care for the needs of older adults—enabled by bundled payment systems—can be achieved through segmentation.

Courtesy of Dana Barnes MPH, Kaiser Permanente.

yield meaningful groups of patients who can be placed prospectively into care pathways early in their trajectory of illness. For older adults, segmentation algorithms might be designed on the basis of medical conditions, functional limitations, and prior utilization (Kelley et al., 2017).

With access to data on the total health of individuals, further segmentation based on social and nonmedical needs would add valuable insight, and could illuminate subgroups that would benefit from specialized services such as the following:

- In-home, nonclinical supportive caregiving and/or caregiver respite
- Community-based strategies to address social needs (e.g., food insecurity, housing instability, financial stress, isolation, transportation needs)
- Consultation from multidisciplinary palliative care teams to address symptom management, plan for end of life, and coordinate treatment plans across multiple specialties (Kelley et al., 2017)

▶ Summary

Porter and Lee (2013) believe that "transformation to value based care is well underway." Many systems and payers are recognizing the value agenda and organizing care accordingly. The evolution of TJRs is one example of these efforts to center care planning on what matters most to patients.

Payment reform and the accompanying system transformation hold the promise of radically improving care, quality, and value for all patients, including older adults. Nevertheless, many challenges remain to be overcome on the road to change. Payment reforms "challenge the status quo" and will require providers to reframe their perspective from expecting reimbursement for units of service delivered to managing risk and focusing on value (Burke, 2013). There are potential challenges to implementing quality-linked payment, such as the temptation to cherry pick lower risk patients; payment models

will require careful design with adequate risk adjustment to protect against these issues (Hood, 2007). Payers—and patients—will also face changing roles and responsibilities (Burke, 2013). Despite the depth of change that will be needed to realize the value equation, we believe that it is not only necessary but also possible. Other industries have embraced a value-delivery framework, leveraging a deep understanding of individuals' needs and habits to shape customized offerings and deliver convenient and customer-centered experiences. Health care is at the edge of this reform, and a cascade of services will be transformed in the model of the TJR evolution in the decade to come.

▶ Acknowledgments

We wish to thank the many front-line orthopedic surgeons, anesthesiologists, nurses, allied health providers, and administrators who collaborated to rethink how we could deliver better, more affordable care to our members who require total joint replacement surgery and who deliver this care every day. We also wish to acknowledge our leadership teams for their tenacity in championing this work. The graphics in this chapter were created by Dana C. Barnes, MPH.

References

Berwick, D. M., Nolan, T. W., & Whittington, J. (2008). The Triple Aim: Care, health, and cost. *Health Affairs*, *27*(3), 759–769.

Burke, G. (2013). *Moving toward accountable care in New York*. United Hospital Fund. Retrieved from https://www.uhfnyc.org/assets/1091

Burwell, S. M. (2015). Setting value-based payment goals: HHS efforts to improve US health care. *New England Journal of Medicine, 372*(10), 897–899.

Centers for Medicare and Medicaid Services (CMS). (2015). Comprehensive Care for Joint Replacement (CJR) model. Retrieved from https://www.cms.gov/Newsroom/MediaReleaseDatabase/Fact-sheets/2015-Fact-sheets-Items/2015-11-16.html

Centers for Medicare and Medicaid Services (CMS). (2017). Bundled Payments for Care Improvement (BPCI) initiative: General information. Retrieved from https://innovation.cms.gov/initiatives/bundled-payments/

Chimento, G. F., & Thomas, L. C. (2017). The perioperative surgical home: Improving the value and quality of care in total joint replacement. *Current Reviews in Musculoskeletal Medicine, 10*(3), 365–369.

Davis, A. C., & Long, P. (2013). *Multi-sector health care payment reform in California: Framing report for California's State Innovation Model Design Grant Workgroup.* Retrieved from http://www.calhospital .org/sites/main/files/file-attachments/cmmi_report.pdf

Delbanco, S. (2014). The payment reform landscape: Overview. *Health Affairs Blog.* Retrieved from https://www .healthaffairs.org/do/10.1377/hblog20140206.037019/full/.

Delbanco, S. F., Anderson, K. M., Major, C. E., Kiser, M. B., & Toner, B. W. (2011). *Promising payment reform: Risk-sharing with accountable care organizations.* Commonwealth Fund. Retrieved from http://www .commonwealthfund.org/~/media/files/publications /fund-report/2011/jul/1530delbancopromisingpayment reformrisksharing-2.pdf

Evans, R. G. (1974). Supplier-induced demand: Some empirical evidence and implications. In M. Perlman (Ed.), *The economics of health and medical care* (pp. 162–173). London, UK: Palgrave Macmillan UK.

Ginsburg, P. B., & Patel, K. K. (2017). Physician payment reform—progress to date. *New England Journal of Medicine, 377*(3), 285–292.

Hood, R. G. (2007). Pay-for-performance—financial health disparities and the impact on healthcare disparities. *Journal of the National Medical Association, 99*(8), 953–958.

Ibrahim, M. S., Alazzawi, S., Nizam, I., & Haddad, F. S. (2013). An evidence-based review of enhanced recovery interventions in knee replacement surgery. *Annals of the Royal College of Surgeons of England, 95*(6), 386–389.

Kelley, A. S., Covinsky, K. E., Gorges, R. J., McKendrick, K., Bollens-Lund, E., Morrison, R. S., & Ritchie, C. S. (2017). Identifying older adults with serious illness: A critical step toward improving the value of health care. *Health Services Research, 52*(1), 113–131.

Koh, H. K., & Sebelius, K. G. (2010). Promoting prevention through the Affordable Care Act. *New England Journal of Medicine, 363*(14), 1296–1299.

Kremers, H. M., Larson, D. R., Crowson, C. S., Kremers, W. K., Washington, R. E., Steiner, C. A., ... Berry, D. J. (2015). Prevalence of total hip and knee replacement in the United States. *Journal of Bone and Joint Surgery: American, 97*(17), 1386–1397.

Loewenstein, G., Asch, D. A., & Volpp, K. G. (2013). Behavioral economics holds potential to deliver better results for patients, insurers, and employers. *Health Affairs, 32*(7), 1244–1250.

Mouille, B., Higuer, C., Woicehovich, L., & Deadwiler, M. (2016). How to succeed in bundled payments for total joint replacement. *NEJM Catalyst.* Retrieved from http://catalyst.nejm.org/how-to-succeed-in-bundled -payments-for-total-joint-replacement/

Murray, R. (2009). Setting hospital rates to control costs and boost quality: The Maryland experience. *Health Affairs, 28*(5), 1395–1405.

Navathe, A. S., Troxel, A. B., Liao, J. M., Nan, N., Zhu, J., Zhong, W., & Emanuel, E. J. (2017). Cost of joint replacement using bundled payment models. *JAMA Internal Medicine, 177*(2), 214–222.

Offord, N., Harriman, P., & Downes, T. (2017). Discharge to assess: Transforming the discharge process of frail older patients. *Future Hospital Journal, 4*(1), 30–32.

Porter, M. E. (2009). A strategy for health care reform— toward a value-based system. *New England Journal of Medicine, 361*(2), 109–112.

Porter, M. E., & Lee, T. H. (2013). The strategy that will fix health care. *Harvard Business Review, 91*(12), 24.

Proudfoot, S., Bennett, B., Duff, S., & Palmer, J. (2017). Implementation and effects of Enhanced Recovery After Surgery for hip and knee replacements and fractured neck of femur in New Zealand orthopaedic services. *New Zealand Medical Journal, 130*(1455), 77–90.

Shah, N. R., Garofalo-Wright, L. M., Navarro, R., & Kanter M. (2017). Health care providers must stop wasting patients' time. *Harvard Business Review.* Retrieved from https://hbr.org/2017/05/health-care -providers-must-stop-wasting-patients-time

Song, Z., Safran, D. G., Landon, B. E., Landrum, M. B., He, Y., Mechanic, R. E., ... Chernew, M. E. (2012). The "Alternative Quality Contract," based on a global budget, lowered medical spending and improved quality. *Health Affairs, 31*(8), 1885–1894.

Talmo, C. T., Aghazadeh, M., & Bono, J. V. (2012). Perioperative complications following total joint replacement. *Clinics in Geriatric Medicine, 28*(3), 471–487.

Thaler, R. H., & Sunstein, C. R. (2009). *Improving decisions about health, wealth, and happiness.* London, UK: Penguin.

Westphal, E. C., Alkema, G., Seidel, R., & Chernof, B. (2016). How to get better care with lower costs? See the person, not the patient. *Journal of the American Geriatrics Society, 64*(1), 19–21.

CHAPTER 6

The VA Health System for Older Adults

Kenneth Shay, Thomas Edes, and Richard M. Allman

CHAPTER OBJECTIVES

1. Illustrate the overall enrollment growth in the Veterans Health Administration.
2. Describe the early integration of geriatric evaluation in Veterans Affairs care, and review its impact on older adults.
3. Review current sites in which geriatric evaluation is provided and examine its mainstream development and implementation.

KEY TERMS

Community living centers (CLCs)

Geriatric evaluations

home-based primary care (HBPC)

Longitudinal care

Veteran

Veterans Affairs (VA)

▶ Introduction

The U.S. Department of **Veterans Affairs (VA)** began as a National Asylum in 1865 at the order of President Abraham Lincoln "to care for Disabled Volunteer Soldiers"; it evolved to be called the **Veterans** Bureau, and then was consolidated into the Veterans Administration by President Herbert Hoover in 1930. President George H. W. Bush established the Cabinet-level Department of Veterans Affairs in 1989.

In World War II, over the years 1941 through 1945, nearly 16 million Americans, mostly male, were inducted into military service. Following the German and Japanese surrenders in the European and Asian-Pacific theaters, respectively, the system of care for **veterans**—which had developed in the early 1930s in response to demands for health and support services by veterans of the Spanish–American War and World War I—was initially incapable of addressing the needs presented by the expansion of the veteran population from about 5 million to more than 20 million former soldiers, sailors, marines, and airmen.

In response, President Harry S. Truman signed Public Law 79-293 into law on December 7, 1945. It transitioned the VA's Medical Service into the Department of Medicine and Surgery and initiated a 10-year plan to increase the number of VA medical facilities and beds by 50% (from 91 to 137 hospitals; from 82,000 to 120,000 beds) (Adkins, 1967, pp. 210–214). To help increase the number of physicians staffing both the existing and newly built facilities, VA physicians were exempted from many obstructive civil service hiring regulations and salary caps. The legislation also established authority for medical schools and VA hospitals to enter into partnerships under which VA would support thousands of medical residency positions, with those whose training had been interrupted by military service receiving preferential selection. The medical faculty supervising the residents further supplemented the VA physician workforce in exchange for access to resources for conducting biomedical research. As a result of these measures, the number of full-time physicians employed by VA grew from about 2500 on June 30, 1945, to nearly 4000 one year later (Adkins, 1967, pp. 218–219).

As early as the late 1950s, VA leaders recognized that the aging of the surviving veterans of World War II, combined with the 20th century's dramatic increase in life expectancy, would, by the end of the 1970s and thereafter, challenge their system with an unprecedented predominance of demand for health care and services encountered among people of advanced age (Adkins, 1967, p. 263). As an example, in 1980, 10.5% of the 28.6 million veterans in America were age 65 or older; by 2000, 37% of the 24.3 million veterans were age 65 or older;

and by 2017, 46% of the 20.0 million veterans were in that age group. While only 839,000 veterans were age 75 or older in 1980 (Veterans Administration, 1984, pp. 3–5), veterans in that age group numbered more than 4 million by 2017.

To prepare for these changes, beginning in 1976 VA developed, and in 1980 Congress authorized the establishment of, a system of Geriatric Research, Education, and Clinical Centers (GRECCs) to investigate the causes and potential management strategies for aging and the diseases associated with it, and to share lessons learned with the clinical workforce and those training in VA. From an initial cadre of 6 GRECCs in 1976, the number of GRECCs expanded to 20 by the beginning of the current millennium.

Today, the Veterans Health Administration (VHA) is the largest integrated healthcare system in the United States, providing care at 1243 healthcare facilities, including 170 medical centers and 1063 outpatient sites of care. Care sites include 134 VA community living centers. **Geriatric evaluation** is offered in outpatient, inpatient, and home- and community-based settings across the system.

Approximately 9 million people, representing approximately 40% of all veterans, are enrolled in VHA each year. Nearly half of the enrolled veterans are age 65 years or older. VHA anticipates that the number of veterans enrolled from this age group will continue to exceed 4 million for at least the next 20 years, and the number of enrollees age 75 or older is projected to increase 36% from 1.9 million in 2016 to 2.6 million veterans in 2037.

The Rise, Fall, and Integration of Geriatric Evaluation in VA

One early and visible GRECC contribution to clinical geriatric practice was described in the *New England Journal of Medicine* by Rubenstein et al. in 1984. Adapted from an approach that had been developed by Dr. Marjory Warren in "geriatric hospitals" in Great Britain in the early 1940s (Warren, 1946), investigators working at the Sepulveda (California) GRECC reported on a trial of a "geriatric evaluation unit" (GEU) among older veterans. After one year of follow-up, patients randomized to the GEU had lower mortality (23.8% versus 48.3%) and were less likely to be discharged to a nursing home (12.7% versus 30.0%) or to have spent any time in a nursing home (26.9% versus 46.7%). Moreover, patients in the geriatric unit were significantly more likely to have improvement in functional status and morale than controls.

All of the first GRECCs developed GEUs, and by 1984 an equal number of non-GRECC programs were in operation as well. VA had initiated Interdisciplinary Team Training in Geriatrics (ITTG) programs in 1979, and by 1984, there were 12 in existence, 3 of which were co-located with GRECCs (Veterans Administration, 1984, pp. 51–52). ITTGs were responsible for locally, regionally, and nationally providing VA staff with on-site training in the team building, interdisciplinary dialogue, and care planning that characterized GEUs. In 1990, VA secured Congressional funding to implement Geriatric Evaluation and Management (GEM) programs at approximately 50 self-selected sites, with funds distributed to underwrite 50% of the first 2 years' support of one physician, one social worker, and one nurse per site. Programs were administratively and geographically located within nursing home care, acute care, intermediate care, inpatient psychiatry, and rehabilitation units, and as an outpatient service.

After the initial period of funding, however, many GEM and ITTG programs gradually lost staff and disappeared—a fate largely attributable to three factors: new internal accounting rules within VA that served as powerful disincentives to providing nursing home care in general and to implementing interdisciplinary team meetings specifically; adoption across all long-term care settings of standardized data sets that dictated details of care planning and resource allocation; and a diminishing supply of clinicians with advanced trained in geriatric care.

In November 1999, the Veterans Millennium Benefits Act, Public Law 106-180 (the "Mill Act"), was signed into law by President Bill Clinton. A sweeping endorsement for VA providing long-term care to veterans in need of such services, the Mill Act committed VA to providing or purchasing nursing home care to a particular subset of veterans who had been deemed disabled above a particular threshold; it also committed VA to make available, to all veterans who would stand to benefit from them, several non-institutional extended care services for supporting frail and dependent elders who sought to remain in their homes with optimal health, safety, and independence. These services included geriatric evaluation, adult day health care, homemakers/home health aides, respite care, and **home-based primary care (HBPC)** (Congress of the United States, 1999). Three years later, the General Accountability Office (GAO) observed that many VA sites were still not providing all of the required non-institutional services, and recommended that VA institute means for compelling and tracking adherence to the Mill Act. Because geriatric evaluation was not exclusively provided in an eponymous program and, therefore, was more challenging for GAO to document in its survey, the recommendation did not address activity in geriatric evaluation.

Anticipating that such guidance would eventually be forthcoming, VA instituted a means for recording geriatric evaluation workload, regardless of the clinical setting in which it was provided. Included in that workload was every new HBPC patient, because of the interdisciplinary assessment-based care that is the mainstay of that program. Geriatric evaluation tracking reflected that the service was being provided, but at a rate less than 10% of what would be expected, based on several studies. An American study (Saliba, 2001) and an Irish study (McGee, 2008) found strikingly similar rates (32–33%) of indication for geriatric evaluation among community-dwelling elders older than age 75 using the Vulnerable Elder Survey VES-13 screening instrument. Based on those rates, more than 335,000 veterans age 75 years and older should be receiving geriatric evaluation on an annual basis, but the actual numbers remains less than 35,000. Most of that activity occurs in outpatient clinic settings—an observation that provided some of the impetus for a multisite VA comparison of inpatient to outpatient geriatric evaluation; this review found diminished impact of geriatric evaluation when provided for an outpatient cohort (Cohen, 2002). One interpretation of this finding was that, in outpatient settings, the interdisciplinary teams' recommendations were left to be fulfilled by primary care teams who were unable or unwilling to follow the geriatricians' recommendations.

A recent evidence review of the impact of geriatricians on the outcomes of older adults showed that patients receiving care in special geriatric units where **geriatric evaluations** were conducted by a team including a geriatrician have better function at discharge and are more likely to be discharged to home than patients receiving standard hospital care. Including a geriatrician in inpatient evaluations and rehabilitation resulted in lower nursing home admissions, improved function, and lower mortality after up to 1 year of follow-up compared to usual care. In the outpatient settings, interventions in which geriatricians have direct patient contact are more likely to result in better outcomes than interventions where the interaction is limited to supporting other clinicians. Moreover, geriatricians as primary care providers provide more effective medication management than other clinicians (Totten et al., 2012).

In response, many outpatient GEM programs began to offer continuity care in addition to filling their assessment and care planning roles, so as to ensure that the gains accruing to the comprehensive geriatric assessment would not be lost. When VA's copayment structure for primary and specialty cares levied a higher rate for "GEM clinic" care, sites renamed the service "geriatric primary care" (GPC).

VA implemented the patient-centered medical home model of primary care in 2010, under the name "Patient-Aligned Care Teams" (PACT), and undertook a system-wide reeducation of primary care teams in care management, integration with community resources, patient-centered

care, and team-based function. In an unintended twist, the rollout of this approach did not obviate the need for GPC; in fact, the growing workload expectations for primary care teams put at elevated risk for poor outcomes the complex, frail, and cognitively impaired elderly patients whose extensive medical histories and multiple interacting chronic conditions were nearly impossible to review and addressed in the course of a 30-minute appointment.

In 2012, VA deemed that all primary care services should conform to the PACT model and GPC was renamed "GeriPACT." GeriPACT is presently offered at more than half of VA's medical centers and a growing number of freestanding outpatient clinics, where GeriPACT represents a "safety valve" to PACTs struggling to meet access needs for patients in a timely manner.

▶ Present State of Geriatric Evaluation in VA

The dominant provider of geriatric evaluation conducted in VA is GeriPACT, which targets the most complex and frail 1–3% of PACT-covered patients at the more than 80 sites where it is presently offered. Between October 2016 and September 2017, nearly 60,000 veterans had 158,870 visits to GeriPACT—an average of 2.77 visits per individual. Geriatric evaluation is likely completed for most of these veterans, suggesting that the frequency of geriatric evaluation in VHA is under-reported since, as noted earlier, current administrative data suggest that only approximately 35,000 veterans receive geriatric evaluations annually.

The benefits of GeriPACT to patients, as well as to the healthcare system, are still being characterized and analyzed, but a recent retrospective analysis of data from 2012–2013 compared VA and Centers for Medicare and Medicaid Services (CMS) expenses of care for more than 2,000 GeriPACT-treated patients. These were contrasted to expenses for propensity-matched counterparts cared for in PACT (Shay et al., 2017). Costs of care for relatively high-functioning patients—those with Jen Frailty Index [JFI] scores of 0 to 2—were equivalent for PACT and GeriPACT, as they were for those highly impaired veterans with JFI scores of 6 or greater. For the moderately impaired (i.e., those with JFI scores of 3 to 5), however, GeriPACT management was associated with an overall annual total healthcare cost of $6000 to $6800 less than required for the similarly impaired PACT-covered patients.

Another frequent provider of geriatric evaluations in the VA is home-based primary care (HBPC), which was introduced to VA in the late 1970s. HBPC became part of the suite of services that all VA facilities were obligated to provide to eligible veterans under the Mill Act. HBPC is presently offered through all VA medical centers and approximately 300 of the more than 1000 community-based outpatient clinics operated by VA. HBPC provides comprehensive **longitudinal care** in the home not only for home-bound individuals, but also for home-dwelling veterans whose physical status and medical fragility are not effectively managed without providing comprehensive care directly in the home. HBPC is provided by a physician-directed interdisciplinary team that includes nurses, nurse practitioners or physician assistants, social workers, mental health professionals, dietitians, rehabilitation therapists, and pharmacists, all of whom meet as a team and create a single unified care plan for the patient. Home visits are made by individual team members depending on the specific needs of each veteran. Nearly 60,000 veterans received HBPC services between October 2016 and September 2017. Analysis of several different patient cohorts both in and beyond VA, covering the period from 2011 to the present, has consistently demonstrated approximately a 15% net cost savings with HBPC compared to usual care among high-risk veterans as well as a significant reduction in hospital admissions, readmission after discharge, and use of emergency departments (Edes et al., 2014).

The strong success of VA's HBPC as a model of interdisciplinary geriatric evaluation and management for a population with arduous access challenges contributed substantially to the development and implementation of Medicare's HBPC demonstration program. Lessons from VA's HBPC experience were applied to shape the program characteristics, standards, target population, clinical outcome measures, and economic structure that was envisioned as sustainable in Medicare. VA's demonstration that enrollment in its HBPC program resulted in significant reductions in hospital days and in total costs of care, both in VA and in Medicare, led to strong Congressional support for this model and approval of the Independence at Home demonstration project in 2010. Corroborating the VA experience, this Medicare HBPC demonstration program, which was based on the principles of geriatric evaluation, improved access to higher-quality care while reducing the total cost of care by more than $2000 per patient per year.

The third most common site in which geriatric evaluation is provided is VA's nursing homes, which are termed **community living centers (CLCs)**. The CLC daily census in VA is approximately 10,000, although the number of veterans receiving such care in a given year is approximately triple that number. An overarching theme of the extended care programs in VA is that individuals should be able to reside in the least-restrictive setting that is safe for them. As such, a significant amount of effort in CLC is devoted not only to addressing a resident's daily care needs, but also to identifying and implementing management strategies to optimize function and well-being. For many veterans, CLCs play an integral role in the safe and effective transition from hospital to home. At heart, this was the original motivation behind geriatric evaluation. As long-term care practice has migrated from a custodial to a life optimization function, geriatric evaluation has become mainstreamed in the development and implementation of care plans. Although some sites include specific subunits within CLC that are devoted expressly to geriatric evaluation, much as occurred in the original GEMs, the amount of actual activity in CLCs devoted to that end is unquestionably far greater than is reflected in the geriatric evaluation workload figures.

▶ Summary

VA geriatric evaluation has made significant advances in care for persons facing the challenges of aging, disability, and serious chronic disease, but there remain tremendous opportunities to expand access to geriatric evaluation. Early clinical geriatric evaluation investigations were sufficiently promising that deliberate efforts were undertaken to disseminate geriatric evaluation system-wide. As incentives driving choices and sites of care have changed, geriatric evaluation has changed as well, going from a service offered in a limited number of settings to one that has become infused throughout all settings of care. Although workload numbers reflect relatively limited provision of geriatric evaluation in VA, its underlying principles of interdisciplinary team-based care are well integrated into VA's nursing home and home care approaches. Nearly a decade of experience with the expanding Geri-PACT program, in which nearly all patients new to the program do, in fact, receive assessment and care planning consistent with "comprehensive geriatric assessment," suggests that the geriatric evaluation workload as reported in that program is a significant under-representation of actual services provided and needed. The interdisciplinary models of geriatric evaluation not only improve health and function for those individuals who receive their care through these models, but also provide unique interdisciplinary training experiences that will be needed for the future healthcare workforce in all disciplines to meet the care needs of the expanding population of older Americans.

References

Adkins, R. (1967, April). *Medical care of veterans.* Washington, DC: U.S. Government Printing Office.

Cohen, H. J., Feussner, J. R., Weinberger, M., Carnes, M., Hamdy, R. C., Hsieh, F., . . . Lavori, P. (2002). A controlled trial of inpatient and outpatient geriatric assessment and management. *New England Journal of Medicine, 346,* 905–912.

Congress of the United States. (1999, November 30). *Public Law 106-117: The Veterans Health Care and Benefits Act.* Washington, DC: U.S. Government Printing Office. Retrieved from https://www.gpo.gov/fdsys/pkg/GPO-CDOC-106sdoc13/pdf/GPO-CDOC-106sdoc13-2-17-1.pdf

Edes, T., Kinosian, B., Vuckovic, N. H., Nichols, L. O., Becker, M. M., & Hossain, M. (2014). Better access, quality and cost for clinically complex veterans with home based primary care. *Journal of the American Geriatrics Society, 62,* 1954–1961.

McGee, H. M., O'Hanlon, A., Barker, M., Montgomery, A., Conroy, R., & O'Neill, D. (2008). Vulnerable elderly people in the community: Relationship between the Vulnerable Elderly Survey and Health Service Use. *Journal of the American Geriatrics Society, 56,* 8.

Rubenstein, L. Z., Josephson, K. R., Wieland, G. D., English, P. A., Sayre, J. A., & Kane, R. L. (1984). Effectiveness of a geriatric evaluation unit: A randomized clinical trial. *New England Journal of Medicine, 311,* 1664–1670.

Saliba, D., Elliott, M., Rubenstein, L. Z., Solomon, D. H., Young, R. Y., Kamberg, K. J., . . . Wenger, N. S. (2001). The Vulnerable Elders Survey: A tool for identifying vulnerable older people in the community. *Journal of the American Geriatrics Society, 49,* 1691–1696.

Shay, K., Phibbs, C., Intrator, O., Kinosian, B., Scott, W., Dally, S., & Allman, R. (2017). Evaluation of the costs for veterans receiving care in geriatric medical homes *(GeriPACT)* [Abstract]. *Innovation in Aging, 1*(suppl. 1), 1329.

Totten, A., Carson, S., Peterson, K., Low, A., Christensen, V., & Tiwari, A. (2012). *Evidence brief: Effect of geriatricians on outcomes of inpatient and outpatient care.* VA-ESP Project 2012; #09-199. Portland, OR: Department of Veterans Affairs, Veterans Health Administration, Office of Research and Development, Quality Enhancement Research Initiative.

Veterans Administration. (1984). *Caring for the older veteran.* Washington, DC: U.S. Government Printing Office.

Warren, M. W. (1946). Care of the chronic aged sick. *Lancet, i,* 841–843.

CHAPTER 7

Following the Assessment Data—Whose Data Is It: Open Notes in Real Time

C. T. Lin

CHAPTER OBJECTIVES

1. Describe the rapidly growing demographic of geriatric patients who have access to an electronic health records patient portal.
2. Describe the available tools for geriatric patients and their caregivers within patient portals.
3. Describe the concept of Open Notes, and the potential risks and benefits for geriatric patients with this tool.

KEY TERMS

Electronic health record	Open Notes	Physician–patient
Online patient portal		communication

▶ Introduction

The use of the Internet for direct patient care dates back to the 1970s, when patients and physicians would occasionally send email to each other. The emergence of this means of communication prompted the development of patient and physician guidelines for the use of email (Kane & Sands, 1998). Over the past 30 years, online tools have matured substantially.

Patient portals, with secure communication tools, were developed in the 1990s. Many were not linked to a healthcare provider's **electronic health record**, such as Google's Personal Health Record (PHR) (Google Health, 2017) or Microsoft's HealthVault (2017), among others (Archer, Fevrier-Thomas, Lokker, McKibbon, & Straus, 2011). Since then, a growing number of patient portals have been introduced as built-in modules within a specific healthcare provider's electronic health record (EHR) system (Archer et al., 2011). Many patients can now see their own demographic information, insurance information, diagnoses, medications, medical allergies, and immunizations (Archer et al., 2011). Increasingly, patients can see their own test results, including laboratory tests, radiology tests, and pathology reports (Archer et al., 2011).

In the past 15 years, a growing movement has sought to give patients access to progress notes written by their physician (Open Notes, 2017; Ross et al., 2005). Despite a substantial cultural pushback from physicians, who tend to see the patient's medical record as the exclusive purview of clinicians, the Open Notes movement has succeeded in giving more than 15 million patients access to their Open Notes medical records (Open Notes, 2017).

Open Notes is not a commercial product, but rather a cultural agreement about information transparency with patients with the goal of improving communication, patient satisfaction, and clinical outcomes. Although most EHRs have a patient portal setting to "turn on" Open Notes, the details of how that is done are crucial. When done well, patient trust, adherence to therapy, empowerment, and satisfaction can improve, while nurse and clinician impacts are minimal to none. Open Notes thus lays the foundation for further innovative care and information transparency with patients.

This chapter describes the importance, best practices, and challenges of opening up the patient's medical record via Open Notes for the use of patients, including geriatric patients.

▶ Trends in Geriatric Access to Electronic Patient Portals

Older adults, defined as those older than age 65, are the fastest-growing demographic among patients using electronic patient portals. Twenty percent of patients age 60 or older have experience with using an **online patient portal**, and this percentage is expected to increase in the future (Lober et al., 2006; Turner et al., 2015).

Geriatric patients often have difficulty with mobility, hearing, remembering conversations with their physician, and remembering the importance of their medications and treatments. The patient portal allows for convenient, asynchronous communication among patients and their clinicians (e.g., physicians, nurses). Traditional telephone calls may be hard to hear, and travel to and from the clinic can impose a hardship on some older patients. Those who do not have a good memory can use the patient portal to review content such as their diagnoses, medications, and allergies.

Some organizations have added other tools to the patient portal. Many organizations release test results to patients online (Centers for Medicare and Medicaid Services, 2016; Irizarry, DeVito, & Curran, 2015). Our organization, the University of Colorado Health system, uses the following rules to release results: All blood and urine laboratory tests are released to patients immediately (no delay), which means that in some cases patients will see the results before their clinician does. Despite initial fears by clinicians, research and experience have shown that such "immediate release policies" improve patient trust and are not anxiety-provoking for patients (Ball & Lillis, 2001; Earnest, Ross, Wittevrongel, Moore, & Lin, 2004; Pillemer et al., 2016; Ross, Moore, Earnest, Wittevrongel, & Lin, 2004; Tang et al., 2003). Similarly, our organization releases plain-film radiology, ultrasound, mammogram, and echocardiogram results immediately. Complex radiology results, such as those involving computed tomography (CT) scan, magnetic resonance imaging (MRI), and positron electron tomography (PET) scans are delayed for 7 days and pathology/biopsy results are delayed for 14 days to allow clinicians to prepare treatment plans, if needed, for new cancer diagnosis (Sprague, Pell, & Lin, 2013).

More recently, some organizations have expanded the scope of what patients can see in their patient portal. Those patients who have a patient portal that incorporates Open Notes can view their clinicians' progress notes and recommendations, and recall conversations with their clinician. In one study among patients age 65 and older, as much as 50% of the information imparted to a patient at hospital discharge was forgotten by the patient within 5 days. Furthermore, family members of geriatric patients are often not immediately available either in person or by phone to hear the advice of clinicians (Albrecht et al., 2014; Earnest et al., 2004; Flacker, Park, & Sims, 2007), so such Open Notes access enables them to review this information at their convenience.

▶ Current Best Practices

In clinics and healthcare facilities that effectively use EHRs and patient portals with Open Notes, physicians routinely invite *all* patients, including geriatric patients, to sign up for, and communicate using, the patient portal. Some examples follow.

Presbycusis

Older patients who are hard of hearing can easily ask questions online. In our otolaryngology clinic for patients with sensorineural hearing loss (a common condition among older adults), use of the portal is quite popular and typically replaces telephone calls. Additionally, seeing Open Notes allows patients to review the progress note written by their physician and recall

any items they had not understood or had not heard properly (Earnest et al., 2004).

Coordination with Caregivers and Family Members

Often family members cannot travel to attend conversations between patients and physicians. This is partly why the use of proxy access to the patient portal is high in the geriatrics clinic at our organization. Proxy access allows a family member or caregiver to access the online patient portal on behalf of the patient and communicate with the clinic, as well as to view test results and Open Notes. Some family members reside out of state, so sharing such information such as Open Notes can help with coordinating care and ensuring all care team members are well informed.

Coordination Between Physicians Using Different EHRs

Older patients often have primary care physicians and specialists who use disparate EHRs or paper medical record systems. Notes from one clinician often do not reach the next clinician in time to impact the patient's care. Patients and their caregivers with access to Open Notes can serve a crucial role by delivering clinician notes in these cases, and can improve the coordination of their own care (Earnest et al., 2004).

Patient Satisfaction Measures

Use of Open Notes can effect a significant change in clinical practice, in that patients are more likely to report that doctors did a good job of listening to their concerns and questions (Ross et al., 2004). In one case, a patient stated:

> I told my doctor that I could no longer cross-country ski because of my heart failure symptoms. Instead of responding, he went on to ask additional questions

about my symptoms. Later, when I read his notes about our visit, he wrote that "what is important to the patient is her inability to cross-country ski, and this will be a goal of our treatment." I have never felt closer to my doctor than at that moment.

Patient-Friendly Terminology

In one study, some patients liked the idea of a special patient-friendly form of the record, but all preferred that the official, untranslated medical record be available to them (Earnest et al., 2004). One patient stated:

> I would rather have the doctors just write what they write and me work to understand it, than them writing it for me and leaving something out that I would like to know.

Other Patient Perceptions

In one study, focus groups of patients benefited from (1) learning more about their condition, (2) learning about medical decision making, (3) increasing patient participation in medical care, and (4) confirming normal results and accuracy of the record (Earnest et al., 2004). One patient noted: "My doctor works very hard on my behalf; I had no idea." Another noted: "I don't always read my doctors' notes, but the fact that you offer it means I can trust you."

Improved Adherence to Treatment

Patients with access to Open Notes tend to renew their prescriptions at a higher rate than control patients (Wright et al., 2015).

Obtaining Test Results

Nurses have noted that patients ask better questions when they have access to Open Notes. In one study, prior to the implementation of Open Notes, cardiology patients would call primarily to get the results of their most recent echocardiogram (heart imaging study), and find out their ejection fraction result. A detailed telephone discussion of what that meant would then follow. After they gained access to Open Notes, cardiology patients would look up their own echocardiogram results, study the ejection fraction, do additional reading online about heart failure medicines and treatments, and then call the nurse with a more sophisticated question: "So, I see that my ejection fraction has increased. Is that due to my digoxin (heart medicine)?" (Earnest et al., 2004).

▶ Future Possibilities

OurNotes is a grant-funded initiative at Beth Israel Deaconess Medical Center (2015) that seeks to include patients in the shared documentation of clinical notes—namely, reviewing their most recent Open Notes prior to the next appointment, and adding a list of topics or questions they would like to discuss at their upcoming appointment. This could further improve **physician–patient communication**, engagement, and possibly shared decision making and outcomes (Open Notes, 2017).

Patient-reported outcome measures (PROMs) allow patients to document blood sugars, vital signs, pedometer steps, and symptom scores. Patients could contribute these data to the EHR by automated device readings as well as through manual entry. Many treatments and medication combinations have unknown symptoms and outcomes, especially among older patients who have multiple conditions and are taking multiple medications. Having patients record and report blood sugars for diabetes monitoring, blood pressure for hypertension monitoring, weights for patients with congestive heart failure or respiratory failure, and pedometer steps to track activity in patients with heart disease, lung disease, and diabetes or other metabolic illnesses, can all be ways that patients can contribute knowledge to their own care. Imagine a diverse population of patients regularly reporting symptoms, activities, and vital signs. This rich source of data could be searched for effective medication combinations and relatively ineffective treatments (Black, 2013; Wagle, 2016).

At the moment, EHRs are still in their infancy. As we learn how to best capture data from clinicians as well as patients, we will have an increasingly robust data set that can be explored to find patterns among symptoms, diagnoses, treatments, and outcomes. Not only can clinicians access these data, but patients should have access to the data as well. At present, data sharing with patients is primarily in the format of narrative text, but some patients are now requesting their data in codified reports. Newer data-exchange formats such as FHIR (fast healthcare interoperable resources; Mandel, Kreda, Mandl, Kohane, & Ramoni, 2016) and health information exchange organizations (Walker et al., 2005) may eventually enable clinicians and patients to send and receive data between organizations, between websites, and perhaps via smartphone applications. Imagine patients exporting their codified health data (diagnoses, medications, medical allergies, past medical history, family history, vital signs, lab results, and radiology results) and being able to share those data with an app from another organization. The availability of such data could allow patients to shop for the lowest-cost pharmacy for their medications or find the least expensive health insurance plan tailored to the type of care they need. It could also allow patients to see whether the American Heart Association has recommendations for the "best practice treatment" for their heart condition, or enable patients to search national databases for the best "clinical trial" to treat a rare disease (deBronkart, 2013).

▶ Challenges

Physician Resistance

Physician resistance to Open Notes has been well documented (Earnest et al., 2004; Leventhal, 2017; Miliard, 2015; Ross et al., 2004, 2005).

Overcoming this resistance will require a combination of visionary leadership, strong communication, and committed support from executive and clinical leaders. It is important that clinically respected leaders are visible champions for this cause. Only then will the display of research reports as well as local trials of Open Notes help prove that such access does not cause unexpected disruptions in patients' care or in clinicians' lives.

Technical Savvy

Geriatric patients often are not comfortable using computers (Turner et al., 2015). Although the percentage of older patients who are not comfortable with computers is declining, which may be a cohort effect, there persists a significant fraction of patients who are not "online" (Lober et al., 2006). Nevertheless, many older patients have children or grandchildren who can set up computers or access online resources on their behalf.

Communication Problems

Some patients, regardless of age, do not understand the limitations of using an online portal for messages. Very infrequently (less than once a month, among 250,000 patients using the patient portal for the University of Colorado Health system), patients may send inappropriately urgent messages. There are disclaimers on the site indicating that users who send messages may not receive a response for 2 business days, and advising them to make a phone call, schedule an urgent appointment, or go to an urgent care or emergency department if the question is urgent. Our website requires the patient to answer a question: When would you like a response to this question? Options are "Sooner than 2 business days" or "Two or more business days." If the patient chooses the former, the *only* option that follows is "Please call us at XXX phone number." In contrast, if they choose "Two or more business days," the system permits them to ask their question online.

Understanding Terminology

Both clinicians and patients have been concerned about the ability of patients to understand medical terminology. They have voiced fears that use of medical terms in EHRs would lead to confusion or, even worse, to anxiety and misunderstanding. Nevertheless, in 2017, despite most physician offices having an online patient portal, a small but growing minority of patients have access to physician-written reports and documentation (Open Notes, 2017).

Traditionally, paper medical records were stored in locked archives in physician offices. Access to and viewing of these charts was highly restricted. Additionally, fewer than 1% of patients request their paper records, possibly due to the cost (dozens of dollars), the time delay (up to a month), and the inconvenience (having to visit a separate office and sign a release form for each request) associated with this process (K. Adams, personal communication, July 15, 2017). As a result, clinicians have typically expected that the audience for their writing in paper medical records was almost exclusively other clinicians.

With Open Notes, clinicians have anticipated that they might face more patient phone calls, more anxious patients, and lawsuits about use of pejorative terms in records. At worst, they have worried that clinicians would hide important facts because they feared patients reading and misunderstanding the notes. The medical terms used in EHRs can be difficult to understand—for example, "venous thromboembolism" and "diastolic dysfunction." Other terms could be medically useful, yet considered pejorative: "obese patient," "noncompliant patient," "smelling of alcohol," or "drug-abuser" (Earnest et al., 2004). Clinicians feared that exposing patients to such documentation could result in litigation.

In reality, research findings have largely allayed these fears (Delbanco et al., 2012; Earnest et al., 2004; Ross et al., 2004). The vast majority of patients have no issue with Open Notes. One stated:

I was able to ask questions of the medical people I have in my family, and when I didn't, I was able to go on the Internet and type in what I didn't understand, and then probably find out more than I ever wanted to know. So, with a little research I was able to understand. (Earnest et al., 2004)

Still others noted that they valued being able to take their clinician's notes to the next provider of care, and being the conduit and manager of their own medical information. One patient stated:

I lost my medications in my airline luggage on a trip. Do you know how difficult it is to convince an urgent care physician that you REALLY DO take Vicodin? Imagine instead, walking into that office and saying, "If you have a web browser, I can give you my medical record. Could I have a prescription for 3 days of my pills?" It is a very different conversation. (Earnest et al., 2004)

Most physicians do not need to change their documentation at all for Open Notes. However, white paper with guidelines by this chapter's author (Lin, 2016) offers suggestions on how physicians can improve their documentation in progress notes. A psychiatrist best describes the goals for Open Notes documentation by physicians:

When we think about our patients in a kind of language that WE deem inappropriate or potentially offensive to the uninitiated, who is to say that our own attitudes toward our patients are not affected by that language? Wouldn't we be closer to our patients' experience if we got into the habit of thinking about them in language they would find meaningful and useful? (Cassandra Cook, cited in Kahn, Bell, Walker, & Delbanco, 2014)

Psychiatry/Behavioral Health Issues

In some cases, physicians may be reluctant to share Open Notes with older patients who are threatening, who disagree about treatment, who are opiate-seeking, who have a psychiatric illness, and who have strained family relationships, or at other visits where the conversation is difficult. Clinicians, when writing about such challenging interactions, could still be respectful:

> The patient and I disagreed about how best to reach the goal of pain control; he would like more narcotic medications, and I believe that opiates are not a good solution in this case.

In our organization, the academic faculty and resident psychiatry practices have adopted the Open Notes policy since February 2017 (5 months at this writing) without difficulty.

Hiding or Suppressing Notes

In some rare cases, clinicians may find sharing notes with patients via Open Notes to be potentially harmful to patient care. For example, a patient may be a victim of domestic abuse and may not be able to keep her patient portal login secure from her partner. Rather than expose documentation of that physician–patient encounter to a potential interloper, the physician may choose "DO NOT SHARE" with the patient to suppress that note from being seen by the patient or other party. There may also be other instances in which a clinician deems it inappropriate to share the note. The experience at our organization is that less than 5% of all notes are not shared with patients.

Privacy and Security Concerns

Patients have long expressed concerns about the privacy and security of EHRs. It is helpful to recall that even paper medical records have security and privacy risks. Security tools to protect electronic medical records, such as encryption and firewalls, are strong and improving. Nevertheless, recent ransomware and other attacks from cybercriminals (Perlroth, 2017; Sanger, Chan, & Scott, 2017) continue to worry patients. This applies to all EHRs, regardless of an organization's stance on Open Notes. Despite such concerns, the further spread of EHRs and efforts toward improving information transparency for patients are unlikely to be affected.

▶ Practical Application

The deployment of Open Notes, like with any major change in policy and culture at a large organization, requires leadership, communication, and persistence (Leventhal, 2017). Having the unanimous support of the chief medical officers and all other clinical leaders is crucial to the successful deployment of this technology change. It is far easier to make technology changes than it is to effect the cultural acceptance required for such initiatives.

In our organization, some clinical departments had major reservations and objections to the Open Notes policy. They indicated that their patient populations were particularly challenging. From a leadership perspective, we agreed to revisit each of the concerned departments a month after the go-live point in case there were substantial complaints from patients and/or clinicians. No significant issues have since been raised. Aside from excluding 6 out of 8 psychiatry practices from Open Notes at go-live, no other departments have since opted out. The remainder of all specialties throughout our 400-clinic, 21-emergency-department, 7-hospital organization agreed to use Open Notes and have been successfully sharing notes with patients since May 2016.

▶ Summary

Open Notes is a cultural agreement between clinicians and patients, in which patients are engaged to read their clinicians' notes online. Despite initial anxieties, clinicians have found that Open Notes does not result in more work, more phone calls, or more lawsuits. Instead, patients are very appreciative and use the notes to better understand their conditions and treatments, to coordinate future care, and to inform family members. For patients, this results in better adherence to therapy, better patient–physician communication, and more trust in their clinicians.

Older patients, with greater need for careful coordination of care, may have the most to gain from Open Notes. This approach is an easy way for a patient or caregiver to manage complex medical information and share it with all appropriate parties.

The future of Open Notes will involve shared documentation and further information transparency. We see a day when patients and their clinicians co-author the patient's medical narrative, set shared goals, better capture patient symptoms and outcomes, and use these data to further improve care.

References

Albrecht, J., Gruber, A., Hirshon, J., Brown, C., Goldberg, R., Rosenberg, J., . . . Furuno, J. (2014). Hospital discharge instructions: Comprehension and compliance among older adults. *Journal of General Internal Medicine, 29*(11), 1491–1498. doi: 10.1007/s11606-014-2956-0

Archer, N., Fevrier-Thomas, U., Lokker, C., McKibbon, K., & Straus, S. (2011). Personal health records: A scoping review. *Journal of the American Medical Informatics Association, 18*(4), 515–522. https://doi.org/10.1136/amiajnl-2011-000105

Ball, M., & Lillis, J. (2001). E-health: Transforming the physician/patient relationship. *International Journal of Medical Informatics, 61*(1), 1–10. https://doi.org/10.1016/S1386-5056(00)00130-1

Beth Israel Deaconess Medical Center. (2015, January 23). BIDMC receives Commonwealth Fund grant to develop OurNotes. Retrieved from https://www.opennotes.org/news/bidmc-receives-commonwealth-fund-grant-to-develop-ournotes/

Black, N. (2013). Patient reported outcome measures could help transform healthcare. *British Medical Journal, 346*. doi: http://dx.doi.org/10.1136/bmj.f167

Centers for Medicare and Medicaid Services. (2016, March). EHR incentive programs in 2015 through 2017: Patient electronic access. Retrieved from https://www.cms.gov/Regulations-and-Guidance/Legislation/EHRIncentivePrograms/Downloads/2016_PatientElectronicAccess.pdf

deBronkart, D. (2013). How the e-patient community helped save my life: An essay by Dave deBronkart. *BMJ, 346*, f1990.

Delbanco, T., Walker, J., Bell, S. K., Darer, J. D., Elmore, J. G., Farag, N., . . . Leveille, S. G. (2012). Inviting patients to read their doctors' notes: A quasi-experimental study and a look ahead. *Annals of Internal Medicine, 157*, 461–470. doi: 10.7326/0003-4819-157-7-201210020-00002

Earnest, M., Ross, S., Wittevrongel, L., Moore, L., & Lin, C. (2004). Use of a patient-accessible electronic medical record in a practice for congestive heart failure: Patient and physician experiences. *Journal of the American Medical Informatics Association, 11*, 410–417. doi: 10.1197/jamia.M1479

Flacker, J., Park, W., & Sims, A. (2007). Hospital discharge information and older patients: Do they get what they need? *Journal of Hospital Medicine, 2*, 291–296. doi: 10.1002/jhm.166

Google Health. (2017). *Wikipedia*. Retrieved from https://en.wikipedia.org/wiki/Google_Health

Irizarry, T., DeVito, A., & Curran, C. (2015). Patient portals and patient engagement: A state of the science review. *Journal of Medical Internet Research, 17*(6), e148. doi: 10.2196/jmir.4255

Kahn, M. W., Bell, S. K., Walker, J., & Delbanco, T. (2014). Let's show patients their mental health records. *Journal of the American Medical Association, 311*(13), 1291–1292. doi: 10.1001/jama.2014.1824

Kane, B., & Sands, D. (1998). Guidelines for the clinical use of electronic mail with patients. *Journal of the American Medical Informatics Association, 5*(1), 104–111. https://doi.org/10.1136/jamia.1998.0050104

Leventhal, R. (2017, March 16). UCHealth's Open Notes journey: From a few docs to enterprise-wide acceptance. *Healthcare Informatics*. Retrieved from https://www.healthcare-informatics.com/article/patient-engagement/uchealth-s-opennotes-journey-few-docs-enterprise-wide-acceptance

Lin, C. (2016, April). *Open Notes: Words that tatter. Documentation tips*. [White paper for UCHealth internal files].

Lober, W., Zierler, B., Herbaugh, A., Shinstrom, S., Stolyar, A., Kim, E., & Kim, Y. (2006). Barriers to the use of a personal health record by an elderly population. *AMIA Annual Symposium Proceedings, 2006*, 514–518. PMCID: PMC1839577

Mandel, J. C., Kreda, D. A., Mandl, K. D., Kohane, I. S., & Ramoni, R. B. (2016). SMART on FHIR: A standards-based, interoperable apps platform for electronic health records. *Journal of the American Medical Informatics Association, 23*(5), 899–908. doi: 10.1093/jamia/ocv189

Microsoft HealthVault. (2017). Home page. Retrieved from https://www.healthvault.com/en-us/

Miliard, M. (2015, January 8). Open Notes: This is not a software package, this is a movement. A lot of doctors told us to go to hell. *Healthcare IT News.* Retrieved from http://www.healthcareitnews.com/news/opennotes-not-software-package-movement

Open Notes. (2017). Home page. Retrieved from http://www.opennotes.org

Perlroth, N. (2017, May 13). With new digital tools, even nonexperts can wage cyberattacks. *New York Times.* Retrieved from https://www.nytimes.com/2017/05/13/technology/hack-ransomware-scam-cyberattacks.html

Pillemer, F., Anhang, R., Paone, S., Martich, D., Albert, S., Haidari, L., . . . Mehrotra, A. (2016). Direct release of test results to patients increases patient engagement and utilization of care. *PLoS One, 11*(6), e0154743. doi: 10.1371/journal.pone.0154743

Ross, S. E., Moore, L. A., Earnest, M. A., Wittevrongel, L., & Lin, C. (2004). Providing a Web-based online medical record with electronic communication capabilities to patients with congestive heart failure: Randomized trial. *Journal of Medical Internet Research, 6*(2):e12. http://www.jmir.org/2004/2/e12/

Ross, S. E., Todd, J., Moore, L. A., Beaty, B. L., Wittevrongel, L., & Lin, C. (2005). Expectations of patients and physicians regarding patient-accessible medical records. *Journal of Medical Internet Research, 7*(2), e13. Retrieved from http://www.jmir.org/2005/2/e13/

Sanger, D., Chan, S., & Scott, M. (2017, May 14). Ransomware's aftershocks feared as U.S. warns of complexity. *New York Times.* Retrieved from https://www.nytimes.com/2017/05/14/world/europe/cyberattacks-hack-computers-monday.html?_r=0

Sprague, J., Pell, J., & Lin, C. T. (2013). Divergent care team opinions about online release of test results to an ICU patient. *Journal of Participatory Medicine, 5*, e24.

Tang, P., Black, W., Buchanan, J., Young, C., Hooper, D., Lane, S., . . . Burnbull, J. (2003). PAMF Online: Integrating ehealth with an electronic medical record system. *AMIA Annual Symposium Proceedings, 2003*, 644–648.

Turner, A., Osterhage, K., Hartzler, A., Joe, J., Lin, L., Kanagat, N., & Demiris, G. (2015). Use of patient portals for personal health information management: The older adult perspective. *AMIA Annual Symposium Proceedings, 2015*, 1234–1241.

Wagle, N. (2016, November 17). Implementing patient-reported outcome measures. *NEJM Catalyst.* Retrieved from http://catalyst.nejm.org/implementing-proms-patient-reported-outcome-measures/

Walker, J., Pan, E., Johnston, D., Adler-Milstein, J., Bates, D. W., & Middleton, B. (2005). The value of health care information exchange and interoperability. *Health Affairs, 24*, W5-10 W5-18.

Wright, E., Darer, J., Tang, X., Thompson, J., Tusing, L., Fossa, A., . . . Walker, J. (2015). Sharing physician notes through an electronic portal is associated with improved medication adherence: Quasi-experimental study. *Journal of Medical Internet Research, 17*(10), e226. doi: 10.2196/jmir.4872

CHAPTER 8

Assessment and Care Plans That Support Goals That Matter to the Person

Gretchen Alkema and Amy Berman

CHAPTER OBJECTIVES

1. Set the contextual frame for providers to engage in an assessment and care-planning process that elicits and supports goals that matter to the person.
2. Define person-centered care in the context of assessment and care planning for older adults.
3. Describe the process of ascertaining a person's goals in the assessment process and using the goals as a basis for care planning.
4. Identify factors that may affect goal elicitation and use of person-centered goals as the frame for assessment and care planning.

KEY TERMS

Person-centered care

▶ Introduction

Imagine that you are seeing a patient for the first time. She is 84 years old and accompanied by her daughter. The patient has multiple chronic health conditions—some well controlled, such as her high blood pressure and diabetes, and some poorly controlled, such as her chronic obstructive pulmonary disease (COPD). She also has mild cognitive impairment and has come to you with pain in the hip that she lives with on a daily basis. Her previous doctor closed his practice, but the daughter informs you that her mother was considering a hip replacement with that physician.

As a clinician, you review the medical record, vital signs, and the medically oriented problem list collected and synthesized by the nurse. You begin to gather clinical information using open-ended and problem-focused questions such as "What brings you in today?" and "What is troubling you?" Based on the patient's and daughter's initial responses, you begin the standard assessment processes for her overall health, the unstable COPD, and the condition of her hip. You ask her a series of questions that delve deeper and are more disease focused, performing relevant screening exams and tests. Given her mother's mild cognitive impairment, you ask the daughter to confirm and elaborate on what may be happening. As a clinician, you then filter and synthesize all of the responses through medically oriented guidelines and clinical experience into a decision tree as you deliver your professional opinion on care and treatment. You lay out a course of action and interventions and referrals (e.g., pharmaceutical, surgical, rehabilitative).

While this process and outcome are technically appropriate as guideline-informed care, they failed to identify and incorporate the person's goals and values—that is, what she is trying to achieve and avoid. This is the most critical information to ensure that care is concordant with the person's goals. The missing information includes knowing what matters most to this older adult and the reasons underlying her health issues. Goals often expressed by older adults include maintaining independence and function, along with freedom from troubling pain and/or symptoms. Other goals may be longevity, such as being able to be present for a future family event. Clinicians can obtain this information only by asking their patients about their needs, values, and preferences for care in an attempt to understand how they seek to live life every day and what they hope to avoid.

In this case, the older woman wanted to remain at home—that was the single most important thing to her. Her daughter helped her shop, cook, and manage her bills, so living at home had been a good option for her.

Sadly, she was not asked what mattered most to her and was referred to a surgeon to evaluate her hip. She developed delirium in the hospital following the hip replacement and was sent to a nursing home for post-acute rehabilitation. The change of setting caused further deterioration of her cognitive state. She was unable to benefit from rehabilitation and fell in the nursing home, suffering a hip fracture. She never returned to her home, and both her overall health and cognitive state declined rapidly. She died, in constant pain, within a year.

A conscious and deliberate inquiry into "what matters" is at the heart of a **person-centered care** approach to clinical practice, particularly when caring for older adults with complex medical and social needs. This attention to person-centeredness by the clinician can ensure that the interventions included in a jointly created care plan will have a much greater chance of achieving the health outcomes of your patients and their families.

This chapter outlines the contextual frame that allows providers to engage in an assessment and care-planning process that support goals that matter to the person. It also defines person-centered care in the context of assessment and care planning for older adults, and describes the process of ascertaining their goals. Finally, it articulates how this information can be used as the basis for care planning and identify factors that may impact goal elicitation.

▶ Contextual Frame of Older Adults with Complex Health and Social Care Needs

Older adults who seek medical attention generally do so because some component of their everyday functioning has changed for the worse, and they (or family members) do not feel as if they can manage this new daily living challenge on their own. A change can come in the form of various physical symptoms—for example, increased joint pain, decreased vision, difficulty breathing, or confusion—as well as the distal impact of the symptoms, such as an injury from a fall. Increased physical distress over time may signal a more significant health event, such as cardiac arrest or a stroke.

When older adults have a significant medical condition that needs immediate attention, they generally seek help because of the problematic symptoms and functional decline they experience (e.g., "I am having trouble breathing and feel pain in my arm"), not because they are aware of the underlying condition (e.g., "I am experiencing a myocardial infarction"). While the elements of, and solution to, the underlying medical problem are vital, what is generally most important to the older adult in distress is that he or she can return to a state of being where the least amount of medical intervention is needed in daily life.

Older adults may have unreasonable expectations in part because clinicians may not discuss the prognosis (i.e., the likely course of the disease) within the context of overall health, as opposed to just the specific health issue being addressed. Without a clear understanding of prognosis, coupled with treatment options that fit with a person's goals and values, care may unrealistically be seen as fixing the medical problem so the person can get on with the business of living well. Yet when clinicians work with an older adult living with multiple chronic health conditions, the idea of "fixing the health problem" and returning to a pre-illness state is often not the goal.

A survey of frail, older adults at senior centers on what mattered most to them found that their health goals fit into four key domains: (1) independence, which included the ability to live at home and not be a burden on others; (2) improved function, which included being able to do and enjoy specific activities; (3) management of pain and symptoms; and (4) length of life, meaning maximized longevity. In this study, the focus on longevity was the least popular response by far (Fried et al., 2011). These four outcomes are predicated on a clear sense of what the older adult wants as care outcomes and what the idea of "matters most" means in a personal way. However, the goals of care may not be immediately self-evident to the older adult, the family, or the clinician, and hence require dedicated dialogue to elicit and utilize them in a useful manner. For older people with multiple chronic conditions and associated functional limitations, asking about a person's goals in the assessment process has an even deeper meaning and necessity given that treatment protocols across disease states can be often unclear, contradictory, or simply nonexistent.

Historically, adults did not live into old age and experience significant comorbidities coupled with functional impairment. The advent of antibiotics, modern technology, effective public health interventions, and a series of socioeconomic forces have contributed to the U.S. population now having an average life expectancy of 79 years (National Center for Health Statistics, 2017). However, long life does not mean that people live well through the end of their life. As of 2015, *healthy* life expectancy was only 69 years in the United States (World Health Organization, 2016). Why the difference? Because half of all Americans turning 65 today will one day find themselves needing a high level of help with basic daily activities such as walking, eating, getting out of bed in the morning, and bathing (Favreault & Dey, 2015).

At the same time, the number of aging Americans with significant healthcare and daily living needs is projected to grow from 6 million to almost 16 million over the next several decades (Favreault & Dey, 2015). This trend toward greater disability in old age has significant implications for healthcare delivery. Research has shown that the costliest 5% of older Medicare beneficiaries account for nearly 40% of that federal program's annual spending. Older adults with daily living needs coupled with chronic health conditions cost Medicare roughly twice as much as those living with chronic conditions alone (Rodriguez, Munevar, Delaney, Yang, & Tumlinson, 2014).

At a macro level, health systems and federal policy efforts continue to strive for new system transformations to improve care while lowering costs, particularly for those with high healthcare utilization. Taking a bold step, the Centers for Medicare and Medicaid Services (CMS) instituted the "Triple Aim" framework, which calls for better population health, better care for individuals, and lower per capita costs through system improvement. This trend has continued, with CMS announcing its intention to shift from largely fee-for-service payment to value-based purchasing arrangements focused on both costs of care and quality outcomes.

With the advent of value-based payment, how can the healthcare system support older adults with complex health and daily living needs and foster the right kind and amount of care so as to improve cost and quality of care? Increasingly, health systems and leaders are rethinking the care delivery to older adults with these kinds of complex medical, functional, and social care needs, with the aim of better aligning that care delivery with their goals. Connecting the right population with the right set of interventions is critical. The key, however, is meeting the needs of older adults who live with complex care needs where they are and seeing them as whole people, *not just as patients*, through the assessment and care planning process.

▶ What Is Person-Centered Care and How Does It Relate to Assessment and Care Planning?

Healthcare providers and advocacy group of various types have published several definitions of "patient-centered" or "person-centered" care over the last 25 years (Kogan, Wilber, & Mosqueda, 2015). While varying in depth, focus, and utility, a key omission in these definitions is apparent: none has focused on the group of older adults with the most complex and expensive care needs, those also at risk for the greatest harms caused by the care itself (e.g. polypharmacy), and those living with multiple chronic conditions coupled with functional impairment. To meet this challenge, the American Geriatrics Society (AGS) convened a national expert panel in 2015 to clarify the meaning and implementation of person-centered care when serving older adults with multiple chronic conditions and functional limitations. AGS published the following statement:

> Person-centered care means that individuals' values and preferences are elicited and, once expressed, guide all aspects of their health care, supporting their realistic health and life goals. Person-centered care is achieved through a dynamic relationship among individuals, others who are important to them, and all relevant providers. This collaboration informs decision-making to the extent that the individual desires. (American Geriatrics Society Expert Panel on Person-Centered Care, 2015)

The AGS expert panel also articulated eight essential elements to operationalizing person-centeredness for an older adult population with complex medical and daily living needs. Two of the essential elements are as follows (American Geriatrics Society Expert Panel on Person-Centered Care, 2015):

- *An individualized, goal-oriented care plan based on the person's preferences.* A thorough medical, functional, and social assessment provides a foundation for the person and family to consider their goals. For some people, the assessment should be conducted in their place of residence.
- *Ongoing review of the person's goals and care plan.* Reassessing the care plan on a regular basis helps to determine the plan's effectiveness, to address the person's evolving health and life goals, and to address changes in the person's medical, functional, psychological, or social status.

The AGS definition seeks to move the locus of control from the clinician and health system to older adults, basing care on their own needs, values, preference, and personal goals. It defines quality and value, not simply through technical measures of care, but through dignity, respect of personal choices, and life goal achievement.

Person-centered care starts with gathering information about the personal needs, values, and preferences of care of older adults with complex medical and daily living needs, with input from family support if desired. This information, in combination with a comprehensive medical and functional assessment, is used to help the older adult person articulate and shape clear, specific, measurable goals that focus on improved or retained functioning rather than a medically defined clinical outcome. All of this information is synthesized into a single plan of care and shared with the appropriate team of providers and community supports. The person's goals in the care plan serve as the guiding vision of success, and the care plan and implementation strategy are updated as the older person's unique circumstances change.

▶ Timing and Nuance of Ascertaining Goals in the Assessment Process

As clinicians provide care and support to an older adult with complex needs, they must demonstrate at least three professional characteristics when ascertaining the older adult's goals during the assessment process: ability to know when and how often to ask about the person's needs, values, and preferences for care; an inquisitive nature balanced with good judgment; and, most importantly, professional courage to ask tough questions that do not have easy medically oriented answers.

Clinicians often wonder when and how often to broach conversations about what matters most to the older adults whom they are treating. While each case may be different, it is prudent to begin any assessment process with questions that elicit the person's needs, values, and preferences for care and daily living. All healing relationships are built on trust, engagement, and patience, and a key to starting this process and moving it in a positive direction is to remember an old social work maxim: "Assessment is intervention." Simply asking a question to another person begins the relationship-forming process and opens up new perspectives of engagement between the older adult, clinician, and support persons involved.

The beginning questions set the tone for the care experience, and inherently shape all future discussions between the provider and the person receiving care. Starting with what matters most to the older adult fosters a relationship of honor and respect so that the individual's clinical, functional, and social assessment information can be placed in context of his or her life and unique personal circumstances.

Drs. Mary Tinetti of Yale University and Caroline Blum of New York University have spearheaded efforts to elicit persons' values and goals, and then translate them into tailored care and treatment though an initiative known as Patient Priorities Care. Following are some suggested questions that they developed, in collaboration with Aanand Naik and Lillian Dindo of Baylor College of Medicine, and that should be considered as part of the initial and ongoing assessment process (Gerontological Society of America, 2016; Naik, Martin, Moye, & Karel, 2016):

- What brings you the most enjoyment or pleasure in life? (Addresses enjoying life)
- When taking care of yourself, what is most important to you now? (Addresses function)
- Which relationships or connections are most important to you? (Addresses connecting)
- What do you hope your care can do for you? (Addresses managing health)

Two additional key questions are:

- Who else should be part of this conversation with us? If needed, who will help you put in place any care plan that you and I develop together?
- What else should I be asking you?

▶ Using Assessment Information for Care Planning

Once identified, the person's goal becomes the "true north" of their care and ideally is shared with other members of the healthcare team so that they, too, can provide goal-concordant care. The next step is to establish meaningful and measurable health goals. For example, if we were to review what matters to the older woman with hip pain described at the beginning of the chapter, we might consider her risk for delirium and poor outcomes before referring her to the surgeon, given that her number one priority was to remain independent.

Care planning can be driven by the older adult's goals in the context of the clinical and functional profile as opposed to being driving solely by clinical indication and guidelines alone. For example, if an older adult says that she wants the most active life possible and is willing to tolerate pain to achieve that lifestyle, then a clinician can discuss treatment options that minimize the risk of functional decline and support mobility while managing pain. In contrast, if an older adult's goal is to attend a time-bound event such as a family wedding six months from the time of assessment, then the clinician can guide the care plan toward interventions that may delay necessary burdensome treatment and focus on stabilizing the person for travel so as to make attendance at the wedding possible.

While each circumstance is unique, older adults with significant clinical and functional decline rely on personal relationships for support and active help in achieving daily living goals. Their support networks could consist of family, friends, neighbors, members of religious or socially oriented communities, paid personal care providers, and the like. These individuals provide the vast majority of supportive care and are usually key members of the implementation team for the care plan developed by the older adult and clinical providers. Therefore engagement with these personal relationships alongside the older adult can be the difference between success and failure of the care plan.

Additionally, older adults may benefit from receiving a range of community-based supports and services that can help an individual maximize independence, such as Meals on Wheels and chronic disease self-management programs. An assessment process that focuses on the whole person will help uncover needs beyond the medical realm that provide critical support for health and well-being. **FIGURE 8-1** shows potential sources of daily living support for people with substantial daily living needs that can complement clinical services (Gitlin, Szanton, & DuGoff, 2011). Sources of support generally fall into two categories: those bolstering an older person's social environment and those focused on the physical environment. While not an exhaustive list in each category, meaningful access

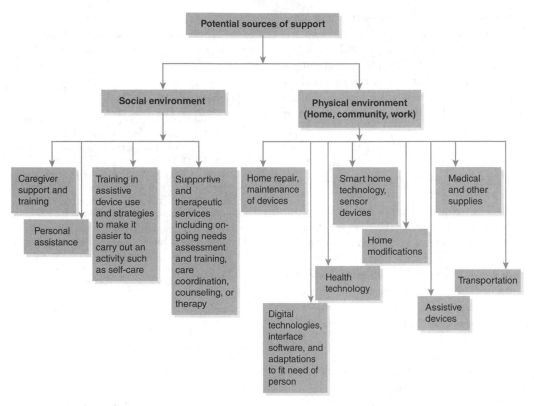

FIGURE 8-1 Potential sources of support for individuals with disability challenges.

Reproduced from Gitlin, L., Szanton, S., & DuGoff, E., The Scan Foundation. (2011). Supporting individuals with disability across the lifespan at home: Social services, technologies, and the built environment. CLASS Technical Assistance Brief Series, 1, 1-8.

to items such as caregiver support and training, home modifications, and transportation can make or break a well-intentioned medically oriented care plan if not considered or effectively addressed in their absence.

Clinicians face a number of critical challenges in implementing assessment and care planning processes to support goals that matter to the older person. First, structural and process issues in the care delivery environment can create tremendous challenges for clinicians who seek to treat their older adult patients in a person-centered manner. The short time frame of appointments, pressures to maintain high volume of visits, and barriers in record keeping that can be shared across care providers—even within electronic health record systems—all create barriers to engaging in a person-centered dialogue. Careful system planning through the application

of human-centered design that incorporates the perspectives of older adults and their families can help mitigate structural and process barriers.

Second, there may be clinical barriers or perceived clinical barriers to providing person-centered care. Cognitive decline or behavioral health issues may create challenges related to the person's active participation in elicitation of goals. It may be a cultural preference not to participate in conversations about goals of care. After extending an invitation to discuss these issues, the clinician should respect the person's preferences on this front. When and if the person is unable or unwilling to participate in such dialogue, the clinician can ask the family or paid caregiver for any pertinent information that may help in tailoring care.

Family and other significant others may offer differing views about goals and preferences;

they may contradict the older adult or another member of the family. When conflicts arise that cannot be talked through, a referral to social services or behavioral health might be appropriate. When the conflict revolves around goals of care in advanced illness or at the end of life, a member of the palliative care would also be an effective resource.

Last, and most importantly, clinicians must overcome their own knowledge deficits and bias regarding engagement in person-centered discussions with older adults with complex care needs. The culture of health, and the history of clinical training programs, has focused squarely on clinical assessment and treatment, to the exclusion of the person. Older adults living with chronic health conditions, which by their very nature will not be ameliorated, fundamentally change conversation dynamics and can leave cure-focused clinicians feeling helpless and hopeless. Engaging in a person-centered dialogue is a skill to be actively acquired and practiced. It requires a keen sense of self-awareness of one's own training and biases in relation to multimorbid diagnosis, treatment, and ideas of successful intervention. Personal attributes for clinician leaders that incline them toward person-centered assessment and care planning include patience, good listening and questioning skills, a willingness to tolerate significant ambiguity in the face of unsolved problems, and, above all, humility about both the process and outcomes of care.

▶ Summary

The most important member of the healthcare team is the older adult in partnership with the family and friends who make up the personal support network of the person's own choosing. Taking a person-centered approach to assessment and care planning ensures that the older adult gets goal-concordant care, receives the right interventions at the right time by the right providers, avoids unwanted care, and is supported in terms of his or her overall goals for health.

References

American Geriatrics Society Expert Panel on Person-Centered Care. (2015). Person-centered care: A definition and essential elements. *Journal of the American Geriatrics Society, 64* (1), 16–18.

Favreault, M., & Dey, J. (2015). *Long-term services and supports for older Americans: Risks and financing research brief.* Retrieved from http://aspe.hhs.gov /basic-report/long-term-services-and-supports-older -americans-risks-and-financing-research-brief

Fried, T., Tinetti, M., Iannone, L., O'Leary, J., Towle, V., & Van Ness, P. (2011). Health outcome prioritization as a tool for decision making among older persons with multiple chornic conditions. *Archives of Internal Medicine, 171*(20), 1854–1856.

Gerontological Society of America. (2016). *Patient-centered medical homes and the care of older adults.* Retrieved from https://www.johnahartford.org/images/uploads /reports/PCMH_Roadmap2016.pdf

Gitlin, L., Szanton, S., & DuGoff, E. (2011). *Supporting individuals with disability across the lifespan at home: Social services, technologies, and the built environment.* 2011. Retrieved from http://www.thescanfoundation. org/sites/thescanfoundation.org/files/TSF_CLASS_TA _No1_Supporting_Individuals_At_Home_FINAL.pdf

Kogan, A., Wilber, K., & Mosqueda, L. (2015). Person-centered care for older adults with chronic conditions and functional impairment: A systemic literature review. *Journal of the American Geriatrics Society, 64*(1), e1–e7.

Naik, A., Martin, L., Moye, J., & Karel, M. (2016). Health values and treatment goals of older, multimorbid adults facing life-threatening illness. *Journal of the American Geriatrics Society, 64*(3), 625–631.

National Center for Health Statistics. (2017). *Health, United States, 2016: With chartbook on long-term trends in health.* Retrieved from https://www.cdc.gov/nchs/data /hus/hus16.pdf#015

Rodriguez, S., Munevar, D., Delaney, C., Yang, L., & Tumlinson, A. (2014). *Effective management of high-risk Medicare populations.* Retrieved from http:// avalere-health-production.s3.amazonaws.com/uploads /pdfs/1411505132_AH_WhitePaper_TSF.pdf

World Health Organization. (2016). *Healthy life expectancy at birth (years), 2000–2015.* Retrieved from http:// gamapserver.who.int/gho/interactive_charts/mbd /hale_1/atlas.html

CHAPTER 9

Self-Care Self-Management

Shirley M. Moore, Carol M. Musil, and Sarah Givens

CHAPTER OBJECTIVES

1. Define self-care and self-management.
2. Describe the significance of self-management in the care of older adults.
3. Review current practices and challenges in the assessment of self-management capabilities and behaviors in older adults.
4. Provide an exemplar of assessment of the older adult's self-management capabilities and behaviors.

KEY TERMS

Assessment
Older adults

Self-care
Self-management

▶ Introduction

Self-care and **self-management** are two closely related terms, and the source of debate in the literature as to whether self-care includes self-management, or vice versa. For the purpose of this chapter, self-management is viewed as a component of the broader concept of self-care. On the one hand, self-care refers to the ability to care for oneself as well as the ability to carry out activities needed to achieve, maintain, and promote optimal health (Richard & Shea, 2011). On the other hand, self-management is the ability of an individual to collaborate with family, community, and healthcare professionals to monitor perceived health and implement strategies to manage symptoms, treatments, lifestyle changes, and the psychosocial, cultural, and spiritual consequences of both acute and chronic health conditions (Richard & Shea, 2011; Wilkinson & Whitehead, 2009). A distinguishing feature of self-management is the emphasis on a collaborative care approach in which self-management education is part of the patient–provider partnership paradigm (Bodenheimer, Lorig, Holman, & Grumbach, 2002). The term "self-management" is used throughout this chapter because of its emphasis on the use of collaborative approaches. Self-management is thought to include both the maintenance of wellness and the management of acute and chronic illness (Grady & Gough, 2014; Moore et al., 2016).

Self-management can be viewed as either a process or an outcome, or as both of these. The processes of self-management (e.g., self-monitoring, symptom management, decision making) usually occur on a daily basis, and require confidence to regulate and take action that result in specific self-management behaviors and health outcomes (Moore et al., 2016). Self-management encompasses formal patient education that teaches the skills needed for the individual to have a functional life, including use of medications, health behavior changes, and emotional support needed to manage a condition.

Self-management is particularly important for people living with a chronic condition. In chronic illness management, the purpose of self-management support is to help patients be informed about their condition(s) and able and willing to take an active role in their treatment. Effective self-management incorporates collaboration between the clinician and the patient in defining the problem, setting targets and goals, planning interventions, and maintaining active and sustained follow-up. This process includes collaborative decision making regarding medications (Does the patient agree to take what is recommended and prescribed?), diagnostic tests, procedures, and the health-related goals that the patient will pursue. Clinicians tend to define health problems in terms of a diagnosis and a treatment, whereas patients tend to define problems by the symptoms, their interference with normative functioning, difficulties they have with the treatment, and emotional concerns related to the problem (Patel, Shafazand, Schaufelberger, & Ekman, 2007). Self-management support,

therefore, is driven by a philosophy and a set of activities in which patients and healthcare providers form a partnership to assist an individual to be actively engaged in his or her own care.

▶ Self-Management and Older Adults

Self-management is a particularly important aspect of care for **older adults** because they often have multiple chronic conditions (MCC). Two out of three older Americans, including 21.4 million Medicare beneficiaries (Centers for Medicare and Medicaid Services, 2012), have at least two chronic physical or behavioral health conditions, and 14% have six or more MCC. The prevalence of MCC increases with age and is greater in women (Lochner, 2013). The existence of MCC confers a compounding burden on overall health status, functional ability, and quality of life—all of which require self-management to achieve optimal outcomes. The effects of multiple existing conditions in older adults are further compounded if acute conditions are present, instead of just chronic or permanent ones. Additionally, the inclusion of common risk factors, such as obesity, or pre-symptomatic conditions, such as low bone density, increases the prevalence of multimorbidity and the need for self-management.

As chronic conditions have become more prevalent, there has been a shift in health care toward encouraging older adults to participate in their health care through self-management programs (Wilkinson & Whitehead, 2009). Self-management education is an effective way to enable older adults to manage these chronic conditions and ultimately live healthier lives (Marks, Allegrante, & Lorig, 2005). Self-management has been shown to be effective for the most frequently occurring chronic conditions, including chronic obstructive pulmonary disease (COPD), diabetes, asthma, arthritis, hypertension, depression, and heart failure (Bourbeau et al., 2003; Gibson et al., 2002; Jaarsma, Cameron, Riegel, & Stromberg,

2017; Lorig & Holman, 2003; Marciniuk et al., 2011; McManus et al., 2010; Norris, Lau, Smith, Schmid, & Engelgau, 2002). Self-management interventions have been shown to reduce in-hospital admissions, emergency room visits, number of physician visits, and costs of chronic illness care (Bourbeau et al., 2003; Lorig, Mazonson, & Holman, 1993; Lorig, Ritter, Laurent, & Fries, 2004). Studies of the effects of self-management also have shown decreases in bothersome symptoms (e.g., pain, shortness of breath; Gibson et al., 2002; Lorig, Ritter, & Plant, 2005), reduction in depressed mood, and changes in important health status indicators, such as HbA1c levels (Norris et al., 2002).

▶ Self-Management Best Practices

A hallmark of self-management support by healthcare providers is the encouragement of patients to take an active role in decision making and the assumption of more of a coach or advocate role (Funnell & Anderson, 2004). The patient–provider dyad should look more like a partnership, rather than a student–teacher relationship. Using active listening, the provider should assess the patient's concerns, opinions, fears, questions, and progress toward the patient's individualized goals. These factors should also be taken into consideration when working with the patient to create a plan of care. As a plan is created, the provider should assist the patient in problem solving, and help the patient identify areas of self-management that can be encouraged by all members of the healthcare team (Funnell & Anderson, 2004). Family members who are involved in the care of the older person are included in this care partnership as well.

A major goal in self-management support is that patients gain an understanding of their condition, be able to monitor their condition at home (including the self-assessment of symptoms), obtain regular medical **assessment** by a clinician, and be able to engage in collaborative planning (Gibson et al., 2002). Self-management support also aims to help patients shift their thinking to maintain wellness as their focus, and tailor their plan accordingly (Lorig & Holman, 2003). The definition of wellness may vary from patient to patient, and their priorities may not be the same as providers' priorities. The patient's definition of wellness should be defined and used as the focus of care.

For providers interested in implementing a self-management education program, many resources and standards exist. For example, the National Standards for Diabetes Self-Management Education was designed to assist diabetes educators in providing the best self-management education and support to their clients (Haas et al., 2012). These standards are an excellent resource for providers caring for patients with diabetes and prediabetes. Like other self-management programs, the main goal is to "support informed decision making, self-care behaviors, problem solving, and active collaboration with the health care team to improve clinical outcomes, health status, and quality of life" (Haas et al., 2012, p. 620).

Stanford Medicine offers a Chronic Disease Self-Management Program, as well as programs for diabetes, chronic pain, cancer survivors, and HIV (Stanford University School of Medicine, 2017). Its website has numerous resources for clinicians and patients, including helpful self-management tools such as guides for symptom monitoring and goal setting.

There also are assessment tools that clinicians can incorporate in their practice for self-care and self-management. For example, the National Alliance for Mental Illness (NAMI, 2017) has developed a Self-Care Inventory that includes the domains of physical, psychological, emotional, spiritual, and workplace/professional self-care. Clinicians have also created symptom "checklists" to assist patients with monitoring their condition and then making subsequent decisions based on this assessment.

A variety of technological tools can facilitate self-management as well. Healthcare providers should work with patients to determine which type of role they would like to take in their own self-management program, and assist them in choosing tools accordingly (Barrett, 2005). Tools can range from those that relieve the patient of most of the need to perform self-management (e.g., monitoring devices, such as cameras, and implanted technology, such as pacemakers) to those that incorporate more structured roles requiring some, though limited, participation by the patient (e.g., telemedicine consultation or home blood pressure monitoring devices). Tools that support collaborative roles for patients require patients to draw on their own knowledge and to make a decision along with their provider. They include chronic disease management tools, such as a glucometer or a mobile app (Sjostrom, Lindholm, & Samuelsson, 2017). In the most autonomous patient role in self-management, patients take their care into their own hands with minimal involvement from the provider, such as with an online patient support group (Barrett, 2005). The Stanford Chronic Disease Self-Management Program is an example of an evidence-based, peer-led, group-based self-management program (Bodenheimer et al., 2002; Holman & Lorig, 2004; Lorig et al., 2005). It has also been shown to be effective when delivered over the internet (Lorig, Ritter, Laurent, & Plant, 2006).

EXEMPLAR: ASSESSMENT OF SELF-MANAGEMENT CAPABILITIES AND BEHAVIORS IN OLDER ADULTS

Assessment of Self-Management Capabilities

Assessment of self-management capabilities refers to the capacity or the ability of someone to engage in self-management processes and behaviors. It refers to the competencies, attitudes, knowledge, skills, experience, and resources of an individual to carry out self-management activities. A major role of the geriatric healthcare provider is to assess the self-management capabilities of the older adult. The following assessment domains are of particular importance in the assessment of self-management capabilities of older adults:

- Confidence to perform self-management activities
- Motivation to engage in self-management
- Cognition (memory, judgment, decision making, attention, self-evaluation)
- Mood/emotions (depression, anxiety, anger)
- Sensory abilities (hearing, sight, smell, fine motor, taste)
- Physical function ability
- Understanding of health-promoting behaviors
- Experience in performing health-promoting behaviors
- Communication skills
- Knowledge of health care and healthcare system resources
- Social support (family, friends, community)
- Patient–provider relationship
- Complexity of health problems and treatment regimens

Assessment of Self-Management Behaviors

Self-management behaviors consist of the actions and activities that an individual performs to monitor, treat, change or maintain their health condition. The following assessment domains of self-management behaviors are important for older adults:

- Medication taking
- Oral care

- Activity/fatigue level
- Eating and drinking patterns
- Sleeping patterns
- Engagement in social activities
- Goal setting
- Symptom monitoring
- Communicate needs and goals to clinicians and others
- Garner social support

These assessment domains are a broad, but essential set of self-management behaviors. These assessment domains of self-management behaviors should be used in conjunction with assessment of behaviors specific to a particular condition, such as heart failure (Bryant, 2017) or diabetes (Haas et al., 2012), or a specific geriatric syndrome, such as urinary incontinence (Wagg et al., 2015).

▶ Practice Challenges

When older persons have multiple conditions, those conditions interact to produce a complex and challenging dynamic for both older adults and clinicians regarding self-management. For example, depression may be present in combination with other chronic illnesses in as many as 60% of patients (Sheps, Freedland, Golden, & McMahon, 2003) and is a side effect of medications for treatment of some chronic illnesses. Likewise, arthritis interferes with the ability to exercise for cardiovascular disease and obesity.

Another challenge in supporting self-management in older adults is that self-management is often inadequate or not feasible for a person with dementia. Because of their impaired memory, judgment, and reasoning ability, older adults with dementia often cannot manage or direct their own care. They have difficulty engaging in self-management activities commonly associated with chronic illness management, such as medication taking, recognizing symptoms that may reflect changes in their health status, following diet and exercise regimens prescribed by their clinicians, and engaging with their clinicians in decision making about their health care. Engaging family as part of the care partnership is important in this situation.

Finally, it is important to remember that the self-care self-management paradigm may not be appropriate for all older adults. Cultural considerations must be taken into account regarding the extent to which individuals expect to take personal responsibility for care decisions and be actively involved in their treatment. Expectations about roles of patients and providers vary across cultures and should be part of the discussion in forming a patient–provider partnership.

▶ Summary

Given the large number of older adults who currently have multiple chronic conditions and the expected increase in this subpopulation in the future due to the aging of the overall population, self-management is an important component of care. Healthcare professionals increasingly must develop multidimensional and effective strategies to maintain or improve health status and quality of life of older adults. To achieve that goal, healthcare professionals need to become experts in understanding the philosophy and skills of self-management support to assist older adults in taking active roles in their care. This support includes assessment of the older adult's self-management capabilities and behaviors, engagement in collaborative patient–provider relationships to support joint decision making regarding treatment goals and care planning, and the use of behavioral techniques to enhance the engagement and adherence of patients to treatment regimens.

References

Barrett, M. J. (2005). Patient self-management tools: An overview. California Healthcare Foundation. Retrieved from http://www.chcf.org/publications/2005/06/patient-selfmanagement-tools-an-overview

Bodenheimer, T., Lorig, K., Holman, H., & Grumbach, K. (2002). Patient self-management of chronic disease in primary care. *Journal of the American Medical Association, 288*(19), 2469–2475.

Bourbeau, J., Julien, M., Maltais, F., Rouleau, M., Beaupre, A., Begin, R., . . . Chronic Obstructive Pulmonary Disease Axis of the Respiratory Network Fonds de la Recherche en Sante du Quebec. (2003). Reduction of hospital utilization in patients with chronic obstructive pulmonary disease: a disease-specific self-management intervention. *Archives of Internal Medicine, 163*(5), 585–591.

Bryant, R. (2017). Heart failure: Self-care to success: Development and evaluation of a program toolkit. *Nurse Practitioner, 42*(8), 1–8. doi: 10.1097/01.NPR.0000520833.22030.d0

Centers for Medicare and Medicaid Services (CMS). (2012). *Chronic conditions among Medicare beneficiaries, chartbook, 2012 edition.* Baltimore, MD: Author.

Funnell, M. M., & Anderson, R. M. (2004). Empowerment and self-management of diabetes. *Clinical Diabetes, 22*(3), 123–127.

Gibson, P. G., Powell, H., Wilson, A., Abramson, M. J., Haywood, P., Bauman, A., . . . Roberts, J. J. L. (2002). Self-management education and regular practitioner review for adults with asthma. *Cochrane Database of Systematic Reviews, 3*, CD001117. doi: 001110.001002/14651858.CD14001117

Grady, P. A., & Gough, L. L. (2014). Self-management: A comprehensive approach to management of chronic conditions. *American Journal of Public Health, 104*(8), e25–e31. doi: 10.2105/AJPH.2014.302041

Haas, L., Maryniuk, M., Beck, J., Cox, C. E., Duker, P., Edwards, L., . . . Youssef, G. (2012). National standards for diabetes self-management education and support. *Diabetes Educator, 38*(5), 619–629. doi: 10.1177/0145721712455997

Holman, H., & Lorig, K. (2004). Patient self-management: A key to effectiveness and efficiency in care of chronic disease. *Public Health Reports, 119*(3), 239–243.

Jaarsma, T., Cameron, J., Riegel, B., & Stromberg, A. (2017). Factors related to self-care in heart failure patients according to the middle-range theory of self-care of chronic illness: A literature update. *Current Heart Failure Reports, 14*(2), 71–77. doi: 10.1007/s11897-017-0324-1

Lochner, K. A. (2013). Prevalence of multiple chronic conditions among Medicare beneficiaries, United States, 2010. *Preventing Chronic Disease, 10.*

Lorig, K., & Holman, H. (2003). Self-management education: History, definition, outcomes, and mechanisms. *Annals of Behavioral Medicine, 26*(1), 1–7.

Lorig, K. R., Mazonson, P. D., & Holman, H. R. (1993). Evidence suggesting that health education for self-management in patients with chronic arthritis has sustained health benefits while reducing health care costs. *Arthritis & Rheumatology, 36*(4), 439–446.

Lorig, K., Ritter, P., Laurent, D., & Fries, J. (2004). Long-term randomized controlled trials of tailored-print and small-group arthritis self-management interventions. *Medical Care, 42*(4), 346–354.

Lorig, K., Ritter, P., Laurent, D., & Plant, K. (2006). Internet-based chronic disease self-management: A randomized trial. *Medical Care, 44*(11), 964–971.

Lorig, K., Ritter, P. L., & Plant, K. (2005). A disease-specific self-help program compared with a generalized chronic disease self-help program for arthritis patients. *Arthritis & Rheumatology, 53*(6), 950–957.

Marciniuk, D. D., Goodridge, D., Hernandez, P., Rocker, G., Balter, M., Bailey, P., . . . Canadian Thoracic Society, COPD Committee Dyspnea Expert Working Group. (2011). Managing dyspnea in patients with advanced chronic obstructive pulmonary disease: A Canadian Thoracic Society clinical practice guideline. *Canadian Respiratory Journal, 18*(2), 69–78.

Marks, R., Allegrante, J. P., & Lorig, K. (2005). A review and synthesis of research evidence for self-efficacy–enhancing interventions for reducing chronic disability: Implications for health education practice (part II). *Health Promotion Practice, 6*(2), 148–156.

McManus, R. J., Mant, J., Bray, E. P., Holder, R., Jones, M. I., Greenfield, S., . . . Hobbs, F. D. (2010). Telemonitoring and Self-Management in the Control of Hypertension (TASMINH2): A randomised controlled trial. *Lancet, 376*(9736), 163–172. doi: 10.1016/S0140-6736(10)60964-6

Moore, S. M., Schiffman, R., Waldrop-Valverde, D., Redeker, N. S., McCloskey, D. J., Kim, M. T., . . . Grady, P. (2016). Recommendations of common data elements to advance the science of self-management of chronic conditions. *Journal of Nursing Scholarship, 48*(5), 437–447. doi: 10.1111/jnu.12233

National Alliance for Mental Illness (NAMI). (2017). Self-care inventory. Retrieved from https://www.nami.org/getattachment/Extranet/Education,-Training-and-Outreach-Programs/Signature-Classes/NAMI-Homefront/HF-Additional-Resources/HF15AR6SelfCare.pdf

Norris, S. L., Lau, J., Smith, S. J., Schmid, C. H., & Engelgau, M. M. (2002). Self-management education for adults with type 2 diabetes: A meta-analysis of the effect on glycemic control. *Diabetes Care, 25*(7), 1159–1171.

Patel, H., Shafazand, M., Schaufelberger, M., & Ekman, I. (2007). Reasons for seeking acute care in chronic heart failure. *European Journal of Heart Failure, 9*(6–7), 702–708. doi: 10.1016/j.ejheart.2006.11.002

Richard, A. A., & Shea, K. (2011). Delineation of self-care and associated concepts. *Journal of Nursing Scholarship, 43*(3), 255–264. doi: 10.1111/j.1547-5069.2011.01404.x

Sheps, D. S., Freedland, K. E., Golden, R. N., & McMahon, R. P. (2003). ENRICHD and SADHART: Implications for future biobehavioral intervention efforts. *Psychosomatic Medicine, 65*(1), 1–2.

Sjostrom, M., Lindholm, L., & Samuelsson, E. (2017). Mobile app for treatment of stress urinary incontinence: A cost-effectiveness analysis. *Journal of Medical Internet Research, 19*(5), e154. doi: 10.2196/jmir.7383

Stanford University School of Medicine. (2017). Chronic Disease Self-Management Program (CDSMP). Retrieved from http://patienteducation.stanford.edu/programs /cdsmp.html

Wagg, A., Gibson, W., Ostaszkiewicz, J., Johnson, T. 3rd, Markland, A., Palmer, M. H., . . . Kirschner-Hermanns, R. (2015). Urinary incontinence in frail elderly persons: Report from the 5th International Consultation on Incontinence. *Neurourology and Urodynamics, 34*(5), 398–406. doi: 10.1002/nau.22602

Wilkinson, A., & Whitehead, L. (2009). Evolution of the concept of self-care and implications for nurses: A literature review. *International Journal of Nursing Studies, 46*(8), 1143–1147. doi: 10.1016/j.ijnurstu.2008.12.011

CHAPTER 10

The Family Context

Susan C. Reinhard

CHAPTER OBJECTIVES

1. Describe the growing complexity of the family caregiver's role in supporting older adults.
2. Discuss how policy and payment changes affect family caregiving.
3. Identify potential resources for incorporating family caregiving into practice.

KEY TERMS

CARE Act	Family caregiver	Medical/nursing tasks

▶ Introduction

Family caregivers (FCs) are the main providers of care and support for older adults, particularly for those who have multiple chronic conditions. Their job description is multidimensional and becoming excessively complex, as they are expected to perform more medical and nursing tasks. Current policy and payment trends are shifting even more caregiving expectations to FCs, heightening the need to focus on the family context of care. For their part, family caregivers look to nurses and other professionals to guide them in how to do their jobs, especially complex care tasks. These professionals should consider the person and family as a unit and embrace the concepts of person- and family-centered care. To ensure effective and high-quality care, healthcare professionals need to determine which family caregivers are willing and able to execute complex caregiving responsibilities, and provide the necessary instruction and support so that FCs can perform these tasks with confidence.

▶ Who Are the Family Caregivers of Older Adults and What Do They Do?

A key component of both acute health care and long-term services and supports (LTSS) is the role of the family caregiver. According to the National Academy for Sciences, Engineering, and Medicine (2016), millions of Americans provide care and support to an older adult—a parent, spouse, friend, or neighbor—who needs help because of a limitation in physical, mental, or cognitive functioning. Caregivers include both traditional relatives and individuals without a legally defined relationship (e.g., a neighbor) to the individual. Family caregivers provide invaluable and often vital support to people across an almost unlimited range of emotional, functional, and complex care support.

An estimated 40 million American adults provide unpaid support to an adult who has limitations in his or her daily activities (National Alliance for Caregiving & AARP Public Policy Institute, 2015). Collectively, this group provides a total of 37 billion hours of care annually, valued at more than $470 billion per year (Reinhard, Feinberg, Choula, & Houser, 2015). For the sake of comparison, the value of unpaid family caregiving is greater than that of the entire Medicaid program, which serves more than 70 million people at an annual cost of $450 billion. Clearly, one cannot overstate the importance of family caregiving to health care.

The demand for family caregivers is growing, but the pool of available family caregivers for older adults is shrinking. There were approximately seven potential family caregivers for each adult age 80 or older in 2010. By 2030, there will be just four potential family caregivers for each adult in that age group; by 2050, this care gap will widen further to just three potential family caregivers (Redfoot, Feinberg, & Houser, 2013). Family caregivers should be viewed as dwindling resources that need to be respected and supported.

Who Are Family Caregivers of Older Adults?

Family caregivers of older adults play an especially critical role. Indeed, most family caregivers (33.4 million) provide support to an adult age 50 or older. Nearly half (47%) of these family caregivers support a parent, and an additional 11% support a spouse or partner (Reinhard & Hunt, 2015).

Family caregivers are a diverse group. Although the average caregiver is a Caucasian woman in her 40s caring for her aging mother, the reality is that 40% of caregivers are men, and 1 in 5 (21%) is a millennial younger than the age of 34. In addition, more than one-third of family caregivers of older adults have multicultural identities, including Hispanic (16%), African American (13%), and Asian American (7%). The income levels of family caregivers also vary, with a nearly even split between family caregivers with household incomes greater than $50,000 (54%) and those with household incomes below that threshold (46%) (Reinhard & Hunt, 2015). Most family caregivers are employed, with more than 6 out of 10 family caregivers facing the dual pressures of employment and family caregiving (Feinberg, 2016).

Clearly, family caregiving of older adults is becoming a normative experience, cutting across gender, race, economic status, and relationship to the person. Recognizing the family context of care is crucial to successful clinical practice, as anyone can potentially be a family caregiver. Identifying the appropriate family caregiver(s) for any particular patient will help professionals better meet the needs of both the family caregiver and the patient.

Which Functions Do Family Caregivers of Older Adults Perform?

The most common types of tasks that family caregivers perform include activities of daily living (ADLs), instrumental activities of daily living

(IADLs), and **medical/nursing tasks**. ADLs include transfers in and out of beds and chairs (45% of family caregivers of the age 50-plus care recipients), help with getting dressed (32%), and transfers to and from the toilet (28%). IADLs include transportation (78%), shopping (76%), and help with housework (72%) (Reinhard & Hunt, 2015).

Historically, these ADLs and IADLs were considered "traditional" tasks performed by family caregivers. Today, however, family caregivers are doing much more. They often serve as ad hoc care managers, coordinating care across providers, practitioners, and insurance companies. In addition, they are increasingly being called upon to perform complex care tasks that are typically considered to be in the province of healthcare professionals, especially nurses.

Family Caregivers Routinely Perform Complex, Medical/Nursing Tasks

In recent years, research identifying the types of tasks that family caregivers perform has revealed more complex, difficult tasks being assumed by such caregivers. Key among these is medical/nursing tasks—that is, procedures that extend beyond traditional ADLs and IADL support. The first national survey of U.S. family caregivers examining their role in performing medical/nursing tasks, known as the *Home Alone* study, found that almost half (46%) of the respondents shouldered such responsibilities. These tasks involved medication administration (including injections and intravenous fluids); care of wounds, catheters, colostomies, and ventilators; preparing special diets; and help with mobility tasks and assistive devices such as canes and walkers, among other tasks (Reinhard, Levine, & Samis, 2012).

In addition to identifying the frequency with which family caregivers perform these complex tasks, the *Home Alone* study provided evidence that family caregivers often do not receive support or instruction from healthcare

professionals about this role. Among family caregivers performing medication management functions, for example, 61% indicated that they "learned on [their] own" how to perform these tasks. They did not consistently receive instruction on how to perform wound care. In many cases, this lack of guidance left the family caregiver feeling stressed and concerned about making a mistake (Reinhard et al., 2012). Combined with the caregivers' lack of formal preparation, this uneasiness about performing complex, but necessary, medical/nursing tasks could have a negative impact on patients. This aspect of caregiving can be addressed by more active engagement and inclusion of family caregivers during hospital stays and other interactions with professionals.

The gap between what family caregivers are expected to do and which resources and support are available to them is a major concern that healthcare systems and individual clinicians need to address. For example, family caregivers can often make the difference between a successful hospital discharge and an unplanned hospital readmission (Rodakowski et al., 2017). As the population continues to age and more people need support from family caregivers, the frequency with which these tasks are performed by family members will likely increase, highlighting the importance of bridging this gap and providing more adequate support to family caregivers filling this role. Demand for support from family caregivers performing ADL and IADL tasks is also likely to occur.

In the face of this current and growing demand for family caregiver support, it is important for professionals from all disciplines to be prepared to actively engage and support family caregivers. This outreach will improve care for the patient, provide relief to the family, and lead to better outcomes for all parties. It is also important to support family caregivers of individuals who have both lower and higher acuity. Even inpatient cases with relatively minor post-discharge needs will need at least some degree of family caregiver support.

▶ Value-Based Purchasing and Implications for Family Caregivers

In addition to the implications for quality and health outcomes, the role and engagement of family caregivers will likely have financial implications for health systems as healthcare financing evolves. New payment models are already changing how healthcare systems interact with family caregivers; such changes will continue as the shift toward value-based purchasing (VBP) expands throughout health care. In VBP, payers link payments to providers and individual healthcare professionals with quality measures and patient outcomes. A key driver of this shift, especially among older adults, is the Medicare program. Value-based purchasing has long been part of certain portions of the Medicare program, and in recent years the Centers for Medicare and Medicaid Services (CMS) has accelerated this trend across settings and services. The resulting increased focus on quality and outcomes will have implications for family caregivers and the ways in which clinicians interact with and engage families.

Bundled Payment Models

One type of VBP is bundled payment ("bundles"). In this arrangement, hospitals and health systems receive a predefined reimbursement rate to pay for the entirety of a given clinical episode, such as a hip replacement surgery. All expenses associated with that episode must be covered by that payment (from surgery through post-acute care), and participating providers are able to retain a portion of any funds saved compared to a nonbundled episode cost (Ciarametaro & Dubois, 2016). When this payment approach is used, health systems are more incentivized to discharge patients to home rather than to more expensive and resource-intensive subacute

facilities, even for short postdischarge stays. At the same time, they will need to ensure quality to meet bundling program requirements.

This shift in discharge patterns will necessarily affect family caregivers, increasing the amount of time over which they are expected to provide care and expanding the scope of which tasks they are expected to perform as part of that care. Individual professionals providing care to patients served through a bundle will need to ensure that families are adequately engaged throughout the care process and are prepared and trained to perform any postdischarge tasks they are asked to carry out.

Accountable Care Organizations

Another model emerging in VBP is the accountable care organization (ACO). Implemented across Medicare, Medicaid, and private insurance plans, ACOs are networks of hospitals, health systems, physician groups, and other healthcare providers that share responsibility for patient care and payment accountability for that care (Gold, 2015). The payment structure of ACOs requires increased and improved care coordination across settings, which should necessitate increased family caregiver engagement by participating providers.

Medicare and Value-Based Purchasing

In the context of Medicare, both bundled payment and ACO models are key components of the CMS Quality Payment Program (QPP), an effort to transition the Medicare fee-for-service program from volume-based to value-based payments. Most physicians and nurse practitioners participating in Medicare are required to participate in the QPP and often do so through participating in an alternate payment model (APM) such as a bundling model or an ACO (Findlay, 2017). As the QPP moves forward and more providers and clinicians are engaged in value-based care, there will be an increased emphasis on the family caregiver. In the context of hospital stays, this trend underscores the need for professionals across disciplines to involve families throughout the care and discharge planning processes and to provide adequate and timely support to family caregivers.

In addition to VBP, other policy levers are currently in place that will increase the emphasis and importance of family caregivers.

▶ Hospital Readmissions and the Family Caregiver

The Patient Protection and Affordable Care Act, more simply known as the Affordable Care Act (ACA), raised the stakes associated with hospital discharge trends by tying readmission rates to payment. Specifically, the ACA established the Hospital Readmissions Reduction Program, through which Medicare assesses penalties to hospitals with 30-day readmission rates that exceed the national average 30-day readmission rate, adjusted for the age and acuity of a hospital's case mix. A hospital with an older and/or sicker case mix, for example, has greater leeway in this program than a hospital that serves younger and relatively healthier patient populations (Boccutti & Colissas, 2017).

For hospitals with excessive readmission rates, Medicare reduced the base payments on all Medicare inpatient admissions, starting at 1% in 2013 and increasing to 3% in 2015 and subsequent years (Boccutti & Colissas, 2017). In response to this policy, hospitals and health systems across the United States prioritized readmission reduction efforts so as to keep discharged patients, especially those covered by Medicare (e.g., older adults), at home and out of the hospital (Rennke & Ranji, 2015).

While several approaches have shown promise for—or even evidence of—reducing the hospital readmission rate, engagement of family caregivers has been found to have a marked impact on keeping older adults out of the hospital once discharged. A 2017 meta-analysis revealed that integrating the family caregiver(s) in discharge planning was associated with a 25% readmission reduction at 90 days, and a 24% reduction at 180 days. While this analysis did not include the 30-day span most relevant to Medicare payments, it does show the impact of family caregiver engagement in the discharge planning process (Rodakowski et al., 2017).

Both health systems and state and local governments have adopted various policy approaches to reduce Medicare inpatient readmissions. While it is difficult to definitively prove that one or two of these approaches were the "silver bullet" behind reduced rates, the 2017 meta-analysis documents that policies that encourage family caregiver support and engagement could have a positive impact. One policy—a state law known as the Caregiver Advise, Record, and Enable (CARE) Act—seeks to codify this approach into practice by requiring hospitals to identify and offer instruction to family caregivers.

▶ The CARE Act Brings Policy into Practice

In response to the *Home Alone* research and subsequent increased awareness of the role of family caregivers in performing complex care tasks, AARP translated the research findings into model state legislation to better support family caregivers. The model **CARE Act** includes the following core provisions:

- Hospitals must ask all admitted patients if they want to identify a family caregiver.
- If the patient identifies a family caregiver, that person must be included in the medical record in accordance with the patient's decision.
- The designated family caregiver must be notified of the patient's discharge plans.
- Hospitals must offer the designated family caregiver instruction on how to perform medical/nursing tasks that they need to perform.

In 2014, Oklahoma became the first state to sign this model into law, followed shortly by New Jersey. As of December 2017, 39 states and territories have enacted their own versions of the CARE Act, and more states are considering it. Similar to changes in payment policies, the CARE Act will require providers and individual health professionals to more actively engage family caregivers.

Clearly, the shifting policy environments at both the federal and state levels are putting the family caregiver at center stage. With that in mind, practice challenges and examples of promising practices are important to examine and understand.

▶ Family Caregivers and Healthcare Professionals: Practice Challenges and Resources

As the role of family caregivers increasingly becomes a part of public and policy conversations, these individuals' needs must be considered. The first step is addressing a common experience faced by family caregivers: feeling invisible. In busy hospitals and other healthcare settings, nurses and other clinicians may focus only on the needs of the patient. While this is clearly the priority, it is also important to acknowledge and engage the family members who are helping the patient both during hospital stays and after discharge.

Often families are acknowledged only when it is time to make a major care decision or when it is time to discharge the patient. At that point, many family caregivers report that they suddenly become visible. The focus of these conversations is often where to send the patient and when. The family caregivers' capacity to provide care post discharge is not always a substantial part of the discussion, despite the responsibilities they

may be expected to assume. Family caregivers are rarely asked, "How are you doing?" or "How are you managing?" Inadequate communication between family caregivers and healthcare and social services professionals not only risks turning family caregivers into patients themselves, but also threatens the quality of care provided to older adults (Reinhard & Choula, 2011).

These situations are problematic for those family caregivers who provide intensive levels of help, especially for those who manage complex chronic care. They can exacerbate caregivers' sense of insecurity, stress, and burnout. More active support and engagement from healthcare professionals can help alleviate these negative outcomes.

In today's healthcare environment, people are hospitalized only for serious conditions that typically require posthospital treatment and care—often at home. Family caregivers need guidance from professionals across settings—clinician offices, hospitals, outpatient surgical centers, home care, rehabilitation and nursing homes, and other locations. The increased interest in reducing readmissions raises the stakes for making sure both the patient and the family are well prepared to perform all the posthospital instructions so the patient does not require readmission.

Many resources and tools are available to professionals to help support these family caregivers, such as the "Ask Me Too" tool. Meant to be analogous to the widely used "Ask Me 3" tool for promoting better patient–provider communication, "Ask Me Too" includes scripted questions to ask family caregivers; these questions can help hospital staff ensure consistent communication with family caregivers:

- What questions do you have regarding care today?
- What questions do you have about care at home?

One important aspect of these questions is the focus on how the family caregiver is doing as an individual. In addition, these questions provide a structured approach for accurate communication between families and the clinical team. These questions are meant to stimulate dialogue between the healthcare professional and the family caregiver.

The process of family engagement starts on admission and/or the first interaction with the family, at which time the family caregiver is given a communication notebook. This technique is similar to the "whiteboard" method that has been promoted by the Agency for Healthcare Research and Quality (2013), but reduces the concerns over patient privacy when a board is visible to anyone entering the room. The notebook creates a forum for all care participants to communicate with each other throughout the hospital stay. It provides consistency in communication and serves as a "checklist" of tasks and questions to be answered throughout the stay. The notebook goes home with the patient and family as a reference for postdischarge care (Reinhard, Capezuti, Bricoli, & Choula, 2017).

Other emerging tools include evidence-based videos and articles that are available for professionals to use in supporting and instructing family caregivers who are asked to perform complex care tasks. Through its Home Alone Alliance^SM effort, AARP recently produced multiple series of instructional videos designed to teach family caregivers how to complete certain medical/nursing tasks, including medication management, mobility assistance, and wound care. Example titles of these videos include *What to Do When Someone Falls* and *Getting from a Car to a Wheelchair* (Reinhard, 2017). Development of more videos is in progress, including additional videos on medication management. These videos are accompanied by consumer- and family caregiver–focused resource guides that provide written instruction to family caregivers. Both can be employed by health professionals to help train family caregivers on these tasks.

In addition, in May 2017 the *American Journal for Nursing* published a series of articles for health professionals that provide detailed guidance and evidence on how to instruct and support family caregivers performing medication management tasks. These include managing complex medication regimens (Harvath, Lindauer, & Sexson, 2017), administering subcutaneous injections (Sexson, Lindauer, & Harvath, 2017a), discharge planning and teaching (Sexson, Lindauer, & Harvath, 2017b), medication management for people with dementia (Lindauer, Sexson, & Harvath, 2017a), and administering eye drops, transdermal patches, and suppositories (Lindauer, Sexson, & Harvath, 2017b).

▶ Summary

Most patients in the hospital setting will need some sort of family caregiving support after discharge, not just those patients considered to be at high risk for readmission. Regardless of the patient's acuity or condition, family caregivers are asked to step in as care coordinators and direct providers of care tasks. For family caregivers of older patients, the time after discharge can be difficult or even frightening, as the tasks or support they are expected to provide are often unfamiliar or new to them and to the patient. Nurses and other professionals can help alleviate the uncertainty associated with these responsibilities by more actively offering support and communicating with family caregivers of all patients, particularly older adults.

References

Agency for Healthcare Research and Quality. (2013, June). *Guide to patient and family engagement in hospital quality in safety strategy 2: Communicating to improve quality.* Retrieved from http://www.ahrq.gov/sites/default/files/wysiwyg/professionals/systems/hospital/engagingfamilies/strategy2/Strat2_Implement_Hndbook_508.pdf

Boccutti, C., & Colissas, G. (2017, March 10). *Aiming for fewer hospital U-turns: The Medicare Hospital Readmission Reduction Program.* Retrieved from http://www.kff.org/medicare/issue-brief/aiming-for-fewer-hospital-u-turns-the-medicare-hospital-readmission-reduction-program/

Ciarametaro, M., & Dubois, R. (2016, April 20). *Designing successful bundled payment initiatives.* Retrieved from http://healthaffairs.org/blog/2016/04/20/designing-successful-bundled-payment-initiatives/

Feinberg, L. F. (2016, May 2). *The dual pressures of family caregiving and employment.* Retrieved from https://www.aarp.org/ppi/info-2016/the-dual-pressures-of-family-caregiving-and-employment.html

Findlay, S. (2017, March 27). *Implementing MACRA.* Retrieved from http://www.healthaffairs.org/healthpolicybriefs/brief.php?brief_id=166

Gold, J. (2015, September 14). *Accountable care organizations, explained.* Retrieved from http://khn.org/news/aco-accountable-care-organization-faq/

Harvath, T. A., Lindauer, A., & Sexson, K. (2017, May). Managing complex medication regimens. *American Journal of Nursing, 117*(5), S3–S6. Retrieved from http://journals.lww.com/ajnonline/Fulltext/2017/05001/Managing_Complex_Medication_Regimens.2.aspx

Lindauer, A., Sexson, K., & Harvath, T. A. (2017a, May). Medication management for people with dementia. *American Journal of Nursing, 117*(5), S17–S21. Retrieved from http://journals.lww.com/ajnonline/Fulltext/2017/05001/Medication_Management_for_People_with_Dementia.5.aspx

Lindauer, A., Sexson, K., & Harvath, T. A. (2017b, May). Teaching caregivers to administer eye drops, transdermal patches, and suppositories. *American Journal of Nursing, 117*(5), S11–S16. Retrieved from http://journals.lww.com/ajnonline/Fulltext/2017/05001/Teaching_Caregivers_to_Administer_Eye_Drops,.4.aspx

National Academies of Sciences, Engineering, and Medicine. (2016). *Families caring for an aging America.* Washington, DC: National Academies.

National Alliance for Caregiving & AARP Public Policy Institute. (2015). *Caregiving in the United States 2015.* Retrieved from http://www.aarp.org/ppi/info-2015/caregiving-in-the-united-states-2015.html

Redfoot, D., Feinberg, F., & Houser, A. (2013, August). *The aging of the baby boom and the growing care gap: A look at future declines in the availability of family caregivers.* Retrieved from http://www.aarp.org/home-family/caregiving/info-08-2013/the-aging-of-the-baby-boom-and-the-growing-care-gap-AARP-ppi-ltc.html

Reinhard, S. (Producer). (2017, March). *What to do when someone falls* [Video file]; *Getting from a car to a wheelchair* [Video file]. Retrieved from http://www.aarp.org/nolongeralone

Reinhard, S., Capezuti, E., Bricoli, B., & Choula, R. (2017). Feasibility of a family-centered hospital intervention. *Journal of Gerontological Nursing, 43*(6). Retrieved from http://www.healio.com/nursing/journals/jgn/2017-6-43-6/%7Bc1836043-acfa-41fc-9adb-ec8946c0255d%7D/feasibility-of-a-family-centered-hospital-intervention?utm_source=selligent&utm_medium=email&utm_campaign=nursing%20journals&m_bt=1737610567129

Reinhard, S., & Choula, R. (2011) Lifting the cloak of invisibility: Nurses and social workers supporting family caregivers. *AARP International: The Journal.* Retrieved from http://journal-archive.aarpinternational.org/a/b/2011/08/Lifting-the-Cloak-of-Invisibility-Nurses-and-Social-Workers-Supporting-Family-Caregivers

Reinhard, S., Feinberg, L. F., Choula, R., & Houser, A. (2015). *Valuing the invaluable 2015 update: Undeniable progress, but big gaps remain.* Retrieved from http://www.aarp.org/ppi/info-2015/valuing-the-invaluable-2015-update.html

Reinhard, S., & Hunt, G. (2015). *Caregivers of older adults: A focused look at those caring for someone age 50+.* Retrieved from http://www.aarp.org/content/dam/aarp/ppi/2015/caregivers-of-older-adults-focused-look.pdf

Reinhard, S., Levine, C., & Samis, S. (October 2012). *Home alone: Family caregivers providing complex chronic care.* Retrieved from http://www.aarp.org/home-family/caregiving/info-10-2012/home-alone-family-caregivers-providing-complex-chronic-care.html

Rennke, S., & Ranji, S. (2015). Transitional care strategies from hospital to home. *Neurohospitalist, 5*(1), 35–42. Retrieved from http://journals.sagepub.com/doi/10.1177/1941874414540683

Rodakowski, J., Rocco, P., Ortiz, M., Folb, B., Schulz, R., Morton, S., . . . James, A. E. (2017). Caregiver integration during discharge planning for older adults to reduce resource use: A meta-analysis. *Journal of the American Geriatrics Society, 65*(5). Retrieved from https://www.ncbi.nlm.nih.gov/pubmed/28369687

Sexson, K., Lindauer, A., & Harvath, T. A. (2017a, May). Administration of subcutaneous injections. *American Journal of Nursing, 117*(5), S7–S10. Retrieved from http://journals.lww.com/ajnonline/Fulltext/2017/05001/Administration_of_Subcutaneous_Injections.3.aspx

Sexson, K., Lindauer, A., & Harvath, T. A. (2017b, May). Discharge planning and teaching. *American Journal of Nursing, 117*(5), S22–S24. Retrieved from http://journals.lww.com/ajnonline/Fulltext/2017/05001/Discharge_Planning_and_Teaching.6.aspx

CHAPTER 11

The Social Determinants of Health

John Auerbach and Karen DeSalvo

CHAPTER OBJECTIVES

1. Understand how the social determinants of health influence healthcare outcomes.
2. Describe issues of access to comprehensive healthcare services.
3. Describe examples of selective approaches for addressing social determinants of health.

KEY TERMS

Social determinants

▶ Introduction

Patty Edwards, who recently turned 70, sat in an examining room of her newly selected doctor. She listened politely as the doctor explained that Patty had prediabetes. The doctor patiently informed her of the dangers associated with diabetes and counseled her to make changes in her lifestyle. Patty needed to eat a healthier diet—ideally one filled with more vegetables and fruits—and she needed to exercise. The doctor prescribed medicine for her asthma, which had been acting up since Patty moved a few years ago. She suggested Patty review the pamphlet she handed her, which listed the environmental triggers for asthma that she should avoid.

Patty tried to look like she was seriously taking in all this information. But she was thinking:

> If she only knew! I can barely make rent every month, and I just spent $20 that I needed for this week's groceries on the co-pay for this visit. How am

I supposed to exercise when it isn't safe to even walk in my neighborhood? How am I supposed to afford those pricey health foods? I buy what's on sale and what I know my husband likes. And maybe this medicine will help with my asthma but I think there's something in our apartment that's making me sick. I didn't have this problem before we moved. Fat chance the landlord's likely to do something about that.

When the visit ended, Patty thanked the doctor and told her she would be sure to follow her advice. Both she and her doctor knew the odds were against it.

This scenario will sound familiar to many clinicians and caregivers. The patient either has or is at risk of developing one or more chronic conditions. The physician does everything within his or her power to diagnose, treat, and counsel the patient. But even the best quality clinical intervention can achieve only so much. While access to affordable, quality health care is necessary to improving health, especially for those patients with chronic medical conditions, it is a relatively weak determinant of population health (McGinnis & Foege, 1993; Mokdad, Marks, Stroup, & Gerberding, 2004).

Clinicians understandably focus on the traditional clinical factors that are within their control, primarily the diagnosis and treatment of illness and injury. That is what they are trained to do. Identifying—let alone addressing—the socioeconomic factors affecting their patients usually seems beyond the scope of their practice. Clinicians who try to grapple with these issues—either alone or in conjunction with others in their practice, such as social workers or nurses—often find it difficult to intervene in productive ways. Fortunately, there are increasing efforts and a growing number of tools to help even busy clinicians gain a fuller understanding of the conditions in patients' lives that contribute to their health and to assist those patients in meeting some of their unmet **social determinants** of health.

The U.S. Department of Health and Human Services' *Healthy People 2020* initiative defines social determinants of health as "conditions in the environments in which people are born, live, learn, work, play, worship, and age that affect a wide range of health, functioning, and quality-of-life outcomes and risks" (Centers for Disease Control and Prevention [CDC], 2017). These social determinants of health comprise social and economic factors beyond the reach of the typical clinician and clinical environment, and are recognized as major contributors to global health. With that perspective, the World Health Organization (WHO) adds to the *Healthy People* definition: "The social determinants of health . . . are shaped by the distribution of money, power and resources at global, national and local levels. The social determinants of health are mostly responsible for health inequities—the unfair and avoidable differences in health status seen within and between countries." In the last several years, there has been a deepening of the understanding of what these factors are, how they contribute to health, and what can be done to ameliorate their potential negative impact (Adler & Newman, 2002; Braveman, 2006; Marmot, 2007; Norman, Kennedy, & Kawachi, 1999; Saegert & Evans, 2003; Walker, Keane, & Burke, 2010; Williams, Costa, Odunlami, & Mohammed, 2008).

This chapter identifies several of the primary social determinants of health (SDOH), discusses their impact on health, and highlights some of the effective efforts to address them as a component of patients' care plans and community-wide efforts.

▶ Access to Comprehensive Health Services

It may seem odd to consider access to affordable, comprehensive health care to be a social determinant of health. In fact, considerable evidence shows that it is strongly related to such factors as income, geography, and social status. While nearly 99% of Americans who were 65 years or older had health insurance according to the 2015 census (Barnett & Vornovitsky, 2016), there continue to be obstacles to comprehensive and affordable, high-quality care for older adults. Most elderly adults enrolled in Medicare purchase some form supplemental insurance, but the ability to purchase and the quality of the supplemental insurance are often dependent on income, as it can be costly for low-income older adults who are not eligible for Medicaid (National Academy of Social Insurance, n.d.). Prior to the passage of the Patient Protection and Affordable Care Act, one in three families with older adults spent at least 10% of after-tax household income on health care (Bieber, 2017).

Even when individuals are insured, the benefits covered may not be comprehensive. For example, Medicare does not cover the routine cost of dental care, hearing aids, or vision care for people with a chronic condition such as Alzheimer's disease. This omission is problematic because the cost of a full-time home health aide—whose services may be needed to avoid a costly acute episode—is almost $50,000 per year, far outside the budget of most Americans (Schulz & Eden, 2016). Even small copayments of as little as a few dollars have been shown to discourage the filling of a prescription for low-income persons (Ku, Deschamps, & Hilman, 2004).

Furthermore, services are not always accessible for a variety of reasons, including but not limited to geography, language access, and service availability. In rural areas, for example, medical services may be available only for those individuals who are able to travel long distances by car (Oregon State University, 2015; Stanford Medicine, n.d.). For those with limited English proficiency, healthcare access may be physically available but out of reach because of an inability to communicate. Moreover, services may be unavailable due to the healthcare provider's hours or operation, which may coincide with the working hours of patients.

▶ Poverty and Economic Stability

The case presented in the opening scenario is an example of the importance of income as a key determinant of health. Put simply, if you are poor, you are more likely to be ill (Schoeni, Martin, Andreski, & Freedman, 2005). People with low incomes have higher rates of preventable chronic and infectious diseases and a greater likelihood of dying prematurely (Chen et al., 2006). In fact, mortality rates increase in direct proportion to poverty levels. This is dramatically illustrated when comparing the disparities in life expectancy in the same city. The differences in life expectancy between the richer and poorer neighborhoods—sometimes only a mile or two apart—can be more than 20 years (Robert Wood Johnson Foundation, 2013).

The correlation between poverty and poor health is particularly problematic for the elderly, because they are more likely than younger adults to have limited, fixed incomes. Approximately one-third of older adults in the United States and half of those on Medicare have low incomes—below 200% of the federal poverty level (Jacobson, Huang, Neuman, & Smith, 2014; O'Brien, Wu, & Baer, 2010). People age 65 or older who did not graduate from high school—a marker for poverty—are twice as likely as college graduates to have diabetes and coronary heart disease, and much less likely to be vaccinated against both flu and pneumonia (Robert Wood Johnson Foundation, 2013). In addition, older adults with less than a high school education have higher rates of physical limitations than their more highly educated counterparts (Holmes, Griner, Lethbridge-Cejku, & Heyman, 2009).

What is there about poverty that leads to poor health? Poverty is associated with several other SDOHs, each of which, by itself, can contribute to deterioration of good health. In other words, numerous social and economic conditions within low-income communities contribute to poorer health outcomes (Braveman, 2006; Saegert & Evans, 2003; Walker et al., 2010).

Lower-income neighborhoods are more likely to have pollution from certain types of businesses or from traffic, to have obstacles to outdoor exercise, to have lower-quality housing, and to lack stores with affordable and healthy food. A few examples that illustrate these factors follow (Robert Wood Johnson Foundation, n.d.; Wallace, 2015).

▶ Food Insecurity

Nearly 3 million households including seniors age 65 and older lack a sufficient quantity of affordable, nutritious food (Coleman-Jensen, Rabbitt, Gregory, & Singh, 2016)—a condition sometimes referred to as food insecurity. In 2014, 5.7 million older Americans (9% of this subpopulation) were food insecure. That number is projected to increase by 50% when the youngest members of the baby boom generation reach age 60 in 2025 (Ziliak & Gundersen, 2009, 2016). Poorer adults are less likely to have access to healthier foods. More than one-fifth of poor and near-poor older adults report such difficulties due to income limitations (O'Brien et al., 2010, pp. 7, 44).

An additional barrier to realizing food security may be a lack of stores that sell healthy foods. The U.S. Department of Agriculture estimates that 40% of all U.S. households do not have easy access—that is, access within 1 mile of their residence—to supermarkets and large grocery stores. Access is often especially problematic among residents of rural, lower-income, and predominantly minority communities compared to residents of other communities (Berke, Koepsell, Moudon, Hoskins, & Larson, 2007; Cress et al., 2004; Physical Activity Guidelines Advisory Committee, 2008). A CDC disparities report in 2013 found that neighborhoods where seniors accounted for 14% or more of the population were less likely to have a healthier food retailer than those with fewer seniors (CDC, 2013, p. 24). Moreover, low-income communities are more likely to have convenience stores and fast-food restaurants than supermarkets selling fresh produce (Meyer, Yoon, & Kaufmann, 2013, p. 22).

Food-insecure seniors are at increased risk for chronic health conditions, even when controlling for other factors such as income. They are approximately 50% more likely to have depression, report a heart attack, or develop asthma (Feeding America and National Foundation to End Senior Hunger, 2014).

▶ Housing and Neighborhood Settings

For many people, putting a roof over their head can be a challenge. Poor older adults spend as much as 60% of their annual household income on housing—a much higher percentage than the non-poor (O'Brien et al., 2010, p. 7). They are more likely to rent rather than own their home. This arrangement leaves them with fewer assets to draw upon and less security in their continued domicile, putting the condition of the housing in the hands of others (O'Brien et al., 2010, p. 40). Of course, even those older adults who own their home are likely to have difficulties with upkeep if they have a limited income.

Subpar housing may be associated with environmental conditions that put the health of older adults at risk for a variety of injuries and illnesses. Poorly maintained or lit stairways may put older adults at risk of a fall. In addition, because of the physical changes that accompany aging, older adults may be more susceptible to environmental toxins and extreme temperature changes in the environment (Fernandez, Byard, Lin, Benson, & Barbera, 2002; Geller & Zenick, 2005). Temperature control in the winter or summer may be problematic for elderly individuals' health. Windows or walls that have mold or mildew may exacerbate asthma and other respiratory illnesses.

The physical activity necessary to stay healthy and remain independent may be discouraged by the conditions in the community environment in which one lives (Blazer, Yaffe, &

Liverman, 2015; Lee et al., 2012), including the general quality of the air and water or the proximity to highways and polluting businesses. For example, there is increasing evidence that air pollution is associated with cognitive performance among middle-aged and older adults (Ailshire & Clarke, 2014; Ailshire & Crimmins, 2014; Fonken et al., 2011). Lack of exercise may also be related to the physical or safety conditions in the immediate neighborhood in which a person lives. Elevated crime rates and physical barriers such as sidewalks and street lighting in need of repair may impede even simple physical activities such as walking or shopping (Harvard T. H. Chan School of Public Health, n.d.).

Transportation options may also be more limited in poor communities. Lower-income individuals are less likely to own cars, and using public transportation may be a challenge. Indeed, more than 15 million older adults in the United States live in areas where there is little or no public transportation. Each year, an estimated 4 million missed or delayed medical appointments for older adults are attributed to transportation issues (Syed, Gerber, & Sharp, 2013; Transportation for America, n.d.).

In part due to the distances over which they need to travel, the dependence on the automobile, and the lack of public transportation, the more than 7 million older adults living in U.S. rural communities face elevated health risk. They can experience significant challenges to maintaining their health and well-being compared to their counterparts in more urban or suburban settings, resulting in great risk of chronic disease and obesity (Durazo et al., 2011; Grantmakers in Aging, 2015).

▶ Discrimination Based on Race and Ethnicity

An additional social determinant of health is discrimination. Experiences of discrimination have been shown to contribute to increased stress and unhealthy adaptive behaviors that can

have a negative impact on health, increasing the prevalence of chronic disease and contributing to premature death (Zarit & Pearlin, 2005).

Discrimination—including that based on gender, sexual orientation, and gender identity—can have chilling effects on older adults. For example, the number of poor older women is more than twice the number of poor older men not only because women live longer, but also because they are likely to have earned less during their lifetimes. Approximately 70% of older adults living in poverty are women compared with 30% who are men (O'Brien et al., 2010). Lesbian, gay, and bisexual older adults have higher rates of disability, cardiovascular disease, obesity, and depression than heterosexual older adults (Aging with Pride, n.d.; Institute of Medicine, 2011; Meeks & Prucho, 2017).

An obvious form of such discrimination is racism and ethnic prejudice. A growing body of evidence documents that the experience of racial discrimination can have a negative physiological impact of health. Multiple negative experiences can diminish coping mechanisms and damage the immune system (Juster, McEwen, & Lupien, 2010; Lu & Halfon, 2003; McEwen & Seeman, 1999; Saban, Mathews, DeVon, & Janusek, 2014). Discrimination has been shown to increase the risk of stress, hypertension, and cardiovascular disease through the increase of physical and emotional stressors (Silverstein, 2013).

In addition, such discrimination may limit educational, job, and income opportunities, thereby contributing to an intensified impact from the types of harmful conditions related to poverty mentioned earlier. The poverty rates for older minorities are significantly higher than those for older whites. For example, in populations that are age 65 and older, Latinos are three times and African Americans are two and a half times more likely to be poor compared to whites (Cubanski, Casillas, & Damico, 2015). Older women of color are especially likely to live in poverty. One-third of older women who are black or Hispanic are poor or near poor (i.e., have incomes less 125% of the federal poverty line) (O'Brien et al., 2010). Older adults who are a racial or ethnic minority or have a lower socioeconomic status are more likely to experience chronic diseases. Whites also live longer: In 2014 life expectancy was 75.6 years for blacks and 79 years for whites—a difference that was smaller than in past years but still significant (Beckles & Truman, 2013; Louie & Ward, 2011; National Center for Health Statistics, 2015; Tavernise, 2016).

The negative health effects of racism and ethnic discrimination are due in part to the impact of segregated housing. Evidence shows that predominantly minority neighborhoods have greater exposure to environmental contaminants, even when controlling for income. For example, the CDC (2013, p. 50) cites a greater risk of exposure to traffic-related air pollution in minority communities than in poor communities, which already had a higher risk than that within higher-income communities.

The impact of this elevated prevalence will become more obvious in the coming years due to changing demographics. By 2060, the percentage of people of color among the older U.S. adult population will have notably increased: more than 40% of the older adult population will be members of a minority group. Specifically, 12% of the U.S. population will be black, 9% will be Asian, and 22% will be Hispanic (Colby & Ortman, 2015).

▶ Social Isolation

Several studies have shown that social isolation and loneliness are associated with a wide range of negative health effects, including cognitive decline, high blood pressure, and heart disease (Holwerda et al., 2013; O'Luanaigh et al., 2012; Shankar, Hamer, McMunn, & Steptoe, 2013; Tilvis et al., 2004; Wilson et al., 2007). This deterioration of health may lead to further reductions in social engagement, resulting in a downward spiral of social isolation and illness.

These risks are particularly acute for older adults, as 20% of men and 36% of women age 65 and older lived alone in 2015. Whether living alone leads to social isolation is dependent in no small part on the conditions in an individual's life (Healthypeople.gov, 2017). As indicated earlier, low-income neighborhoods may have conditions that discourage routine travel to carry out the activities of daily living, such as shopping in a store or going to the library. This issue intensifies the likelihood of social isolation. Older adults who live in walkable communities are more likely to engage in physical activity than those who do not, while those who live in neighborhoods without benches, parks, or pedestrian-friendly sidewalks are at a higher risk for disability (Keysor et al., 2010).

A striking example of the impact of neighborhood conditions on health can be seen with the 1995 heat wave that hit Chicago, Illinois, resulting in hundreds of deaths. According to Eric Klinenberg, the author of the definitive study of this occurrence, the elevated rate of death among the elderly was associated with isolation exacerbated by poverty-related neighborhood abandonment by stores, businesses, and services (University of Chicago Press, 2002).

Older adults can avoid the health risks associated with isolation by participating in regular, organized social interactions. Those who are employed or involved in community organizations have better health than do those who do not (Hinterlong, 2006; Young & Glasgow, 1998). Volunteering by older adults has been shown to contribute to better mental and physical function and reduced risk of death (Brown, Nesse, Vinokur, & Smith, 2003; Gottlieb & Gillespie, 2008; Hao, 2008).

▶ Addressing the Social Determinants of Health

Healthcare System Approaches

Of particular note to busy clinicians may be the increasing number of initiatives designed to link clinical practices to services that address patient

		Yes / No
○	In the last 12 months*, did you ever **eat less than you felt you should** because there wasn't enough money for food?	Y N
💡	In the last 12 months, has the **electric, gas, oil, or water company threatened to shut** off your services in your home?	Y N
🏠	Are you worried that in the next 2 months, you **may not have stable housing**?	Y N
👥	Do problems getting **child care make it difficult for you to work** or study? *(leave blank if you do not have children)*	Y N
$	In the last 12 months, have you needed to see a doctor, **but could not because of cost?**	Y N
🚗	In the last 12 months, have you ever had to go without health care because you didn't have **a way to get there?**	Y N
👤	Do you ever need help **reading hospital materials?**	Y N
✚	I often feel that **I lack companionship.**	Y N
✎	**Are any of your needs urgent?** For example: I don't have food tonight, I don't have a place to sleep tonight	Y N
💬	If you checked YES to any boxes above, **would you like to receive assistance** with any of these needs?	Y N

*time frames can be altered as needed

FIGURE 11-1 The HealthLeads program's healthcare system.
Courtesy of Healthleads.

social determinants of health. A starting point for making such connections is, of course, the identification of the circumstances in patients' lives that may be negatively affecting their health. To make that determination, screening instruments have been developed and tested. Several tools are being piloted in practice. One such tool—known as PRAPARE—was developed by the National Association of Community Health Centers (2017) in consultation with others; it aligns with Meaningful Use measures and clinical coding under ICD-10.

Another example of a relatively simple form currently in use was developed by the Health-Leads program (**FIGURE 11-1**). HealthLeads is designed to utilize the information gathered through systematic patient screening. Trained college student volunteers assist patients with needs such as paying for healthy food and utility bills or finding a job or receiving assistance

for housing. Kaiser Permanente, the largest integrated health delivery organization in the United States, has effectively incorporated HealthLeads into both SDOH screening and access to needed social services into its model of care. Its Total Health initiative targets its members' unmet social needs as part of their overall health care. Among the components of Kaiser Permanente's response is a call center that proactively reaches out to high-risk patients to inquire about their unmet social needs and aid in seeking appropriate services (Shah, Rogers, & Kanter, 2016; Tuso, 2014).

These types of structured approaches are demonstrating that addressing social needs can improve health outcomes and decrease cost (Berkowitz, Hulberg, Standish, Reznor, & Atlas, 2017; Edwards, Levine, Cullinan, Newbern, & Barnes, 2015; HealthLeads, n.d.). For example, a study of patients at Massachusetts General

Hospital (2016) who had access to HealthLeads found that participation in the service led to lower blood pressure and cholesterol levels.

Payment Models That Address the Social Determinants of Health

The Centers for Medicare and Medicaid Services (CMS) has developed a model pilot program known as the Accountable Health Community (AHC) initiative that provides funds to large clinical practices in scores of sites across the United States to screen patients for the social determinants of health. The goal is to assess whether the systematic identification of social needs and referral to services will result in improved patient healthcare utilization and lower costs.

CMS's AHC model also provides funds that allow clinical sites to refer patients to certain community services and jointly collaborate with community partners to ensure that the services are available and responsive to patient needs (CMS, 2017). AHC aims to identify and address beneficiaries' health-related social needs in such areas as housing instability, food insecurity, utility needs, interpersonal violence, and transportation at the community, as well as the individual level (CMS, 2017).

Broader Policy Changes

Sir Michael Marmot, the long-time chair of the Commission on Social Determinants of Health at the World Health Organization and a renowned expert on the barriers to good health, has encouraged the development of broad policy and systems efforts to address such factors rather than a focus on individual-level solutions.

> If the major determinants of health are social, so must be the remedies. . . . While social determinants can be addressed on an individual basis, addressing these social factors at the policy, environment and systems level is critical. (Marmot, 2005)

Fortunately, there are already a wide array of programs to assist poor older adults. Some of them have been in place for many years—such as Social Security and Medicare Part D—and been shown to be effective in reducing negative health effects. In addition, programs that address the conditions associated with poverty—such as those that subsidize healthy foods or offer free and safe places to exercise—can be effective in achieving this goal. Notable short-term health outcomes have resulted from such income-related programs as tax credits for low-income individuals and home repair and improvement programs for low-income community members (CDC, 2016).

There are also innovative initiatives across the United States that seek to keep older adults healthy by changing policies, laws, and regulations at the municipal level. The CDC's Health Impact in Five Years or Less (HI-5) initiative identified 14 evidence-based policies that have been shown to improve the health and well-being of community residents in a relatively short period. Several of these have relevance to the health needs of older adults. For example, HI-5 highlights the efficacy of public transportation, alcohol and tobacco pricing, low-income tax credits, and low-income home improvements (CDC, 2016). Such efforts promote mobility, community connectivity, and physical activity among older adults by improving access to transportation, healthy food, and safe housing.

▶ Summary

The U.S. Surgeon General's report entitled *Healthy Aging in Action* presents a multifaceted model for promoting health among older adults. This model is linked to the National Prevention Strategy through four components: clinical and community prevention services, the elimination of health disparities, healthy and safe community environments, and empowered people (U.S. Surgeon General, 2016) (**FIGURE 11-2**). Within the report, 23 action steps are suggested to support healthy,

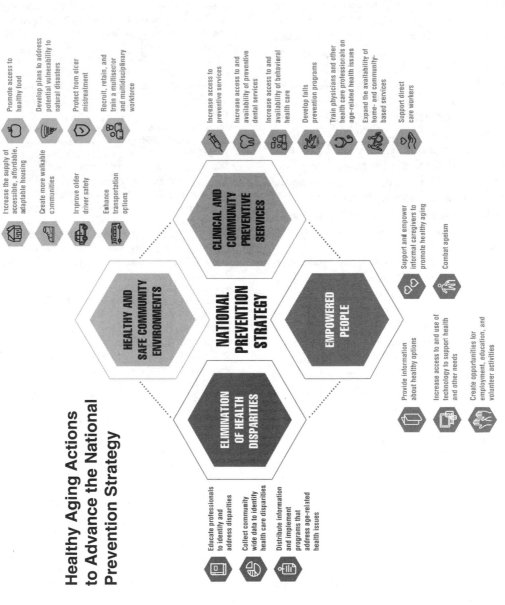

FIGURE 11-2 Healthy aging actions to advance the National Prevention Strategy.

well-informed older adults with both high-quality health services and social conditions designed for optimal well-being. Many federally funded programs already exist that can assist patients in reaching these steps. Among those cited in the report are the Seniors Corps, which provides opportunities for older adults to volunteer in schools, nonprofits, and other community organizations, and the Active Aging Initiative, which addresses barriers to physical activity among older adults (U.S. Surgeon General, 2016).

Unfortunately, a substantial share of low-income adults do not benefit from these efforts and programs despite their eligibility to participate in them. Sometimes lack of participation is due to a lack of awareness about the programs themselves; sometimes it is due to a need for assistance in completing the application processes; and sometimes it is due to a reluctance to seek help from such programs. Clinicians and caregivers can help elderly individuals overcome these barriers. Where such programs either do not exist or are insufficient to meet the demand, clinicians can also assist their patients by demonstrating the need for them and drawing the connections between such programmatic efforts and improved health, and can participate in multisector community efforts. By applying what is known about SDOH, clinicians can not only improve individual and population health but also advance health equity (Healthypeople. gov, 2017; Secretary's Advisory Committee, 2010; WHO, 2017).

References

Adler, N. E., & Newman, K. (2002). Socioeconomic disparities in health: Pathways and policies. *Health Affairs, 21*(2), 60–76.

Aging with Pride. (n.d.). National health, aging, and sexuality/gender study. Retrieved from http://age-pride.org/

Ailshire, J. A., & Clarke, P. (2014). Fine particulate matter air pollution and cognitive function among US older adults. *Journals of Gerontology Series B: Psychological Sciences and Social Sciences, 70*(2), 322–328.

Ailshire, J. A., & Crimmins, E. M. (2014). Fine particulate matter air pollution and cognitive function among older US adults. *American Journal of Epidemiology, 180*(4), 359–366.

Barnett, J., & Vornovitsky, M., Health insurance coverage in the United States: 2015. *Current Population Reports.* Retrieved from https://www.census.gov/content/dam/Census/library/publications/2016/demo/p60-257.pdf

Beckles, G. L., & Truman, B. I. (2013, November 22). Education and income—United States, 2009 and 2011. *Morbidity and Mortality Weekly Report, 62*(3), 9–19. Retrieved from https://www.cdc.gov/mmwr/preview/mmwrhtml/su6203a3.htm?s_cid=su6203a3_w

Berke, E. M., Koepsell, T. D., Moudon, A. V., Hoskins, R. E., & Larson, E. B. (2007). Association of the built environment with physical activity and obesity in older persons. *American Journal of Public Health, 97*(3), 486492. doi: 10.2105/ AJPH.2006.085837

Berkowitz, S. A., Hulberg, A. C., Standish, S., Reznor, G., & Atlas, S. J. (2017). Addressing unmet basic resource needs as part of chronic cardiometabolic disease management. *JAMA Internal Medicine, 177*(2), 244–252.

Bieber, C. (2017, March 12). Trumpcare could send seniors' insurance rates skyrocketing. *The Motley Fool.* Retrieved from https://www.fool.com/retirement/2017/03/12/trumpcare-could-send-seniors-insurance-rates-skyro.aspx

Blazer, D. G., Yaffe, K., & Liverman, C. T. (Eds.). (2015). *Cognitive aging: Progress in understanding and opportunities for action.* Washington, DC: National Academies Press.

Braveman, P. (2006). Health disparities and health equity: Concepts and measurement. *Annual Review of Public Health, 27*, 167–194.

Brown, S. L., Nesse, R. M., Vinokur, A. D., & Smith, D. M. (2003). Providing social support may be more beneficial than receiving it: Results from a prospective study of mortality. *Psychological Sciences, 14*(4), 320–327.

Centers for Disease Control and Prevention (CDC). (2013, November 22). CDC health disparities and inequalities report—United States, 2013. *Morbidity and Mortality Weekly Report, 62*(3 Suppl.). Retrieved from https://www.cdc.gov/mmwr/pdf/other/su6203.pdf

Centers for Disease Control and Prevention (CDC), Office of the Associate Director for Policy. (2016, October 21). *Health impact in 5 years.* Retrieved from https://www.cdc.gov/policy/hst/hi5/

Centers for Disease Control and Prevention (CDC). (2017, July 28). Social determinants of health: Know what affects health. Retrieved from https://www.cdc.gov/socialdeterminants/

Centers for Medicare and Medicaid Services (CMS). (2017, September 5). *Accountable health communities model.* Retrieved from https://innovation.cms.gov/initiatives/ahcm/

Chen, J. T., Rehkopf, D. H., Waterman, P. D., Subramanian, S. V., Coull, B. A., Cohen, B., . . . Krieger, N. (2006). Mapping and measuring social disparities in premature mortality: The impact of census tract poverty within and across Boston neighborhoods, 1999–2001. *Journal of Urban Health, 83*(6), 1063–1084.

Colby, S. L., & Ortman, J. M. (2015). Projections of the Size and Composition of the US Population: 2014 to 2060. Population Estimates and Projections. Current Population Reports. P25–1143. US Census Bureau.

Coleman-Jensen, A., Rabbitt, M. P., Gregory, C., & Singh, A. (2016). *Household food security in the United States in 2015* (Table 2). Washington, DC: U.S. Department of Agriculture, Economic Research Service.

Cress, M., Buchner, D., Prohaska, T., Rimmer, J., Brown, M., Macera, C., . . . Chodzko-Zajko, W. (2004). Physical activity programs and behavior counseling in older adult populations. *Medicine & Science in Sports & Exercise, 36*(11), 1997–2003.

Cubanski, J., Casillas, G., & Damico, A. (2015, June 10). *Poverty among seniors: An updated analysis of national and state level poverty rates under the official and supplemental poverty measures.* Henry J. Kaiser Family Foundation. Retrieved from https://www.Kff.org/report-section /poverty-among-seniors-issue-brief

Durazo, E. M., Jones, M. R., Wallace, S. P., Van Arsdale, J., Aydin, M., & Stewart, C. (2011). *The health status and unique health challenges of rural older adults in California.* Los Angeles, CA: UCLA Center for Health Policy Research. Retrieved from https://www.ncbi.nlm .nih.gov/pubmed/21688692

Edwards, P. K., Levine, M., Cullinan, K., Newbern, G., & Barnes, L. (2015). Avoiding readmissions: Support systems required after discharge to continue rapid recovery? *Journal of Arthroplasty, 30,* 527–530.

Feeding America and National Foundation to End Senior Hunger. (2014). *Spotlight on senior health: Adverse health outcomes of food insecure older Americans.* [PDF file]. Retrieved at http://www.feedingamerica.org/research /senior-hunger-research/or-spotlight-on-senior-health -executive-summary.pdf

Fernandez, L. S., Byard, D., Lin, C., Benson, S., & Barbera, J. A. (2002). Frail elderly as disaster victims: Emergency management strategies. *Prehospital Disaster Medicine, 17,* 67–74.

Fonken, L. K., Xu, X., Weil, Z. M., Chen, G. Sun, Q., Rajagopalan, S., & Nelson, R. J. (2011). Air pollution impairs cognition, provokes depressive-like behaviors and alters hippocampal cytokine expression and morphology. *Molecular Psychiatry, 16*(10), 987–995. doi:10.1038/mp.2011.76

Geller, A. M., & Zenick, H. (2005). Aging and the environment: A research framework. *Environmental Health Perspectives, 113*(9), 1257–1262. doi:10.1289/ehp.7569

Gottlieb, B. H., & Gillespie, A. A. (2008). Volunteerism, health, and civic engagement among older adults. *Canadian Journal of Aging, 27*(44), 399–406.

Grantmakers in Aging. (2015). *Rural aging.* Retrieved from http://www.giaging.org/programs-events/rural -aging-initiative/

Hao, Y. (2008). Productive activities and psychological wellbeing among older adults. *Journals of Gerontology,*

Series B: Psychological Sciences and Social Sciences, 63B(2), S64–S72.

Harvard T. H. Chan School of Public Health. (n.d.). *Obesity prevention source: Environmental barriers to activity.* Retrieved from https://www.hsph.harvard.edu/obesity -prevention-source/obesity-causes/physical-activity -environment/

HealthLeads. (n.d.). Home page. Retrieved from https:// healthleadsusa.org

Healthypeople.gov. (2017, November 21). Social determinants of health. Retrieved from https://www.healthypeople .gov/2020/topics-objectives/topic/social-determinants-of -health

Hinterlong, J. (2006). Racial disparities in health among older adults: Examining the role of productive engagement. *Health & Social Work, 31,* 275–288.

Holmes, J., Griner, E. P., Lethbridge-Cejku, M., & Heyman, K. (2009). *Aging differently: Physical limitations among adults aged 50 years and over: United States, 2001–2007.* NCHS Data Brief No. 20. Hyattsville, MD: National Center for Health Statistics.

Holwerda, T., Deeg, D., Beekman, A., Tilburg, T., Stek, M., Jonker, C., & Schoevers, R. (2013). Feelings of loneliness, but not social isolation, predict dementia onset: Results from the Amsterdam Study of the Elderly (AMSTEL). *Journal of Neurology, Neurosurgery and Psychiatry, 85,* 133–134. Retrieved from http://jnnp.bmj.com/content /early/2012/11/06/jnnp-2012-302755

Institute of Medicine, Committee on Lesbian, Gay, Bisexual, and Transgender Health Issues and Research Gaps and Opportunities. (2011). *The health of lesbian, gay, bisexual, and transgender people: Building a foundation for better understanding.* Washington, DC: National Academies Press. Retrieved from https://www.ncbi.nlm.nih.gov /books/NBK64800/

Jacobson, G., Huang, J., Neuman, T., & Smith, K. (2014, January). *Incomes and assets of Medicare beneficiaries—2013–2030.* Kaiser Family Foundation. Retrieved from https://kaiserfamilyfoundation.files .wordpress.com/2014/01/8540-income-and-assets-of -medicare-beneficiaries-2013-e28093-20301.pdf

Juster, R. P., McEwen, B. S., & Lupien, S. J. (2010). Allostatic load biomarkers of chronic stress and impact on health and cognition. *Neuroscience & Biobehavioral Reviews, 35*(1), 2–16.

Keysor, J. J., Jette, A. M., LaValley, M. P., Lewis, C. E., Torner, J. C., Nevitt, M. C., & Felson, D. T. (2010). Community environmental factors are associated with disability in older adults with functional limitations: The MOST study. *Journals of Gerontology, Series A: Biological Sciences and Medical Sciences, 65A,* 393–399.

Ku, L., Deschamps, E., & Hilman, J. (2004, November 2). *The effects of copayments on the use of medical services and prescription drugs in Utah's Medicaid program.* Center on Budget and Policy Priorities. Retrieved from http://www.cbpp.org/research/the-effects-of

-copayments-on-the-use-of-medical-services-and-prescription-drugs-in-utahs

Lee, I. M., Shiroma, E. J., Lobelo, F., Puska, P., Blair, S. N., & Katzmarzyk, P. T. (2012). Effect of physical inactivity on major non-communicable diseases worldwide: An analysis of burden of disease and life expectancy. *Lancet, 380*(9838), 219–229.

Louie, G. H., & Ward, M. M. (2011). Socioeconomic and ethnic differences in disease burden and disparities in physical function in older adults. *American Journal of Public Health, 101*(7), 1322–1329.

Lu, M. C., & Halfon, N. (2003). Racial and ethnic disparities in birth outcomes: A life-course perspective. *Maternal and Child Health Journal, 7*(1), 13–30.

Marmot, M. (2005). Social determinants of health inequalities. *Lancet, 365*(9464), 1099–1104.

Marmot, M.; Commission on Social Determinants of Health. (2007). Achieving health equity: From root causes to fair outcomes. *Lancet, 370*(9593), 1153–1163.

Massachusetts General Hospital. (2016, December 12). *Meeting patients' socioeconomic needs can improve cardiovascular risk factors.* Retrieved from http://www .massgeneral.org/about/pressrelease.aspx?id=2022

McEwen, B. S., & Seeman, T. (1999). Protective and damaging effects of mediators of stress: Elaborating and testing the concepts of allostasis and allostatic load. *Annals of the New York Academy of Sciences, 896,* 30–47.

McGinnis, M. J., & Foege, W. H. (1993). Actual causes of death in the United States. *Journal of the American Medical Association, 270*(18), 2207–2212.

Meeks, S., & Prucho, R. (2017). Practice concepts will become intervention research effective January 2017. *Gerontologist, 57*(2), 151–152. Retrieved from https://academic.oup.com /gerontologist/search-results?f_TocHeadingTitle=Editorial

Meyer, P. A., Yoon, P. W., & Kaufmann, R. B. (2013, November 22). Introduction: CDC health disparities and inequalities report—United States, 2013. *Morbidity and Mortality Weekly Report, 62*(3 Suppl.). Retrieved from https://www .cdc.gov/mmwr/preview/mmwrhtml/su6203a2.htm

Mokdad, A., Marks, J. S., Stroup, D. F., & Gerberding, J. L. (2004). Actual causes of death in the United States 2000. *Journal of the American Medical Association, 291*(10), 1238–1245.

National Academies of Sciences, Engineering, and Medicine. (2016). *Families caring for an aging America.* Washington, DC: National Academies Press. https://doi .org/10.17226/23606

National Academy of Social Insurance. (n.d.). *Gaps in Medicare.* Retrieved from https://www.nasi.org/learn /medicare/gaps-medicare

National Association of Community Health Centers. (2017). *What is PRAPARE?* Retrieved from http://www.nachc .org/research-and-data/prapare/

National Center for Health Statistics. (2015). *Health, United States, 2014: With special feature on adults aged 55–64.*

Hyattsville, MD: Author. Retrieved from http://www .cdc.gov/nchs/data/hus/hus14.pdf

Norman, D., Kennedy, B., & Kawachi, I. (1999). Why justice is good for our health: The social determinants of health inequalities. *Daedalus, 128,* 215–251.

O'Brien, E., Wu, K. B., & Baer, D. (2010). *Older Americans in poverty: A snapshot.* AARP Public Policy Institute. Retrieved from http://assets.aarp.org/rgcenter/ppi /econ-sec/2010-03-poverty.pdf

O'Luanaigh, C., O'Connell, H., Chin, A., Hamilton, F., Coen, R., Walsh, C., . . . Lawlor, B. (2012). Loneliness and cognition in older people: The Dublin Healthy Ageing study. *Aging & Mental Health, 16*(3), 347–352. https:// doi.org/10.1080/13607863.2011.628977

Oregon State University. (2015, November 12). *Barriers to health care increase disease, death risk for rural elderly.* Retrieved from http://oregonstate.edu/ua/ncs/archives/2015/nov /barriers-health-care-increase-disease-death-risk-rural -elderly

Physical Activity Guidelines Advisory Committee. (2008). *Physical Activity Guidelines Advisory Committee report, 2008.* Washington, DC: U.S. Department of Health and Human Services.

Robert Wood Johnson Foundation. (n.d.). *Improving the health of all Americans by focusing on communities.* Retrieved from http://www.rwjf.org/content/dam/farm /reports/reports/2013/rwjf406483

Robert Wood Johnson Foundation. (2013). *Overcoming obstacles to health in 2013 and beyond.* Retrieved from https://www.rwjf.org/content/dam/farm/reports /reports/2013/rwjf406474

Saban, K. L., Mathews, H. L., DeVon, H. A., & Janusek, L. W. (2014). Epigenetics and social context: Implications for disparity in cardiovascular disease. *Aging and Disease, 5*(5), 346–355.

Saegert, S., & Evans, G. W. (2003). Poverty, housing niches, and health in the United States. *Journal of Social Issues, 59*(3), 569–589.

Schoeni, R. F., Martin, L. G., Andreski, P. M., & Freedman, V. A. (2005). Persistent and growing socioeconomic disparities in disability among the elderly: 1982–2002. *American Journal of Public Health, 95*(11), 2065–2070.

Secretary's Advisory Committee on Health Promotion and Disease Prevention Objectives for 2020. (2010, July 26). *Healthy people 2020: An opportunity to address the societal determinants of health in the United States.* Retrieved from https://www.healthypeople.gov/sites /default/files/SocietalDeterminantsHealth.pdf

Shah, N. R., Rogers, A. J., & Kanter, M. H. (2016, April 13). Health care that targets unmet social needs. *NEJM Catalyst.* Retrieved from http://catalyst.nejm.org/health -care-that-targets-unmet-social-needs/

Shankar, A., Hamer, M., McMunn, A., & Steptoe, A. (2013). Social isolation and loneliness: Relationships with cognitive function during 4 years of follow-up in the English

Longitudinal Study of Ageing. *Psychosomatic Medicine, 75*(2), 161–170. doi:10.1097/PSY.0b013e31827f09cd

Silverstein, J. (2013, March 12). How racism is bad for our bodies. *The Atlantic.* Retrieved from https://www.theatlantic.com/health/archive/2013/03/how-racism-is-bad-for-our-bodies/273911/

Stanford Medicine, eCampus Rural Health. (n.d.). *Healthcare disparities & barriers to healthcare.* Retrieved from http://ruralhealth.stanford.edu/health-pros/factsheets/disparities-barriers.html

Syed, S. T., Gerber, B. S., & Sharp, L. K. (2013). Traveling towards disease: Transportation barriers to health care access. *Journal of Community Health, 38*(5), 976–993. doi:10.1007/s10900-013-9681-1

Tavernise, S. (2016, May 8). Black Americans see gains in life expectancy. *New York Times.* Retrieved from https://www.nytimes.com/2016/05/09/health/blacks-see-gains-in-life-expectancy.html

Tilvis, R. S., Kähönen-Väre, M. H., Jolkkonen, J., Valvanne, J., Pitkala, K. H., & Strandberg, T. E. (2004). Predictors of cognitive decline and mortality of aged people over a 10-year period. *The Journals of Gerontology, 59*(3), M268–M274. https://doi.org/10.1093/gerona/59.3.M268

Transportation for America. (n.d.). Seniors and transit. Retrieved from http://t4america.org/maps-tools/seniors mobilitycrisis2011//

Tuso, P. (2014). Physician update: Total health. *The Permanente Journal, 18*(2), 58–63. doi:10.7812/TPP/13-120

University of Chicago Press. (2002). *Dying alone: An interview with Eric Klinenberg.* Retrieved from http://www.press.uchicago.edu/Misc/Chicago/443213in.html

Walker, R. E., Keane, C. R., & Burke, J. G. (2010). Disparities and access to healthy food in the United States: A review of food deserts literature. *Health & Place, 16*(5), 876–884.

Wallace, S. P. (2015). Equity and social determinants of health among older adults. *Generations: Journal of the American Society on Aging.* Retrieved from http://www.asaging.org/blog/equity-and-social-determinants-health-among-older-adults

Williams, D. R., Costa, M. V., Odunlami, A. O., & Mohammed, S. A. (2008). Moving upstream: How interventions that address the social determinants of health can improve health and reduce disparities. *Journal of Public Health Management & Practice, 14*(Suppl.), S8.

Wilson, R. S., Krueger, K. R., Arnold, S. E., Schneider, J. A., Kelly, J. F., Barnes, L. L., . . . Bennet, D. A. (2007). Loneliness and risk of Alzheimer disease. *Archives of General Psychiatry, 64*(2), 234–240.

World Health Organization (WHO). (2017). Social determinants of health. Retrieved from http://www.who.int/social_determinants/sdh_definition/en/

Young, F. W., & Glasgow, N. (1998). Voluntary social participation and health. *Research on Aging, 20,* 339–362.

Zarit, S. H., & Pearlin, L. I. (2005). Special issue on health inequalities across the life course. *Journals of Gerontology Series B: Psychological Sciences and Social Sciences, 60*(Special_Issue_2), S6-S6.

Ziliak, J., & Gundersen, C. (2009). *Senior hunger in the United States: Differences across states and rural and urban areas.* Retrieved from http://www.mowaa.org/document.doc?id=193

Ziliak, J. P., & Gundersen, C. (2016). *The state of senior hunger in America 2014: An annual report, supplement.* Alexandria, VA: National Foundation to End Senior Hunger.

CHAPTER 12

Multiculturalism and Geriatric Assessment

Charles Mouton

CHAPTER OBJECTIVES

1. Discuss the heterogeneity of older ethnic minority groups.
2. Understand measurement issues related to assessment of older minority persons.
3. Recognize appropriate communication strategies with diverse older adults.

KEY TERMS

Beliefs and attitudes   Diversity   Ethnic minorities

▶ Introduction

The proportion of the population of the United States that is older than age 65 years is increasing rapidly. At the same time, the number of older adults from minority groups, such as Hispanics, African Americans, and Asian Americans, continues to increase (Agree & Freedman, 1999). Given the **diversity** of the aging population, a text on geriatric assessment should highlight cultural issues in the assessment of older persons and seek to improve the cultural competence of

its readers (Lavizzo-Mourey & Mackenzie, 1996). Cultural competence in health care encompasses at least three components: (1) knowledge of the prevalence, incidence, and risk factors (epidemiology) for diseases in different ethnic groups; (2) understanding of how the illness presentation, disease assessment, and response to medications and other treatments vary with ethnicity; and (3) discussion of **beliefs and attitudes** toward illness, treatment, and the healthcare system. Cultural competence includes an appreciation that patient assessments must be sensitive to changes in meaning and circumstances that were not intended by the developers of a test. This chapter highlights some clinical considerations in the assessment of older adults from diverse ethnic groups. In doing so, we focus on aspects applicable to the largest minority groups identified by the U.S. Census.

A description of the epidemiology of medical conditions across different ethnic groups would likely require a book of its own (Mouton & Espino, 1999). Nevertheless, the reality is that in some cases we simply do not have solid information about the prevalence, incidence, and risk factors of disease, even for some common disorders of late life (Gallo & Lebowitz, 1999). For example, there are few credible community-based estimates of the prevalence of Alzheimer's disease (AD) and related dementias in various **ethnic minorities** in the United States. Estimates of the prevalence of dementia and AD in minorities from the community-based studies that have been done reveal substantial disease burden in the African American and Hispanic communities, with rates of AD in minorities several times higher than those observed in whites (Hendrie et al., 1995; Tang et al., 1998). In addition to more data on prevalence, more scientific evidence is needed regarding how the effects of medications used to treat AD vary among ethnic minorities, especially for the elderly. Examples of medications for which differences in response according to ethnicity have been documented include antihypertensives (Prisant & Mensah, 1996) and antidepressants (Pi, Wang, & Gray, 1993; Sramek & Pi, 1996).

In this chapter, we focus on assessment in relation to the domains of function, cognitive impairment, depression, and social and economic issues. Before making specific comments about these areas, we make some general comments regarding (1) the heterogeneity of ethnic groups; (2) the reliability, validity, and use of assessment instruments for persons of a different cultural background from the population with which the instruments were developed and tested; (3) enhancing communication between professional caregivers and older adults of diverse ethnic backgrounds; and (4) eliciting beliefs and attitudes about illness.

▶ Heterogeneity Within Older Ethnic Minority Groups

To develop cultural competence, healthcare providers must confront and question their casual conceptions of "race," ethnicity, and culture. When socioeconomic factors are considered, many apparent differences between older persons from minority groups and other older persons disappear or narrow for many important outcomes. Differences in health and habits ascribed to "race" reflect *social* more than *genetic* differences (Cooper & David, 1986; Lillie-Blanton, Anthony, & Schuster, 1993). Older adults are a diverse group, even *within* ethnic categories. It is just as important to understand that the heterogeneity *within* ethnic groups is often greater than that *between* ethnic groups (Whitfield, 1996). For example, some African Americans were brought to the United States against their will from Africa, but others migrated from the Caribbean. Hispanic Americans are a heterogeneous group, with cultural origins in Mexico, Puerto Rico, South and Central America, Cuba, and other Spanish-speaking countries. Asian Americans from China, Japan, Korea, and Southeast Asia have differing health practices and beliefs. Native American elders derive from more than 500 tribes, which collectively speak more than 150 languages.

Because of this heterogeneity within cultural groups, clinicians should not lose sight of the need to evaluate each older person as an *individual* who has a cultural and personal contextual background that suffuses into every aspect of assessment and care. Clinicians should construe the comments presented in this chapter as broad *general guidelines* for assessment of older persons from minority groups, rather than as firm rules to follow when assessing older adults from specific ethnic groups.

▶ Reliability, Validity, and Use of Instruments for Ethnic Minorities

Any assessment procedure is subject to error. Error in measurement can arise because the instrument is inconsistent (poor reliability) or because it does not measure what we think it is measuring (poor validity). For decades, researchers have questioned the assumption that the same construct is measured when instruments developed among whites are applied to African Americans or other minority ethnic groups (Neighbors & Lumpkin, 1990). At one level, differing idioms and colloquialisms can cause a translated instrument to have meanings different from those intended by the original developers. Even within ethnic groups, older persons who are recent immigrants may interpret items differently from older persons who have lived in the United States for some time. In addition to issues with entire scales, individual items in each instrument may display racial/ethnic bias. Differential item functioning has emerged as a tool that researchers can use to modify assessment instrument to adjust for bias in certain populations.

At a more subtle level, some constructs may be so different across cultures as to be quite different or even irrelevant. Depressive disorder provides an example of cultural heterogeneity in expression that has drawn attention from anthropologists and medical researchers concerned with detection and treatment of depression (Kleinman, 1980; Kleinman & Good, 1985). Some cultures do not have concepts that are equivalent to a Western notion of "depression." The Hopi Indians of Arizona, for example, describe an illness similar to major depression but without dysphoria (Manson, Shore, & Bloom, 1985). The Flathead people of Montana express depression as a social phenomenon of loneliness—the feeling that "no one cares for you" (O'Nell, 1996). Neurasthenic patients in China deny dysphoria, but do exhibit the other symptoms of depression, such as psychomotor retardation and somatic complaints (Kleinman, 1980). Older African Americans tend to deny sadness but are more likely to report thoughts of death than older whites (Gallo, Cooper-Patrick, & Lesikar, 1998).

In the domain of functional assessment, the willingness to report difficulty taking care of oneself may be powerfully related to fear of admitting one's dependence on others by older persons from certain groups. Observed differences in functional status across ethnic groups may represent true differences, but could result from measurement error stemming from the instrument used in the assessment of physical function. Physical function assessments generally employ self-report instruments that rely on the subjective response of patients. Although performance-based measures provide more objective measures of function, they are more difficult to carry out in the clinical setting and may not always relate directly to performance at home (Guralnik, Branch, Cummings, & Curb, 1989; Guralnik, Reuben, Buchner, & Ferrucci, 1995). The choice of method generally relates to the time constraints on the clinician, the training of the clinician (and staff), and the need for the most reliable and valid information. A number of instruments are discussed in this chapter, but unfortunately most instruments have not been specifically assessed for their performance in older adults from minority groups. Even the meaning of the term *elderly* has different interpretations across cultures.

As a last comment in this section, we point out that literacy and level of educational attainment may be important considerations when assessing all older adults, but especially older adults from ethnic minorities who historically have had fewer opportunities to advance in school. Older women, in particular, grew up in an historical period in which it was uncommon for girls to finish high school and attend college.

The association of ethnic grouping with functional decline and other important health outcomes probably has more to do with level of educational attainment than "race." At the age of 65 years, persons with 12 or more years of schooling have an active life expectancy (i.e., life spent without reported functional disability) that is 2 to 4 years longer than older adults with less education, regardless of ethnic grouping (Guralnik, Land, Blazer, Fillenbaum, & Branch, 1993). Closely tied to educational level attained is literacy, referring to the ability to understand and use written information. In one study conducted among 144 African Americans older than age 65 years living in New York City, half of the participants had a reading level that was below the eighth grade (Albert & Teresi, 1999), suggesting that materials designed for older persons must be evaluated for reading level. It remains to be seen whether improved educational opportunities for persons from ethnic minorities will result in older persons with diminished rates of functional impairment when compared to the current cohort of older persons. In clinical work, consideration of the educational level of patients who may not be used to the type of questions that are asked in many functional and cognitive tests is important.

We are not suggesting that clinicians need to develop their own instruments for assessment of depression, function, or other domains to properly assess older adults from different ethnic groups. Instead, when interpreting results from assessment, clinicians should be aware of the reliability and validity of the instruments employed. For example, an instrument developed for use with urban hospitalized patients in the northeastern United States may not be applicable to a border community in rural southern Texas. The selection of instruments and other aspects of assessment should be tailored to the known demographic profile of the practice in which the questionnaires are to be used. As researchers and clinicians become more keenly aware of the need to consider the cultural context of assessment, more information may become available to make good decisions about geriatric assessment procedures that are most appropriate to different ethnic groups.

▶ Enhancing Communication with Ethnically Diverse Older Adults

The assessment of older adults who do not speak or read English well, and who have a different worldview and goals than the healthcare professional, can be a difficult and arduous task. Additionally, social distance, racism, unconscious fears, biases, and similar concerns on the behalf of patients and professionals may contribute to further problems in assessment and diagnosis of older adults from different ethnic groups (Brangman, 1995). Early attention to building rapport will go a long way toward facilitating such cross-cultural communication. In many cultures, such as China and Mexico, rapport begins through exchange of pleasantries or chit-chat before beginning the business of medical history taking and physical examination (Elliott, Di Minno, Lam, & Tu, 1996; Gallagher-Thompson, Talamantes, Ramirez, & Valverde, 1996). Older Hispanic Americans often expect healthcare personnel to be warm and personal while still treating them with dignity (Villa, Cuellar, Gamel, & Yeo, 1993).

As a sign of respect, older persons should be addressed by their last name. Gesturing should be avoided because seemingly benign body or hand movements may have adverse connotations in other cultures. Take care to evaluate whether questions or instructions have been understood, because some persons will nod "yes" even when they do not really comprehend. Outright questioning of authority is taboo in some cultures, so encourage the patient to ask questions freely. Tell the patient that you realize that some things are not normally discussed, but that it is necessary so that the best care can be planned.

▶ Eliciting Beliefs and Attitudes About Illness

When caring for older adults, make an attempt to elicit their beliefs and attitudes about illness. Eliciting beliefs and attitudes about illness that may be rather different from one's own requires maintaining an accepting attitude and putting the family and patient at ease—that is, reassuring them that their ideas are valued in developing the care plan. Ask patients what they think is wrong or causing the problem. Ask if they think that there may be some ways to get better that doctors may not know about, and whether anyone else has been asked to help with the problem. To draw out beliefs about illness, ask patients what worries them most about their illness, and why they think they are ill now.

Time devoted to getting into the "assumptive world" (Frank & Frank, 1991) of the patient is time well spent. First, doing so can uncover useful information about over-the-counter medications or home remedies that might interfere with prescribed medicines. For example, older persons within traveling distance of Mexico often obtain pharmacologically active compounds that are not always equivalent to medications bought in the United States (Greene & Monahans, 1984). In addition, traditional folk remedies play a central role in health for older Mexican Americans (Espino, 1988). In many cases, standard prescriptions may be more acceptable if traditional remedies can continue to be taken. Second, assessing cultural beliefs about illness includes asking about diet. For example, dietary prescriptions are often a component of traditional healing practices in Native Americans (McCabe & Cuellar, 1994). Third, failure to elicit ideas about illness can result in poor communication, lack of adherence to prescribed therapy, or refusal to undergo tests or therapeutic procedures. For example, the idea that illness is punishment for past deeds may inhibit participation in preventive or therapeutic procedures (McBride, Morioka-Douglas, & Yeo, 1996). Finally, asking and listening about the cultural beliefs of the patient helps establish rapport, shows respect for the older person, and can be one of the most interesting aspects of caring for older adults.

▶ Selected Domains of Geriatric Assessment

Subsequent sections of this chapter highlight specific considerations in the multidimensional evaluation of older persons from ethnic minority groups. We focus our attention on features of assessment related to ethnicity, with the understanding that the reader will refer to other chapters for further information on each individual area of assessment.

Functional Assessment

In general, the functional ability of older African Americans declines more rapidly than that of other Americans. In the North Carolina Established Populations for Epidemiologic Studies of the Elderly (EPESE), 9.6% of African Americans older than 65 reported difficulty with two or more activities of daily living (ADLs), and 19% reported two or more difficulties on instrumental activities of daily living (IADLs) (Foley, Fillenbaum, & Service, 1990; Miles & Bernard, 1992). Older African Americans are 1.38 times more likely to have trouble getting around and more than 1.5 times more likely to be confined to their homes than whites (Edmonds, 1993). In advanced age (the ninth and tenth decades of life), older African Americans appear to function better than whites, probably because only the most hardy individuals survive (Miles & Bernard, 1992).

Hispanic Americans also have significant burden of functional impairment as assessed by ADLs and IADLs (Andrews, 1989). Markides and colleagues (1996) reported that functional impairment among Hispanics was related to specific medical conditions such as diabetes mellitus, stroke, myocardial infarction, arthritis, and hip fracture. Rates of functional impairment due to medical conditions were greater in older Hispanic Americans than in whites (Chiodo, Karren, Gerety, Mulrow, & Cornell, 1994; Espino, Neufeld, Mulvhill, & Libow, 1988; Markides et al., 1996; Rudkin, Markides, & Espino, 1997).

Among Asian Americans, comparative data on function impairment and disability are insufficient to draw firm conclusions. Asian Americans of high socioeconomic status or who came from earlier immigrant groups probably have rates of disability similar to those for whites (Lum, 1995).

Cognitive Function Assessment

A number of assessment instruments are available to evaluate cognitive function; many have application across cultures. One purpose of evaluating cognitive status in older persons is to detect and manage mild cognitive impairment, dementia, and delirium. Assessing older adults from ethnic minorities for cognitive impairment, dementia, and delirium presents a number of challenges, however, including finding suitable translators when patients' command of English is poor, the variable beliefs related to cognitive loss with age in different cultures, and the best way to approach the decision to institutionalize patients (Yeo & Gallagher-Thompson, 1996). Typically, a cutpoint score on various assessment instruments is employed as a way to standardize evaluation and determine when cognitive impairment is significant. In this section, we focus on some instruments commonly used to assess cognitive status with respect to ethnicity: (1) the Mini-Mental State Examination (MMSE); (2) the Short Portable Mental Status Questionnaire (SPMSQ); (3) the Montreal Cognitive Assessment (MoCA); and (4) formal neuropsychological testing.

African Americans and people from other ethnic groups, especially with less than 8 years of formal education, tend to be falsely identified as possibly cognitively impaired when using the MMSE (Anthony, LeResche, Niaz, Von Korff, & Folstein, 1982; Baker, 1996; Yeo & Gallagher-Thompson, 1996). Among older African Americans, Hispanic Americans, and

persons with educational attainment less than high school, a lower threshold score for determination of cognitive impairment has been recommended (less than 18 out of a possible 30 points) to improve sensitivity (82%) and specificity (99%) for the diagnosis of dementia (Crum, Anthony, Bassett, & Folstein, 1993; Tangalos et al., 1996). In other words, using a standard cutpoint of 23 points or less on the MMSE to determine cognitive impairment tends to overestimate the number of African Americans and Hispanics with true impairment of cognitive function. Increasing functional difficulty with decreasing MMSE scores has not been found among African American women, suggesting that the MMSE not be a valid predictor of subsequent decline (Leveille et al., 1998).

The Hispanic Established Populations for Epidemiologic Studies in the Elderly (EPESE) indicated that when the standard MMSE threshold score of 23 was used, 22.3% of Mexican American older adults were classified as cognitively impaired, but this high rate may reflect a lack of education rather than actual cognitive impairment (Royall, Espino, Polk, Palmer, & Markides, 2004). Like African Americans and Hispanic Americans, Asian American elders also show a decline in MMSE score with lower education and older age (Ishizaki et al., 1998).

Some of the ethnic variation noted in the MMSE is related to differential items functioning (DIF)—that is, the statistical demonstration that group differences in correct responses to a test item are independent of underlying ability. While the MMSE has been used in numerous racial/ethnic groups and translated into more than 17 languages, it is recognized that the MMSE has the potential for bias across cultures (Ramirez, Teresi, Holmes, Gurland, & Lantigua, 2006; Steis & Schrauf, 2009). In an examination for bias in the items of the MMSE, Ramirez and colleagues (2006) found that 10 of the 20 items on the MMSE show DIF for either ethnicity, education, or language. Some have suggested eliminating the biased items from the MMSE and making a scoring adjustment based on education (Marshall, Mungas, Weldon, Reed, & Haan, 1997; Teresi, Holmes, Ramirez, & Lantigua, 2001). Others suggest that the modified Mini-Mental State Examination (3MS), which adjusts for these items, may offer greater reliability, sensitivity, and validity than the MMSE. Normative tables for African American elders, stratified by age with adjustments for education and gender, are available for the MMSE (Brown, Schinka, Mortimer, & Graves, 2003).

Issues also arise in the translation of the MMSE into other languages. Even in a single language, idiomatic nuances can allow bias to be introduced. Comparison of Spanish translations of the MMSE in various regions has revealed different wording of items across versions (Ramirez et al., 2006). Also, as with any translation, the psychometric properties of this brief assessment become challenging when layered with linguistic and cultural issues and, therefore, the tool needs adaptation.

The Clock Drawing Test (CDT) has also been used as a brief measure of cognitive impairment (Lin et al., 2013). This instrument has been used in a number of clinical settings as a rapid assessment of visuoconstructive and visuospatial skill, semantic memory, conceptual abilities, and executive functioning (Hubbard et al., 2008). The CDT seems to function well in multiethnic elders (Borson et al., 1999), showing acceptable sensitivity in this group. Nevertheless, it is still significantly affected by education level (Borson et al., 1999; Hubbard et al., 2008).

The Mini Cog test is a brief screen for cognitive impairment using a three-item recall and a simple for the CDT. The Mini Cog has been found to be less biased by low education and low literacy than the MMSE (Aiken Morgan et al., 2010; Borson, Scanlan, Watanabe, Tu, & Lessig, 2005).

The Montreal Cognitive Assessment (MoCA) is a brief cognitive screening instrument assessing cognitive and executive function. It assesses 11 domains and takes approximately 10 minutes to administer. The MoCA has been translated and validated in a Chinese population, retaining a Receiver Operator Characteristic curve (ROC) for mild cognitive impairment of 0.93 (95% confidence interval [CI], 0.894–0.965) (Hubbard et al., 2008), and a Japanese population, with ROC 0.95 (95% CI, 0.9–1.0) (Borson et al., 1999). While formal studies in multiethnic

populations have not been performed to assess bias in the MoCA, this instrument has been successfully used in multiethnic populations. Some test variation has been noted, suggesting some small variation based on racial/ethnic groups (Rossetti, Lacritz, Cullum, & Weiner, 2011) that is mainly driven by education.

The SPMSQ has been specifically validated in older African American and Hispanic American samples; it shows excellent sensitivity and specificity (Baker, 1996; Miles & Bernard, 1992; Pfeiffer, 1975).

▶ Depression Assessment

Although the prevalence and incidence rates of depression in African Americans appear to be lower than the corresponding rates in whites (Gallo, Royall, & Anthony, 1993), it is not clear to what extent this finding relates to a tendency of older African Americans to assent to somatic symptoms related to depression but not sadness or other symptoms thought to be characteristic of depression (Gallo et al., 1998). In clinical samples, as many as 11% to 33% of older African American patients were found to be depressed (Rosenthal, Goldfarb, Carlson, Sagi, & Balaban, 1987).

We know little about depression rates in older Hispanic Americans, who present significant methodological issues when measuring depression (Wagner, Gallo, & Delva, 1999). The lifetime prevalence of major depression among Mexican American adults in California has been reported to be 7.8%, although this study did not include adults older than 54 years (Vega et al., 1998). In other studies using symptom scales, rates of depression in Mexican Americans were reported to be as high as 20% to 28% (Black, Markides, & Miller, 1998; Kemp, Staples, & Lopez-Aqueres, 1987; Munoz, 1988).

Suicide rates among older persons tend to be highest in white men and lowest in African American women. Older Chinese women have a suicide rate that is estimated to be as much as seven times higher than that in white women (Liu & Yu, 1985; Lum, 1995). Japanese women also have higher suicide rates than white women (Lum, 1995).

Because recognition of depression is problematic, standardized assessment instruments have been developed to facilitate its diagnosis. In most cases, there is little information on how these instruments perform for older adults from ethnic minority groups. We discuss three instruments with regard to ethnicity: (1) the Centers for Epidemiologic Studies Depression Scale (CES-D); (2) the Geriatric Depression Scale; and (3) the Patient Health Questionnaire Depression Module (PHQ-9).

The CES-D is a 20-item questionnaire designed to measure depressive symptoms in a community-based sample (Radloff, 1977). Reliability estimates for the CES-D are high, ranging from 0.84 to 0.92. Studies of this instrument in samples of African Americans and other diverse groups have shown that the CES-D can usefully measure depression (Mouton, Johnson, & Cole, 1995). The CES-D has a sensitivity of 75% in older African Americans and 94% in older whites (Torres, 2012).

The GDS has good sensitivity and specificity in most samples, although it appears to have poorer performance among African Americans when compared to whites (Baker, 1991; Torres, 2012). Among Hispanic Americans, the GDS also appears to be less sensitive to significant depression (Baker & Espino, 1997; Baker, Espino, Robinson, & Stewart, 1993).

The PHQ-9 is a validated depression module from the Patient Health Questionnaire that measures depression severity. It includes the nine *Diagnostic and Statistical Manual of Mental Disorders, Fourth Edition* (*DSM-IV*) criteria to diagnose major depressive disorders. While not typically used in older populations, the PHQ-9 works well in African American and Hispanic American patients (Huang, Chung, Kroenke, & Spitzer, 2006).

▶ Social and Economic Issues in Assessment

Frequently, it is the family who brings the patient into the clinical appointment. The quality and density of the family's social environment is a critical factor in maintenance of independent living at home. Indeed, adequate social support and interaction are significant predictors of morbidity and mortality in older adults (Blazer, 1982; Seeman, Kaplan, Knudsen, Cohen, & Guralnik, 1987). Many cultures have strong traditions of family care for the elderly. For example, among Hispanic Americans, this concept is called *familismo* (Villa et al., 1993); in Japanese families, the concept of filial piety and obligation is called *koko* (McBride et al., 1996). Resistance to accepting help may reflect an unwillingness to transfer these family obligations to healthcare professionals.

Families of older adults from ethnic minorities may have a great need to participate in the care of their older relative. African American caregivers report performing more caregiving activities and caring for persons with greater functional and cognitive impairment than do whites; however, white caregivers report significantly more burden from such caregiving (Fredman, Daly, & Lazur, 1995). In addition to social support from the family, the church is an important source of social and emotional support for older African Americans (Chadiha, Morrow-Howell, Darkwa, & Berg-Weger, 1996; Chatters & Taylor, 1998).

At the same time, healthcare professionals should realize that caring family members may shield their relative from intrusive questions or procedures or may cover up deficiencies in the older patient's performance. Family members must be made aware that adequate assessment of older adults requires that they act as clear translators of questions and answers, not only of assessment instruments, but also in relation to recommended treatment. Family members may be able to suggest ways that the medical treatment can be integrated with the cultural beliefs and practices of the older person.

Minority elders tend to show greater levels of financial strain than other Americans (Commonwealth Fund, 1995; Jackson, Chatters, & Taylor, 1993). Older minorities often face "double jeopardy"—that is, the combined effect of age and minority status leads to greater illness burden and greater limitation on financial resources (Cantor, 1979; Dowd & Bengston, 1978; Ferraro, 1987; Jackson, Kolody, & Wood, 1982; Reed, 1990). Physicians need to consider the financial constraints of older minority patients as recommendations for treatment are developed. While direct questioning about finances may be offensive to some older adults, presenting the possibility of a less expensive but equally effective treatment shows a depth of understanding that is often appreciated by older persons.

▶ Summary

Geriatric assessment forms an important component of clinical practice that can be carried out over a number of visits. Since older adults from ethnic minorities are bound to make up a large proportion of the patients seen, clinicians should pay special attention to the cultural factors that modify aspects of assessment, including the suitability of specific assessment instruments. When this approach is combined with sensitivity to cultural issues and clinical judgment, the health and function of all older adults can be enhanced through careful considerations of the domains of geriatric assessment.

References

Agree, E. M., & Freedman, V. A. (1999). Implications of population aging for geriatric health. In J. Gallo, J. Busby-Whitehead, P. V. Rabins, R. Silliman, & J. Murphy (Eds.), *Reichel's care of the elderly: Clinical aspects of aging* (5th ed., pp. 659–669). Baltimore, MD: Lippincott Williams & Wilkin.

Aiken Morgan, A. T., Marsiske, M., Dzierzewski, J. M., Jones, R. N., Whitfield, K. E., Johnson, K. E., & Cresci, M. K. (2010). Race-related cognitive test bias in the active study: A mimic model approach. *Experimental Aging Research, 36*(4), 426–452. doi: 10.1080/0361073X.2010.507427

Albert, S. M., & Teresi, J. A. (1999). Reading ability, education, and cognitive status assessment among older adults in Harlem, New York City. *American Journal of Public Health, 89,* 95–97.

Andrews, J. (1989). *Poverty and poor health among elderly Hispanic Americans.* Baltimore, MD: Commonwealth Fund Commission.

Anthony, J. C., LeResche, L., Niaz, U., Von Korff, M., & Folstein, M. E. (1982). Limits of the "MiniMental State" as a screening test for dementia and delirium among hospital patients. *Psychological Medicine, 12,* 397–408.

Baker, F. M. (1991). A contrast: Geriatric depression versus depression in younger age groups. *Journal of the National Medical Association, 83,* 340–344.

Baker, F. M. (1996). Issues in assessing dementia in African American elders. In G. Yeo & D. Gallagher-Thompson (Eds.), *Ethnicity and the dementias* (pp. 59–76). Washington, DC: Taylor & Francis.

Baker, F. M., & Espino, D. V. (1997). A Spanish version of the geriatric depression scale in Mexican American elders. *International Journal of General Psychiatry, 12,* 21–25.

Baker, F. M., Espino, D. V., Robinson, B. H., & Stewart, B. (1993). Assessing depressive symptoms in African-American and Mexican-American elders. *Clinics in Gerontology, 14,* 15–21.

Black, S. A., Markides, K. S., & Miller, T. Q. (1998). Correlates of depressive symptomatology among older community-dwelling Mexican Americans: The Hispanic EPESE. *Journals of Gerontology, Series B: Psychological Sciences and Social Sciences, 53,* S198–S208.

Blazer, D. G. (1982). Social support and mortality in an elderly community population. *American Journal of Epidemiology, 115,* 684–694.

Borson, S., Brush, M., Gil, E., Scanlan, J., Vitaliano, P., Chen, J., ... Roques, J. (1999) The Clock Drawing Test: Utility for dementia detection in multiethnic elders. *Journal of Gerontology, 54*(11), M534–M540.

Borson, S., Scanlan, J. M., Watanabe, J., Tu, S. P., & Lessig, M. (2005). Simplifying detection of cognitive impairment: Comparison of the Mini-Cog and Mini-Mental State Examination in multiethnic sample. *Journal of the American Geriatrics Society, 53*(5), 871–874.

Brangman, S. A. (1995). African-American elders: Implications for health care providers. *Clinics in Geriatric Medicine, 11,* 15–23.

Brown, L., Schinka, J., Mortimer, J., & Graves, A.B. (2003). 3MS normative data for elderly African Americans. *Journal of Clinical and Experimental Neuropsychology, 25,* 234–241.

Cantor, M. (1979). The informal support system of New York's inner-city elderly: Is ethnicity a factor? In D. E. Gelfand & A. J. Kutsik (Eds.), *Ethnicity and aging: Theory, research, and policy* (pp. 153–175). New York, NY: Springer.

Chadiha, L., Morrow-Howell, N., Darkwa, O. K., & Berg-Weger, M. (1998). Support systems of African American family caregivers of elders with dementing illness. *African American Research Perspectives, 9,* 104–114.

Chatters, L. M., & Taylor, P. J. (1998). Religious involvement among African Americans. *African American Research Perspectives, 4,* 8.

Chiodo, L. K., Karren, D. W., Gerety, M. B., Mulrow, C. D., & Cornell, J. E. (1994). Functional status of Mexican-American nursing home residents. *Journal of the American Geriatrics Society, 42,* 293–296.

Commonwealth Fund. (1995). *National comparative survey of minority health care.* New York, NY: Author.

Cooper, R., & David, R. (1986). The biological concept of race and its application to public health and epidemiology. *Journal of Health Politics, Policy, and Law, 11,* 97–116.

Crum, R. M., Anthony, J. C., Bassett, S. S., & Folstein, M. E. (1993). Population-based norms for the Mini-Mental State examination by age and educational level. *Journal of the American Medical Association, 269,* 2386–2391.

Dowd, J., & Bengston, V. L. (1978). Aging in minority populations: An examination of the double jeopardy hypothesis. *Journal of Gerontology, 33,* 427–436.

Edmonds, M. K. (1993). Physical health. In J. S. Jackson, I. M. Chatters, & R. J. Taylor (Eds.), *Aging in black America* (pp. 151–167). Newbury Park, CA: Sage.

Elliott, K. S., Di Minno, M., Lam, D., & Tu, A. M. (1996). Working with Chinese families in the context of dementia. In G. Yeo & D. Gallagher-Thompson (Eds.), *Ethnicity and the dementias* (pp. 89–108). Washington, DC: Taylor & Francis.

Espino, D. V. (1988). Medication usage in elderly Hispanics: What we need to know. In M. Sotomayor & N. R. Ascencio (Eds.), *Proceedings on improving drug use among Hispanic elderly* (pp. 7–11). Washington, DC: National Hispanic Council on Aging.

Espino, D. V., Neufeld, R. R., Mulvhill, M. K., & Libow, I. S. (1988). Hispanic and non-Hispanic elderly on admission to the nursing home: A pilot study. *Gerontologist, 28,* 821–824.

Ferraro, K. E. (1987). Double jeopardy to health for African-American older adults? *Journal of Gerontology, 42*(5), 528–533.

Foley, D. J., Fillenbaum, G., & Service, C. (1990). Physical functioning. In J. D. Cornoni-Huntley, A. M. Ostfeld, J. O. Taylor, et al. (Eds.), *Established populations for the epidemiologic studies of the elderly: Resource data book* (pp. 34–50). Publication no. 90-495. Washington, DC: National Institute on Aging, National Institute of Health, U.S. Public Health Service.

Frank, J. D., & Frank, J. B. (1991). *Persuasion and healing: A comparative study of psychotherapy.* Baltimore, MD: Johns Hopkins University Press.

Fredman, L., Daly, M. P., & Lazur, A. M. (1995). Burden among white and black caregivers to elderly adults. *Journals of Gerontology, Series B: Psychological Sciences and Social Sciences, 50,* S1104118.

Gallagher-Thompson, D., Talamantes, M., Ramirez, R., & Valverde, I. (1996). Service delivery issues and recommendations for working with Mexican American family caregivers. In G. Yeo & D. Gallagher-Thompson (Eds.), *Ethnicity and the dementias* (pp. 137–152). Washington, DC: Taylor & Francis.

Gallo, J. J., Cooper-Patrick, L., & Lesikar, S. (1998). Depressive symptoms of whites and African Americans aged 60 years and older. *Journals of Gerontology: Psychological Sciences, 53B,* 277–286.

Gallo, J., & Lebowitz, B. D. (1999). The epidemiology of common late-life mental disorders in the community: Themes for a new century. *Psychiatric Services, 50*(9), 1158–1166.

Gallo, J., Royall, D. R., & Anthony, J. C. (1993). Risk factors for the onset of major depression in middle age and late life. *Social Psychiatry and Psychiatric Epidemiology, 28,* 101–108.

Greene, V. L., & Monahans, D. J. (1984). Comparative utilization of community-based longterm care services by Hispanic and Anglo elderly in a case management system. *Journal of Gerontology, 39,* 730–735.

Guralnik, J. M., Branch, L. G., Cummings, S. R., & Curb, J. D. (1989). Physical performance measures in aging research. *Journal of Gerontology, 44,* M141–M146.

Guralnik, J. M., Land, K. C., Blazer, D. G., Fillenbaum, G. G., & Branch, L. G. (1993). Educational status and active life expectancy among older blacks and whites. *New England Journal of Medicine, 329,* 110–116.

Guralnik, J. M., Reuben, D. B., Buchner, D. M., & Ferrucci, L. (1995). Performance measures of physical function in comprehensive geriatric assessment. In L. Z. Rubenstein, D. Wieland, & R. Bernabei (Eds.), *Geriatric assessment technology: The state of the art* (pp. 59–74). New York, NY: Springer.

Hendrie, H. C., Osuntokun, B. O., Hall, K. S., Ogunniyi A. O., Hui S. L., Unverzagt, F. W., . . . Musick, B. S. (1995). Prevalence of Alzheimer's disease and dementia in two communities: Nigerian African and African Americans. *American Journal of Psychiatry, 152,* 1485–1492.

Huang, F. Y., Chung, H., Kroenke, K., & Spitzer, R. L. (2006). Racial and ethnic differences in the relationship between depression severity and functional status. *Psychiatric Services, 57*(4), 498–503.

Hubbard, E. J., Santini, V., Blankevoort, C. G., Volkers, K. M., Barrup, M. S., Byerly, L.,... Stern, R. A. (2008). Clock drawing performance in cognitively normal elderly. *Archives of Clinical Neuropsychology, 23*(3), 295–327. doi: 10.1016/j.acn.2007.12.003

Ishizaki, J., Meguro, K., Ambo, H., Shimada, M., Yamaguchi, S., Hayasaka, C., . . . Yamadori, A. (1998). A normative, community-based study MiniMental State in elderly adults: The effect of age and educational level. *Journals of Gerontology: Social Sciences, 53,* 359–363.

Jackson, J. S., Chatters, L. M., & Taylor, R. J. (1993). *Aging in African-American America.* Newbury Park, CA: Sage.

Jackson, M., Kolody, B., & Wood, J. L. (1982). To be old and African-American: The case for the double jeopardy on income and health. In R. C. Manuel (Ed.), *Minority aging: Sociological and social psychological issues* (pp. 427-436). Westport, CT: Greenwood Press.

Kemp, B. S., Staples, F. R., & Lopez-Aqueres, W. (1987). Epidemiology of depression and dysphoria in the elderly Hispanic population. *Journal of the American Geriatrics Society, 35,* 920–926.

Kleinman, A. (1980). *Patients and healers in the context of culture: An exploration of the borderland between anthropology, medicine, and psychiatry.* Los Angeles, CA: University of California Press.

Kleinman, A., & Good, B. (1985). *Culture and depression: Studies in the anthropology and cross cultural psychiatry of affect and disorder.* Los Angeles, CA: University of California Press.

Lavizzo-Mourey, R., & Mackenzie, E. R. (1996). Cultural competence: Essential measurements of quality for managed care organizations. *Annals of Internal Medicine, 124,* 919–921.

Leveille, S. G., Guralnik, J. M., Ferrucci, L., Corti, M. C., Kasper, J., & Fried, L. P. (1998). Black/white differences in the relationship between MMSE scores and disability: The Women's Health and Aging Study. *Journals of Gerontology: Psychological Sciences and Social Sciences, 53,* 201–208.

Lillie-Blanton, M., Anthony, J. C., & Schuster, C. R. (1993). Probing the meaning of racial/ethnic group comparisons in crack cocaine smoking. *Journal of the American Medical Association, 269,* 993–997.

Lin, J. S., O'Connor, E., Rossom, R. C., Perdue, L. A., Burda, B. U., Thompson, M., & Eckstrom, E. (2013). *Screening for cognitive impairment in older adults: An evidence update for the US Preventive Services Task Force.* Evidence Report No. 107. AHRQ Publication No. 14-05198-EF-1. Rockville, MD: Agency for Healthcare Research and Quality.

Liu, W. T., & Yu, E. (1985). Asian/Pacific American elderly: Mortality differentials, health status, and the use of health services. *Journal of Applied Gerontology, 4,* 35–64.

Lum, O. M. (1995). Health status of Asians and Pacific Islanders. *Clinics in Geriatric Medicine, 11,* 53–69.

Manson, S. M., Shore, J. H., & Bloom, J. D. (1985). The depressive experience in American Indian communities: A challenge for psychiatric theory and diagnosis. In A. Kleinman & B. Good (Eds.), *Culture and depression: Studies in the anthropology and cross cultural psychiatry of affect and disorder* (pp. 331–368). Los Angeles, CA: University of California Press.

Markides, K. S., Stroup-Benham, C. A., Goodwin, J. S., Perkowski, L. C., Lichtenstein, M., & Ray, L. A. (1996). The effect of medical conditions on the functional limitations of Mexican-American elderly. *Annals of Epidemiology, 6,* 386–391.

Marshall, S., Mungas, D., Weldon, M., Reed, B., & Haan, M. (1997). Differential item functioning in the Mini-Mental State Examination in English and Spanish speaking older adults. *Psychology and Aging, 12,* 718–725.

McBride, M., Morioka-Douglas, N., & Yeo, G. (1996). *Aging and health: American Indian/Alaska Native elders* (2nd ed.). Palo Alto, CA: Stanford Geriatric Education Center.

McCabe, M., & Cuellar, J. (1994). *Aging and health: American Indian/Alaska Native elders* (2nd ed.). Palo Alto, CA: Stanford Geriatric Education Center.

Miles, T. P., & Bernard, M. A. (1992). Morbidity, disability, and the health status of black American elderly: A new look at the oldest-old. *Journal of the American Geriatrics Society, 40,* 1047–1054.

Mouton, C. P., & Espino, D. V. (1999). Ethnic diversity of the aged. In J. Gallo, J. Busby-Whitehead, P. V. Rabins, R. Silliman, & J. Murphy (Eds.), *Reichel's care of the elderly: Clinical aspects of aging* (5th ed., pp. 595–608). Baltimore, MD: Lippincott Williams & Wilkins.

Mouton, C. P., Johnson, M. S., & Cole, D. R. (1995). Ethical considerations with African American elders. *Clinics in Geriatric Medicine, 11,* 113–129.

Munoz, E. (1988). Care for the Hispanic poor: A growing segment of American society. *Journal of the American Medical Association, 260,* 2711–2712.

Neighbors, H. W., & Lumpkin, S. (1990). The epidemiology of mental disorder in the black population. In D. S. Ruiz (Ed.), *Handbook of mental health and mental disorder among black Americans* (pp. 55–70). Westport, CT: Greenwood Press.

O'Nell, T. D. (1996). *Disciplined hearts: History, identity, and depression in an American Indian community.* Los Angeles, CA: University of California Press.

Pfeiffer, E. (1975). A short portable mental status questionnaire for the assessment of organic brain deficit in elderly patients. *Journal of the American Geriatrics Society, 23,* 433–441.

Pi, E. H., Wang, A. L., & Gray, G. E. (1993). Asian/non-Asian transcultural tricyclic antidepressant psychopharmacology: A review. *Progress in Neuro-Psychopharmacology and Biological Psychiatry, 17,* 691–702.

Prisant, L. M., & Mensah, G. A. (1996). Use of beta-adrenergic receptor blockers in blacks. *Journal of Clinical Pharmacology, 36*(10), 867–873.

Radloff, I. S. (1977). The CES-D Scale: A self-report depression scale for research in the general population. *Applied Psychological Measurement, 1,* 385–401.

Ramirez, M., Teresi, J., Holmes, D., Gurland, B., & Lantigua, R. (2006). Differential item functioning (DIF) and the Mini-Mental State Examination (MMSE). *Medical Care, 44,* S95–S104. doi: 10.1097/01.mlr.0000245181.96133.db

Reed, W. (1990). Health care needs and services. In A. Harel, E. A. McKinney, & M. Williams (Eds.), *African-American aged: Understanding diversity and service needs* (pp. 100–113). Newbury Park, CA: Sage.

Rosenthal, M. P., Goldfarb, N. J., Carlson, B. L., Sagi, P. C., & Balaban, D. J. (1987). Assessment of depression in a family practice. *Journal of Family Practice, 25,* 143–148.

Rossetti, H., Lacritz, L. H., Cullum, C. M., & Weiner, M. F. (2011). Normative data for the Montreal Cognitive Assessment (MoCA) in a population-based sample. *Neurology, 77*(13), 1272–1275. doi: 10.1212/WNL.0b013e318230208a

Royall, D. R., Espino, D. V., Polk, M. J., Palmer, R. E., & Markides, K. S. (2004). Prevalence and patterns of executive impairment in community dwelling Mexican Americans: Results from the Hispanic EPESE study.

International Journal of Geriatric Psychiatry, 19(10), 926–934.

Rudkin, L., Markides, K. S., & Espino, D. V. (1997). Functional limitations in elderly Mexican Americans. *Topics in Geriatric Rehabilitation, 12,* 38–46.

Seeman, T. E., Kaplan, G. A., Knudsen, L., Cohen, R., & Guralnik, J. (1987). Social network ties and mortality among the elderly in the Alameda County study. *American Journal of Epidemiology, 126,* 714–723.

Sramek, J., & Pi, E. H. (1996). Ethnicity and antidepressant response. *Mount Sinai Journal of Medicine, 63,* 320–325.

Steis, M., & Schrauf, R. (2009). A review of translations and adaptations of the Mini-Mental State Examination in languages other than English and Spanish. *Research in Gerontological Nursing, 2*(3), 214–221. doi: 10.3928/19404921-20090421-06

Tangalos, E. G., Smith, G. E., Ivnik, R. J., Petersen, R. C., Kokmen, E., Kurland, L.T., . . . Parisi, J. E. (1996). The Mini-Mental State examination in general medical practice: Clinical utility and acceptance. *Mayo Clinic Proceedings, 71,* 829–837.

Tang, M. X., Stern, Y., Marder, K., Bell, K., Gurland, B., Lantigua, R., . . . Mayeux, R. (1998). The APOE-epsilon-4 allele and the risk of Alzheimer's disease among African Americans, whites, and Hispanics. *Journal of the American Medical Association, 279,* 751–755.

Teresi, J. A., Holmes, D., Ramirez, M., & Lantigua, R. (2001). Performance of cognitive test among different racial/ethnic and education groups: Finding of differential item functioning and possible test bias. *Journal of Mental Health and Aging, 7,* 79–90.

Torres, E. R. (2012). Psychometric properties of the Center for Epidemiologic Studies Depression Scale in African-American and black Caribbean Adults. *Issues in Mental Health Nursing, 33*(10), 687–696. doi: 10.3109/01612840.2012.697534

Vega, W. A., Kolody, B., Aguilar-Gaxiola, S., Alderete, E., Catalano, R., & Caraveo-Anduaga, J. (1998). Lifetime prevalence of *DSM-III-R* psychiatric disorders among urban and rural Mexican Americans in California. *Archives of General Psychiatry, 55,* 771–778.

Villa, M. L., Cuellar, J., Gamel, N., & Yeo, G. (1993). *Aging and health: Hispanic-American elders* (2nd ed.). Palo Alto, CA: Stanford Geriatric Education Center.

Wagner, F. A., Gallo, J., & Delva, J. (1999). Depresión en la edad avanzada: Problema oculto de salud poeblica para México? *Salud Publica Mexico, 41,* 189–202.

Whitfield, K. E. (1996). Studying cognition in older African-Americans: Some conceptual considerations. *Journal of Aging and Ethnicity, 1,* 41–52.

Yeo, G., & Gallagher-Thompson, D. (Eds.). (1996). *Ethnicity and the dementias.* Washington, DC: Taylor & Francis.

CHAPTER 13

Vulnerable Populations

Stephen A. Somers and Alexandra Kruse

CHAPTER OBJECTIVES

1. Recognize the characteristics and circumstances of low-income, vulnerable older adults.
2. Describe the practice challenges that exist when addressing the diverse needs of these individuals.

KEY TERMS

Dually eligible individuals
Economic security

Social determinants of health
Vulnerable older adults

▶ Introduction

Many older adults are at higher risk for poor outcomes (e.g., lower health status, quality of care, or satisfaction with care; higher rates of service utilization or costs of care) because of socioeconomic and health-related factors (e.g., having very low incomes, being medically complex, having unmet needs). Professionals and clinicians practicing in a variety of settings should be aware of the unique characteristics and circumstances that make these older adults more vulnerable to poor health outcomes than their healthier and wealthier peers. They should also recognize the specific challenges and opportunities associated with assessment and care management for this population.

This chapter examines vulnerability in low-income older adults through a number of lenses, including financial well-being as well as social and clinical needs. These factors can affect a patient's ability to access care and independently manage day-to-day needs. **Vulnerable older adults** must navigate a largely uncoordinated system of federally funded health care and state-based long-term services and supports (LTSS) programs that will likely be affected by shifting state and federal policies. This fragmented system of care magnifies the vulnerability of this population.

▶ Defining Vulnerability

A growing subset of the United States' low-income older adult population faces significant health and economic challenges. These patients—and their caregivers—struggle with day-to-day management of complex medical and functional needs; mounting bills; and inadequate housing, nutrition, and transportation. These individuals may also have a high incidence of functional impairment, cognitive impairment, and depression that may affect their ability to keep medical appointments or self-manage their care (Centers for Medicare and Medicaid Services [CMS], 2016; Medicare Payment Advisory Commission & Medicaid and CHIP Payment and Access Commission [MedPAC/MACPAC], 2017).

The vulnerability of low-income older adults may derive from not only visible complex clinical care needs, but also unmet social support needs that may be less apparent to healthcare providers. Professionals and clinicians will encounter individuals with some or all of these vulnerabilities in a variety of aging, health care, and social services practice settings. While there is no definitive measure of the prevalence of "vulnerability" among older adults, it is possible to roughly gauge the numbers of individuals having certain economic and clinical/functional characteristics and those affected by other **social determinants of health** that may make them vulnerable to poor outcomes.

Economic Characteristics

Many older adults experience a high degree of economic insecurity, despite recent declines in overall poverty rates among the U.S. elderly population (Anzick & Weaver, 2001). More than 4.2 million Americans age 60 and

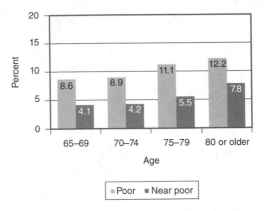

FIGURE 13-1 Poverty status among older adults in the United States, 2014.

Source: Social Security Administration, 2016.

older live at or below the federal poverty level (Proctor, Semega, & Kollar, 2016; U.S. Department of Health and Human Services, 2017),[1] and 1 in 3 older adults lives above the poverty level but at an income level below that required to live with **economic security** (Mutchler, Li, & Xu, 2016). The level of economic insecurity is higher in some subsets of the older adult population, including nonmarried women, minorities, individuals living alone, and those older than age 74 (**FIGURE 13-1**) (Social Security Administration, 2016). Additionally, approximately 11.4 million low–income individuals are dually eligible for Medicare and Medicaid in the United States (Kaiser Family Foundation, n.d.; U.S. Department of Health and Human Services, Centers for Medicare and Medicaid Services [U.S. DHHS, CMS], 2017). Their coverage is administered by the federal Medicare program and by state-based Medicaid programs. For those who qualify, Medicaid programs assist these Medicare beneficiaries with out-of-pocket Medicare costs and long-term care needs.

---

1 For 2017, the federal poverty level was $12,060 for a one-person household and $16,240 for a two-person household (U.S. Department of Health and Human Services, 2017).

Clinical and Functional Characteristics

Sixty-eight percent of all older adults in the United States have multiple chronic conditions (CMS, 2016), meaning that they have clinical and functional needs that require the involvement of multiple professionals and clinicians. **Dually eligible individuals** age 65 and older have an even higher prevalence of multiple chronic conditions than their Medicare-only counterparts. These low-income individuals also have a greater incidence of functional impairment and often require LTSS, with three times as many experiencing deficits in three to six activities of daily living (**FIGURE 13-2**). Ongoing assessment is essential for this population to ensure that their clinical and functional needs are being addressed.

An often unrecognized health issue in assessing low-income older adults is their behavioral health status. According to one estimate, 25% of Medicare beneficiaries age 65 and older have a behavioral health condition such as depression, anxiety, and medication or alcohol misuse (Older Americans Behavioral Health Technical Assistance Center, 2012). Older adults are less likely to receive behavioral health care than younger

adults, and many older adults with behavioral health issues simply do not receive the treatment they need (Older Americans Behavioral Health Technical Assistance Center, 2012). Fragmented care and lack of coordination between providers of behavioral health and physical health services are also significant issues for this population.

Older adults with intellectual and developmental disabilities (I/DD) are yet another vulnerable subpopulation that needs specialized assessment. Advances in medical care and a greater array of services and supports are helping individuals with I/DD to live longer. Estimates suggest that while there were approximately 650,000 adults age 60 and older with I/DD and related conditions in 2000, this number will double by 2030 (Heller, Janicki, Hammel, & Factor, 2002).

Social Determinants of Health

Assessing a patient's social determinants of health, such as level of community engagement and access to transportation or nutritious meals, is often as critical as assessing medical needs for vulnerable older adults. Both the health status and the level of frailty of low-income older adults can be

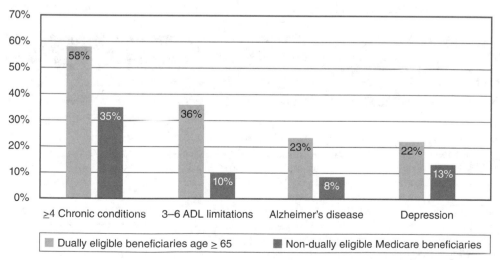

FIGURE 13-2 Prevalence of chronic conditions and functional limitations among dually eligible individuals, 2015.

Source: CMS, 2016.

affected by a number of social, environmental, and behavioral factors (McGinnis, Williams-Russo, & Knickman, 2002). Affordable and accessible housing can influence an older adult's ability to stay mobile, access medical care, and engage in community activities. In fact, when community-dwelling vulnerable older adults have access to supportive services and affordable housing, they are less likely to enter a nursing home or go to a hospital than their peers without similar services (Castle & Resnick, 2014). Some vulnerable older adults may have unstable housing arrangements or experience homelessness as they transition between care settings, so that they can be hard to contact, particularly if the professional doing the assessment is relying on outdated information. Despite these factors' impact on health status, professionals and clinicians rarely address social determinants of health, although attention to these issues is growing.

▶ Understanding How Vulnerable Older Adults Get Their Care

Professionals and clinicians should understand the system of care that vulnerable older adults must navigate. In the United States, it comprises a mix of public and private institutions and state and federal programs, which are often supplemented by unpaid caregiving as well as out-of-pocket spending on LTSS.

As mentioned earlier, many of the most vulnerable older adults in the United States are dually eligible for Medicare and Medicaid—these individuals account for more than 20% of all Medicare beneficiaries (Kaiser Family Foundation, n.d.; U.S. DHHS, CMS, 2017). The federally administered Medicare program and state-based Medicaid programs provide essential services and supports to this population (**TABLE 13-1**). Although Medicare and Medicaid were established at the same time, they were not designed to work together. In most communities, therefore, dually eligible individuals must navigate two separate and uncoordinated systems of care: Medicare for the coverage of most preventive, primary, and acute healthcare services and prescription drugs, and Medicaid for the coverage of LTSS, certain behavioral health services (e.g., treatment of serious mental illness, substance use disorders), and help with Medicare premiums and cost sharing. For these individuals, determining the distinct roles and coverage details of each program can be confusing, both at enrollment and when accessing care.

TABLE 13-1 Which Program Pays for Which Services?

Medicare	Medicaid	Older Americans Act
▪ Hospital care ▪ Physician and ancillary services ▪ Skilled nursing facility care (up to 100 days) ▪ Home health care ▪ Hospice ▪ Prescription drugs ▪ Durable medical equipment (DME) ▪ Limited behavioral health treatment	▪ Medicare cost sharing ▪ Nursing home care (once Medicare benefits are exhausted) ▪ Wide array of home- and community-based services (HCBS) ▪ Hospital care once Medicare benefits are exhausted ▪ Some prescription drugs and DME not covered by Medicare ▪ Most treatments for substance abuse disorders and serious mental illness	▪ Access to services (care management, transportation) ▪ Nutrition (meals, nutrition counseling and education) ▪ Limited HCBS (home care, adult day care, family caregiver support) ▪ Disease prevention and health promotion (physical fitness, chronic disease management) ▪ Vulnerable elder rights protection (ombudsman, abuse and neglect)

Misalignments in Medicare and Medicaid create significant barriers to effective care coordination and person-centered care for dually eligible individuals. These patients typically visit multiple providers that do not communicate with one another, and they may experience significant gaps in care when no one professional or organization is responsible for delivering and coordinating their care. A common care gap is a lack of effective discharge planning and at-home support when older adults transition between hospital and community settings.

A number of emerging or growing programs (e.g., Medicaid managed LTSS programs, Medicare Advantage Dual Eligible Special Needs Plans, the Medicare–Medicaid Financial Alignment Initiative demonstrations, and PACE programs) are striving to blend and align Medicare and Medicaid administrative processes, policies, and care management practices to make them work together more effectively. Professionals and clinicians may increasingly encounter these programs that offer opportunities to improve care for dually eligible beneficiaries.

In addition to the services provided by Medicare and Medicaid, vulnerable older adults receive services through the federally funded Older Americans Act, which supports a range of home- and community-based services such as home-delivered meals and other nutrition programs, in-home services, transportation, legal services, elder abuse prevention, and caregiver supports (Table 13-1). These services are provided at the local level through a national network of 56 state agencies on aging, 629 area agencies on aging, and nearly 20,000 service providers. Older Americans Act funding represents just a fraction of the budget for the Medicare and Medicaid programs, so the demand for these services exceeds their availability.

Health care spending for dually eligible individuals with multiple chronic conditions and/or functional needs is significantly higher than that for other populations. This subpopulation accounts for a disproportionately large share of expenditures in both the Medicare and Medicaid programs compared to the overall enrollment. In 2012, they accounted for 20% of Medicare enrollees, yet were targeted by 34% of the program's spending. The same individuals account for 15% of Medicaid enrollees nationwide, but 35% of spending (MedPAC/MACPAC, 2017).

Medicaid is the dominant source of payment for LTSS in the United States, followed by out-of-pocket payments by individuals and families (**FIGURE 13-3**) (O'Shaughnessy, 2012). Publicly financed LTSS coverage under Medicaid includes payment for both institutional and home- and

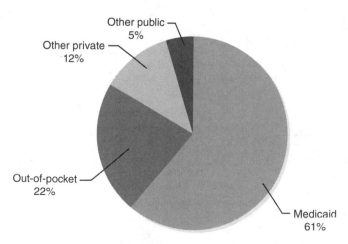

FIGURE 13-3 Long-term services and supports (LTSS) expenditures by source, 2012.

Source: O'Shaughnessy, C.V., National Health Policy Forum. (2014). National spending for long-term services and supports (LTSS), 2012. Washington, DC: National Health Policy Forum. Retrieved from http://www.nhpf.org/library/the-basics/Basics_LTSS_03-27-14.pdf

community-based care, although the latter is optional and varies by state. There is a growing focus on increasing the amount of care provided in home and community settings, which is the setting most preferred by those receiving care. This individual preference is captured in assessment tools for publicly funded LTSS programs.

In recent years, there has been a greater reliance on managed care arrangements under both the Medicare and Medicaid programs, with the goal of improving care delivery while reducing costs to state and federal governments. This trend has broadened the field of assessment beyond the primary care office to health plan–driven assessments and care planning processes that aim to include physicians, social services, and other providers. Given the health and long-term care spending patterns of vulnerable older adults, these arrangements are expected to increase in the future.

▶ Using Assessment Data for Policymaking and Program Planning

Beyond the professionals and clinicians who conduct assessments to develop a care plan or other intervention for an individual patient, a variety of other stakeholders use assessment data to inform policy and program development and allocate resources. Health plans, providers, community agencies, consumers, and state and federal policymakers are all involved in developing and using assessment tools and data (**TABLE 13-2**).

The level of standardization of assessment tools, content of the tools, assessment processes, and uses of the data collected vary significantly across the states. Policymakers are increasingly

TABLE 13-2 Assessment Types and Purposes

Assessing Entity	Type of Assessment	Purpose
Professional or clinician	Provider- or practice-driven assessment tools	■ Medical history and development of treatment plan
Nursing facility	Minimum Data Set	■ Development of a care plan ■ Payment ■ Reporting of quality data and ratings
Medicare or Medicaid managed care organization	Comprehensive assessment for Medicaid LTSS and health risk assessment for Medicare	■ Stratification of members into risk groups ■ Development of a care plan ■ Service authorizations
Medicaid eligibility staff or contractors	State-selected comprehensive, LTSS assessment	■ Determination of functional eligibility ■ Policy and program development
Medicaid LTSS care coordinators (typically employed by a local aging or disability agency)	State-selected comprehensive LTSS assessment	■ Development of a care plan ■ Service authorizations

Abbreviation: LTSS, long-term services and supports.

using Medicare and Medicaid assessment data to establish reimbursement rates that match payment to the acuity or service utilization of the population served. Professionals and clinicians should understand how assessment data are used and the relevant stakeholders that may be involved in assessment of vulnerable older adults in their state or community.

▶ Programmatic Issues and Practice Challenges

As described in this chapter, vulnerable older adults have unique circumstances and needs, and often must access their care through fragmented, uncoordinated delivery systems that can create gaps in care. Professionals and clinicians conducting assessments of this population should be aware of several practice challenges and considerations:

- *Social support needs may take precedence over clinical needs.* Unmet social support needs or a lack of financial resources may hinder a patient's ability to self-manage chronic conditions or follow recommended treatment plans. When these needs are uncovered during the assessment process, referrals can be made to care coordinators or community agencies that will help determine the individual's eligibility for relevant public assistance programs. Local Aging and Disability Resource Centers and Centers for Independent Living operate information and referral services that can link patients to needed programs. The assessment of social support needs can also assist overburdened caregivers by linking them to respite programs and support groups.
- *The diverse needs of older adults require varied solutions.* The varied clinical and functional needs of older adults may not fit into one program design, so multiple programs or referrals may be needed; however, funding

for these programs may be limited as the population of vulnerable older adults grows. In addition, concentrated populations of particular ethnic or linguistic groups may require care providers to develop assessment instruments that reflect the cultural needs and preferences of multiple groups.

- *Interdisciplinary care teams offer both opportunities and challenges.* Professionals and clinicians are increasingly being asked to coordinate care for vulnerable older adults across many dimensions. This has led to the development of both interdisciplinary team approaches and physician practice–based care management. Although this more coordinated approach is a positive change, there are corresponding needs to identify timely and cost-effective ways to share assessment data with other parties, and ensure that there is an organized process for determining who makes final decisions and communicates with the individuals being assessed.
- *An individual's ability to access care may vary by location.* Professionals and clinicians working in in rural areas may encounter difficulty finding LTSS providers for their patients. Also, a lack of medical specialists, primary care physicians, or behavioral health providers may hinder the clinician's ability to manage an individual's complex physical or behavioral health conditions. In urban settings, the higher prevalence of low-income older adults may also result in access challenges when the need for services exceeds the supply of providers or funding.
- *Assessment processes affect both patients and providers.* When deciding which assessment tools they will use, professionals and clinicians may want to select tools and design assessment processes that will reduce redundancy and avoid overwhelming the individual patient. Since the patient may be assessed by multiple parties, efforts should be made to share assessment data and become familiar with the different assessments used at the federal, state, or health plan level, including

the accessibility and timeliness of the data collected via those means. Professionals and clinicians may be required by programs or health plans to complete assessments for certain patients within a defined time frame. Sometimes, however, patients may decline the assessment, be difficult to locate or engage, or have significant physical or cognitive impairments that complicate the assessment process.

■ *Additional considerations may arise in relation to state and local policies.* Increasingly, the entity conducting an assessment must be independent from the entity providing or paying for the service, particularly in managed care arrangements. In addition, regardless of the needs identified in an assessment, funding for medical, behavioral, or social services may be insufficient to meet demands. Professionals and clinicians should be aware of program constraints (e.g., budget and staffing shortfalls in local programs; Medicaid waitlists for home and community-based services) as well as state and local efforts under way to address them.

▶ Summary

Although the planning, financing, and delivery of health care, long-term care, and social services for vulnerable older adults often occurs in isolation today, solutions that better integrate care are emerging. Today's healthcare system is focused on improving care for this and other populations with complex needs, which requires a dramatic shift in how care is delivered. Instead of managing a single disease, there is now a movement toward simultaneously managing multiple diseases and cognitive and/or functional impairments, while creating solutions that address unmet needs and serve individuals in their preferred settings. Accordingly, our collective understanding of and approach to caring for these vulnerable older adults needs to change, all the way from the front-line assessor

to the policymaker. Innovative state and federal agencies are partnering with stakeholders to use assessment results to understand the needs of vulnerable older adults and create responsive programs. For professionals and clinicians serving these older adults, ensuring comprehensive and accurate assessment of patient needs can improve care for the individual, while supporting these broader efforts.

References

Anzick, M. A., & Weaver, D. A. (2001). Reducing poverty among elderly women. Social Security Office of Policy. ORES Working Paper No. 87. Retrieved from https://www.ssa.gov/policy/docs/workingpapers/wp87.html

Castle, N., & Resnick, N. (2014). Service-enriched housing: The Staying at Home Program. *Journal of Applied Gerontology, 35*(8), 1–21.

Centers for Medicare and Medicaid Services (CMS). (2016). Multiple chronic conditions. Prevalence state level: All beneficiaries by Medicare-Medicaid enrollment and age, 2007–2015 [data table]. Retrieved from https://www.cms.gov/Research-Statistics-Data-and-Systems/Statistics-Trends-and-Reports/Chronic-Conditions/Downloads/MCC_Prev_State_County_All.zip

Heller, T., Janicki, M., Hammel, J., & Factor, A. (2002). *Promoting healthy aging, family support, and age-friendly communities for persons aging with developmental disabilities: Report of the 2001 Invitational Research Symposium on Aging with Developmental Disabilities.* Chicago, IL: Rehabilitation Research and Training Center on Aging with Developmental Disabilities, Department of Disability and Human Development, University of Illinois at Chicago.

Kaiser Family Foundation. (n.d.). *Total number of Medicare beneficiaries, 2015* [data set]. Menlo Park, CA: Kaiser Family Foundation. Retrieved from http://www.kff.org/medicare/state-indicator/total-medicare-beneficiaries/?currentTimeframe=0&sortModel=%7B%22colId%22:%22Location%22,%22sort%22:%22asc%22%7D

McGinnis, J. M., Williams-Russo, P., & Knickman, J. (2002). The case for more active policy attention to health promotion. *Health Affairs, 21*(2), 78–93.

Medicare Payment Advisory Commission (MedPAC) & Medicaid and CHIP Payment and Access Commission (MACPAC). (2017). Beneficiaries dually eligible for Medicare and Medicaid: Data book. Retrieved from http://www.medpac.gov/docs/default-source/publications/jan17_medpac_macpac_dualsdatabook.pdf?sfvrsn=0

Mutchler, J. E., Li, Y., & Xu, P. (2016). *Living below the line: Economic insecurity and older Americans insecurity in the states 2016.* Paper 13. Boston, MA: University of

Massachusetts. Center for Social and Demographic Research on Aging Publications. Retrieved from http://scholarworks.umb.edu/demographyofaging/13

O'Shaughnessy, C. V. (2014). *The basics: National spending for long-term services and supports (LTSS), 2012.* Washington, DC: National Health Policy Forum. Retrieved from http://www.nhpf.org/library/the-basics/Basics_LTSS_03-27-14.pdf

Older Americans Behavioral Health Technical Assistance Center. (2012). Older Americans behavioral health needs: Series overview. U. S. Administration on Aging and Substance Abuse and Mental Health Services Administration. Retrieved from https://www.ncoa.org/wp-content/uploads/Series-Overview-Issue-Brief-1.pdf

Proctor, B. D., Semega, J. L., & Kollar, M. A. (2016). *Income and poverty in the United States: 2015.* Current Population Reports, P60-256. Washington, DC: U.S. Government Printing Office. Retrieved from https://www.census.gov/library/publications/2016/demo/p60-256.html

Social Security Administration. (2016). Income of the aged chartbook, 2014. SSA Publication No. 13-11727. Washington, DC: Social Security Administration. Retrieved from https://www.ssa.gov/policy/docs/chartbooks/income_aged/2014/iac14.pdf

U.S. Department of Health and Human Services. (2017). Annual update of the HHS poverty guidelines. *Federal Register, 82*(19), 8831–8832. Retrieved from https://www.gpo.gov/fdsys/pkg/FR-2017-01-31/pdf/2017-02076.pdf

U.S. Department of Health and Human Services (DHHS), Centers for Medicare and Medicaid Services (CMS). (2017). Medicare–Medicaid Coordination Office fiscal year 2016 report to Congress. Retrieved from https://www.cms.gov/Medicare-Medicaid-Coordination/Medicare-and-Medicaid-Coordination/Medicare-Medicaid-Coordination-Office/Downloads/MMCO_2016_RTC.pdf

CHAPTER 14

Targeting Older Persons for Optimal Team Care Outcomes

Jan Busby-Whitehead and Kathryn Hyer

CHAPTER OBJECTIVES

1. Define population aging as a public health challenge with profound implications for providers and systems of health care.
2. Specify the epidemiological comorbidity challenges associated with demographic changes.
3. Identify healthcare system changes that encourage population-based patient management and collaborative care.
4. Describe characteristics of older adults who would most likely benefit from interprofessional care.

KEY TERMS

Collaborative care/
 interprofessional care (IPC)
Comorbidity

Long-term supports
 and services

Palliative care

▶ Introduction

As efforts to improve population health for seniors while managing costs escalate, it is important to target the group of older persons most likely to benefit from team-based care.

This chapter first discusses the epidemiological challenges from the demographic changes facing the United States. It provides data on rates of chronic disease, functional limitations, and the need for home- and community-based supports to provide a rationale for why one primary care provider cannot manage the multiple needs of older adults without the assistance of other providers as part of a team. As our definition of team care, we use the terms **collaborative care** and **interprofessional care (IPC)** interchangeably when the following four components are present: (1) a multiprofessional approach to patient care, (2) structured management plans, (3) scheduled patient follow-ups, and (4) enhanced interprofessional communication. Collaborative care can be delivered by a multitude of providers across time and settings if these elements of collaboration are present.

This chapter also provides a brief discussion of the context in which IPC is provider—that is, the changing healthcare system. Our overview includes the incentives to coordinate care as the Medicare system moves from a fee-for-service approach to more "managed care" and accountable care organizations. These new systems of care have an infrastructure that include electronic health records accessible by providers, education modules for patients, and reimbursement models that all work to reinforce collaborative care approaches.

The chapter concludes by describing the characteristics of patients who would most likely benefit from participation in an evidence-based model of geriatric care, such as that discussed in the *Evidence-Based Models in Action That Work* chapter.

▶ Epidemiological Challenges of Demographic Changes

The aging of the U.S. population is expected to continue for the next 50 years: After the baby boomers turn 65 years of age, they will be followed on this path by the baby boom echo, the millennials. However, it is the demographic prospect of the increased numbers of the "oldest old"—adults older than 85 years—that will create more demand for geriatric team-based care.

Gerontologists teach that aging increases variability. Thus, some older adults surviving into old age will enjoy longevity without disability, whereas others are likely to have multiple chronic conditions with related disability and frailty. Those who need support to remain independent in the community will almost certainly require that multiple professionals work together and communicate effectively to provide optimal care.

The Rand Corporation (Buttorff, Ruder, & Bauman, 2017) has reported 60% of American adults have at least one chronic condition, and 42% have more than one condition. Among those 65 and older, 81% have multiple chronic conditions. The co-occurrence of multiple chronic conditions, termed **comorbidity**, occurs most often as adults age because the risk of acquiring most diseases increases with age. Statistics published by the Centers for Medicare and Medicaid Services (CMS, 2016) provide another view of comorbidity, presented in **FIGURE 14-1**. This figure provides ample evidence of the complexity of many older adults with comorbidity, but also demonstrates the clustering of multiple chronic conditions, especially heart disease.

Both the prevalence and the severity of chronic conditions increase with advancing age. The heterogeneous decline in all organ function that comes with greater age also affects the efficacy of treatments for these conditions. For example, patients experience changes in medication clearance rates owing to liver- and kidney-related changes, as well as changes in digestion and absorption of nutrients from foods. It is the age-related interactions that create the solo practitioner's challenge in medically managing the comorbidities, encouraging active patient self-management, determining how physical and functional changes affect the quality of life and treatments, and continuously adjusting referrals for community resources and for patient and caregiver support.

Comorbidity increases older adults' difficulties with functioning in the community—namely, the ability to continue to perform personal care

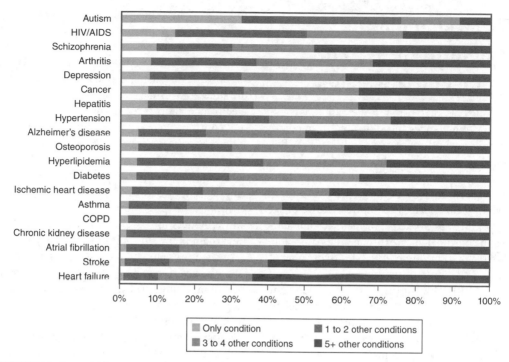

FIGURE 14-1 Comorbidity among chronic conditions.

Reproduced from Centers for Medicare & Medicaid Services. (2016). Chartbooks and charts. Retrieved from https://www.cms.gov/research-statistics-data-and-systems/statistics-trends-and-reports
/chronic-conditions/chartbook_charts.html

tasks or basic activities of daily living (BADLs; e.g., bathing and grooming) and instrumental activities of daily living (IADLs; e.g., difficulty shopping and cooking). Compromised functional ability is another hallmark of patients who likely require a team approach to care. As the number and severity of conditions increase, the patient may request help, or admit during a visit that the weight loss occurs because of an inability to get to the supermarket. Medical complexity may be difficult to manage, but many primary care providers do help patients coordinate their medical issues. However, as patients request help to remain in their community while facing disease progression and myriad psychological, social, and financial challenges, no one single practitioner can address those needs. When multiple providers are working with the same patient, a collaborative approach is required if the patient is to have a structured management plan, scheduled patient follow-ups, and enhanced interprofessional communication.

One chronic condition that dramatically increases with age—Alzheimer's dementia and related disorders—is especially burdensome for single practitioners. Figure 14-1, which displays data related to comorbidity among chronic conditions, shows that, in 2015, 50% of Medicare fee-for-service beneficiaries with Alzheimer's disease had at least five other medical conditions. Because Alzheimer's disease decreases cognitive functioning and limits the patient's ability to make decisions about care, it can take considerable time to help a patient and his or her family cope with the diagnosis. As the illness progresses, the person with dementia requires substantial help—initially with cognitive tasks, and ultimately with all personal care. This progressive decline generally precludes the person's ability to live alone independently and creates considerable challenges for a medical practitioner to manage as a sole provider because of the need to coordinate social and **long-term supports and services** for the patient and/or the patient's family.

▶ The Changing Healthcare System and Practice Model

The longevity revolution (Butler, 2008) is a testimony to advances in public health, medical technology, and increased wealth. Nevertheless, studies of the healthcare costs associated with large numbers of sick and disabled individuals have raised questions about the value of some healthcare expenditures (Rowe et al., 2016). CMS has worked to increase accountability and coordinated care through the Affordable Care Act and multiple initiatives to encourage home- and community-based care.

FIGURE 14-2 highlights the movement away from a fee-for-service payment model, in which practitioners are paid for every service separately, and toward a value-based model with more bundled payments for outcomes of service (Conway, 2015). The fee-for-service system encourages fragmentation, has incentives for volume rather than value, and is becoming a less common method of payment. As the U.S. healthcare system has struggled to increase value, avoid bad outcomes, and enhance the patient's voice

in care, providers have moved into larger group practices such as medical homes and accountable care organizations. The evolving healthcare model of the future encourages large provider groups and, increasingly, systems where patients are situated within a managed care system with electronic health records and more integrated and coordinated care. This emphasis on value, integrated care, and outcomes has created new models of care that segment older adults into different groups requiring different types of collaborative care. Ultimately, segmentation may encourage the provision of healthcare coaches and providers for older adults who are well to help them maintain their healthy lifestyle.

Medicare's annual wellness visit and chronic care management payments exemplify the new payment model and the movement toward population health. Both recognize the need to create baseline data and to manage both the population of active older adults who are well and those who need routine monitoring. This approach also moves the patient from a passive model of care where the patient receives information to an active model that emphasizes patient accountability/responsibility for care. Again, larger organizations can create more patient-centered knowledge through adoption

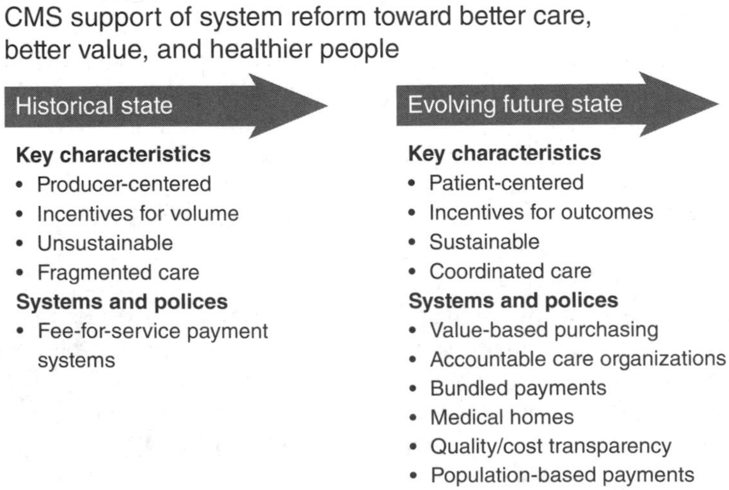

CMS support of system reform toward better care, better value, and healthier people

Historical state

Key characteristics
- Producer-centered
- Incentives for volume
- Unsustainable
- Fragmented care

Systems and polices
- Fee-for-service payment systems

Evolving future state

Key characteristics
- Patient-centered
- Incentives for outcomes
- Sustainable
- Coordinated care

Systems and polices
- Value-based purchasing
- Accountable care organizations
- Bundled payments
- Medical homes
- Quality/cost transparency
- Population-based payments

FIGURE 14-2 Changing practice model.

of electronic health records (EHRs) and development of patient educational materials. The elements that are essential to our definition of collaborative care—multiple professionals working on one coordinated plan of care, actively engaged with the patient, using electronic medical records to maintain "real-time records"—require interprofessional communication.

The need for a new paradigm of care of patients with complex medical conditions has led to the development of multiple models of geriatric, interprofessional team care. In the *Evidence-Based Models in Action That Work* chapter, examples of hospital-based, community-based, long-term care–based models as well as care transitions models are discussed. Models that focus on outcomes such as reduction in hospitalizations, emergency department visits, and nursing home admissions seem to be the most successful. Targeting those patients who will benefit the most from a chosen model can be challenging, yet is critical to the success of the program. No specific set of inclusion criteria has yet been validated for predicting the best results for any model. Of note, several models have been implemented primarily in the Veterans Administration system (e.g., Geriatric Evaluation and Management, GRACE, Home-Based Primary Care).

▶ Older Adults Most Likely to Benefit from Team Care

As the saying goes, "If you've seen one 75-year-old, you've seen one 75-year-old." The aging-related physiologic changes that occur with respect to body composition, organ decline and function, and illness burden are unique to each person. The 90-year-old patient with hypertension and no other comorbidities will not need the services of an interprofessional geriatrics team. How, then, to best target those elders who would benefit the most from participation in a geriatrics care model?

Elders with complex healthcare needs constitute a modest but growing proportion of the U.S. population that is generally responsible for a large percentage of healthcare costs. Most of the older adults in this group are Medicare beneficiaries with multiple chronic conditions, frequent hospitalizations, and difficulties performing BADLs and IADLs due to physical, mental, and/or psychosocial issues.

Studies (Buttorff et al., 2017; Meier, McCormick, Arnold, & Savarese, 2017) suggest that people with five or more chronic conditions and people at the end of life are particularly vulnerable and require more healthcare services and social supports as well as community resources if they are to remain safely in the community. A proxy for multiple comorbidities is the number of medications a person is taking. If that number is ten or more, the patient is at high risk for adverse drug events.

Other markers for at-risk elders include frequent visits to the emergency department and frequent hospitalizations. These events are more likely to occur with patients who have certain medical conditions, such as congestive heart failure, chronic obstructive pulmonary disease, renal failure, and certain types of cancer. Multiple falls, especially with injury, should be a red flag for the need for an interprofessional approach to an elder's care.

Dementia is another medical condition that should raise concern and encourage the provider to work with a team of professionals, especially if the older adult lives alone or with an aging spouse. The team of providers with knowledge of the patient's multiple needs can work to match those needs with long-term supports and services to meet them. The goal is to develop a coordinated care plan based on the home assessment, patient and caregiver abilities, the environment, and financial resources to enable the older adult to remain in the community as long as it is appropriate. Some programs have highlighted poor financial resources and difficulty with access to care due to living in a rural area as markers for elders who could benefit from team care. Disability requiring use of an assistive device and difficulty with driving are also markers for frailty. Elders who have any one or more of these conditions can be identified more easily now through the electronic health record.

Older adults who are living with serious illness or who are unlikely to benefit from acute care interventions are also prime targets for team-based care. Such a team is generally composed of doctors, nurses, social workers, and chaplains, but may have additional members depending upon the **palliative care** and/or hospice model delivering the care (Meier et al., 2017). Older adults or disabled individuals who are appropriate candidates for this care have agreed that the goal of care is to improve quality of life and relieve suffering while living with serious illness.

When working with patients, teams need to recognize the nonmedical issues that can contribute to poor health outcomes. Socioeconomic factors play an undisputed role in health, with those individuals who face a lifetime of racial discrimination and economic deprivation being at disproportionate risk for adverse health outcomes. Limited income and decreasing assets are common with increasing age; indeed, many older adults may be perceived as poorly adhering to medication regimens or having an appearance of self-neglect when the issue is actually limited finances. Severe financial stress and poverty place many older adults at risk for a myriad of other problems as well, including inadequate housing, limited access to food, poor transportation, and isolation from social services. Recognizing the interaction of financial well-being with health is critical for teams targeting older adults at risk for poor outcomes.

Another well-established component of elder well-being is maintaining meaningful relationships and social interactions. Loneliness or perceived social isolation is associated with poor physical health and increased depressive symptoms, including cognitive decline. Encouraging social engagement, increasing access to community services, and supporting strong social networks has been proven to have many physical and mental benefits. Those elderly persons living alone in the community are at increased risk for poor health outcomes and social isolation, especially if the older adult has limited finances and has a limited network of friends and family.

Finally, teams need to recognize the presence or potential for caregiver stress and attempt to support the many unpaid caregivers who assist elderly patients. At the same, they must recognize that many older adults may be at risk for elder abuse or financial exploitation from family or paid caregivers. All team members need to assess older adults for signs or symptoms of abuse and neglect and to be alert to this possibility when targeting adults at risk for poor outcomes.

▶ Summary

While achieving some success in dissemination, most of the geriatric interprofessional models of care have not yet been widely adopted. This hesitation among providers suggests that research to more clearly identify the older patients who will benefit the most and have better outcomes from coordinated team care is needed. Healthcare professionals who have practiced in interprofessional teams can attest to the benefits that accrue to individual patients and their own professional satisfaction in delivering coordinated care. As our healthcare system evolves toward a more population-based approach, the need for team care will grow.

References

Butler, R. N. (2008). The longevity revolution: The benefits and challenges of living a long life. *Public Affairs*, *1*, 576.

Buttorff, C., Ruder, T., & Bauman, M. (2017). *Multiple chronic conditions in the United States.* Santa Monica, CA: Rand. Retrieved from https://www.rand.org/content/dam/rand/pubs/tools/TL200/TL221/RAND_TL221.pdf

Centers for Medicare and Medicaid Services (CMS). (2016). *Chronic conditions among Medicare beneficiaries.* Retrieved from https://www.cms.gov/Research-Statistics-Data-and-Systems/Statistics-Trends-and-Reports/Chronic-Conditions/Downloads/2012Chartbook.pdf

Conway, P. (2015). Transforming health care delivery through the CMS innovation center: Better care, healthier people, and smarter spending. Centers for Medicare and Medicaid Services. Retrieved from https://blog.cms.gov/2017/01/05/transforming-health-care-delivery-through-the-cms-innovation-center/

Meier, D. E., McCormick, E., Arnold, R. M., & Savarese, D. M. (2017). Benefits, services, and models of subspecialty palliative care. Retrieved from http://www.uptodate.com /contents/benefits-services-and-models-of-subspecialty -palliative-care#H549034646

Rowe, J. W., Berkman, L., Fried, L., Fulmer, T., Jackson, J., Naylor, M., . . . Stone, R. (2016). *Preparing for better health and health care for an aging population. Vital Directions for Health and Health Care Series.* Washington, DC: National Academy of Medicine. Retrieved from https://nam .edu/wp-content/uploads/2016/09/Preparing-for-Better -Health-and-Health-Care-for-an-Aging-Population.pdf

CHAPTER 15

Developing and Managing a High-Functioning Interprofessional Team

Paul Andrew Jones and Eugenia L. Siegler

CHAPTER OBJECTIVES

1. Describe an interprofessional team and present evidence for its effectiveness.
2. Discuss the team-building process and resources needed to help build and maintain teams.
3. Examine the impact of technology on the interprofessional team.

KEY TERMS

Interprofessional team   Team formation   Virtual team

▶ Introduction

Because comprehensive geriatric assessment encompasses so many domains, providers with varied areas of expertise and different assessment skills often struggle to shape their observations into a complete picture of the individual patient.

The format that seems to best meld disparate points of view is the **interprofessional team**. Although formal interprofessional team training is the ideal means of ensuring high-quality care (Montagnini et al., 2014), there are many opportunities to learn team skills on the job, and with recent advances in patient safety, hospitals offer many opportunities to learn about and participate in teams. The *Community Team-Based Geriatric Care* chapter discusses team-based comprehensive geriatric assessment in the community; this chapter focuses on hospital-based teams.

CASE VIGNETTE

Daily rounds commence at 10:00 a.m.; this morning the geriatric physician assistant presents the case of a 94-year-old woman who fell at home and was brought in by her family overnight. Present are the attending physician, resident physician, primary nurse, nurse manager, physical therapist, care coordinator, social worker, and registered dietician. Each member of the team presents findings based on personal evaluation of the patient and/or interviews with family. The medical plan of care is presented by the resident and endorsed by the attending physician. The care coordinator and social worker lead a lively discussion of the patient's home environment and functional status based on the physical therapist's assessment, and the team plans her discharge based on these recommendations in concert with the patient's and family's wishes. All parties agree on an estimated day of discharge and the discussion moves to the next patient.

▶ What Are Teams?

Although we have granted the interprofessional team an almost mythic status, its very size and diversity often preclude it from functioning as efficiently or effectively as the one depicted in the preceding vignette. Nonetheless, teams offer the best opportunity to combine the expertise of multiple health professionals, and when they do work, they provide not just a forum for case discussion, but also emotional support for those who are caring for very needy patients.

Teams, which are described in both the medical and business literature, have been defined as "a small number of people with complementary skills who are committed to a common purpose, set of performance goals, and approach for which they hold themselves mutually accountable" (Katzenbach & Smith, 2005). Teams can be composed of members from one profession or several. We tend to reserve the term "interprofessional" for those multidisciplinary teams that show healthy—and even contentious—interactions when problem solving and that foster shared decision making (Siegler & Whitney, 1994). Although in casual usage, the two terms are interchangeable, "interprofessional" has more recently replaced "interdisciplinary"

to reflect the difference between the discipline, which is academic, and the profession, which denotes the actual practice (Parse, 2015). For consistency, we will use the term "interprofessional" in this chapter.

Interprofessional teams have been likened to marriages, in that they represent a union of different individuals and require attention and energy to maintain that union. Unlike married couples (ideally), members of teams come and go; although this turnover can add life and new ideas, it is inherently destabilizing and one of the greatest challenges to a team's growth and function.

▶ Evidence for the Effectiveness of Teams

Healthcare teams are most useful when they are responsible for patients with complex medical and social problems. Unfortunately, studies demonstrating that teams improve patient outcomes are notoriously difficult to conduct; proving the team is responsible for a positive effect may be nearly impossible when variables, such as mortality, may not be sensitive to measure teams' functionality (Pannick et al., 2015). In addition, the literature on interprofessional teams lacks consistent terminology and methods, and measured outcomes may be poorly chosen (Mosher & Kaboli, 2015).

A recent Cochrane review examined interprofessional collaboration (IPC) and the effects of practice-based interventions on professional practice and healthcare outcomes. After examining collaborative efforts such as interprofessional rounds, meetings, and similar interactions, three studies found some improvements in patient care and length of stay, while two other studies showed mixed results (Zwarenstein, Goldman, & Reeves, 2009). Two Cochrane reviews of collaborative, postoperative rehabilitation of patients who had experienced hip fractures were inconclusive because the studies in this area were sparse and subject to bias (Handoll, Cameron, Mak, & Finnegan, 2009; Smith et al., 2015). A systematic review of team-based care interventions on general medical units failed to show improvements in quality measures such as length of stay (LOS), mortality, or readmissions (Pannick et al., 2015).

Of the areas especially germane to inpatient geriatric teams, ACE (acute care for elders) units include interprofessional team rounds among their distinguishing features; other features include a prepared environment, patient-centered care, discharge planning, medical director review, and oversight of patient care (Boaden & Leaviss, 2000). ACE units appear to reduce costs, length of stay, readmission rates, delirium, and polypharmacy (Ahmed & Pearce, 2015) despite increased patient acuity, as measured by a case mix index (CMI) (Ahmed, Taylor, McDaniel, & Dyer, 2012).

Creating and Maintaining a Team

Healthcare teams are not a recent phenomenon. Those interested in the history of teams can consult a number of sources; Tsukuda (2000), in particular, offers an insightful view of teams' progress over the last century. She describes certain themes that, although not necessarily evidence based, recur throughout the literature (p. 33):

- Team care improves the quality of care.
- Successful teams must be developed; they do not just happen.
- Teamwork is difficult, requiring active learning and practice of specific knowledge and skills.
- Team development takes time.
- Teams need administrative and financial support to succeed.
- Team education must take place at all levels.

Practically speaking, although every team is unique and has its own life and history, team growth and development are to some degree predictable. Because teams are dynamic, understanding group process increases the likelihood that members can form and maintain a healthy team. Drinka and Clark (2000, pp. 18–27) described five phases of **team formation**:

- Forming: A team begins, and all participants are on good behavior.
- Norming: The team develops goals and a sense of purpose.
- Confronting: Conflicts that have been suppressed begin to surface; individuals begin to exert
- more power and to debate in a constructive manner.
- Performing: The team is at its most effective, efficient, and creative.
- Leaving: Individual members may depart or the team may disband.

These phases are neither unidirectional nor monolithic; teams can move back and forth between different phases, and individual team members may be in a different phase from the rest of the team. Such dynamics are essential, as teams work best if their members relate well to each other. In one example, a study of physician inpatient teams determined that teams with high relationship scores had lower complication rates and that trust and mindfulness were associated with fewer unnecessary LOS days (McAllister et al., 2014).

Team maintenance requires considerable effort, and clinicians must first determine whether a team will be a helpful addition to patient care. Once planned, creating the team and its forum for interaction requires a number of steps.

Determine the Purpose of the Team

Reasons to form teams include, but are not limited to, (1) development or modification of care plans, (2) teaching, (3) development of creative solutions for difficult problems, and (4) quality improvement and patient safety. Teams may have more than one purpose; many interprofessional teams serve both educational and care management functions. Participants must clearly understand the team's purpose(s) if they are to understand their own roles and to monitor the team's effectiveness.

Determine Whether a Team Is Necessary

Too often, we form teams because that is what geriatric specialists are supposed to do. Before starting a team, ask whether it is truly necessary. Keep in mind that teams are expensive. If an eight-member team meets weekly for an hour, can its members honestly say the team has accomplished the equivalent of a day's worth of work?

Determine the Team Membership in Advance

The purpose of the team should determine its membership. There is no advantage to including representatives from every discipline if they will not be active participants. Unlike outpatient assessment teams, which often have fixed membership and are composed of professionals, inpatient care teams often have rotating members, many of whom are trainees. A patient may receive care from multiple overlapping teams, including primary medical and consultative teams, a frequently changing nurse–intern dyad, and the interprofessional team that coordinates

care and prepares the patient for discharge. The latter team can include the unit patient care director (PCD; i.e., nurse manager), social worker, care coordinator, and dietician, along with the medical attending physician, resident, intern, physician assistant, physical therapist, and chaplain. Interprofessional rounds may end up with several dozen participants if all stay to hear every patient discussed.

Decide on the Frequency, Timing, Location, Structure, and Etiquette of Meetings

Convenience and a comfortable setting promote team effectiveness. Excessive informality does not.

Designate One Individual to Be Responsible for the Meetings

The organizer must determine which cases will be presented, who will present them, and which materials (charts, consultants' notes) must be available. This can be a responsibility designated to one individual, or it can rotate among individual team members.

Devote Some Meetings to the Team Itself

Like our relationships, gardens, or automobiles, teams require ongoing maintenance. Teams are composed of people who must devote real effort to create something that is useful, exciting, and fun. People can also be lazy, angry, tired, bored, uninterested, or even pathologic; such counterproductive behaviors can destroy any team. Only if time is devoted to self-examination can the team learn to identify its problems, solve them before they become intractable, and function well again. Because the PCD, social worker, and care coordinator may be the only fixed presences on an inpatient interprofessional team, they are often tasked with team maintenance functions; this responsibility can be especially challenging when physician teams may be under time pressures or fail to share the same priorities.

Technology's Role in Changing Teamwork

Although geographic localization is more conducive to team building and facilitates communication between team members, patients in a busy hospital are often boarded on a unit other than their home team's unit, necessitating creation of a **virtual team**. How do the virtual teams work together? Technology has affected team communication and promoted *virtual* teamwork in two major ways: through the electronic health record (EHR) and by promoting real-time communication via mobile technologies.

As part of the American Recovery and Reinvestment Act, eligible hospitals and providers qualified for financial incentives if they were able to demonstrate "meaningful use" of electronic health records to improve patient safety and quality of care, decrease health disparities, and increase patient and family engagement (Centers for Medicare and Medicaid Services, 2017). The EHR, which was originally designed to facilitate billing and order entry, has changed the way health professionals share information, evolving into a platform for communication that generates handoffs, information about quality measures, and general documentation about the patient's progress. Not surprisingly, the quality of those communications depends on the quality of the input.

Technology has also facilitated real-time communication through electronic devices, combining the convenience of mobile phones with the Health Insurance Portability and Accountability Act (HIPAA) compliance requirements for beepers (Patel, Siegler, Stromberg, Ravitz, & Hanson, 2016). With these applications, members of the interprofessional team can communicate, update, and touch base with each other throughout the day. Some preliminary data demonstrate improved outcomes with these modalities (Patel, Patel, et al., 2016), but they have not solved the problem of excessive interruptions and will not replace face-to-face discussion (Vaisman & Wu, 2017).

▶ Team Training

Ultimately, no technology can replace real teamwork, but training can certainly enhance even basic communication between teammates. Formal training in use of a structured communication tool for patient handoffs improves content and clarity of communication during telephone referrals (Marshall, Harrison, & Flanagan, 2009). A recent randomized controlled trial (RCT) simulation, which implemented an escalation of care training program for post graduate year 1 and post graduate year 2 (PGY1 and PGY2) surgeons, suggests formal training can decrease morbidity and mortality and increase recognition of errors (Johnston et al., 2016). Nevertheless, setting aside time for team process and training, although necessary, is not sufficient if team members do not know how to work together. Team skills are not intuitive; healthcare professionals must learn them.

A number of options for training and evaluation are available. **TABLE 15-1** summarizes the programs and gives information on how to access them.

Interprofessional Education

Not necessarily designed for team training, interprofessional education models build respect and collaborative skills by having students of different professions learn with and teach each other (Keijsers, 2016). The clinical impact of classroom-based team-building training has yet to be demonstrated. A systematic review examining the impact of interprofessional education (IPE) on professional practice, however, found some studies yielded improvements in the culture of emergency rooms and operating rooms and increased patient satisfaction. Other studies in the review reported mixed results or no impact of IPE (Reeves, Perrier, Goldman, Freeth, & Zwarenstein, 2013).

TABLE 15-1 Examples of Resources for Team Building and Effectiveness Assessment

Topic	Resource	URL
Team curricula, in-person training, online training	TeamSTEPPS (Agency for Healthcare Quality and Research)	https://www.ahrq.gov/teamstepps/index.html
Veterans Affairs On-Site Team Training	Rural Interdisciplinary Team Training Program	https://www.ruralhealth.va.gov/RITT-program.asp
	Veterans Affairs Clinical Team Training Program	https://www.patientsafety.va.gov/professionals/training/team.asp
Geriatric Team Training: Written Materials	Geriatric Interdisciplinary Team Training (GITT) Program (Hartford Institute for Geriatric Nursing, New York University)	https://consultgeri.org/education-training/e-learning-resources/geriatric-interdisciplinary-team-training-program-gitt
Team Training Simulation	Simulation Scenario Building Tools from University of Washington Center for Health Sciences Interprofessional Education, Research, and Practice	https://collaborate.uw.edu/ipe-teaching-resources/simulation-scenario-building/
Team Care Resource Center (e.g., articles, webinars, assessment tools)	National Center for Interprofessional Practice and Education (University of Minnesota)	https://nexusipe.org/informing/resource-center/
Train-the-Trainer Courses in Communication	Institute for Healthcare Communication	http://healthcarecomm.org/training/faculty-courses/
Journals	*Journal of Interprofessional Education & Practice* (Elsevier)	https://www.journals.elsevier.com/journal-of-interprofessional-education-and-practice
	Journal of Interprofessional Care (Taylor and Francis)	http://www.tandfonline.com/toc/ijic20/current
	Health and Interprofessional Practice (Pacific University Libraries)	http://commons.pacificu.edu/hip/
	Journal of Research in Interprofessional Practice and Education (Canadian Institute for Studies in Publishing Press)	http://www.jripe.org/index.php/journal

Team-Building Programs

Needless to say, formal team training is expensive and logistically cumbersome. Even when there is institutional support and time for training, gaining buy-in from all parties may be difficult. The experiences of the Geriatric Interdisciplinary Team Training (GITT) program reflect this; Reuben et al. (2004) documented that the "disciplinary split" (the "tradition, culture, and regulatory requirements" unique to each profession) remains a serious barrier to team training, with physicians, in particular, demonstrating the least enthusiasm for the process.

Finding ways to educate trainees in a cost-effective and efficient manner remains one of the greatest challenges for those who teach and work in teams. Table 15-1 lists a number of options. One of them, TeamSTEPPS, is an evidence-based teamwork system designed for healthcare professionals to improve communication and teamwork. The Department of Defense's Patient Safety Program developed TeamSTEPPS in partnership with the Agency for Healthcare Research and Quality (U.S. Department of Health and Human Services, 2017).

Measuring Team Effectiveness

Choosing the appropriate outcome measures to measure team effectiveness is difficult, and it requires a true understanding of exactly what the team is trying to improve. Reliable process measures are available to measure teamwork skills, and focusing on process may be an easier place to start (Havyer et al., 2016). Many of the programs listed in Table 15-1 provide information about measurement tools.

▶ Summary

Assessment tools are most useful when they guide subsequent decision making. The patient with complex healthcare needs who requires assessment in multiple domains presents special challenges; the identified needs may come into conflict or may be too overwhelming for a single provider to manage. By working together, providers may be able to devise solutions that none alone could have foreseen or implemented. That is the idea and the ideal behind the interprofessional team. Even experienced and motivated clinicians must expend significant energy creating and maintaining these teams, but those of us who love this kind of collaboration feel that we have been amply rewarded.

References

Ahmed, N. N., & Pearce, S. E. (2010). Acute care for the elderly: A literature review. *Population Health Management, 13*, 219–225.

Ahmed, N., Taylor, K., McDaniel, Y., & Dyer, C. B. (2012). The role of an acute care for the elderly unit in achieving hospital quality indicators while caring for frail hospitalized elders. *Population Health Management, 15*, 236–240.

Boaden, N., & Leaviss, J. (2000). Putting teamwork in context. *Medical Education, 34*, 921–927.

Centers for Medicare and Medicaid Services. (2017). Electronic health records (EHR) incentive programs. Retrieved from https://www.cms.gov/Regulations-and-Guidance/Legislation/EHRIncentivePrograms/index.html?redirect=/EHRIncentivePrograms/

Drinka, T. J. K., & Clark, P. G. (2000). *Health care teamwork: Interdisciplinary practice and teaching.* Westport, CT: Auburn House.

Handoll, H. H. G., Cameron, I. D., Mak, J. C. S., & Finnegan, T. P. (2009). Multidisciplinary rehabilitation for older people with hip fractures [Review]. *Cochrane Database of Systematic Reviews, 4*. Retrieved from http://onlinelibrary.wiley.com.proxy.wexler.hunter.cuny.edu/doi/10.1002/14651858.CD007125.pub2/epdf

Havyer, R. D., Nelson, D. R., Wingo, M. T., Comfere, N. I., Halvorsen, A. J., McDonald, F. S., & Reed, D. A. (2016). Addressing the interprofessional collaboration competencies of the association of American Medical Colleges: A systematic review of assessment instruments in undergraduate medical education. *Academic Medicine, 91*(6), 865–88.

Johnston, M. J., Arora, S., Philip, P. H., McCartan, N., Reissis, Y., Chana, P., & Darzi, A. (2016). Improving escalation of care: A double-blinded randomized controlled trial. *Annals of Surgery, 263*(3), 421–425.

Keijsers, C. J. P. W., Dreher, R., Tanner, S., Forde-Johnston, C., Thompson, S., & Education, T. S. I. G. (2016). Interprofessional education in geriatric medicine. *European Geriatric Medicine, 7*(4), 306–314.

Katzenbach, J. R., & Smith, D. K. (2005). The discipline of teams. *Harvard Business Review, 83*(7/8), 162–171.

Marshall, S., Harrison, J., & Flanagan, B. (2009). The teaching of a structured tool improves the clarity and content of interprofessional clinical communication. *Quality and Safety in Health Care, 18*, 137–140.

McAllister, C., Leykum, L. K., Lanham, H., Reisinger, H. S., Kohn, J. L., Palmer, R., . . . McDaniel, R. R. Jr. (2014). Relationships within inpatient physician housestaff teams and their association with hospitalized patient outcomes. *Journal of Hospital Medicine, 9*(12), 764–771.

Montagnini, M., Kaiser, R. M., Clark, P. G., Dodd, M. A., Goodwin, C., Periyakoil, V. S., . . . OngChansanchai, L. C. (2014). Position statement on interdisciplinary team training in geriatrics: An essential component of quality health care for older adults. *Journal of American Geriatrics Society, 62*(5), 961–965.

Mosher, H. J., & Kaboli, P. J. (2015). Inpatient interdisciplinary care: Can the goose lay some golden eggs? *JAMA Internal Medicine, 175*(8), 1298–1300.

Pannick, S., Davis, R., Ashrafian, H., Byrne, B. E., Beveridge, I., Athanasiou, T., Wachter, R. M., & Sevdalis, N. (2015). Effects of interdisciplinary team care interventions on general medical wards: A systematic review. *JAMA Internal Medicine, 175*(8), 1288–1298.

Parse, R. P. (2015). Interdisciplinary and interprofessional: What are the differences? Nursing Science Quarterly *28*(1), 5–6.

Patel, M. S., Patel, N., Small, D. S., Rosin, R., Rohrbach, J. I., Stromberg, N., . . . Asch., D. A. (2016). Change in length of stay and readmissions among hospitalized medical patients after inpatient medicine service adoption of mobile secure text messaging. *Journal of General Internal Medicine, 31*(8), 863–870.

Patel, N., Siegler, L. E., Stromberg, N., Ravitz, N., & Hanson, C. W. (2016). Perfect storm of inpatient communication needs and an innovative solution utilizing smartphones and secured messaging. *Applied Clinical Informatics Journal, 7*(3), 777–789.

Reeves, S., Perrier, L., Goldman, J., Freeth, D., & Zwarenstein, M. (2013). Interprofessional education: Effects on professional practice and healthcare outcomes (update) [Review]. *Cochrane Database of Systematic Reviews, 6*. Retrieved from http://onlinelibrary.wiley.com.proxy.wexler.hunter.cuny.edu/doi/10.1002/14651858.CD002213.pub3/epdf/abstract

Reuben, D. B., Levy-Storms, L., & Yee, M. N. (2004) Disciplinary split: A threat to geriatrics interdisciplinary team training. *Journal of American Geriatrics Society, 52*, 1000–1006.

Siegler, E. L., & Whitney, F. W. (1994). What is collaboration? In *Nurse–physician collaboration: Care of adults and the elderly* (pp. 3–10). New York, NY: Springer; 1994.

Smith, T. O., Hameed, Y. A., Cross, J. L., Henderson, C., Sahota, O., & Fox, C. (2015). Enhanced rehabilitation and care models for adults with dementia following hip fracture surgery [Review]. *Cochrane Database of Systematic Reviews, 6*. Retrieved from http://onlinelibrary.wiley.com.proxy.wexler.hunter.cuny.edu/doi/10.1002/14651858.CD010569.pub2/epdf

Tsukuda, R. A. (2000). A perspective on health care teams and team training. In E. L. Siegler, K. Hyer, T. Fulmer, & M. Mezey (Eds.), *Geriatric interdisciplinary team training* (pp. 21–37). New York, NY: Springer.

U.S. Department of Health and Human Services, Agency for Healthcare Research and Quality. (2017). Team STEPPS. Retrieved from https://www.ahrq.gov/teamstepps/index.html

Vaisman, A., & Wu, R. C. (2017). Analysis of smartphone interruptions on academic general internal medicine wards: Frequent interruptions may cause a "crisis mode" work climate. *Applied Clinical Informatics Journal, 8*(1), 1–11.

Zwarenstein, M., Goldman, J., & Reeves, S. (2009). Interprofessional collaboration: Effects of practice-based interventions on professional practice and healthcare outcomes [Review]. *Cochrane Database of Systematic Reviews, 3*. Retrieved from http://onlinelibrary.wiley.com.proxy.wexler.hunter.cuny.edu/doi/10.1002/14651858.CD000072.pub2/epdf

CHAPTER 16

Building on Geriatric Interdisciplinary Team Training (GITT)

Ellen Flaherty and Stephen J. Bartels

CHAPTER OBJECTIVES

1. Describe the Geriatric Interdisciplinary Team Training (GITT) program.
2. Describe the Geriatric Interprofessional Team Transformation in Primary Care (GITT-PC) model.
3. Recognize current challenges in primary care across the United States.
4. Define characteristics of effective high-functioning teams in primary care.

KEY TERMS

Geriatric Interdisciplinary
  Team Training
  (GITT)

Geriatric Interprofessional
  Team Transformation in
  Primary Care (GITT-PC)

Interprofessional
Quadruple Aim
Team transformation

▶ Introduction

The **Geriatric Interprofessional Team Transformation in Primary Care (GITT-PC)** is a model developed to deliver optimal care to older adults in primary care. This goal is accomplished through the implementation of practice change by assembling teams of health professionals in partnership with community service providers to meet the needs and preferences of patients and their families. These newly composed teams include patients, families, nurses, physicians, advanced practice nurses, physician assistants, clinical assistants, and community partners providing social services and supports.

To maximize uptake, this model focuses on systems and culture change in primary care, capitalizing on the role of nursing and other team members. Specifically, GITT-PC addresses four core components of high-quality geriatric care: (1) health promotion and prevention, (2) chronic disease management, (3) end-of-life care, and (4) dementia care. Emphasizing systems change and sustainability, the GITT-PC model advocates transformation corresponding to Medicare-reimbursable visits, including the annual wellness visit (AWV), chronic care management (CCM), advance care planning (ACP), and dementia care (DC). The successful implementation of these billable visits enables practices to provide evidence-based geriatric care while realizing a significant return on investment. This chapter describes the evolution of the GITT program from an academic training program to a sustainable model geared toward improving the care of older adults through a systematic **team transformation** process that makes a clear business case for primary care.

GITT-PC is an expansion of the John A. Hartford **Geriatric Interdisciplinary Team Training (GITT)** program, which was funded from 1994 to 1997 (Fulmer, Flaherty, & Hyer, 2003). GITT was designed to create training models to reflect the needs of the changing healthcare system and the challenge of caring for older adults with complex conditions. GITT trained more than 2500 students in medicine, nursing, and social work at eight academic medical centers across the United States in the 1990s in key team constructs (Fulmer et al., 2005). The foundation of the GITT-PC model builds on the lessons learned from GITT and the development of curricula and training materials is based on best practices.

GITT-PC focuses on transforming traditional primary care to embrace a new culture of **interprofessional**, team-based care of older adults. One of the tenets of this model is that to transform the work of primary care around geriatrics, it is necessary to first develop effective teams. Building these teams begins with team assessment and includes the restructuring of roles, task reallocation, and maximization of the skill sets of all team members. In addition, the implementation of the model requires an understanding of the process of improvement. The model then builds on the expertise of the high-functioning team to develop systems and processes in the practice of using Medicare reimbursement codes. Such a model is appealing to primary care practices that want to ensure best practices with regard to their geriatric patients but lack the capacity to transform the team without additional resources.

The three main components of the GITT-PC model are (1) team and quality improvement (QI) training; (2) subject content training in applying Medicare codes using a comprehensive toolkit that includes playbooks, checklists, and other materials; and (3) ongoing practice support, either in an elbow-to-elbow manner or through a learning collaborative. Training is delivered both face to face and through a web-based learning management system; it is broken into brief modules so that it is accessible to learners who need to be able to incorporate training within busy primary care environments. Modules include multimedia content, such as videos, reflective questions, interactive content, and competency quizzes, as well as a toolkit that functions as a playbook to walk practices through the changes necessary to effectively deliver and bill for services that are a proxy for good care for older adults.

While the motto of GITT was "Good teams don't just happen," the motto for GITT-PC is "Making it easy to do the right thing."

▶ Why GITT-PC?

The intention of the GITT-PC model is to support the transformation of primary care teams by helping them overcome the inherent challenges faced by primary care practices in caring for older adults. These challenges include (1) financial models that support a fee-for-service structure with rewards for procedures rather than preventive care and risk reduction for older adults; (2) critical workforce issues, especially in rural areas that lack primary care providers; (3) limited capacity to develop systems that support the delivery and reimbursement of Medicare-code services designed to support best geriatric practice in primary care; and (4) moving from a physician-centric model to a team-based approach to care.

Financial Challenges

The financial challenges of primary care contribute to the inability of practices to engage in practice transformation. Implementing substantive practice change requires an investment in staff time for team and quality improvement training that supports systems redesign. Additional support may be needed to enhance the capacity within the electronic medical records system to provide necessary data, coding, and auditing expertise. Implementing a person-centered model such as GITT-PC also requires the active participation of patients and families.

The financial challenges faced in primary care stem from an outdated fee-for-service payment system that is based primarily on the quantity of services delivered, not on the quality of care. Reimbursement based on volume (not value) forces practices into a frenzy of activity, booking schedules beyond their capacity, threatening practitioners' work–life balance, and contributing to team burnout. Primary care processes that rely on the physician, nurse practitioner, or physician assistant to see all patients are inefficient and lead to rushed office visits, causing patient dissatisfaction that cascades into frustration on the part of all team members. The GITT-PC model focuses on helping practices to maximize their revenue through team development, leading to task reallocation and maximizing revenues through the Medicare codes, while striving to bring joy back into the work of primary care.

Workforce Challenges

The many competing demands and suboptimal reimbursement in primary care have led to a significant shortage in this part of the U.S. healthcare workforce. Health professions students in both medicine and nursing are now choosing to practice in subspecialty care, rather than in primary care. For 2001, the data reflect the career plans for all third-year internal medicine residents, including categorical, primary care, medicine–pediatrics, and other tracks. Data for all other years reflect the career plans of third-year residents enrolled in categorical and primary care internal medicine programs. Data for 1998 through 2003 are from Garibaldi et al. Data for 2004 and 2005 are from Carol Popkave, American College of Physicians. NA denotes not applicable. These trends are concerning given the growing need for primary care for an aging population with an increased prevalence of chronic disease (Bodenheimer & Mason, 2017). Currently, in the United States, there is a gap between the population's need for primary care and the capacity of primary care to meet that need. The rate at which primary care physicians are entering the workforce is not matching the pace of retiring primary care physicians (Berra, 2011). The burden of caring for complex patients in the current models of care is resulting in widespread burnout in nursing, medicine, and other disciplines.

The GITT-PC model begins to address some of these workforce issues by improving staff satisfaction through team development and maximizing the role of all team members. Improving revenue streams by ensuring that Medicare codes match essential geriatric services also provides an opportunity to hire additional personnel, thereby helping to reduce burnout.

Medicare Codes

The Centers for Medicare and Medicaid Services provides reimbursement for primary care practices to deliver preventive and chronic care services including the following:

- The annual wellness visit focusing on health promotion and prevention
- Chronic care management supporting non-face-to-face time to monitor and coach Medicare recipients with two or more chronic conditions
- Advance care planning facilitating the implementation and documentation of conversations with patients leading to defined goals of care, including the development of advance directives and provider/clinician orders for life-sustaining treatments (physician orders for life-sustaining treatment [POLST], clinician orders for life-sustaining treatment [COLST], or medical orders for life-sustaining treatment [MOLST], depending on the state-specific documents)
- Dementia care focusing on the development of a comprehensive plan of care for patients with dementia

These codes were intended to provide added revenues to practices offering these evidence-based services to patients. However, the implementation and successful billing for these codes is challenging. Each of these codes has very specific components that require comprehensive documentation. Meeting the documentation requirements for these visits can be an overwhelming burden for practices that are not using standardized tools and templates. While some electronic health records (EHRs) have the capacity to support required documentation, other EHRs have competing requirements that unintentionally provide additional barriers to implementing and billing for these visits.

The GITT-PC model provides comprehensive support to practices enabling the implementation of and successful billing for these Medicare-reimbursable services. In addition to the team development, on-site training, and coaching, the playbooks and checklists embedded into the toolkit provide a path for practice transformation.

Teams

A wealth of evidence demonstrates the effectiveness of team-based care. Team-based care offers many potential advantages, including expanded access to care through more hours of coverage and shorter wait times. Team-based care can also be a more effective and efficient approach to deliver additional services that are essential to providing high-quality care, such as patient education, behavioral health, self-management support, and care coordination. Finally, team-based care is associated with increased job satisfaction, and an environment in which all medical and nonmedical professionals are encouraged to perform work matched to their abilities (Institute of Medicine, 2011). Fundamental to this approach is the belief that, when practices draw on the expertise of a variety of provider team members, patients are more likely to receive the care they need. In addition, a larger provider team might support quality improvement; with effective intrateam communication and problem solving, practices can engage in data-driven, continuous quality improvement.

Better understanding of how to accelerate good team practice is an urgent need given the demographic imperative and the changing nature of healthcare delivery. Principles of team-based health care include shared goals, clear roles, mutual trust, effective communication, and measurable processes and outcomes. By fulfilling the expectations of effective teams, a practice can ensure that care goals and care planning emphasize the particular needs of an individual older adult.

While the evidence suggests that effective team care improves patient outcomes and overall staff satisfaction, creating and sustaining highly effective teams is challenging. As previously described, workforce issues may contribute to burnout and high rates of staff turnover, leading to poor team performance. Most team members have not engaged in formal team training. Moreover, teams are often created through a process of hiring and co-locating individuals without consideration of their work behavior styles.

Development of highly effective teams necessitates going beyond traditional team training. Team transformation requires an initial readiness assessment and training that focuses on improving communication, reducing conflict resolution, and defining roles and responsibilities so as to facilitate good teaming. GITT-PC provides practical tools and templates for effective team meetings, including agendas and process tools to help define roles such as timekeepers and facilitators. Before applying the GITT-PC model, however, primary care practices that are motivated to create high-functioning teams must assess their readiness to change, communication styles, and role development and must have an effective leader who is willing to rethink the systems of culture of the practice.

Moving away from traditional training, the GITT-PC model focuses on culture change to empower primary care teams to achieve best practices in geriatrics. The structure of this model begins with a focus on "teaming up" through didactic training, online self-paced interactive modules, and in-person team coaching that focuses on improving the effectiveness of primary care teams. Using the latest techniques in instructional design and professional case-based videos, teams learn and practice together to embed systematic change in practice while implementing the four Medicare reimbursement codes described earlier. The structure is designed to be practical, and includes team-based and practice assessments for busy primary care teams focusing on the principles of good teamwork while implementing a team-based approach to care.

▶ Implementation of GITT-PC

Successful adoption of the GITT-PC model requires (1) readiness and commitment to transform care, focusing on role expansion and task reallocation; (2) participation in day-long training sessions, including an initial kickoff and boot camps that focus on a step-by-step approach to implementing the four Medicare codes (AWV, CCM, ACP, and DC); and (3) participation in ongoing practice support through either elbow-to-elbow on-site coaching or participation in a learning collaborative lead by the Dartmouth Geriatrics Workforce Enhancement Program (GWEP) faculty from the Dartmouth Centers for Health and Aging. The model is built on the premise that primary care practices will achieve the best outcomes if they are engaged with patients and families to successfully implement and bill for specific Medicare visits. The following subsections outline the four Medicare reimbursement codes implemented through the GITT-PC model representing evidence-based best practice in geriatrics.

Annual Wellness Visit

Prevention services provided through the AWV are valuable for maintaining the quality of life and wellness of older adults. The foundation of geriatrics care is prevention that focuses on reducing risk factors associated with developing chronic health conditions and preventing adverse events associated with common health conditions. Payment for AWVs has been tied to addressing specific clinical content and implementing a health risk assessment (HRA) that covers 34 required elements, including demographics, health status, psychosocial and behavioral risk factors, activities/instrumental activities of daily living, and the development of a personalized health plan (Medicare Learning Network, 2017). When the Affordable Care Act (ACA) incorporated systematic financial support for team-based longitudinal health planning and prevention in AWVs, it created a long-awaited opportunity for primary care practices to re-engineer their practices.

Implementing AWVs with a registered nurse (RN)–run model provides a potential opportunity for achieving an enhanced return on investment, as the reimbursement for the RN-run visit is equal to the reimbursement when a physician or advanced practice nurse conducts the visit. The GITT-PC model supports practice transformation focusing on team development with task reallocation and role development to implement the RN AWV, thereby allowing providers to manage patients in need of a higher level of decision making and resulting in visits with higher revenue generation (Medicare Learning Network, 2017).

Chronic Care Management

The Centers for Medicare and Medicaid Services (CMS) recognizes chronic care management as an essential component of primary care that contributes to better coordination of care for individuals with two or more chronic conditions. CCM focuses on non-face-to-face communication with patients to monitor and support patients in their management of chronic conditions in between office visits. It addresses continuity of care, with the goal of reducing patient costs and number of hospitalizations and emergency care visits, and is implemented using a team approach.

The GITT-PC model supports the implementation of CCM using a team-based model. Team members (including registered nurses, licensed practical nurses, and medical assistants) provide the non-face-to-face communication with the patients, families, and community-based organizations in collaboration with the providers to execute a plan of care that is developed by the team (Medicare Learning Network, 2016b).

Advance Care Planning

On January 1, 2016, CMS began to reimburse for advance care planning when delivered as a service for traditional Medicare beneficiaries. The ACP code supports the face-to-face time that a physician or other qualified healthcare professional spends with a patient, family member, or surrogate to explain and discuss advance directives. Nurses and social workers on a primary care team are qualified to engage patients and families in these conversations and contribute to the visit that is billed by the provider.

GITT-PC provides support to practices through workflow and standardized documentation to ensure the successful billing of ACP codes. These visits focus on working with patients to establish healthcare proxies, durable power of attorney for health care, living wills, and/or POLST. Successful billing for these codes may include introducing standardized forms that may be completed during or after the visit (Medicare Learning Network, 2016a).

Dementia Care and Coding

Medicare reimbursement for dementia care came into effect on January 1, 2017. This code provides reimbursement to physicians and other eligible billing practitioners for a clinical visit that results in a comprehensive dementia care plan. The documentation for billing requires a multidimensional assessment that includes cognition, function, and safety; evaluation of neuropsychiatric and behavioral symptoms; review and reconciliation of medications; and assessment of the needs of the patient's caregiver. The recommendations for this assessment derive from a broad consensus about good clinical practice, informed by intervention trials and emphasizing validated assessment tools that can be implemented in routine clinical care across the United States (Alzheimer's Association, 2016). These components are central to informing, designing, and delivering a care plan suitable for patients with cognitive impairment and can be conducted through a team approach. Nurses, social workers, and other ancillary staff can provide substantial support for the team in implementing this code. GITT-PC provides the support and structure for primary care practices to implement dementia coding through the development of team-based workflows with templated notes that include the evidence-based assessment tools representing good practice.

▶ Summary

As primary care increasingly demands more efficient and effective use of scarce resources, practices that are designed to rely on physician-delivered services are becoming unsustainable. New models of care are needed that focus on task reallocation, maximizing the capacity of team members' roles, and maximizing revenue. The current and projected healthcare workforce shortage, coupled with the aging of the U.S. population, mandate that care models be as efficient and effective as possible. Managing the complex syndromes experienced by frail older adults requires skills beyond the training of one discipline—it necessitates that multiple clinicians collaborate and communicate to provide optimal integrated care. The GITT-PC model was developed to address four concerns: (1) the urgent need for innovative models of care to meet the challenges of providing evidence-based primary care for older adults with complex conditions that incorporates patients, families, and community-based organizations in shared decision making; (2) strong evidence that highly effective teams are critical to create a needed culture shift in primary care; (3) the reality that highly effective team-based care depends on establishing structure, processes, knowledge, and support to create and sustain high-level function; and (4) an expanding role of nursing and other team members in primary care that is critical to transform primary care. The goal of this transformation is to ensure that the four elements of the **Quadruple Aim** are achieved: (1) improve population health, (2) increase patient and family satisfaction, (3) reduce per capita spending, and (4) improve the experience and meaning in the work of every member of the primary care team.

References

Alzheimer's Association, Expert Task Force. (2016, September 6). *Alzheimer's Association Expert Task Force consensus statement on CMS proposed billing code for the assessment and care planning for individuals with cognitive impairment.* Retrieved from http://act.alz.org/site/DocServer/Taskforce_Consensus_Statement_FINAL.pdf?docID=51841

Berra, A. (2011). Benchmarking clinical support staff in primary care sites. *The Blueprint Blog.* Washington, DC: Advisory Board Company.

Bodenheimer, T., & Mason, D. (2017). *Registered nurses: Partners in transforming primary care.* Proceedings of a conference sponsored by Josiah Macy Jr. Foundation, New York, NY, June 2016.

Fulmer, T., Flaherty, E., & Hyer, K. (2003). The Geriatric Interdisciplinary Team Training (GITT) program. *Gerontology & Geriatrics Education, 24*(2), 3–12.

Fulmer, T., Hyer, K., Flaherty, E., Mezey, M., Whitelaw, N., Jacobs, M., & Pfeiffer, E. (2005). Geriatric Interdisciplinary Team Training Program. *Journal of Aging and Health, 17*(4), 443–470.

Institute of Medicine, Committee on the Robert Wood Johnson Foundation Initiative on the Future of Nursing, at the Institute of Medicine. (2011). Transforming practice. In *The future of nursing: Leading change, advancing health.* Washington, DC: National Academies Press. Retrieved from https://www.ncbi.nlm.nih.gov/books/NBK209871/

Medicare Learning Network. (2016a). *Advance care planning.* ICN 909289. Retrieved from https://www.cms.gov/Outreach-and-Education/Medicare-Learning-Network-MLN/MLNProducts/Downloads/AdvanceCarePlanning.pdf

Medicare Learning Network. (2016b). *Chronic care management services.* ICN 909188. Retrieved from https://www.cms.gov/Outreach-and-Education/Medicare-Learning-Network-MLN/MLNProducts/Downloads/ChronicCareManagement.pdf

Medicare Learning Network. (2017). *The ABCs of the annual wellness visit (AWV).* ICN 905706. Retrieved from https://www.cms.gov/Outreach-and-Education/Medicare-Learning-Network-MLN/MLNProducts/downloads/AWV_chart_ICN905706.pdf

CHAPTER 17

Community Team-Based Geriatric Care

Cheryl Phillips

CHAPTER OBJECTIVES

1. Define team-based geriatric care, its evolution, and the role it plays in coordination of services.
2. Describe examples of community-based models of team-based care.
3. Identify barriers to team-based care in the community.
4. Summarize the potential future and role of community team-based approaches to geriatrics.

KEY TERMS

Alternative payment models
Chronic Care Model
Community care worker

Complex care management
Comprehensive geriatric
  assessment (CGA)

Interdisciplinary teams

▶ Introduction

The role of teams has been a foundational element of geriatrics since the mid-1970s. Although such teams were originally developed to manage the complex assessment and treatment needs of hospitalized psychiatric and rehabilitation patients, the transition to geriatrics, with the comprehensive scope of medical and functional challenges, was a natural one. The importance of community assessment is equally fundamental to geriatric health care. A basic tenet of geriatrics is that older people are not merely the sum of their diseases. Instead, their medical issues, disabilities, and abilities must be viewed in the context of their lives, their families and social networks, their environment, and their community. Older individuals' ability to adapt in the settings where they live greatly impacts their ability to remain independent.

Core to the evolution of the team-based approach was the introduction of the **comprehensive geriatric assessment** (**CGA**; Epstein et al., 1987). The CGA was used to integrate not just the medical issues, but also the formal assessment of function and cognition, behavioral health, and social support needs, and was most often applied to those persons identified as high risk or frail. Such an assessment typically involved the physician, nurse, social worker, and, depending on the presenting problems, a rehabilitation therapist, pharmacist, dietician, or psychiatrist. Other health professionals, such as dentists, podiatrists, and audiologists, were included based on the specific issues and availability of these clinicians.

The CGA was shown to improve care and survival for frail older people by identifying unrecognized syndromes such as incontinence and falls, and anticipating support needs that often delayed nursing home placement (Stuck et al., 1995; Stuck, Siu, Wieland, Adams, & Rubenstein, 1993). However, because of patients' limited access to the full array of health professionals necessary to complete the CGA, its use was primarily limited to teaching hospitals and Veterans Administration (VA) centers. Reimbursement of the nonphysician components to the assessment created even further challenges to the expansion of CGA in the outpatient and community settings.

Even the definition of *teams* has evolved over the past decades. Early hospital-based approaches to assessment often involved multiple health professionals acting independently, within the scope of their specific discipline, to provide contributions to the care management. Eventually, **interdisciplinary teams** emerged, based on the recognized value in having the various health professionals work collaboratively in the identification of problems and the development of a common plan of care to which each contributes. As these teams have matured, many have become *transdisciplinary* teams, in which the boundaries between disciplines are less important, and in which the team members *and*

the patient engage, teach, and learn together to both coordinate care and identify short- and long-term solutions in a holistic approach to the individual and his or her family.

In the early 1990s, a growing awareness recognized that the approach to care for older persons needed to focus more on the long-term needs of people with chronic conditions, rather than the short-term acute care interventions that had dominated health care for decades prior. At that time, the healthcare system revolved around episodic, acute interventions (e.g., hip surgery for fractures, coronary artery grafting for heart disease, or respiratory interventions for chronic lung disease provided in the intensive care unit), but few systems were in place to handle the longitudinal needs for people with those conditions that were not "curable," but rather progressive in nature. This acute care approach was chaotic, fragmented, and very expensive. As one suggested remedy, Wagner, Austin, and Von Korff (1996) described the **Chronic Care Model**, which provided a heuristic approach to the management of chronic illness. Specifically, this model called for a prepared team-based approach to care, and the coordination of community resources needed for support.

Ultimately, it was the rapid growth of Medicare managed care, in the form of Medicare health maintenance organizations (HMOs), that provided the fuel for team-based care for older patients enrolled in Medicare. The Economic and Social Research Institute, funded by the Pew Charitable Trust, published a comprehensive study of interdisciplinary geriatric teams as a strategy to address the rapidly rising medical costs for those beneficiaries with complex chronic care needs enrolled in Medicare Advantage healthcare plans (Regenstein, Meyer, & Bagby, 1998). This study evaluated the impact of these teams in reducing utilization rates and costs, primarily by avoiding hospitalizations and "unnecessary" expensive interventions. Because of the capitated payment structure adopted as part of managed care, a potential financial mechanism was available to cover the costs of the actual team—as long as the health plans could develop a reimbursement model for the team members that did not require traditional fee-for-service payments. Those delivery systems where providers were more likely to be salaried (e.g., the Veterans Administration, Kaiser Permanente in Northern California, and the Program of All-Inclusive Care for the Elderly) were much more likely to embrace this approach to geriatric care.

In recent years, an additional driver for the expansion of the team approach into community settings has been the focus on care transitions and the need to reduce hospital 30-day readmissions. Inspired by the 2009 *New England Journal of Medicine* article by Jencks, Williams, and Coleman, hospitals, health plans, and the Centers for Medicare and Medicaid Services (CMS) have focused on a 20% readmission rate as both a measure of quality and a potentially avoidable cost. Furthermore, Medicare's rapidly rising costs led policymakers to focus on the subpopulation of beneficiaries deemed "high cost and high risk"—that is, those patients with multiple complex chronic conditions who account for a disproportionate share of those costs. Multiple hospital systems and health plans looked to care transition teams as means to decrease the costs associated with those patients, and also developed a myriad of care coordination programs that focused on "**complex care management**" (McCarthy, Ryan, & Klein, 2015).

Evidence for the success of these care coordination teams has been mixed. Smaller provider-based case studies have demonstrated reduced hospitalization rates and reduced costs, particularly when the teams' efforts are targeted toward a very vulnerable or high-risk group—typically older persons with multiple comorbidities and functional limitations. An evaluation of the Medicare Coordinated Care Demonstration found that none of the 11 programs studied saved significant Medicare dollars (Brown et al., 2012). What this study did find, however, was that those programs were more likely to demonstrate benefits in the form of in-person evaluations; in-person meetings involving the coordinator, the patient, and the providers; use

of evidence-based education for the patients; medication management assistance; and comprehensive transitional care after hospitalization.

More recently, the focus of community care management has broadened to identify and coordinate care for not only those patients with complex medical conditions, but also those individuals with behavioral health needs and socioeconomic challenges. Atul Gawande (2011), in his seminal article in *The New Yorker* titled "The Hot Spotters," described the work of Dr. Jeffrey Brenner, who developed the Camden Coalition of Healthcare Providers, through which high-cost "super-utilizers" received team-based care in the community. This care focused on not only on the medical needs, but also the associated social supports—such as transportation, housing, and access to medications or even food—that these individuals needed.

Managed Medicaid plans have begun to realize that by applying this "hot spotting" approach, they can focus resources and teams on a very high-risk and costly population of older persons living in low-income or subsidized housing. These new models of community team-based care, which often include nursing and a service coordinator at the housing community, when collaborating with the primary care team, can reduce avoidable hospitalization and reduce the need for higher levels of care in institutional settings (Sanders et al., 2016).

▶ Targeting and Assessment

Successful community team-based care begins with identifying to whom to provide such care. Because the deployment of such teams is costly, both in dollars and in the workforce impact, at-risk populations must be identified or "targeted." Targeting is the strategy of screening those persons most likely to benefit from the team-based care and, therefore, most likely to demonstrate the sustainable impacts necessary to keep such programs afloat. Targeting is not identical to assessment. That is, targeting tells the organization or healthcare provider which individuals *may* be at risk, with formal assessment then evaluating that risk and identifying which medical or support needs are present. A number of strategies are used to target populations as risk, including specific medical conditions (e.g., heart failure), self-report surveys, provider referrals based on functional limitations (e.g., deficits in activities of living), and defined thresholds of healthcare utilization such as the number of hospitalizations or emergency department visits in the past 12 months, recent nursing home discharge, or even total costs of care over a given time frame.

Effective assessment for community-based teams involves a full evaluation of the whole person—that is, the individual's medical conditions and needs, including medications and nutrition; functional and cognitive status; social supports and environment; behavioral health; barriers to self-care such as limited transportation, poverty, or limited health literacy; and expressed goals of care and wishes (**TABLE 17-1**). In addition, special focus needs to be placed on areas that may be overlooked in busy primary care offices such as incontinence, sexual function, falls, oral care, or loss of hearing or vision. While it may be beneficial to include specific health professionals, such as pharmacists for medication review, dieticians for nutritional assessments, or therapists for specific areas of function, most of the domains of the community-based assessment may be completed by nurses or social workers.

Multiple standardized tools are readily available to assess these domains (Osterweil, Brummel-Smith, & Beck, 2000). It is important to remember that assessment, in and of itself, is not the goal. The purpose of the assessment is to identify opportunities where care and support services can be utilized to address needs, prevent avoidable decline, and develop a care plan with the person and his or her identified care partners. Thus, the assessment becomes the basis for the effective team-based care going forward.

TABLE 17-1 Domains of Community Assessment

Medical

- Problem list of medical issues (acute and chronic)
- Medications (including over-the-counter medications and supplements)
- Allergies
- Nutritional status
- Oral health, dentition

Behavioral Health

- Mood and anxiety
- Past behavioral health history
- Cognition

Function

- Activities of daily living
- Instrumental activities of daily living
- Life roles and activities of importance to the individual
- Fall risk and history
- Incontinence
- Hearing/vision loss
- Ability to self-manage medications

Social

- Need for and adequacy of caregivers
- Access to adequate nutrition
- Social activities and networks of importance to the person, risks for social isolation
- Finances and risk of poverty
- Health literacy

Environment

- Adequate housing, risk of homelessness
- Access to transportation

Self-Direction

- Advance care plans
- Expressed personal goals or preferences or care
- Surrogate decision makers

▶ Models of Effective Community Team-Based Care for Older Adults

A wide variety of community team-based care models have been developed (Boult et al., 2009). They may provide comprehensive primary care, such as the Program of All-Inclusive Care for the Elderly (PACE; Eng, Pedulla, Eleazer, McCann, & Fox, 1997) or Home-Based Primary Care (HBPC; De Jonge et al., 2014). They may work with primary and specialty care, such as the Geriatric Resources for Assessment and Care of Elders (GRACE; Counsell, Callahan, Tu, Stump, & Arling, 2009) or Guided Care (Boult et al., 2011) models. Alternatively, they may involve primary care interdisciplinary teams and nonclinical service providers as in Community Care Teams (Center for Health Care Strategies, 2016) and Vermont's Support and Services at Home (SASH) program (RTI International, 2014).

Nevertheless, all of these community team-based models have several elements in common. Specifically, they involve an interdisciplinary (sometimes transdisciplinary) team, and they utilize assessment approaches that include domains of function, cognition, behavioral health, and social support, in addition to the medical aspects of care alone. They are longitudinal in nature, rather than merely limited to an episode of illness or event. They involve coordination of care and information across settings. Finally, they all engage the individual in the development of the plan of care.

In reviewing several of these models (as well as others), Hong, Siegel, and Ferris (2014) identified common strategies for successful community care teams:

- The need to define case loads
- Use of telephone monitoring, in addition to in-person visits in the primary care office, hospital, emergency room, or home

- Structuring the composition of the team to reflect the needs of the population served
- Adding additional team members (e.g., behavior health providers, pharmacists) based on specific needs of individuals
- Meeting face-to-face as a team on regular intervals, with information technology used to share important information among team members
- Building trusting relationships with the care team and the individuals and their families

New models are also emerging, such as those that include nonclinical and direct care providers as the community focal point. **Community care workers** often align with medical home practices and help individuals navigate their insurance claims process, coordinate community-based services, and support communication with the medical team—all in a more culturally competent manner (Rosenthal et al., 2010). Some health plans are working with trained healthcare coaches in the home; these coaches use hand-held devices that capture answers to a core set of questions, which are then sent to a clinician or primary care provider to identify and triage those patients who may need additional care (Ostrovsky, 2014). The potential for including the unlicensed direct care worker, linked via technology to the clinical care team, further expands the whole concept of community-based team.

▶ Summary

The need for effective, integrated teams that can address the full scope of challenges for at-risk older people in the community is expected to continue to grow. **Alternative payment models**, such as managed care health plans, bundled payments, and accountable care organizations (ACOs), are pushing providers to identify "the right care, for the right patient, at the right time, in the right setting," and requiring that a fragmented delivery model evolve into one that is integrated and person-focused. In an April 2017 policy report, the Bipartisan Policy

Center proposed a number of strategies to better incent non-Medicare-covered community supports through improved risk adjustment, quality measures, waivers, and other means to tailor integrated care for high-risk, high-cost Medicare patients. This transformation will require competent and prepared teams, as well as payment models that support these teams and information systems that can connect them. Furthermore, healthcare delivery and payment models will need to have the flexibility to allow "interventions" that move beyond traditional medical services to include community supports, personal care workers, case managers, coaches, and drivers, just to name a few. All of these resources need to become part of the community care teams focused on person-centered care and goals where people live for the 360 days a year they are not in the hospital.

References

Bipartisan Policy Center. (2017, April). *Improving care for high-need, high-cost Medicare patients.* Retrieved from https://bipartisanpolicy.org/library/improving-care-for-high-need-high-cost-medicare-patients/

Boult, C., Green, A. F., Boult, L., Pacala, J. T., Snyder, C., & Leff, B. (2009). Successful models of comprehensive care for older adults with chronic conditions: Evidence for the Institute of Medicine's "retooling for an aging America" report. *Journal of the American Geriatrics Society, 57*(12), 2328–2337. doi: 10.111/j.1532-5415.2009.02571.x

Boult, C., Reider, L., Leff, B., Frick, K. D., Boyd, C. M., Wolff, J. L., . . . Scharfstein, D. O. (2011). The effect of guided care teams on the use of health services. *Archives of Internal Medicine, 171*(5), 460–466. doi: 10.1001/archinternalmed.2010.540

Brown, R. S., Peikes, D., Peterson, G., Schore, J., & Razafindrakoto, C. M. (2012). Six features of Medicare coordinated care demonstration programs that cut hospital admissions of high-risk patients. *Health Affairs, 31*(6), 1156–1166. doi: 10.1377/hlthaff.2012.0393

Center for Health Care Strategies, State Health Access Data Assistance Center. (2016, March). *Community care teams: An overview of state approaches.* Retrieved from https://www.chcs.org/resource/community-care-teams-overview-state-approaches/

Counsell, S. R., Callahan, C. M., Tu, W., Stump, T. E., & Arling, G. W. (2009). Cost analysis of the geriatric resources for assessment and care of elders care management intervention. *Journal of the American Geriatrics Society, 57*(8), 1420–1426. doi: 10.1111/j.1532-5415.2009.02383.x

De Jonge, K. E., Jamshed, N., Gilden, D., Kubisiak, J., Bruce, S. R., & Taler, G. (2014). Effects of home-based primary care on Medicare costs in high-risk elders. *Journal of the American Geriatrics Society, 62*(10), 1825–1831. doi: 10.111/jgs.12974

Eng, C., Pedulla, J., Eleazer, P. G., McCann, R., & Fox, N. (1997). Program of All-Inclusive Care for the Elderly (PACE): An innovative model of integrated geriatric care and financing. *Journal of the American Geriatrics Society, 54*(2), 223–244. doi: 10.1111/j.1532-5415.1997.tb04513.x

Epstein, A. M., Hall, J. A., Besdine, R., Cumella, E. Jr., Feldstein, M., McNeil, B. J., & Rowe, J. W. (1987). The emergence of geriatric assessment units: The "new technology of geriatrics." *Annals of Internal Medicine, 106*(2), 299–303. doi: 10.7326/0003-4819-106-2-299

Gawande, A. (2011, January 24). The hot spotters: Can we lower medical costs by giving the neediest patients better care? *New Yorker.* Retrieved from http://www.newyorker.com/magazine/2011/01/24/the-hot-spotters

Hong, C. S., Siegel, A. L., & Ferris, T. G. (2014, August). *Caring for high-need, high-cost patients: What makes for a successful care management program?* Retrieved from http://www.commonwealthfund.org/publications/issue-briefs/2014/aug/high-need-high-cost-patients

Jencks, S. F., Williams, M. V., & Coleman, E. A. (2009). Rehospitalizations among patients in the Medicare fee-for-service program. *New England Journal of Medicine, 360*(14), 1418–1428. doi: 10.1056/NEJMsa0803563

McCarthy, D., Ryan, J., & Klein, S. (2015, October). *Models of care for high-need, high-cost patients: An evidence synthesis.* Retrieved from http://www.commonwealthfund.org/publications/issue-briefs/2015/oct/care-high-need-high-cost-patients

Osterweil, D., Brummel-Smith, K., & Beck, J.(2000). *Comprehensive geriatric assessment.* New York, NY: McGraw-Hill.

Ostrovsky, A. (2014, July 30). Community-based health coaches and care coordinators reduce readmissions using information technology to identify and support at-risk Medicare patients after discharge. Retrieved from https://innovations.ahrq.gov/profiles/community-based-health-coaches-and-care-coordinators-reduce-readmissions-using-information

Regenstein, M., Meyer, J. A., & Bagby, N. (1998, March). *Geriatric teams in managed care organizations: A promising strategy for costs and outcomes.* Washington, DC: Economic and Social Research Institute.

Rosenthal, E. L., Brownstein, J. N., Rush, C. H., Hirsch, G. R., Willaert, A. M., Scott, J. R., . . . Fox, D. J. (2010). Community health workers: Part of the solution. *Health Affairs, 29*(7), 1338–1341. doi: 10.1377/hlthaff.2010.0081

RTI International. (2014, September 1). *Support and Services at Home (SASH) evaluation: First annual report.* Prepared for Office of Disability, Aging and Long-Term Care Policy Office of the Assistant Secretary for Planning and Evaluation U.S Department of Health and Human

Services. Retrieved from https://aspe.hhs.gov/execsum /support-and-services-home-sash-evaluation-first -annual-report

Sanders, A., Smathers, K., Patterson, T., Stone, R., Kahn, J., Marshall, J., & Alecxih, L. (2016). *Affordable senior housing plus services: What's the value? Examining the association between available onsite services and health care use and spending.* Retrieved from https://www.leadingage .org/research-projects/senior-housing-plus-services -whats-value

Stuck, A. E., Aronow, H. U., Steiner, A., Alessi, C. A., Büla, C. J., Gold, M. N., . . . Beck, J. C. (1995). A trial of annual in-home comprehensive geriatric assessments for elderly people living in the community. *New England Journal of Medicine, 333*(18), 1184–1189. doi: 10.1056 /NEJM199511023331805

Stuck, A. E., Siu, A. L., Wieland, D., Adams, J., & Rubenstein, L. Z. (1993). Comprehensive geriatric assessment: A meta-analysis of controlled trials. *Lancet, 342*(8878), 1032–1036. doi: 10.1016/0140-6736(93)92884-V

Wagner, E. H., Austin, B. T., & Von Korff, M. (1996). Organizing care for patients with chronic illness. *Millbank Quarterly, 74*(4), 511–544. doi: 10.2307/3350391

CHAPTER 18

Effects of Team Care on Quality and Outcomes

David B. Reuben

▶ Introduction

As the baby-boom generation has aged and people are living longer, the financial and personal costs of chronic disease for individuals, healthcare providers and systems, and insurers has grown. Moreover, multimorbidity (also referred to as multiple chronic conditions) is exceedingly common in the geriatric population,

with more than half of all older adults living with three or more chronic conditions ("Guiding Principles for the Care of Older Adults with Multimorbidity," 2012). Twentieth-century models of solo and small-group practice of medicine cannot meet the complex needs of this population and have become dysfunctional in providing the care that is necessary today. Despite advances in diagnostics and therapeutics, the quality of care for older persons remains poor, fragmented, and often expensive both for the governmental programs that pay for care and for the older patients who must expend personal resources on such care.

Simultaneously, increased administrative work generated by the electronic health record (EHR) and other documentation regulations has reduced the amount of time available to address patient concerns and manage chronic conditions. Although intended to facilitate the quality and efficiency of care, the EHR has proved to be a disruptive technology that consumes more of providers' time than the actual provision of care (Sinsky et al., 2016).

Recognizing the inadequacies of current care of older persons, the Centers for Medicare and Medicaid Services has established the "Triple Aim" of (1) improving individual health, (2) improving population health, and (3) decreasing health care costs (Berwick, Nolan, & Whittington, 2008). In response to this call for better, more effective delivery of health care, **team care** has emerged as a potential solution for improving efficiency and quality of care. At the simplest level, team care entails multiple health professionals or para-professional staff working together to provide high-quality patient care.

Within this broad definition, however, team care can vary in terms of how teams are convened (membership and size) and function (roles, responsibilities, and communication). At one extreme is delegation—that is, the transfer of specified tasks from highly skilled and professionals to other staff. For example, care partners or certified nursing assistants frequently assist hospital nurses in many tasks, pharmacy technicians mix medicines and give patients instructions, and physical therapy assistants implement rehabilitation plans under the supervision of a physical therapist. Delegation often follows a "top down" approach, in which the opinions of assistive personnel may be sought to identify work that they would be able to assume but the specification of tasks and responsibilities usually is determined by managers. At the other extreme,

collaborative team care is characterized by the recognition and contribution of various disciplines in creating and implementing planned care to manage the health care and medical conditions of older persons. Both approaches may use protocols or guidelines to allow team members other than physicians to adjust plans of care, such as titrating blood pressure or diabetes medication dosages in response to preset care parameters. Both approaches have value in improving the quality of care, and some models have also demonstrated better clinical outcomes and lower costs. Moreover, many hybrid models incorporate elements of both delegation and **collaborative care**.

In addition, team care can be based within the health system, in the community, or both. Although successful team care models have been implemented in hospital and post-acute settings (both in the home and in skilled nursing facilities), this chapter focuses on teams in outpatient care and in-home primary care models. The goal of all forms of team care is to have all professionals work at the very top of their license and competencies as part of an interdisciplinary approach geared toward meeting the needs of vulnerable older adults.

▶ Best Practices

In a series of studies, the Assessing Care of Vulnerable Elders (ACOVE) researchers first defined quality for common geriatric conditions and then aimed to improve it and the resulting clinical outcomes through the ACOVE-2 model. This structured intervention includes case finding, delegated clinical data collection, structured visit notes, primary care provider and patient education, and linkage to community resources (Reuben, Roth, Kamberg, & Wenger, 2003). Delegation of specific care processes includes components such as measurement of orthostatic blood pressures and visual testing in persons who report falling as well as cognitive screening. Implementation of this model has improved quality of care for geriatric conditions in primary care (Wenger et al., 2010; Wenger et al., 2009). Moreover, in a pooled analysis of eight studies using ACOVE quality indicators, delegation improved the quality of care provided for three common geriatric conditions—falls, urinary incontinence, and dementia—and a secondary analysis suggested that more delegation is possible and might result in higher quality scores (Lichtenstein et al., 2015).

Another example of delegation has been an effort to reduce the burden of the EHR by using scribes. Although the effects of scribes on quality and clinical outcomes have not been well defined, studies in geriatrics as well as internal medicine practices have demonstrated that they save time and are associated with some increased patient satisfaction (Reuben, Knudsen, Senelick, Glazier, & Koretz, 2014; Reuben, Miller, Glazier, & Koretz, 2016).

In contrast, other models of team-based care which focus on chronic care management, including disease management and care coordination (Berwick et al., 2008; Boyd et al., 2007; Counsell et al., 2007; Unutzer et al., 2002), have been developed to improve quality and outcomes while containing costs. The various models differ with respect to the level of professional (e.g., registered nurses versus nurse practitioners) and the size of teams. Some teams have several members representing a variety of disciplines, whereas others have only two members—a primary care provider (PCP)[1] and another health professional. They also differ in whether the team is advisory or has order-writing capabilities; in this chapter, the latter model is referred to as "**co-management**." In these models, care is often organized around a care plan in which problems and approaches to management are recorded; shared with the healthcare team, patient, and, often, family; and used to implement and monitor management. A history of the development of team care is presented in the

Community Team-Based Geriatric Care chapter. Models are described in the *Evidence-Based Models in Action That Work* chapter, and some paradigm examples are noted here.

Improving Mood–Promoting Access to Collaborative Treatment

Improving Mood–Promoting Access to Collaborative Treatment (IMPACT) is a collaborative care model for the management of older persons with depression (Boyd et al., 2007; Gilbody, Bower, Fletcher, Richards, & Sutton, 2006; Jacob et al., 2012). IMPACT and other collaborative care models for depression include case managers—usually nurses or psychologists—who support PCPs by educating patients, discussing patient preferences for treatment (e.g., antidepressants versus psychotherapy), recommending treatments based on algorithms, following up to monitor adherence to treatment and response, and adjusting treatment plans for patients who do not respond. PCPs are usually responsible for routine screening and diagnosis of depressive disorders, prescribing antidepressants, and referring patients to mental health specialists as needed. Mental health specialists provide clinical advice and decision support to PCPs, often through in-person meetings. Care processes and communication are frequently coordinated and supported by EHRs, telephone support, and provider reminder mechanisms.

The IMPACT model has resulted in higher rates of depression treatment, reductions in depressive symptoms, more satisfaction with depression care, less functional impairment, and better quality of life. A meta-analysis that included trials of collaborative care for depression of persons of all ages found robust effects

---

1 Health professionals other than physicians may provide primary and specialty care; throughout the remainder of the chapter, the term PCP refers to clinicians who may be a primary care or specialty physician or a mid-level clinician providing primary care.

of this model in improving adherence to treatment, depression symptoms, quality of life/functional status, and satisfaction with care (Thota et al., 2012).

More recently, team-based care integrating physical and mental health using process-of-care protocols and a common EHR had benefits on outcomes beyond metal health. Those benefits included improved adherence to diabetes care and better hypertension control as well as fewer emergency department visits and hospital admissions (Reiss-Brennan et al., 2016).

Co-management

With increasing recognition of the specialized knowledge and skills required to effectively manage specific geriatric conditions as well as the need to implement care processes that may be time-consuming (e.g., patient and caregiver education and referrals), models of co-management have emerged. These models usually rely on nurse practitioners or registered nurses. As noted earlier, these models differ from the team care models described previously in that the co-management team members can usually write orders (sometimes using standing order sets or protocols) and are often responsible for making medication adjustments, while keeping PCPs informed.

A meta-analysis of nurse-led management of common medical conditions (not specific to geriatric patients) demonstrated that for the management of hypertension, dyslipidemia, and diabetes mellitus, nurse-managed protocols result in small but significant improvements in secondary outcomes for patients, including blood pressure control, cholesterol levels, and hemoglobin A1c measurements (Shaw et al., 2014). Other geriatrics-specific programs have relied on nurse practitioners to co-manage multiple (Ganz et al., 2010) or single conditions (e.g., dementia). Several of these models have resulted in substantial improvements in quality of care. For example, one study of nurse practitioner co-management of five conditions of care resulted in quality scores for falls, incontinence, and dementia that were 22 to 50 percentage points

higher than in those for patients receiving usual care provided by physicians alone (Reuben, Ganz, et al., 2013).

A nurse practitioner-led dementia co-management program at the University of Indiana includes periodic needs assessment and evaluation of ongoing therapy, self-management tools to manage symptoms and navigate the health care system, pharmacological interventions, and case management and coordination with community resources. This program has demonstrated benefits related to quality, clinical outcomes (Callahan et al., 2006), and costs (Callahan et al., 2011).

Another dementia co-management model, the UCLA Alzheimer's and Dementia Care program, also utilizes nurse practitioner "dementia care managers." This program provides for structured needs assessments of patients and their caregivers, creation and implementation of individualized dementia care plans based on needs assessments, monitoring and revising care plans as needed, and 24/7/365 access to assistance and advice (Reuben, Evertson, et al., 2013). The quality of care for patients in the UCLA program has been very high, with scores exceeding 90% for most dementia quality indicators and overall quality of dementia care (Jennings et al., 2016).

Team care can also be based in the community and extend into the healthcare system. For example, the Benjamin Rose Institute Care Consultation model is a telephone care coaching program for patients with dementia and their family or friend caregivers that is based in the community and relies on bachelor's or master's degree–prepared social workers or nurses. This model has been associated with beneficial changes in psychosocial outcomes for both patients and caregivers (e.g., decreased symptoms of depression), embarrassment about memory problems, various forms of care-related and caregiving strains, and social isolation (Bass, Clark, Looman, McCarthy, & Eckert, 2003; Clark, Bass, Looman, McCarthy, & Eckert, 2004). It has also been implemented in a joint collaboration with the Department of Veterans Affairs health system in which team members are based both within and outside the health system (Bass et al., 2013; Bass et al., 2014).

▶ Practice Challenges

Team care models have not been integrated into most practices. Some barriers to delegation include state and federal regulations about which types of providers can provide specific services. These range from laws specifically prohibiting the provision of some care processes by para-professionals to exclusions from reimbursement (e.g., noncertified staff cannot provide services billed under the Chronic Care Management code). However, much of the lack of adoption of delegated care may be due to reluctance by PCPs, other professionals, and administrators, who may perceive their staff as being unable or too busy to perform additional data-gathering tasks.

An insufficiently prepared workforce is another barrier to team-based care. Historically, healthcare professionals have received little, if any, training in how to work in teams to provide care. In the John A. Hartford Foundation–supported Geriatric Interdisciplinary Team Training initiative, efforts to promote interdisciplinary team training were implemented in nine health systems. An important barrier to team training was "disciplinary split," referring to the attitudinal and cultural traditions of different health professions faculty and students (Reuben et al., 2004).

Chronic care management models also have barriers to diffusion and implementation. They often need to be adapted to fit the culture and resources of the adopting system, including the payer mix. Team members require infrastructure to support them (e.g., answering calls, scheduling) or they are likely to become inefficient, performing tasks that less expensive staff could do. Even in programs that achieve cost savings, an initial upfront investment in hiring and training personnel is required. Organizational readiness, institutional support, and structure have been identified as other key elements of success in geriatrics interdisciplinary team training (Reuben, Yee, et al., 2003).

To be implemented in some health systems, interventions may need to be modified. For example, using registered nurses rather than nurse practitioners as dementia care managers can reduce staffing costs and address access in areas that may lack advanced practice nurses. However, these reduced staff costs must be weighed against the loss of billable income that nurse practitioners can generate. Even the best models of care are rarely "shelf ready," such that modifications need to be made both prior to and after their implementation. Formal coaching by those who developed the models can be valuable in ensuring fidelity to the successful intervention by making certain that the core principles are retained in the adaptation and by providing experience of which modifications might be effective or ineffective (Ganz et al., 2016).

When developing approaches to team care, the following steps are important:

- Identify the problem being addressed. Is it a specific condition (e.g., falls, dementia) or overall care coordination (e.g., preventing readmissions, safe transitions)?
- Decide whether a team is the most effective approach. Sometimes an individual provider who has comprehensive understanding of the patient may be more effective and efficient than a team of providers.
- If team care is to be provided, plan how each member can work to the top of his or her capabilities or license. Think about how to make the care efficient and avoid duplication of effort.
- Get input from stakeholders, especially those who may be skeptical and may impede the program's progress by refusing to refer patients or ignoring the team's recommendations.
- Establish metrics to gauge success. Early on, these are likely to be quality measures. Improved clinical outcomes and reduced costs will take more time to demonstrate success.
- Expect false starts. Regardless of how many hours are spent sitting around a table and planning, no healthcare program ever works exactly as planned. Numerous decisions

must be made that require compromise between the intentions of design and the practicality of implementation. Even when implemented, surveillance is necessary; mid-course correction may turn a failure into success (Peikes, Peterson, Brown, Graff, & Lynch, 2012).

■ Get the word out about the program. Publish the results, and present them at every opportunity.

▶ Summary

With the growth of the elderly population, healthcare professionals and systems are having increasing difficulty meeting quality standards and achieving good clinical outcomes while containing costs. Team care approaches are valuable strategies to resolve these problems. The spectrum of team care ranges from delegation of less skilled tasks to comprehensive models that provide ongoing care management, in which multiple disciplines are involved in the design and implementation.

With the continuing desire of health systems to achieve the Triple Aim, it is likely that these models will be increasingly adapted and adopted, and new models will be created. These models will need to be evaluated in clinical trials and other research designs that include comparison groups. Moreover, adopting organizations should monitor implementation to ensure fidelity to the key elements of the intervention and reevaluate the program's effectiveness in their own institutions.

References

Bass, D. M., Clark, P. A., Looman, W. J., McCarthy, C. A., & Eckert, S. (2003). The Cleveland Alzheimer's managed care demonstration: Outcomes after 12 months of implementation. *Gerontologist, 43*(1), 73–85.

Bass, D. M., Judge, K. S., Snow, A. L., Wilson, N. L., Morgan, R., Looman, W. J., . . . Kunik, M. E. (2013). Caregiver outcomes of partners in dementia care: Effect of a care coordination program for veterans with dementia and their family members and friends. *Journal of the*

American Geriatrics Society, 61(8), 1377–1386. doi: 10.1111/jgs.12362

Bass, D. M., Judge, K. S., Snow, A. L., Wilson, N. L., Morgan, R. O., Maslow, K., . . . Kunik, M. E. (2014). A controlled trial of Partners in Dementia Care: Veteran outcomes after six and twelve months. *Alzheimer's Research & Therapy, 6*(1), 9. doi: 10.1186/alzrt242

Berwick, D. M., Nolan, T. W., & Whittington, J. (2008). The Triple Aim: Care, health, and cost. *Health Affairs (Millwood), 27*(3), 759–769. doi: 10.1377/hlthaff.27.3.759

Boyd, C. M., Boult, C., Shadmi, E., Leff, B., Brager, R., Dunbar, L., . . . Wegener, S. (2007). Guided care for multimorbid older adults. *Gerontologist, 47*(5), 697–704.

Callahan, C. M., Boustani, M. A., Unverzagt, F. W., Austrom, M. G., Damush, T. M., Perkins, A. J., . . . Hendrie, H. C. (2006). Effectiveness of collaborative care for older adults with Alzheimer disease in primary care: A randomized controlled trial. *Journal of the American Medical Association, 295*(18), 2148–2157. doi: 10.1001 /jama.295.18.2148

Callahan, C. M., Boustani, M. A., Weiner, M., Beck, R. A., Livin, L. R., Kellams, J. J., . . . Hendrie, H. C. (2011). Implementing dementia care models in primary care settings: The Aging Brain Care Medical Home. *Aging & Mental Health, 15*(1), 512. doi: 10.1080/13607861003801052

Clark, P. A., Bass, D. M., Looman, W. J., McCarthy, C. A., & Eckert, S. (2004). Outcomes for patients with dementia from the Cleveland Alzheimer's Managed Care Demonstration. *Aging & Mental Health, 8*(1), 40–51. doi: 10.1080/13607860310001613329

Counsell, S. R., Callahan, C. M., Clark, D. O., Tu, W., Buttar, A. B., Stump, T. E., & Ricketts, G. D. (2007). Geriatric care management for low-income seniors: A randomized controlled trial. *Journal of the American Medical Association, 298*(22), 2623–2633. doi: 10.1001 /jama.298.22.2623

Ganz, D., Ganz, D. A., Senelick, W., McCreath, H. E., Jew, J., Osterweil, D., . . . Reuben, D. B. (2016). A strategy for identifying and disseminating best practice innovations in the care of patients with multiple chronic conditions or end-of-life care needs. *Managed Care, 25*(7), 43–48.

Ganz, D. A., Koretz, B. K., Bail, J. K., McCreath, H. E., Wenger, N. S., Roth, C. P., & Reuben, D. B. (2010). Nurse practitioner comanagement for patients in an academic geriatric practice. *American Journal of Managed Care, 16*(12), e343–e355.

Gilbody, S., Bower, P., Fletcher, J., Richards, D., & Sutton, A. J. (2006). Collaborative care for depression: A cumulative meta-analysis and review of longer-term outcomes. *Archives of Internal Medicine, 166*(21), 2314–2321. doi: 10.1001/archinte.166.21.2314

Guiding principles for the care of older adults with multimorbidity: An approach for clinicians: American Geriatrics Society Expert Panel on the Care of Older Adults with Multimorbidity. (2012). *Journal of the American Geriatrics Society, 60*(10), e1–e25. doi: 10.1111/j.1532-5415.2012.04188.x

Jacob, V., Chattopadhyay, S. K., Sipe, T. A., Thota, A. B., Byard, G. J., Chapman, D. P., & Community Preventive Services Task Force. (2012). Economics of collaborative care for management of depressive disorders: A community guide systematic review. *American Journal of Preventive Medicine, 42*(5), 539–549. doi: 10.1016/j.amepre.2012.01.011

Jennings, L. A., Tan, Z., Wenger, N. S., Cook, E. A., Han, W., McCreath, H. E., . . . Reuben, D. B. (2016). Quality of care provided by a comprehensive dementia care comanagement program. *Journal of the American Geriatrics Society, 64*(8), 1724–1730. doi: 10.1111/jgs.14251

Lichtenstein, B. J., Reuben, D. B., Karlamangla, A. S., Han, W., Roth, C. P., & Wenger, N. S. (2015). Effect of physician delegation to other healthcare providers on the quality of care for geriatric conditions. *Journal of the American Geriatrics Society, 63*(10), 2164–2170. doi: 10.1111/jgs.13654

Peikes, D., Peterson, G., Brown, R. S., Graff, S., & Lynch, J. P. (2012). How changes in Washington University's Medicare coordinated care demonstration pilot ultimately achieved savings. *Health Affairs (Millwood), 31*(6), 1216–1226. doi: 10.1377/hlthaff.2011.0593

Reiss-Brennan, B., Brunisholz, K. D., Dredge, C., Briot, P., Grazier, K., Wilcox, A., . . . James, B. (2016). Association of integrated team-based care with health care quality, utilization, and cost. *Journal of the American Medical Association, 316*(8), 826–834. doi: 10.1001/jama.2016.11232

Reuben, D. B., Evertson, L. C., Wenger, N. S., Serrano, K., Chodosh, J., Ercoli, L., & Tan, Z. S. (2013). The University of California at Los Angeles Alzheimer's and Dementia Care program for comprehensive, coordinated, patient-centered care: Preliminary data. *Journal of the American Geriatrics Society, 61*(12), 2214–2218. doi: 10.1111/jgs.12562

Reuben, D. B., Ganz, D. A., Roth, C. P., McCreath, H. E., Ramirez, K. D., & Wenger, N. S. (2013). Effect of nurse practitioner comanagement on the care of geriatric conditions. *Journal of the American Geriatrics Society, 61*(6), 857–867. doi: 10.1111/jgs.12268

Reuben, D. B., Knudsen, J., Senelick, W., Glazier, E., & Koretz, B. K. (2014). The effect of a physician partner program on physician efficiency and patient satisfaction. *JAMA Internal Medicine, 174*(7), 1190–1193. doi: 10.1001/jamainternmed.2014.1315

Reuben, D. B., Levy-Storms, L., Yee, M. N., Lee, M., Cole, K., Waite, M., . . . Frank, J. C. (2004). Disciplinary split: A threat to geriatrics interdisciplinary team training. *Journal of the American Geriatrics Society, 52*(6), 1000–1006. doi: 10.1111/j.1532-5415.2004.52272.x

Reuben, D. B., Miller, N., Glazier, E., & Koretz, B. K. (2016). Frontline account: Physician partners: An antidote to the electronic health record. *Journal of General Internal Medicine, 31*(8), 961–963. doi: 10.1007/s11606-016-3727-x

Reuben, D. B., Roth, C., Kamberg, C., & Wenger, N. S. (2003). Restructuring primary care practices to manage geriatric syndromes: The ACOVE-2 intervention. *Journal of the American Geriatrics Society, 51*(12), 1787–1793.

Reuben, D. B., Yee, M. N., Cole, K. D., Waite, M. S., Nichols, L. O., Benjamin, B. A., . . . Frank, J. C. (2003). Organizational issues in establishing geriatrics interdisciplinary team training. *Gerontology & Geriatrics Education, 24*(2), 13–34.

Shaw, R. J., McDuffie, J. R., Hendrix, C. C., Edie, A., Lindsey-Davis, L., Nagi, A., . . . Williams, J. W. Jr. (2014). Effects of nurse-managed protocols in the outpatient management of adults with chronic conditions: A systematic review and meta-analysis. *Annals of Internal Medicine, 161*(2), 113–121. doi: 10.7326/M13-2567

Sinsky, C., Colligan, L., Li, L., Prgomet, M., Reynolds, S., Goeders, L., . . . Blike, G. (2016). Allocation of physician time in ambulatory practice: A time and motion study in 4 specialties. *Annals of Internal Medicine, 165*(11), 753–760. doi: 10.7326/m16-0961

Thota, A. B., Sipe, T. A., Byard, G. J., Zometa, C. S., Hahn, R. A., McKnight-Eily, L. R., . . . Community Preventive Services Task Force. (2012). Collaborative care to improve the management of depressive disorders: A community guide systematic review and meta-analysis. *American Journal of Preventive Medicine, 42*(5), 525–538. doi: 10.1016/j.amepre.2012.01.019

Unützer, J., Katon, W., Callahan, C. M., Williams, J. W. Jr., Hunkeler, E., Harpole, L., . . . Areán, P. A. (2002). Collaborative care management of late-life depression in the primary care setting: A randomized controlled trial. *Journal of the American Medical Association, 288*(22), 2836–2845.

Wenger, N. S., Roth, C. P., Hall, W. J., Ganz, D. A., Snow, V., Byrkit, J., . . . Reuben, D. B. (2010). Practice redesign to improve care for falls and urinary incontinence: Primary care intervention for older patients. *Archives of Internal Medicine, 170*(19), 1765–1772. doi: 10.1001/archinternmed.2010.387

Wenger, N. S., Roth, C. P., Shekelle, P. G., Young, R. T., Solomon, D. H., Kamberg, C. J., . . . Reuben, D. B. (2009). A practice-based intervention to improve primary care for falls, urinary incontinence, and dementia. *Journal of the American Geriatrics Society, 57*(3), 547–555. doi: 10.1111/j.1532-5415.2008.02128.x

CHAPTER 19

Evidence-Based Models in Action That Work

Jonny Macias and Michael L. Malone

CHAPTER OBJECTIVES

1. Describe several unique challenges that lead to geriatrics models of care.
2. Understand the vulnerability of frail older adults with multiple comorbidities.
3. Describe key examples of evidence-based and cost-effective geriatrics models of care.
4. Consider strategies to sustain and disseminate geriatrics models of care, as well as to develop new models, that will meet changes in Medicare payment systems.

KEY TERMS

vulnerable older patients	Models of care	evidence-based best practices
interdisciplinary care	Population health strategies	

▶ Introduction

The population in the United States will dramatically change over the next decades, as its older population will experience significant growth in its numbers. Older adults are the fastest-growing segment of the U.S. population. This expected change in the older population will bring a larger number of older adults with multiple comorbidities into the healthcare arena—creating new challenges for healthcare systems, healthcare providers, and policymakers. The intense focus on new value-based, outcome-oriented payment models supports the development and implementation of evidence-based models that can improve care and lower costs.

Older adults who develop frailty or chronic medical conditions are particularly vulnerable during their illness or injury. Common vulnerabilities among this group include functional decline, adverse drug events in response to medications, hospitalization and institutionalization, readmission to the hospital, delirium, and malnutrition. To address the vulnerabilities and challenges of this particular population, it is imperative to identify evidence-based **models of care** that are designed to meet the unique needs of older adults. Further, geriatrics leaders need to deploy "best practice" models, which can add value to the care of patients within their practice settings. Health system leaders will need to identify why this care is better than standard care and what specifically needs to be done differently.

The key components of geriatrics models of care should focus on the following major goals:

- Enable seniors to remain at home.
- Prevent functional disability,
- Preserve patient quality of life.
- Respect patients' values, preferences, and goals.
- Address the needs of caregivers, psychosocial needs, and patient safety concerns.

Geriatrics models of care focus on early identification of vulnerability. They take into account patients with multiple comorbidities and rely on interdisciplinary teams (instead of individual health providers) to those patients' need. Many of these models use **population health strategies** to identify the needs of older adults as they navigate the continuum of care. Notably, care coordination is an essential component of many of these models.

Most organizations struggle when defining where they should start in implementing such a model. Many different models have been proposed, but organizations typically have only limited resources to commit to implementing best practice strategies. One place to start is by identifying the area of care where the needs are most compelling—that is, by getting a better understanding of the challenges of older patients and their family caregivers within various settings of the healthcare organization (e.g., the

emergency department, inpatient, outpatient, or the transition from the hospital to post-acute care). A patient story can be very powerful in helping to define a compelling need to improve care. Next, the organization should get a feel for the unique needs of the community and the context of the care (e.g., rural setting with long distances to travel for patients and providers; inner city with lack of access to health care for economic reasons). Likewise, it should try to understand the financial impact of the current care, as well as how improving care for that population is consistent with the mission of the organization.

This chapter outlines five different settings of care and "evidence-based models that work" in each site. Although many geriatrics models of care are described in this chapter, we recognize that our list is incomplete. The goal here is to provide the reader with examples of these models in an effort to highlight the key elements of successful **interdisciplinary care**.

▶ Geriatrics Models of Care

Hospital-Based Models
Acute Care for Elders

An Acute Care for Elders (ACE) unit is designed to prevent functional decline in hospitalized older adults. The key elements of the originally described ACE unit include a prepared environment, with the main goal of enhancing safety and independence; patient-centered care; medical care review to assure safe medical care; and interdisciplinary team rounds (**TABLE 19-1**).

Three randomized clinical trials (RCTs) confirmed the benefits of the ACE model of care as compared to usual care. Patients admitted to ACE units are discharged with less disability and a shorter hospital length of stay, and are less likely to transition to a skilled nursing facility. The total cost of hospitalizations is slightly lower on the ACE units (Landefeld, Palmer, Kresevic,

TABLE 19-1 Hospital-Based Models

Model of Care	Goal	Key Components	Findings That Support the Intervention
Acute Care for Elders (ACE)	■ Lessen the chance of functional decline for hospitalized older adults	■ Interdisciplinary team assessment and care ■ Prepared environment ■ Early planning to go home ■ Medical care review (using ACE Tracker report)	Randomized controlled trial (RCT) has shown improvement in activities of daily living (ADL) performance from 2 weeks prior to admission ($p = 0.05$) and admission compared to discharge ($p = 0.009$). RCT has shown nonsignificant reduction in total hospital costs per case ($6608 versus $7240, $p = 0.93$). RCT showed significantly reduced mortality at 3 (12% versus 27%, $p = 0.004$) and 6 months (16% versus 29%, $p = 0.02$) post discharge.
Nurses Improving Care for Healthsystem Elders (NICHE)	■ Prepare nursing staff in care of older adults ■ Train a cohort of geriatric resource nurses to become experts for other nursing staff	■ Nursing skills and competencies ■ Promotes geriatric quality of care ■ Patient safety across the care continuum ■ Benchmarking service	Improved clinical quality at multiple NICHE sites: ■ Improved patient satisfaction ■ Decreased falls ■ Decreased use of high-risk medications ■ Improved use of senior-friendly protocols ■ Improved cultural competency ■ Improved care for older patients who developed delirium during hospital care
Hospital Elder Life Program (HELP)	■ Lessen the chance of new development of delirium in hospital	■ Screening of vulnerable older patients at risk for delirium ■ Trained and supervised volunteers deploying protocols	RCT showed delirium decreased 10% in HELP versus 15% in a control group. Multiple other studies: ■ Decreased reacmissions to hospital ■ Decreased rate of hospital falls ■ Decreased hospital length of stay ■ Decreased sitter use

Fortinsky, & Kowal, 1995). The strength of the ACE unit model is the potential to disseminate this care within an entire hospital or a healthcare system. The ACE Tracker in the electronic health record has changed the ACE paradigm from a unit-based model to a single-page report that identifies **vulnerable older patients** on each medical–surgical unit *throughout* the hospital. This practical tool has been used to bring the ACE model to scale. In addition, mobile ACE teams have been implemented in many hospitals in an effort to disseminate the best practice from one site to multiple nursing units within a medical center.

Hospital Elder Life Program

The Hospital Elder Life Program (HELP) is an evidence-based model of care designed to prevent delirium. This model's multicomponent intervention deploys six standardized protocols that address specific risk factors for delirium: cognitive impairment, sleep deprivation, immobility, visual impairment, hearing impairment, and dehydration. The effectiveness of HELP was demonstrated in a prospective, individual matching strategy study called the Delirium Prevention Trial. The incidence of delirium was significantly lowered in this study (9.9% among patients receiving the HELP intervention, compared to 15% in the control group, $p = 0.02$) (Inouye et al., 1999). Additional studies of this model have shown that those individuals enrolled in this program have lower rates of delirium, less cognitive decline, less functional impairment, and a decreased rate of hospital falls. HELP has been widely disseminated and can be replicated in medical units, surgical units, and skilled nursing facilities. Additional aspects of cognitive assessment are noted in the *Cognitive/Mentation Assessment* chapter.

Nurses Improving Care for Healthsystem Elders

Nurses Improving Care for Healthsystem Elders (NICHE) is a nursing model designed to improve the quality of care for older adult patients in hospitals and healthcare organizations. NICHE implements **evidence-based best practices** into hospital care. This model of care focuses on improving nursing clinical knowledge and nursing skills. At the heart of NICHE is the geriatric nurse specialist, who prepares staff nurses to serve as clinical resources on geriatric issues to other nurses on medical–surgical units.

NICHE promotes the use of interdisciplinary teams and provides practical tools to improve care for older adults. This model of care supports the implementation of evidence-based, geriatric care for multiple geriatric syndromes: management of pain, prevention of pressure ulcers, adverse medication events, delirium, falls, and management of urinary incontinence (Capezuti et al., 2012). NICHE has been widely disseminated in North America.

Care Transitions Models
Care Transition Intervention

The Care Transition Intervention program was designed to empower individuals to understand their health needs and to make decisions to manage their care. The key outcome of this intervention is reduced hospital readmissions of vulnerable older adults. This model features a nurse as a coach, who helps teach and guide the older patient. The patient and family are trained by the transition coach to identify worsening symptoms or "red flags" and effectively communicate with a patient's primary care provider or specialist. The transition coach also assists and trains the patient and family in medication self-management.

The transition coach does not provide direct patient care services, but instead makes home visits in the month following the patient's hospital discharge. An RCT involving hospitalized older adults with at least one risk factor for unplanned readmission demonstrated lower rehospitalization rates among this group when compared to a control group at 30 days (8.3% versus 11.9%, $p = 0.48$) and at 90 days (16.7% versus

22.5%, $p = 0.04$) (Coleman, Parry, Chalmers, & Min, 2006). This model has been widely disseminated, with key components becoming the standard of care in the United States. The reader is encouraged to review further notes on care transitions highlighted in the *Transitions of Care* chapter.

Transitional Care Model

The Transitional Care Model (TCM) is designed to improve the process of comprehensive discharge planning after an acute medical or surgical illness. A nurse practitioner or a registered nurse coordinates early discharge planning with the patient, family, attending physician, and other health professionals. In RCTs, the TCM intervention reduced 30- and 90-day hospital readmissions and total days of readmission, and reduced total costs of care for 90 days following discharge. Patient satisfaction and quality of life were likewise improved in the intervention group (University of Pennsylvania School of Nursing, n.d.). As the title of this chapter suggests, this model works—it has a very strong evidence base (**TABLE 19-2**).

Better Outcomes for Older Adults Through Safe Transitions

The Better Outcomes for Older Adults Through Safe Transitions (BOOST) model of care is a quality improvement project developed by the Society of Hospital Medicine and intended to optimize hospital discharge processes and improve communication among healthcare providers. The Project BOOST developers created a tool for assessing risk of readmission and preparation for transitions of care. Interventions include (1) a list of items demonstrating general assessment of preparedness for the transition from the hospital and (2) a checklist to review during hospitalization to prepare for care transitions. Project BOOST also uses a structured approach for medication reconciliation. Medications are reviewed with the patient

and/or caregiver, and the patient's understanding is assessed through patient "teach-back." Communication with other providers is assured through personal communication and a discharge summary. While evidence basis for this model is not as strong as the two transitions models described earlier, Project BOOST has achieved wide dissemination through the efforts of the Society of Hospitalist Medicine (Society of Hospital Medicine, n.d.).

Community-Based Models
Program of All-Inclusive Care for the Elderly

The Program of All-Inclusive Care for the Elderly (PACE) provides comprehensive primary care for participants age 55 and older. Its main goal is for its participants to be able to continue living in the community. PACE services are provided at a day health center; in addition to medical care, this center provides nursing services, physical and occupational therapy, recreational therapies, meals, nutrition services, social work, and personal care. PACE is a capitated program that coordinates all services to participants covered by Medicare and Medicaid. This basis also enables the PACE program to provide services or medical equipment, which is not typically covered by Medicare or Medicaid (**TABLE 19-3**). The 119 PACE programs are available in 32 states (Halter et al., 2017; Malone, Capezuti, & Palmer, 2015).

Geriatric and Evaluation Management

Geriatric and Evaluation Management (GEM) is an interdisciplinary team of healthcare professionals designed to assess older adults' medical, functional, psychosocial, nutritional, and environmental needs. This model of care develops an overall plan for treatment and follow-up, with the recommendations being submitted to the primary care physician. The interdisciplinary team, which is led by a geriatrician, generally

TABLE 19-2 Care Transitions Model

Model of Care	Goal	Key Components	Findings That Support the Intervention
Care Transitions Program	Reduce hospital readmissions of vulnerable older patients	■ Personal health record for patient to manage across care settings ■ Medication reconciliation and self-management training ■ Patient-scheduled follow-up visits ■ Patient knowledge of clinical symptoms and how to respond	Randomized controlled trial (RCT) showed significantly lower rates of rehospitalization at 30 and 90 days compared to control group. Improved patients' self-management skills and increased patients' confidence in their role during transitions.
Transitional Care Model	Comprehensive discharge planning	■ Discharge planning early in the hospital care ■ Advanced practice nurse: follows patient home; coaches patient and caregiver; focuses on medication management	RCT showed reduced readmissions, reduced total hospital days, reduced costs, and improved patient /caregiver/provider satisfaction.
Project BOOST (Better Outcomes for Older Adults Through Safe Transitions)	Optimize hospital discharge process	■ 8 P risk assessment ■ Generalized assessment of preparedness ■ Teach back ■ Patient-centered discharge instructions ■ Timely follow- up appointment ■ Standardized communication with primary care providers ■ Follow-up call in 48–72 hours	Pre-post assessment of Project BOOST at multiple hospitals showed improved rehospitalization rates when compared to standard care.
Coordinated-Transitional Care Model (C-TraC Program)	Improve transitional care quality and health outcomes	■ In-hospital visit and integration with the inpatient team ■ Intensive 48-hour follow-up phone call by nurse case manager ■ Weekly follow-up calls for 4 weeks ■ Coordination with primary care provider	Patients who received the C-TraC program intervention experienced one-third fewer hospitalizations than the baseline comparison group.

TABLE 19-3 Community-Based Models

Model of Care	Goal	Key Components	Findings That Support the Intervention
Program of All-Inclusive Care for the Elderly (PACE)	■ Comprehensive primary care for individuals age 55 and older ■ Safely continue living in the community	■ Day health center ■ Medical care ■ Nursing services ■ Therapy ■ Meals ■ Personal care ■ Social worker	Lower rates of hospital use. Lower rates of nursing home use. Higher use of adult daycare services. Better reported health status. Lower rates of emergency department use.
Geriatric Evaluation and Management (GEM)	■ Improve health outcomes of at-risk seniors ■ Develop plan of care and specific interventions	■ Comprehensive geriatric assessment ■ Co-management with the primary care provider (PCP)	Randomized trial showed significant reductions in functional decline with inpatient GEM and improvements in mental health with outpatient GEM, with no increase in costs.
Guided Care	Provides primary care coordinated by a nurse	■ Case management ■ Transitional care ■ Caregiver support	Matched-pair, randomized control trial showed higher quality of chronic care. Higher physician's satisfaction in managing chronic care.
Geriatric Resources for Assessment and Care of Elders (GRACE) Program	Improve quality of care for low-income seniors in the community	■ Team members: nurse practitioner, social worker, and PCP ■ Medical and psychosocial evaluation ■ Medication review ■ Functional assessment ■ Advance directives	Randomized controlled trial showed reduced acute care utilization among a high-risk group.
UCLA Alzheimer's and Dementia Care	Provide comprehensive, patient-centered care for individuals with dementia in a large academic practice	■ Dementia registry ■ Structured needs assessments ■ Individualized dementia care ■ Facilitates transitions of care	Preliminary data showed reduced behavioral symptoms and caregiver stress. Cost-effective as a result of reducing emergency department visits, impatient hospitalizations, and readmissions.

consists of nurses, social workers, and geriatricians, but may also include other members, such as an occupational therapist, physical therapist, psychologist, pharmacist, and nutritionist. These members assess the patient based on the patient's needs and the setting.

The goal of the GEM model of care is to develop a comprehensive plan to improve the patient's quality of life and maximize the patient's function. This program also ascertains the patient's goals of care, advance directives, and end-of-life wishes.

The evidence base for this model comes from both inpatient and outpatient settings. When compared to usual care, frail older patients who received care on a GEM unit had a lower mortality rate, were less likely to be discharged to a skilled nursing facility, and had better functional outcomes. The evidence from the outpatient setting shows better mental health scores for patients with the GEM model, but similar costs and clinical outcomes as with the traditional care model. The GEM model is currently applied primarily in Veterans Administration (VA) settings (Cohen et al., 2002).

Guided Care Model

The guided care model is intended to improve the quality of care and efficiency of resources used by older adults with complex health needs. This model includes a registered nurse as a guided care nurse (GCN). The GCN is based in the primary care office to facilitate communication with the primary care physician and office staff. The GCN's clinical activities include assessment of the patient's medical, functional, cognitive, psychosocial, and environmental status. The GCN also develops care planning, promotes the patient's self-management of chronic conditions, monitors the patient's symptoms and adherence, coordinates care with providers across all care settings, and facilitates access to community resources. Patients enrolled in this model (and their family caregivers) report better quality of chronic care when compared to

usual care (Boult et al., 2013). This model has been implemented in Medicare HMO (health maintenance organization) settings.

Geriatric Resources for Assessment and Care of Elders

The Geriatric Resources for Assessment and Care of Elders (GRACE) model is a cost-effective, patient-centered team care model that focuses on improving the health of older adults in their homes. This model of care features a nurse practitioner, a social worker, and an interdisciplinary care team. The key components of the GRACE model are an in-home geriatric assessment, an individualized care plan, an interdisciplinary team conference, and primary care collaboration. The nurse practitioner and the social worker collaborate with the primary care physician to implement the GRACE care plan. The GRACE support team then monitors the care plan implementation of the interdisciplinary team's suggestions (Table 19-3).

Among a group of older patients at high risk for healthcare utilization, the GRACE intervention reduced emergency department visits and hospital admission rates during the second year of the intervention (Counsell et al., 2007). This model has been successfully implemented at Veterans Administration facilities (Indianapolis and Atlanta) as well as at the HealthCare Partners Medical Group in Los Angeles.

UCLA Alzheimer's and Dementia Care

The University of California, Los Angeles (UCLA) Alzheimer's and Dementia Care (ADC) model provides comprehensive, coordinated, patient-centered care for patients with Alzheimer's disease and other dementias. The key components of this model of care consist of patient recruitment, structured needs assessments, creation and implementation of individualized dementia care plans, thoughtful facilitation of transitions in care, and 24/7 access to a geriatrician for assistance and advice. The ultimate goal of this model is to help patients with dementia maintain independence and functioning.

The ADC program has been successfully implemented in a fee-for-service Medicare population in a large medical group at UCLA. Initial evidence shows that individuals who receive this intervention achieve very high quality ratings on ACOVE measures (Jennings et al., 2016). This model received initial funding from the Center for Medicare and Medicaid Innovation. New billing codes for dementia care may make its implementation feasible within the Medicare fee-for-service model.

Home Care Models of Care

Hospital at Home

This home-based model of care provides patient evaluation and management services usually performed in the acute inpatient hospital setting. Selecting appropriate patients with specific medical conditions is critical to the success of Hospital at Home. The following conditions have been treated in this model: community-acquired pneumonia, chronic obstructive pulmonary disease, chronic heart failure, cellulitis, sepsis due to urinary tract infection, complicated urinary tract infection, ischemic cerebrovascular accident, pulmonary embolism, deep venous thrombosis, pancreatitis, Parkinson's disease, and dehydration. Patients receiving Hospital at Home services report greater satisfaction as compared to those patients who receive care in a traditional inpatient setting. Length of stay is generally shorter for Hospital at Home patients, and this model is less expensive than traditional care (Leff et al., 2005). This model of care has been deployed in settings where the care is paid for by Medicare HMOs. In addition, this model is currently under study by the Center for Medicare and Medicaid Innovations Office (**TABLE 19-4**).

Home-Based Primary Care

The Home-Based Primary Care (HBPC) model of care targets veterans with multiple chronic diseases. The HBPC team consists of a nurse, physician, nurse practitioner, social worker, rehabilitation therapist, dietitian, pharmacist, and psychologist. This program's main goal is to provide long-term care for individuals who have chronic and complex disabling diseases, helping them avoid unwanted emergency visits and hospital admissions. This model has been successfully deployed in the VA healthcare system in both urban and rural settings. Studies showed that costs of (Medicare and VA) care in this model were lower than projected costs, and hospitalization rates were lower than during a period without this program (De Jonge et al., 2014). In short, this model has been well received by veterans. The most compelling argument in its favor is that it allows those patients with complex needs to be served in their homes by interdisciplinary teams. Medicare is testing an equivalent model called Independence at Home.

Community Aging in Place—Advancing Better Living for Elders

The Community Aging in Place—Advancing Better Living for Elders (CAPABLE) model of care is a patient-directed, team-based intervention that integrates a registered nurse, an occupational therapist, and a licensed handyman. The main goal of this program is to keep older adults at home, while helping them remain safe and functional. The occupational therapist assists by identifying and prioritizing problematic functional areas, as well as by assessing the patient's safety, difficulty, and efficiency, and the presence of environmental barriers. The occupational therapist determines the need for environmental modifications and assistive devices. The handyman works on home modifications and repairs to achieve the patient's functional goals. A registered nurse assists the patient in identifying areas that can potentially affect daily function

TABLE 19-4 Home Care Models of Care

Model of Care	Goal	Key Components	Findings That Support the Intervention
Hospital at Home	In-home care for older patients who are medically suitable with: ■ Pneumonia ■ Congestive heart failure exacerbation ■ Chronic obstructive pulmonary disease ■ Cellulitis	■ Eligibility criteria ■ Direct nursing care ■ Medical equipment ■ Medicines	Nonrandomized, controlled study showed shorter length of stay. Higher patient and caregiver satisfaction. Lower delirium incidence and lower cost of care.
Home-Based Primary Care (HBPC)	Primary care and care coordination at home	■ Geriatrician, nurse practitioner, and social worker working together ■ Periodic follow-up	Studies demonstrate improved quality of life without added cost.
Independence at Home	Primary care and care coordination at home for frail older adults	■ Assessment within 24–72 hours of hospital discharge ■ Nurse practitioner ■ Home health agency	Case-controlled study showed cost reduction.
Community Aging in Place—Advancing Better Living for Elders (CAPABLE)	Help older adults remain in their homes longer, improve health outcomes, and decrease medical costs	■ Nursing care assessment ■ Occupational therapy assessment ■ Handyman: home repairs based on the assessments	Preliminary findings: ■ Reduced nursing home utilization and hospital admissions ■ Improved functioning and quality of life ■ Reduced healthcare costs

(e.g., pain, depression, strength, balance, medication management, and ability to communicate with the primary care provider). In the initial assessment of this model, those older patients enrolled in this program had lower nursing home utilization, improved functioning and quality of life, and reduced healthcare costs (Szanton et al., 2015).

Long-Term Care–Based Models
Interventions to Reduce Acute Care Transfers Program

The Interventions to Reduce Acute Care Transfers (INTERACT) program focuses on improving the identification, evaluation, and management

TABLE 19-5 Long-Term Care–Based Models			
Model of Care	**Goal**	**Key Components**	**Findings That Support the Intervention**
Interventions to Reduce Acute Care Transfers (INTERACT)	Reduce potentially avoidable hospitalizations from subacute and long-term care facilities	■ Nursing education ■ "Stop and Watch" ■ SBAR (situation–background-assessment–recommendation) communication ■ Improve communication with healthcare providers	Quality improvement studies show reductions in hospital admissions. Decreased readmission rate. Initial analysis suggests savings to Medicare.

of acute changes in the condition of individuals in post-acute and long-term care. It emphasizes the use of quality improvement tools, the use of tools to improve communication, implementation of decision support tools, early identification and evaluation of changes in the patient's condition, management of common changes in the patient's condition, and advance care planning. Effective implementation of the INTERACT program has been associated with reductions in hospitalization of nursing home residents (Ouslander, Bonner, Herndon, & Shutes, 2014). This model has been successfully disseminated to numerous long-term care facilities in the United States (**TABLE 19-5**).

▶ Strategies to Implement, Sustain, and Disseminate Geriatrics Models of Care

A business plan is essential to implementing any geriatrics model of care successfully. The costs of each program are typically those for the personnel who staff the model. For some programs, there is no direct reimbursement through the Medicare or Medicaid fee-for-service model. The key element of the business plan for most of these models is preventing loss of revenue and improving the quality of care for the older adults. Many of these geriatrics models of care will become more relevant as the payment systems change from fee-for-service to value-based payments.

Sustaining these models requires continued efforts to improve care, along with champions who can promote the program. Critical to the survival of these evidence-based models of care is the development of a strategic plan and a communication plan. To ensure success, it is critical to provide data and reports regularly that demonstrate the impact on patients and the financial outcomes. Finally, the organization must be able to describe how the model of care helps to accomplish its mission.

If there is good evidence that these models work, why are they not widely disseminated across U.S. hospitals and healthcare systems? Several reasons explain their slow rollout. Reimbursement by Medicare has traditionally favored providing more care, whereas the implementation of most of these models leads to less utilization of services. Further, many of these geriatrics models of care require providers to critically review their care daily workflow and strive for continuous improvement—a prospect that takes time and effort. Moreover, gaining support of key stakeholders and hospital administrators is essential to develop these evidence-based models of care for vulnerable older adults. Lastly, much of the training of the current U.S. healthcare workforce is directed toward care delivery, instead of toward systems improvement.

▶ Summary

To successfully disseminate geriatrics models of care that work, organizations must keep a few points in mind. First, they must be able to define the needs of a large population of patients who need care. Second, they must define efficiencies that can allow team members to work on the same project across multiple settings (a common healthcare record system, or a common organizational goal). Lastly, they must define a vision in which multiple facilities strive to work on together. A wide range of successful evidence-based models have been developed that are tailored to different care settings. Changes in reimbursement favor these models, which focus on outcomes over utilization.

As the United States moves toward adopting quality payment programs for healthcare professional reimbursement systems, opportunities will arise for many new models of geriatrics practice. The new themes of care will emphasize improved coordination of care and improved value for the care that is delivered. We remain humble in trying to better serve older adults (and their family caregivers) with their healthcare needs.

References

Boult, C., Leff, B., Boyd, C. M., Wolff, J. L., Marsteller, J. A., Frick, K. D., . . . Scharfstein, D. O. (2013). A matched-pair cluster-randomized trial of guided care for high-risk older patients. *Journal of General Internal Medicine, 28*(5), 612–621. Retrieved from https://link.springer .com/article/10.1007%2Fs11606-012-2287-y

Capezuti, E., Boltz, M., Cline, D., Dickson, V. V., Rosenberg, M.-C., Wagner, L., . . . Nigolian, C. (2012). Nurses Improving Care for Healthsystem Elders: A model for optimising the geriatric nursing practice environment. *Journal of Clinical Nursing, 21*(21/22), 3117–3125. https:// doi.org/10.1111/j.1365-2702.2012.04259.x

Cohen, H. J., Feussner, J. R., Weinberger, M., Carnes, M., Hamdy, R. C., Hsieh, F., . . . May, C. (2002). A controlled trial of inpatient and outpatient geriatric evaluation and management. *New England Journal of Medicine, 346*(12), 905–912.

Coleman, E. A., Parry, C., Chalmers, S., & Min, S. (2006). The Care Transitions intervention: Results of a randomized controlled trial. *Archives of Internal Medicine, 166*(17), 1822–1828.

Counsell, S. R., Callahan, C. M., Clark, D. O., Tu, W., Buttar, A. B., Stump, T. E., & Ricketts, G. D. (2007). Geriatric care management for low-income seniors: A randomized controlled trial. *Journal of the American Medical Association, 298*(22), 2623–2633.

De Jonge, E. K., Jamshed, N., Gilden, D., Kubisiak, J., Bruce, S. R., & Taler, G. (2014). Effects of home-based primary care on Medicare costs in high-risk elders. *Journal of the American Geriatrics Society, 62*(10), 1825–1831.

Halter, J., Ouslander, J., Tinetti, M., Studenski, S., High, K., & Asthana, S. (2017). *Hazzard's geriatric medicine and gerontology.* New York, NY: McGraw-Hill.

Inouye, S. K., Bogardus, S. T., Charpentier, P. A., Leo-Summers, L., Acampora, D., Holford, T. R., & Cooney, L. M. (1999). A multicomponent intervention to prevent delirium in hospitalized older patients. *New England Journal of Medicine, 340*(9), 669–676. https://doi.org/10.1056 /NEJM199903043400901

Jennings, L. A., Tan, Z., Wenger, N. S., Cook, E. A., Han, W., McCreath, H. E., . . . Reuben, D. B. (2016). Quality of care provided by a comprehensive dementia care comanagement program. *Journal of the American Geriatrics Society, 64*,(8), 1724–1730. http://dx.doi .org/10.1111/jgs.1425

Landefeld, C. S., Palmer, R. M., Kresevic, D. M., Fortinsky, R. H., & Kowal, J. (1995). A randomized trial of care in a hospital medical unit especially designed to improve the functional outcomes of acutely ill older patients. *New England Journal of Medicine, 332*(20), 1338–1344. https://doi.org/10.1056/NEJM199505183322006

Leff, B., Burton, L., Mader, S. L., Naughton, B., Burl, J., Inouye, S. K., . . . Frick, K. D. (2005). Hospital at Home: Feasibility and outcomes of a program to provide hospital-level care at home for acutely ill older patients. *Annals of Internal Medicine, 143*(11), 798–808.

Malone, M. L., Capezuti, E., & Palmer, R. M. (2015). *Geriatrics models of care: Bringing best practice to an aging America.* Switzerland: Springer.

Ouslander, J. G., Bonner, A., Herndon, L., & Shutes, J. (2014). The Interventions to Reduce Acute Care Transfers (INTERACT) quality improvement program: An overview for medical directors and primary care clinicians in long term care. *Journal of the American Medical Directors Association, 15*(3), 162–170.

Society of Hospital Medicine. (n.d.). Project BOOST: Better Outcomes for Older Adults Through Safe Transitions. Retrieved from http://www.hospitalmedicine.org /BOOST/

Szanton, S. L., Wolff, J. L., Leff, B., Roberts, L., Thorpe, R. J., Tanner, E. K., . . . Bishai, D. (2015). Preliminary data from Community Aging in Place, Advancing Better Living for Elders, a patient-directed, team-based intervention to improve physical function and decrease nursing home utilization: The first 100 individuals to complete a Centers for Medicare and Medicaid Services Innovation project. *Journal of the American Geriatrics Society, 63*(2), 371–374.

University of Pennsylvania School of Nursing, New Courtland Center for Transitions and Health. (n.d.). Transitional Care Model. Retrieved from http://www.nursing.upenn .edu/ncth/transitional-care-model/

CHAPTER 20

Advance Care Planning

Amy Berman, Sheena Thakkar, Nanxing Li, and Maureen Henry

CHAPTER OBJECTIVES

1. Understand the purpose of advance care planning.
2. Identify and describe the types of advance directives.
3. List four key considerations in the advance care planning process.

KEY TERMS

Advance care planning   Advance directive

▶ Introduction

Death is an inevitable part of the human life cycle. The aging process begins at birth and culminates with the dying process. While death may be sudden or expected, and while it may occur in childhood or as an adult, most deaths happen in older age and are preceded by a course of illness and subsequent decline. The nature of the decline may be rapid, or it may be variable, with multiple periods of decline and improvement occurring before the final decline and death. Whatever the final course, death is a fact of life and as such can be anticipated from the moment of birth.

The dying process has changed with the advent of cutting-edge procedures, medications, and technology aimed at delaying death. The emergence of innovations in health care capable of supporting life as the body, mind, and spirit fade has raised ethical issues related to patient autonomy. The question may not be whether we can keep a person alive artificially, but rather what that person would want his or her care to look like and would want to avoid at the end of life. A number of court cases, including those involving Terri Schiavo, Nancy Cruzan, and Shirley Dinnerstein (Devettere, 2016; Sedensky, 2010), prompted and sustained the national conversation about the right to participate in one's own end-of-life decisions by stating or documenting preferences in advance. Out of this conversation came the process we know in the United States as *advance care planning* (Devettere, 2016).

The Patient Self-Determination Act (PSDA) was passed by Congress in 1990 and enacted in 1991. PSDA required hospitals, nursing homes, home health care, and health maintenance organizations (HMOs) accepting Medicare or Medicaid funding to provide a written policy affirming a patient's right, according that state's law, to accept or refuse treatment and the right to complete an advance directive (101st Congress, 1990).

Advance care planning is a process of discussing values and specific wishes about wanted and unwanted care at the end of life. It may occur in the home, in the community, or within a healthcare delivery setting. It can include members of the family, friends, or significant others, as well as members of the healthcare team including physicians, nurses, and social workers. Many discussions occur in the context of the preparation of legal documents such as a will or during consultation with a financial planner.

▶ Advance Directives

An **advance directive** is a document by which a person makes provisions for healthcare decisions in the event that, in the future, he or she becomes incapacitated and unable to make decisions (Patients Rights Council, 2013). Ideally, advance care planning discussions begin before a health crisis occurs. The discussions and documents should be reviewed periodically and as health changes, and should be updated to reflect the patient's current preferences.

Advance directives typically contain one of two components: the documentation of wishes or the designation of a surrogate (Mayo Clinic,

2014). The statement of wishes might be called a *living will* and the designation of a surrogate may be called a *healthcare power of attorney*. A living will provides general guidance about which care or treatment an individual would want or would not want as part of end-of-life care. A healthcare power of attorney designates a specific person who may make decisions on the individual's behalf when he or she is unable to do so because of health issues.

In addition to advance directives, more than half of U.S. states recognize physician orders for life-sustaining treatment (POLST). In contrast to the general guidance provided in advance directives, POLST forms contain specific instructions about specific interventions, including the overall approach to care, intubation, and resuscitation. POLST forms are generally viewed as appropriate for people with a life expectancy of less than one year.

For healthcare providers to act on an advance directive, that document needs to be available to the clinician. It is critically important that (1) advance care planning leads to the documentation of one's end-of-life preferences in a form recognized by that state, (2) the advance directive or a summary of its contents be accessible to the clinical team, (3) the clinical team provides care congruent with the documented wishes of the patient or his or her designee (proxy), and (4) the patient (or proxy) always maintains the right to change his or her preferences.

▶ Why Is Advance Care Planning Important?

Imagine planning for your own death—or more specifically, how you will die. We live in a death-denying culture. While most people have experienced loss, few choose to think about their own death. Some people want aggressive care to the very end in hopes of more days, no matter what the quality of life those days offer. Others want to focus on trying to manage pain or symptoms, and others would not want to delay death if the quality of life were poor. Many people do not die the way they want, and one barrier is the dearth of advance care planning.

Nearly 70% of older adults prefer to die at home, yet most are likely to die in institutional settings. According to the Centers for Disease Control and Prevention (CDC), there were 859,464 deaths of people older than age 85 in the United States in 2015. Most of those deaths took place in a hospital (22%) or nursing home (36%). By comparison, 25% took place at home, and 8% took place in hospices (CDC, 2016). One contributor to the high rates of deaths in hospitals and nursing homes is a lack of advance care planning.

Advance care planning is important not just to the patient, but also to families who make end-of-life care decisions. In one study of family members of patients treated in an intensive care unit (ICU), the risk of moderate to major post-traumatic stress disorder (PTSD) was found in 48.4% of family members who felt information was incomplete, 47.8% of family members who shared in decision making, 50% of family members whose relative died in the ICU, 60% of those whose relative died after someone else made decisions about life-sustaining treatment, and 81.8% who participated in life-sustaining treatment decisions (Azoulay et al., 2005). Advance care planning can help lessen the risk of PTSD and other burdens experienced by surviving family members.

Despite the potential value of advance care planning, this topic is often not discussed or documented. Moreover, disparities in end-of-life planning are significant. One study of adults ages 18 and older showed that, of 7946 respondents, only 26.3% had an advance directive. The most commonly reported reason for not completing an advance directive was lack of awareness. The completion of advanced directives was associated with being older, more educated, and having a higher income; by comparison, it was less frequent among non-white respondents. Individuals who completed advance directives were more likely to report having chronic disease and a care plan (Rao, Anderson, Lin, & Laux, 2014).

A systematic review of studies from 2011 to 2016 led by Katherine Courtright, an instructor of medicine in the division of Pulmonary, Allergy, and Critical Care and the Palliative and Advanced Illness Research (PAIR) Center at University of Pennsylvania, found that among approximately 800,000 Americans, 63% had not completed any advance directive. Fewer than one-third (29.3%) had completed a living will that contained specific end-of-life care wishes, and roughly one-third (33.4%) had designated a healthcare power of attorney (Yadav et al., 2017).

Many healthcare providers who see older adult patients raise the importance of end-of-life discussions and advance care planning with their patients. Yet, clinicians report significant barriers that prevent them from having these discussions with their patients. Nearly half of the physicians in a nationally representative survey conducted by PerryUndem Research and commissioned by The John A. Hartford Foundation, California Health Care Foundation, and Cambia Health Foundation reported that clinicians do not know how to have this kind of conversation (PerryUndem Research/Communication, 2016). This lack of knowledge about how to do advance care planning stood in stark contrast to the 99% of physician respondents who reported that they should be having these conversations with their patients.

Beginning in 2016, Medicare launched new payment codes that provide reimbursement for advance care planning (U.S. Department of Health and Human Services, 2016). In the first year that healthcare providers were allowed to bill for these critical discussions, nearly 575,000 Medicare beneficiaries took part in the conversations, according to *Kaiser Health News*. Nationwide, slightly more than 1% of Medicare beneficiaries received advance care planning talks that were billed under Medicare (Aleccia, 2017). Use of the billing codes for advance care planning varied widely among states, with 0.2% of older Alaskans and 2.5% of older Hawaiians enrolled in Medicare plans participating in advance care planning according the Medicare billing data. This high degree of variability suggests that even within the national context of the generally low rates of advance care planning, there are significant disparities.

▶ Best Practices in Advance Care Planning

The Conversation

Discussing preferences at the end of life and completing an advance directive can be done at any time across the health trajectory, from people who have no known health issues to people experiencing a life-limiting illness. Typically, advance care planning is initiated with an adult population, but even young children experiencing serious illness can document their wishes. That said, advance care planning with a healthy person looks very different from advance care planning with a seriously ill individual. People living with serious illness or disability need information about their condition and its trajectory, as well as treatment options and their outcomes, to fully participate in decisions about care and treatment.

Advance care planning discussions with a patient experiencing serious health challenges should begin with information sharing. As the patient approaches the end of life, the healthcare team identifies the clinical conditions and the likely course of the disease, also known as the *prognosis*. Before sharing emotionally charged information about prognosis, however, providers should ask the patient about preferences for receiving information, because some people do not want such information. With permission, the provider should share information that includes the context of the person's health, options for care and treatment, and the anticipated outcomes based on the choices for care and probable treatment outcomes. It is this critically important sharing of information (prognosis, treatment options, and treatment outcomes) that enables the patient to fully participate in care decisions and advance care planning.

Given the emotionally charged nature of a discussion of health challenges, it is important to affirm the patient's understanding. One structured approach to eliciting the patient's understanding is known as "ask–tell–ask," wherein the provider asks the patient for permission to provide information; then, with permission, tells the patient about prognosis and treatment options and outcomes; then asks the patient to explain what he or she heard (Center to Advance Palliative Care, 2013).

The next step in advance care planning is the discussion of goals of care. Given the person's overall health and health trajectory, what is he or she trying to achieve? Some commonly described goals include independence (e.g., remaining at home), physical function (e.g., going to church), and pain and symptoms management.

The final step is to reach agreement on a care plan that is based on the patient's care goals, and to document the patient's goals in the form of advance directives, where appropriate.

These steps may be repeated several times as a patient's condition worsens. A change in condition or a change in preferences should prompt a discussion. In addition, providers should consider the value of revisiting the conversation at regularly scheduled intervals, such as decade birthdays for healthy patients, annually for older adults, or within shorter time frames for patients with serious illness.

Documentation

Clinicians can provide care congruent with a person's wishes only if they know what those wishes are. Documentation of advance care planning discussions and completion of an advance directive allows members of the healthcare team to understand the care preferences and/or the patient's choice of surrogate in the event the patient is not able to make the necessary decisions. The forms and documentation vary by state. In general, the state-approved living will and healthcare power of attorney forms may be found on each state's department of health website. The patient is advised to keep a copy of any advance directive and provide a copy to the person with the healthcare power of attorney.

While the process of eliciting the patient's end-of-life preferences is key to advance care planning, the forms may not always have designated areas that capture what a patient wants or wishes to avoid. The clinical team can add notes on the form or in an attachment and in the clinical record to support the patient's right to self-determination at end of life.

As people near the end of life and are expected to die within the next year, providers in states where they are offered should discuss physician orders for life-sustaining treatment forms as part of advance care planning. POLST forms are medical orders signed by the patient and the healthcare provider (physician, nurse practitioner, or physician assistant, depending on state law) that lay out the types of medical treatment a patient wishes to receive at the end of life. POLST forms are more likely than advance directives to be followed because they are more specific than advance directives and leave less room for interpretation. The POLST level of specificity can be determined only further along in the disease trajectory, as a patient approaches the end of life. Because they are more likely to be followed, however, creating POLST forms that accurately reflect the patient's goals and preferences is critical.

When a POLST form appropriately reflects the patient's goals and preferences, it can prevent unwanted care and treatments and align care with patient goals and preferences (Coalition for Compassionate Care, 2017). An advantage of the POLST process is its specificity. Some states have a POLST registry or database that allows emergency medical services (EMS) providers, emergency department providers, and other members of the healthcare team to access the content of the POLST form.

As valuable as advance directives might be, no person can be forced to complete an advance directive or POLST form. Indeed, it is against the law to require a patient to have an advance directive (American Bar Association, n.d.).

Tools

A number of tools are available to support clinicians, patients, and families in the process of advance care planning. *The Conversation Project* (https://theconversationproject.org) was launched to encourage the discussions necessary for advance care planning. Its Conversation Starter Kit contains tools and resources for patients and families (The Conversation Project, 2017).

The American Bar Association Toolkit for Health Care Advance Planning (https://www .americanbar.org/groups/law_aging/resources /health_care_decision_making/consumer_s _toolkit_for_health_care_advance_planning .html) contains worksheets that patients and their family can work through as they engage in advance care planning.

Prepare for Your Care (https://preparefor yourcare.org/welcome) is a website where question prompts and videos can be used to engage patients and families in advance care planning.

In addition, the American Geriatrics Society, the American Academy of Hospice and Palliative Care, and the American Academy of Nursing all have guidelines for clinicians in advance care planning.

▶ Practice Challenges

While advance care planning and advance directives provide patients with the opportunity to influence their care when they are unable to make decisions or communicate their preferences, both bring challenges. Advance care planning must be an ongoing process as people move through life and illness because preferences can change with time and in different circumstances, but patients may view it as "once and done." A meta-analysis of studies on preference stability over time suggests that between 11.1% and 37% of patients have unstable preferences about life-sustaining treatments (Auriemma et al., 2014). Another challenge is that advance directives may be signed years before they are used, which may cause discomfort in providers who have to rely on them.

As noted earlier, physicians think advance care planning is important, but nearly half feel unprepared to have the conversation. Trained physicians are critical to ensure that patients with serious illness can receive the information and assistance they need to engage in advance care planning. Training is available to providers through organizations such as VITALtalk, the Ariadne Labs Serious Illness Care programs, the Center to Advance Palliative Care, and Respecting Choices. In addition, online training and resources are publicly available from the Veterans Administration's Life Sustaining Treatment Decisions Initiative.

Advance directive forms are typically authored by state legislators in language that is very broad because it is designed for everyone, from healthy 18-year-olds to frail 95-year-olds. This broad language can be very challenging for providers to interpret and apply in specific clinical scenarios and, in turn, the lack of clarity can diminish the value of advance directives. If clinicians are unclear about the meaning or intent of an advance directive, it may be disregarded or may result in the provision of unwanted care.

▶ Summary

Advance care planning and advance directives have the potential to empower patients and family members and to support patient autonomy and preserve the right to self-determination. Providers play a critical role in supporting their patients' end-of-life preferences by eliciting preferences in advance care planning discussions and documenting them in the form of advance directives. To fulfill that role successfully, providers need to seek training in advance care planning and must initiate these discussions with their patients—especially those living with serious illness.

References

101st Congress. (1990). H.R.4449: Patient Self Determination Act of 1990. Retrieved from https://www.congress.gov/bill/101st-congress/house-bill/4449/text

Aleccia, J. (2017 February 15). Docs bill Medicare for end-of-life advice as 'death panel' fears reemerge. *Kaiser Health News*. Retrieved from https://khn.org/news/docs-bill-medicare-for-end-of-life-advice-as-death-panel-fears-reemerge/

American Bar Association. (n.d.). Law for older Americans. Retrieved from https://www.americanbar.org/groups/public_education/resources/law_issues_for_consumers/patient_self_determination_act.html

Auriemma, C. L., Nguyen, C. A., Bronheim, R., Kent, S., Nadiger, S., Pardo, D., & Halpern, S. D. (2014). Stability of end-of-life preferences: A systematic review of the evidence. *JAMA Internal Medicine, 174*(7), 1085–1092.

Azoulay, E., Pochard, F., Kentish-Barnes, N., Chevret, S., Aboab, J., Adrie, C., . . . Darmon, M. (2005). Risk of post-traumatic stress symptoms in family members of intensive care unit patients. *American Journal of Respiratory and Critical Care Medicine, 171*(9), 987–994.

Center to Advance Palliative Care. (2013). *Palliative care and the human connection: Ten steps for what to say and do* [Video file]. Retrieved from https://www.youtube.com/watch?v=7kQ3PUyhmPQ

Centers for Disease Control and Prevention (CDC). (2016). About underlying cause of death, 1999–2015. Retrieved from https://wonder.cdc.gov/ucd-icd10.html

Coalition for Compassionate Care. (2017). Physician orders for life-sustaining treatment (POLST). Retrieved from http://coalitionccc.org/what-we-do/physician-orders-for-life-sustaining-treatment-polst/

The Conversation Project. (2017). About us. Retrieved from http://theconversationproject.org/about/

Devettere, R. J. (2016). *Practical decision making in health care ethics: Cases, concepts, and the virtue of prudence.* Washington, DC: Georgetown University Press.

Mayo Clinic. (2014). Living wills and advance directives for medical decisions. Retrieved from https://www.mayoclinic.org/healthy-lifestyle/consumer-health/in-depth/living-wills/art-20046303

Patients Rights Council. (2013). Advance directives: Definitions. Retrieved from http://www.patientsrightscouncil.org/site/advance-directives-definitions/

PerryUndem Research/Communication. (2016). *Physicians' views toward advance care planning and end-of-life care conversations.* Retrieved from https://www.johnahartford.org/images/uploads/resources/ConversationStopper_Poll_Memo.pdf

Rao, J. K., Anderson, L. A., Lin, F.-C., & Laux, J. P. (2014). Completion of advance directives among US consumers. *American Journal of Preventive Medicine, 46*(1), 65–70.

Sedensky, M. (2010). 5 years after Schiavo few make end-of-life plans. *Boston.com.* Retrieved from http://archive.boston.com/news/nation/articles/2010/03/30/5_years_after_schiavo_few_make_end_of_life_plans/

U.S. Department of Health and Human Services. (2016). *Advance care planning.* Retrieved from https://www.cms.gov/Outreach-and-Education/Medicare-Learning-Network-MLN/MLNProducts/Downloads/AdvanceCarePlanning.pdf

Yadav, K. N., Gabler, N. B., Cooney, E., Kent, S., Kim, J., Herbst, N., . . . Courtright, K. R. (2017). Approximately one in three US adults completes any type of advance directive for end-of-life care. *Health Affairs, 36*(7), 1244–1251.

CHAPTER 21

Cognitive Assessment

Marsha N. Wittink, Neha Pawar, and Amy Pacos Martinez

The authors wish to acknowledge the significant contributions of the co-author of this chapter in the previous edition of this text, Joseph J. Gallo.

CHAPTER OBJECTIVES

1. Understand the key differences between dementia and delirium.
2. Describe assessment of each domain of cognitive capacity.
3. Identify common standardized initial screening tools for dementia.

KEY TERMS

Delirium   Dementia

▶ Introduction

The number of people affected by cognitive impairment and **dementia** is predicted to double over the next 20 years, leading some to warn of an impending "dementia epidemic" (Prince et al., 2016). The psychological, social, and physical burdens of cognitive decline deeply affect patients and family members, leading to increased healthcare utilization as well as increased morbidity and mortality (Bellelli et al.,

2007; Boustani et al., 2010; Fick, Steis, Waller, & Inouye, 2013). Patients with cognitive impairment have a significantly increased risk of complications related to confusion and functioning. For example, cognitive decline can lead to loss of independence (Francis & Kapoor, 1992; Inouye & Charpentier, 1996), postoperative complications (Marcantonio et al., 1994), and behavioral difficulties (Cooper, Mungas, & Weiler, 1990). Individuals who develop cognitive impairment are highly susceptible to experiencing **delirium** during hospitalization, postoperatively, and after discharge from the hospital (Francis & Kapoor, 1992; Marcantonio et al., 1994; McCartney & Palmateer, 1985), which in turn may lead to increased morbidity and mortality.

Clinicians working in primary care settings, emergency rooms, and hospitals are on the front lines for identifying early cognitive decline and can play an enormous role in helping mitigate the impact of cognitive decline on health. Recognition of this condition can help identify modifiable risk factors and assist patients and family members in preparing for and coping with its potential consequences. Yet early diagnosis, in particular, can be a challenge given the subtle nature of the changes experienced by the affected individual and the fact that some older people may be able to compensate for their symptoms when they are present. Common barriers to recognizing cognitive decline include clinicians' worries about prematurely or inaccurately diagnosing dementia as well as concerns about causing stigma and psychological distress to patients (Lliffe & Manthorpe, 2004). Even with these concerns, several studies suggest that patients and families prefer early disclosure of a diagnosis (van den Dungen et al., 2014).

As the U.S. health system shifts toward emphasizing patient- and family-centered outcomes such as quality of life and incentivizing clinicians to reduce hospital lengths of stay and readmission rates, there are new reasons to pay closer attention to signs of cognitive impairment. In addition, the increased accessibility of brief pragmatic assessment tools and team-based approaches to care could lead to better outcomes for people at risk for dementia.

▶ Defining Dementia and Cognitive Impairment

Dementia is a syndrome that spans a spectrum of patient condition. Given these variations, one useful diagnosis is that from the *Diagnostic and Statistical Manual, Fifth Edition* (*DSM-V*; American Psychiatric Association, 2013), as it can give a useful starting point. *DSM-V* uses the term "major neurocognitive decline" to characterize dementia as a decline of cognitive capacity involving at least one of the following domains:

- Learning and memory
- Language
- Executive function
- Complex attention
- Perceptual-motor function
- Social cognition

Importantly, the deficits must be severe enough to significantly affect daily functioning and not be otherwise explained by delirium or psychiatric disorder (see **BOX 21-1**).

▶ Differential Diagnosis

Before delving into cognitive assessments, it is useful to consider the differential diagnosis of cognitive impairment. Particularly in the acute setting, the initial distinction that must be made by the clinician is between dementia and delirium. At the outset, it must be emphasized that older adults may exhibit delirium superimposed on dementia. The aged central nervous system may be especially vulnerable to dysfunction brought about by metabolic disturbances. A decline in function of persons with dementia should prompt a search for potentially reversible conditions.

At the same time, a diagnosis of delirium warrants further evaluation even after delirium resolves, recognizing the correlation between dementia and delirium. *Delirium*—a term that is interchangeable with the terms *acute confusional state* and *encephalopathy*, is marked by a disturbance in arousal and attention, usually of acute onset (i.e., in hours or days) with fluctuations during the course of a day. This contrasts substantially with the onset of dementia, which is typically more slowly progressive and occurs over a longer period of months to years and with fewer fluctuations. The disturbance in

BOX 21-1 Diagnostic Criteria for Major Neurocognitive Disorder

Major Neurocognitive Disorder
Diagnostic Criteria

A. Evidence of significant cognitive decline from a previous level of performance in one or more cognitive domains (complex attention, executive function, learning and memory, language, perceptual-motor, or social cognition) based on:
   1. concern of the individual, a knowledgeable informant, or the clinician that there has been a significant decline in cognitive function; and
   2. a substantial impairment in cognitive performance, preferably documented by standardized neuropsychological testing or, in its absence, another quantified clinical assessment.
B. The cognitive deficits interfere with independence in everyday activities (i.e., at a minimum, requiring assistance with complex instrumental activities of daily living such as paying bills or managing medications).
C. The cognitive deficits do not occur exclusively in the context of a delirium.
D. The cognitive deficits are not better explained by another mental disorder (e.g., major depressive disorder, schizophrenia).

Reprinted with permission from the *Diagnostic and Statistical Manual of Mental Disorders, Fifth Edition* (Copyright ©2013). American Psychiatric Association. All Rights Reserved.

attention seen in delirium can be described as a change in the person's ability to direct, focus, and sustain his or her attention. Lethargy and drowsiness are easily recognizable signs of a disturbance in arousal; a more subtle sign occurs when a family member notices that the patient is more easily distracted from a task or conversation.

The key aspect of diagnosing delirium is establishing the patient's baseline mental status. It is therefore essential to take a good history from a caregiver or family member when possible. Establishing the rapidity of the changes is key in differentiating delirium from dementia. It cannot be overemphasized, however, that delirium is a syndrome, not a diagnosis. Delirium requires further evaluation for its underlying causes and includes its own wide differential work-up (Inouye, 2006), even if dementia is also present.

Once delirium is definitively ruled out, or when it is recognized and steps are taken to treat the underlying cause, the clinician must then determine whether global cognitive impairment is present. If this is established with the help of history and assessments described later in this chapter, a consideration of the specific

etiology is in order. Concomitant with the differential assessment, it behooves clinicians to consider the diagnosis of depression, either as the exclusive cause of cognitive changes or concomitantly associated with cognitive changes secondary to another etiology. While Alzheimer's disease is the most common form of dementia, the reality is that a broad range of conditions can cause dementia. A thoughtful work-up to evaluate the possibility of an underlying medical condition as the cause of the dementia and developing appropriate management is always the first step.

▸ Pre-assessment Process

Before embarking on assessments, it is essential that the clinician be aware of several key factors related to the patient and the context. For example, it is well known that age, educational attainment, work experience, and literacy can all affect cognitive assessments (Acevedo,

Loewenstein, Agrón, & Duara, 2007; Manly et al., 1999). Other factors, such as the environment in which the assessment takes place, can also play an important role. Thus, there is good reason to delay definitive assessments of patients who are in the hospital when those patients may be more likely to have resolving delirium—while recognizing that such a delay is not always feasible when trying to determine a course of treatment. Less well understood is the effect of culture and other sociodemographic factors.

It is also important to recognize the value that collateral information obtained from a loved one or family member can yield. Concrete, functional real-life examples of the patient's daily experience can provide useful information in the assessment process and serve to elucidate areas of concern. For all these reasons, completing a comprehensive patient history and involving collateral sources in the assessment to obtain supplementary information is the ideal scenario.

▶ Test Selection

Many assessment instruments have been devised to assist clinicians in measuring cognitive function. Some screening instruments for intellectual functioning were devised for the sole purpose of assessing mental status, whereas others form part of a total instrument that includes measures of functional status and/or psychiatric illness. Further information on instruments to assess mental status and dementia symptoms may be found in *Cognitive Assessment for Clinicians* (Hodges, 2007), *Geropsychology Assessment Resource Guide* (National Center for Cost Containment & U.S. Department of Veterans Affairs, 1996), and *Measuring Health: A Guide to Rating Scales and Questionnaires* (McDowell, 2006). When selecting any test measures, it is important to consider patient-specific factors. Understanding the level of severity of a patient's cognitive difficulties can help with identifying appropriate assessment measures.

In addition to simple detection of the demented state, the mental status assessment instruments can stratify persons with regard to the severity of dementia. Many of the instruments designed specifically for this purpose include some assessment of functional ability.

Providers should be aware that mental status assessment instruments may exhibit threshold or ceiling effects. In other words, persons beyond a certain level of severity of dementia may score the same despite some differences in the degree of their impairment. In a population with a predominance of severely demented persons, for example, an instrument would not be useful for following changes if all severely affected individuals performed equally poorly. By the same token, in a population of relatively well older persons, an easy test will be insensitive to mildly demented persons, who may be able to perform well on it, whereas they would have difficulties on a more discriminating test.

▶ The Mental Status Examination

While there remains lack of consensus regarding *routine* screening for cognitive impairment among older adults (Cordell et al., 2013; Moyer, 2014), the general mental status exam has long been regarded as part of the initial assessment of overall health. Combined with clinical cues or "triggers," the mental status exam can be used to prompt further assessment using one or more assessment instruments discussed later in this chapter. The mental status examination samples behavior and mental capability over a range of intellectual functions (**BOX 21-2**). The standardized brief assessments described in this chapter can be used to detect cognitive impairment by testing a range of intellectual functions using one or two questions in each area. If these screens detect impairment, further examination is warranted. In clinical settings,

BOX 21-2 Intellectual Functions

Level of consciousness
    Attention
Language
    Fluency
    Comprehension
    Repetition
Memory
    Short-term memory
    Remote memory
Proverb interpretation
Similarities
Calculations
Writing
Constructional ability

Data from Strub, R. L., & Black, F. W. (1980). The Mental Status Examination in Neurology. FA Davis Company.

this usually means more detailed mental status testing to localize and define the problem. When further characterization of the intellectual functioning is required, neuropsychologic testing may be in order.

Some healthcare professionals take the mental status examination no further than asking a few questions about orientation, having the person perform calculations, and requiring that he or she remember three items. In some situations, however, a thorough assessment can be crucial in an appropriate diagnosis and hence management. A common example is the patient with intracranial hemorrhage who is not making any sense and is mistakenly thought to be psychotic or confused because a specific language disturbance is not recognized. The complete mental status examination encompasses an assessment of the level of consciousness, attention, language, memory, proverb interpretation, similarities (e.g., "How are an apple and an orange alike?"), calculations, writing, and constructional ability (e.g., copying complex figures).

Higher Cognitive Functions

Ideally, the interview could start with questions of significance to the patient, which also gauge his or her memory and may help allay anxiety. Likewise, introductory statements that indicate interest in the older patient as a person (e.g., occupation, children, grandchildren, and hobbies) help determine the patient's current and previous levels of mental and social functioning. General appearance and grooming, posture, behavior, speech, and word choice can speak volumes to the careful observer (Fry, 1986). At the same time, the examiner should be wary of hearing and visual deficits that may mimic cognitive impairment, and should ask the patient if he or she has eyeglasses or hearing aids that can be used before beginning the assessments.

The higher cognitive functions that may be specifically tested include the patient's fund of information and ability to reason abstractly and perform calculations. After some preliminary questions about personal history are discussed, the patient may be asked questions regarding current events in the news (e.g., "Who is the president now?") or commonly known historical information (e.g., "When did World War II end?") to assess the fund of information. In evaluating responses, it is critical to know the level of educational attainment and whether English is the patient's first language.

Assessment of insight and judgment has important implications for considering driving skills and independence. Accidents and burns may be more common among cognitively impaired persons with poor insight and judgment (Feher, Doody, Pirozzolo, & Appel, 1989). Observe the patient's responses to mental status testing and conversation to note whether statements belie a lack of insight into deficits (Feher et al., 1989).

Proverb testing and similarities can shed light on the patient's reasoning ability, intelligence, and judgment. The examiner needs to be careful that the patient is not repeating the meaning of a proverb from memory rather than reasoning what an abstract interpretation might be.

The Cognitive Capacity Screen (Jacobs, Bernhard, Delgado, & Strain, 1977), the Kokmen Short Test of Mental Status (Kokmen, Naessens, & Offord, 1987), and the Saint Louis University Mental Status Exam are examples of screening instruments that include a test of reasoning with similarities—a task requiring the subject to think in abstract categories to discover how two concepts are alike. An example of a similarity is "How are a poem and a novel alike?" It has been suggested that the use of similarities is better than the use of proverb testing for the assessment of abstraction ability.

The ability to perform calculations may be tested with serial 7s (i.e., "take 7 away from 100 and keep subtracting 7 from the answer all the way down"), serial 3s (i.e., "take 3 away from 20 and keep subtracting 3 from the answer all the way down"), or simple math problems. Corrected mistakes should not be counted as errors. Calculation ability also requires substantial memory and concentration ability. Occasionally, patients who have difficulty with serial 7s will handle the subtractions flawlessly if the problem is expressed in dollar terms (i.e., "If you had $100 and took away $7, how much would you have left?").

Memory

Of all of the components of the mental status examination, memory assessment most commonly engenders anxiety—and understandably so. It sometimes puts the patient at ease when the examiner prefaces the evaluation, particularly when using a standard questionnaire, with an explanation such as the following: "I'm going to ask you some questions. Some are easy. Some may be hard. Please don't be offended because it's the same routine I use for everyone." The examiner should give positive reinforcement during the examination with expressions such as "That's OK" or "That's fine."

Memory can be thought of as comprising three components. First and most fleeting is immediate recall, which can be assessed with digit repetition. Normal older persons can correctly recall five to seven digits (Blum, Jarvik, & Clark, 1970; La Rue, 1982).

The second component of memory is short-term memory, ranging over a period of minutes to days. This is usually tested by asking the person to remember three to four objects or abstract terms and then requesting him or her to recall them 5 or 10 minutes later after an intervening conversation or other testing. Examples of words used are "apple," "table," and "penny" (Gallo, Marino, Ford, & Anthony, 1995). The memory of aphasic persons may be tested by asking them to recall where items have been hidden in the room. It has been suggested that older persons do not use mnemonics when given a memory task, and that this in part accounts for their failure to recall items (Blum et al., 1970). Also, some evidence suggests older persons have increased processing time, which may interfere with learning (Eriksen, Hamlin, & Daye, 1973).

The third component of memory is remote or long-term memory. In one study, older adults were able to recall 80% of a catechism that they had learned some 36 years before (Smith, 1963).

In general, older persons' self-reports of memory difficulty correlate poorly with objective measures of memory function. Not uncommonly, persons who complain fervently of memory loss are depressed, whereas someone with Alzheimer's disease may be oblivious to profound memory deficit (Vogel, Waldorff, & Waldemar, 2010). Early in the course of the disease, however, patients with Alzheimer's disease may notice and complain of memory loss (Grut et al., 1993). Normal middle-aged or older persons may complain of memory difficulties, but their memory symptoms are more consistent with age-associated memory impairment (Grut et al., 1993; Kral, 1962), which is usually not associated with functional impairment and has little impact on daily activities.

Attention and Level of Consciousness

Before an examiner can test and comment on the higher intellectual functions of the brain, including memory, some assessment (even if informal) must be made of the patient's level of consciousness. Obviously, functions such as orientation and memory cannot be tested in a comatose patient.

Orientation to surroundings is a fundamental beginning to mental status testing, but unfortunately, in routine clinical situations, the mental status evaluation often ends there. Questions regarding orientation to time, place, person, and situation are basic. Most people continually orient themselves by means of daily routines, clocks and watches, calendars, news media, and social activities. Older persons, particularly those living alone or in nursing homes, may not experience these activities and, as a result, may have poor orientation to time and events (Blazer, 2003; Fry, 1986).

After it is determined by observation that the person is alert enough for mental status testing to proceed, his or her attentiveness is assessed. Assessing attentiveness is important because a person who is easily distracted and unable to attend to the examiner will have poor performance on mental status testing solely because of inattention. Special note must be taken of the person who is inappropriately distracted by environmental noise or talking in the hallway. In such a case, a specific examination for attention deficit indicative of delirium may be warranted. Tests of attention sometimes used include digit repetition and the "A" test of vigilance. The length of a string of digits able to be repeated immediately after presentation tends to remain stable with age. A normal 90-year-old person should be able to repeat four digits, perhaps even seven or eight, after the examiner (La Rue, 1982). In the "A" test, the patient is asked to tap the table when the letter "A" is heard while the examiner presents random letters at a rate of one letter per second. The examiner observes for errors of commission and omission.

Neglect is a form of inattention in which the individual does not attend to stimuli presented from a particular side, and it occurs most commonly with nondominant hemisphere lesions (usually in the right hemisphere). The examiner needs to avoid interviewing such a person from the neglected side if communication is to be effective.

Language

Language should be observed and tested in a comprehensive mental status examination. Spontaneous speech is observed during the initial interview. Does the patient make errors in words or grammatical construction? Persons with dysarthria, who have difficulty in the mechanical production of language, use normal grammar. Do spoken words flow smoothly? Fluency is one of the features that is used to differentiate the aphasias.

A simplified approach to aphasia divides the spoken language functions to be tested into three areas: comprehension, fluency, and repetition. Comprehension can be tested by asking the patient yes-or-no questions. If there is doubt about the responses, the patient may be asked to point to objects in the room. The task may be made more difficult by having the patient try to point to objects in a particular sequence or after the examiner has provided a description of the item rather than the item's name.

Fluency is a characteristic of speech that describes the rate and rhythm of speech production and the ease in initiating speech. Patients may be asked to name objects and their parts, such as a wristwatch and its band, buckle, and face. Repetition is tested with easy expressions (e.g., "ball" or "airplane") progressing to more difficult ones (e.g., "Methodist Episcopal" or "around the rock the rugged rascal ran").

Writing and Construction Ability

The components of the mental status examination discussed to this point can smoothly follow the history interview because it is primarily a verbal examination. At this point in the examination, the patient may be presented with a blank sheet of paper for subsequent tests.

The patient is asked to write his or her name at the top of the page. Although the signature is usually overlearned and can be intact even with writing difficulty for more complex tasks, this action acclimates the patient to the idea that he or she will be asked to do some writing, and the signature is a nonthreatening way to begin. Below the signature, the patient is asked to write a complete sentence, perhaps about the weather.

While the person has the blank sheet of paper and pen in hand, construction ability may be tested. The ability to reproduce the line drawings of the examiner represents construction ability. This can be a very sensitive test of parietal lobe damage and is an early abnormality in dementia. Trouble with construction ability is not something most persons will complain of specifically, but testing constructional ability can be revealing. The testing begins with simple figures such as a triangle or square, and progresses to more complex drawings such as a cube, house, or flowerpot. Difficulty in copying figures is not specific to dementia, however; trouble with this test may also reflect motor incoordination or apraxia (Jacobs et al., 1977).

Asking the patient to draw a clock showing the numerals and time (e.g., "10 minutes past 11 o'clock") can act as a single-item screen for cognitive impairment. The examiner draws a large circle on a blank sheet of paper and asks the patient to fill in the numbers as on a clock. This task is thought to be a sensitive test of parietal lobe dysfunction. Persons with primarily right or nondominant hemisphere dysfunction will write the numbers correctly but plan poorly. Those with primarily left or dominant hemisphere dysfunction will have trouble writing the numbers but execute the general plan of the clock correctly, perhaps placing lines where the numbers should be. Clock drawing has been used to screen for cognitive impairment (Wolf-Klein, Silverstone, Levy, & Brod, 1989) as well as to follow progression of diagnosed Alzheimer's disease. Several scoring methods for the clock-drawing task are available (Ainslie & Murden, 1993; Shuttleworth, 1982; Sunderland et al., 1989; Tuokko, Hadjistavropoulos, Miller, & Beattie, 1992; Watson, Arfken, & Birge, 1993).

▶ Standardized Brief Assessments

The Montreal Cognitive Assessment (MoCA) is a screening test for cognitive impairment that covers major cognitive domains including episodic memory, language, attention, orientation, visuospatial ability, and executive functions, while remaining brief and easy to administer (Nasreddine et al., 2005). It is generally considered superior to the well-established Mini-Mental State Examination (MMSE) screening test, since the MoCA not only assesses executive functioning but also has a higher sensitivity for mild cognitive impairment (Hoops et al., 2009).

The Mini-Cog test combines the clock drawing test with a three-item recall test. The patient is asked to repeat three unrelated words, then to perform the clock drawing test, and finally to recall the three words. The total possible score ranges from 0 to 5, with one point given for each correctly recalled word (only the delayed recall is scored), and two points for a normal clock drawing test. Scores from 0 to 2 are highly suggestive of dementia, whereas scores from 3 to 5 have a low likelihood of dementia (Borson, Scanlan, Watanabe, Tu, & Lessig, 2005). The Mini-Cog takes 2 to 4 minutes to perform, and has a sensitivity of 76% and a specificity of 89% in detecting dementia (positive likelihood ratio = 7.0; negative likelihood ratio = 0.27).

The Folstein Mini-Mental State Examination (MMSE; Folstein, Folstein, & McHugh, 1975) is one of the most widely employed tests of cognitive function and is one of the best studied (Crum, Anthony, Bassett, & Folstein, 1993; Tombaugh & McIntyre, 1992). Five cognitive functions underlie the items in the MMSE: concentration, language, orientation, memory, and attention (Jones & Gallo, 2001). Population-based norms are readily available according to age and educational level (Crum et al., 1993). The MMSE consists of two parts. The first part requires verbal responses only and assesses orientation, memory, and attention. The three words used to test memory are left up to the examiner, leaving the possibility that this question could vary in difficulty. The items "apple, table, penny" were used in the Epidemiologic Catchment Area Program. In addition to serial 7s, the individual is asked to spell "world" backward, and the best score may be taken for calculating the total score. A "chess move" strategy is used to score the "world" item (i.e., the number of transpositions required to spell "DLROW" yields the number of errors) (Gallo et al., 1995). The second part of the MMSE evaluates the ability to write a sentence, name objects, follow verbal and written commands, and copy a complex polygon. The maximum score is 30. A score of 20 to 24 suggests mild dementia, 13 to 20 suggests moderate dementia, and less than 12 indicates severe dementia. The test is not timed. A telephone version of the MMSE is available for special purposes (Brandt, Spencer, & Folstein, 1988).

There is some question as to the adjustment of scores on mental status screening instruments based on the educational level of the subject. A low score may imply more severe intellectual impairment among persons with high educational attainment. As the education level increases, one expects the specificity of an instrument to rise; an abnormal test result probably really is abnormal because one would expect better performance from an educated person.

Lower scores may occur among patients with less education who are not demented (Crum et al., 1993; Uhlmann & Larson, 1991). Among persons with 0 to 4 years of education, a cutoff point of 19 represents the 75th percentile (i.e., 75% of community-dwelling adults with 0 to 4 years of education would score below 19 on the MMSE). Corresponding cutoff points are for persons with 5 to 8 years of schooling, 23 and below; for 9 to 12 years of schooling, 27 and below; for schooling at the college level and beyond, 29 and below (Crum et al., 1993). The person should be asked how much schooling he or she has had to assist in interpreting scores.

It should also be remembered that the MMSE and other mental status instruments serve as only one component in assessment of dementia.

▶ Practical Considerations

Completing a comprehensive evaluation assessing cognition within a geriatric population can be challenging. Clinicians may want to consider the use of a "rolling" assessment over several visits to obtain the necessary information. One school of thought is to focus on one domain at each visit (e.g., function, physical health, cognition, mental health, polypharmacy, and socio-environmental needs/support). This enables the clinician to acquire the relevant information over time and can aid in obtaining a comprehensive profile of the patient to manage the condition, minimize complications, and improve diagnostic accuracy (Elsawy & Higgins, 2011).

Even with the inclusion of screening measures, it can be difficult for the clinician to confirm the presence of dementia. In cases that are challenging, it may be beneficial to consider the option of referring the patient for a neuropsychological evaluation. Neuropsychologists assess brain function and impairment by drawing inferences from a patient's objective test performance. Tests of neuropsychological function are often able to detect subtle cognitive deficits that are undetected by electrophysiologic or imaging methods ("Assessment: Neuropsychological Testing of Adults," 1996). A neuropsychological assessment can be used to facilitate clinical decision making, inform treatment planning, and monitor performance over time. Further, a formal assessment can help guide practical decisions about safety, driving, work appropriateness, and general changes to lifestyle if indicated (Moberg & Rick, 2008).

Once a diagnosis of dementia has been made, attention needs to be turned to addressing goals of care. These goals can reflect a patient's specific medical treatment goals, specific personal health goals, and patient-specific needs/interests. Embedded in the discussion of a patient's goals of care is the understanding that the family plays a central part in the decision-making process (Yaffe, Orzeck, & Barylak, 2008). The family's adjustment and acceptance of the dementia diagnosis is vital (Schulz & Martire, 2004). Research has suggested that directing the patient toward maintaining a sense of self and finding a purpose or focus can improve general adjustment to dementia. Finally, identifying and locating resources (e.g., community support groups, peer support groups) are considered essential in the journey of dementia care (Frank, Feldman, & Schulz, 2011).

▶ Summary

Assessing the cognitive status of patients is important, especially during the initial work-up for an older adult admitted to a hospital or nursing home and whenever behavior, mental status, or level of functioning is a cause for concern. Changes in cognitive state can be more confidently assessed when a baseline has been established. Assessment of cognitive status must be considered within the context of the individual's functional status, the physical examination (especially vision and hearing), the history from an informant, and the total clinical picture.

References

Acevedo, A., Loewenstein, D. A., Agrón, J., & Duara, R. (2007). Influence of sociodemographic variables on neuropsychological test performance in Spanish-speaking older adults. *Journal of Clinical and Experimental Neuropsychology, 29*(5), 530–544. doi: 10.1080/13803390600814740

Ainslie, N. K., & Murden, R. A. (1993). Effect of education on the clock-drawing dementia screen in non-demented elderly persons. *Journal of the American Geriatrics Society, 41*(3), 249–252.

American Psychiatric Association. (2013). *Diagnostic and statistical manual of mental disorders* (5th ed). Washington, DC: Author.

Assessment: Neuropsychological testing of adults. Considerations for neurologists. Report of the Therapeutics and Technology Assessment Subcommittee of the American Academy of Neurology. (1996). *Neurology, 47*(2), 592–599.

Bellelli, G., Frisoni, G. B., Turco, R., Lucchi, E., Magnifico, F., & Trabucchi, M. (2007). Delirium superimposed on dementia predicts 12-month survival in elderly patients discharged from a postacute rehabilitation facility. *Journals of Gerontology Series A: Biological Sciences and Medical Sciences, 62*(11), 1306–1309.

Blazer, D. G. (2003). Depression in late life: Review and commentary. *Journals of Gerontology Series A: Biological Sciences and Medical Sciences, 58*(3), 249–265.

Blum, J. E., Jarvik, L. F., & Clark, E. T. (1970). Rate of change on selective tests of intelligence: a twenty-year longitudinal study of aging. *Journal of Gerontology, 25*(3), 171–176.

Borson, S., Scanlan, J. M., Watanabe, J., Tu, S. P., & Lessig, M. (2005). Simplifying detection of cognitive impairment: Comparison of the Mini-Cog and Mini-Mental State Examination in a multiethnic sample. *Journal of the American Geriatrics Society, 53*(5), 871–874. doi: 10.1111/j.1532-5415.2005.53269.x

Boustani, M., Baker, M. S., Campbell, N., Munger, S., Hui, S. L., Castelluccio, P., . . . Callahan, C. (2010). Impact and recognition of cognitive impairment among hospitalized elders. *Journal of Hospital Medicine, 5*(2), 69–75. doi: 10.1002/jhm.589

Brandt, J., Spencer, M., & Folstein, M. (1988). The telephone interview for cognitive status. *Cognitive and Behavioral Neurology, 1*(2), 111–118.

Cordell, C. B., Borson, S., Boustani, M., Chodosh, J., Reuben, D., Verghese, J., . . . Fried, L. B., for Medicare Detection of Cognitive Impairment Workshop. (2013). Alzheimer's Association recommendations for operationalizing the detection of cognitive impairment during the Medicare Annual Wellness Visit in a primary care setting. *Alzheimer's & Dementia, 9*(2), 141–150. doi: 10.1016/j.jalz.2012.09.011

Crum, R. M., Anthony, J. C., Bassett, S. S., & Folstein, M. F. (1993). Population-based norms for the Mini-Mental State Examination by age and educational level. *Journal of the American Medical Association, 269*(18), 2386–2391.

Elsawy, B., & Higgins, K. E. (2011). The geriatric assessment. *American Family Physician, 83*(1), 48–56.

Eriksen, C. W., Hamlin, R. M., & Daye, C. (1973). Aging adults and rate of memory scan. *Bulletin of the Psychonomic Society, 1*(4), 259–260. doi: 10.3758/bf03333363

Feher, E. P., Doody, R., Pirozzolo, F. J., & Appel, S. H. (1989). Mental status assessment of insight and judgment. *Clinics in Geriatric Medicine, 5*(3), 477–498.

Fick, D. M., Steis, M. R., Waller, J. L., & Inouye, S. K. (2013). Delirium superimposed on dementia is associated with prolonged length of stay and poor outcomes in hospitalized older adults. *Journal of Hospital Medicine, 8*(9), 500–505. doi: 10.1002/jhm.2077

Folstein, M. F., Folstein, S. E., & McHugh, P. R. (1975). Mini-mental state: A practical method for grading the cognitive state of patients for the clinician. *Journal of Psychiatric Research, 12*(3), 189–198.

Francis, J., & Kapoor, W. N. (1992). Prognosis after hospital discharge of older medical patients with delirium. *Journal of the American Geriatrics Society, 40*(6), 601–606.

Frank, C., Feldman, S., & Schulz, M. (2011). Resources for people with dementia: The Alzheimer Society and beyond. *Canaidan Family Physician, 57*(12), 1387–1391, e1460–1384.

Fry, P. S. (1986). *Depression, stress, and adaptations in the elderly: Psychological assessment and intervention.* Rockville, MD: Aspen.

Gallo, J. J., Marino, S., Ford, D., & Anthony, J. C. (1995). Filters on the pathway to mental health care, II. Sociodemographic factors. *Psychological Medicine, 25*(6), 1149–1160.

Grut, M., Jorm, A. F., Fratiglioni, L., Forsell, Y., Viitanen, M., & Winblad, B. (1993). Memory complaints of elderly people in a population survey: Variation according to dementia stage and depression. *Journal of the American Geriatrics Society, 41*(12), 1295–1300.

Hodges, J. R. (2007). *Cognitive assessment for clinicians.* Oxford, UK: Oxford University Press.

Hoops, S., Nazem, S., Siderowf, A. D., Duda, J. E., Xie, S. X., Stern, M. B., & Weintraub, D. (2009). Validity of the MoCA and MMSE in the detection of MCI and dementia in Parkinson disease. *Neurology, 73*(21), 1738–1745. doi: 10.1212/WNL.0b013e3181c34b47

Inouye, S. K. (2006). Delirium in older persons. *New England Journal of Medicine, 354*(11), 1157–1165. doi: 10.1056/NEJMra052321

Inouye, S. K., & Charpentier, P. A. (1996). Precipitating factors for delirium in hospitalized elderly persons: Predictive model and interrelationship with baseline vulnerability. *Journal of the American Medical Association, 275*(11), 852–857.

Jacobs, J. W., Bernhard, M. R., Delgado, A., & Strain, J. J. (1977). Screening for organic mental syndromes in the medically ill. *Annals of Internal Medicine, 86*(1), 40–46.

Jones, R. N., & Gallo, J. J. (2001). Education bias in the Mini-Mental State Examination. *International Psychogeriatrics, 13*(3), 299–310.

Kokmen, E., Naessens, J. M., & Offord, K. P. (1987). A short test of mental status: Description and preliminary results. *Mayo Clinic Proceedings, 62*(4), 281–288.

Kral, V. A. (1962). Senescent forgetfulness: Benign and malignant. *Canadian Medical Association Journal, 86,* 257–260.

La Rue, A. (1982). Memory loss and aging: Distinguishing dementia from benign senescent forgetfulness and depressive pseudodementia. *Psychiatrics Clinics of North America, 5*(1), 89–103.

Lliffe, S., & Manthorpe, J. (2004). The hazards of early recognition of dementia: A risk assessment. *Aging and Mental Health, 8*(2), 99–105. doi: 10.1080/13607860410001649653

Manly, J. J., Jacobs, D. M., Sano, M., Bell, K., Merchant, C. A., Small, S. A., & Stern, Y. (1999). Effect of literacy on neuropsychological test performance in nondemented, education-matched elders. *Journal of the International Neuropsychology Society, 5*(3), 191–202.

Marcantonio, E. R., Goldman, L., Mangione, C. M., Ludwig, L. E., Muraca, B., Haslauer, C. M., . . . Lee, T. H. (1994). A clinical prediction rule for delirium after elective noncardiac surgery. *Journal of the American Medical Association, 271*(2), 134–139.

McCartney, J. R., & Palmateer, L. M. (1985). Assessment of cognitive deficit in geriatric patients: A study of physician behavior. *Journal of the American Geriatrics Society, 33*(7), 467–471.

McDowell, I. (2006). *Measuring health: A guide to rating scales and questionnaires.* Oxford, UK: Oxford University Press.

Moberg, P. J., & Rick, J. H. (2008). Decision-making capacity and competency in the elderly: A clinical and neuropsychological perspective. *NeuroRehabilitation, 23*(5), 403–413.

Moyer, V. A. (2014). Screening for cognitive impairment in older adults: U.S. Preventive Services Task Force recommendation statement. *Annals of Internal Medicine, 160*(11), 791–797. doi: 10.7326/m14-0496

Nasreddine, Z. S., Phillips, N. A., Bedirian, V., Charbonneau, S., Whitehead, V., Collin, I., . . . Chertkow, H. (2005). The Montreal Cognitive Assessment, MoCA: A brief screening tool for mild cognitive impairment. *Journal of the American Geriatrics Society, 53*(4), 695–699. doi: 10.1111/j.1532-5415.2005.53221.x

National Center for Cost Containment & U.S. Department of Veterans Affairs. (1996). *Geropsychology assessment resource guide: Assessment instruments, GRECC programs, geropsychology professionals' network, VA fellowships, other resources.* Washington, DC: National Center for Cost Containment.

Prince, M., Ali, G.-C., Guerchet, M., Prina, A. M., Albanese, E., & Wu, Y.-T. (2016). Recent global trends in the prevalence and incidence of dementia, and survival with dementia. *Alzheimer's Research & Therapy, 8*(1), 23. doi: 10.1186/s13195-016-0188-8

Schulz, R., & Martire, L. M. (2004). Family caregiving of persons with dementia: Prevalence, health effects, and support strategies. *American Journal of Geriatric Psychiatry, 12*(3), 240–249.

Shuttleworth, E. C. (1982). Memory function and the clinical differentiation of dementing disorder. *Journal of the American Geriatrics Society, 30*(6), 363–366.

Smith, M. E. (1963). Delayed recall of previously memorized material after fifty years. *Journal of Genetic Psychology, 102,* 3–4.

Sunderland, T., Hill, J. L., Mellow, A. M., Lawlor, B. A., Gundersheimer, J., Newhouse, P. A., & Grafman, J. H. (1989). Clock drawing in Alzheimer's disease: A novel measure of dementia severity. *Journal of the American Geriatrics Society, 37*(8), 725–729.

Tombaugh, T. N., & McIntyre, N. J. (1992). The Mini-Mental State Examination: A comprehensive review. *Journal of the American Geriatrics Society, 40*(9), 922–935.

Tuokko, H., Hadjistavropoulos, T., Miller, J. A., & Beattie, B. L. (1992). The clock test: A sensitive measure to differentiate normal elderly from those with Alzheimer disease. *Journal of the American Geriatrics Society, 40*(6), 579–584.

Uhlmann, R. F., & Larson, E. B. (1991). Effect of education on the Mini-Mental State Examination as a screening test for dementia. *Journal of the American Geriatrics Society, 39*(9), 876–880.

van den Dungen, P., van Kuijk, L., van Marwijk, H., van der Wouden, J., Moll van Charante, E., van der Horst, H., & van Hout, H. (2014). Preferences regarding disclosure of a diagnosis of dementia: A systematic review. *International Psychogeriatrics, 26*(10), 1603–1618. doi: 10.1017/s1041610214000969

Vogel, A., Waldorff, F. B., & Waldemar, G. (2010). Impaired awareness of deficits and neuropsychiatric symptoms in early Alzheimer's disease: The Danish Alzheimer Intervention Study (DAISY). *Journal of Neuropsychiatry and Clinical Neurosciences, 22*(1), 93–99. doi: 10.1176/jnp.2010.22.1.93

Watson, Y. I., Arfken, C. L., & Birge, S. J. (1993). Clock completion: An objective screening test for dementia. *Journal of the American Geriatrics Society, 41*(11), 1235–1240.

Wolf-Klein, G. P., Silverstone, F. A., Levy, A. P., & Brod, M. S. (1989). Screening for Alzheimer's disease by clock drawing. *Journal of the American Geriatrics Society, 37*(8), 730–734.

Yaffe, M. J., Orzeck, P., & Barylak, L. (2008). Family physicians' perspectives on care of dementia patients and family caregivers. *Canadian Family Physician, 54*(7), 1008–1015.

CHAPTER 22

Depression Assessment and Other Mental Illnesses

Brenna N. Renn, Diane Powers, Jürgen Unützer, and Patricia A. Areán

CHAPTER OBJECTIVES

1. Review the role of assessment in the care of depressed older adults.
2. Describe commonly used measures for assessing late-life depression.
3. Discuss challenges, best practices, and recommendations for depression screening in older adults.

KEY TERMS

Assessment
Late-life depression

Older adults
Screening

▶ Introduction

Depression is a pressing public health problem. According to the World Health Organization (2017), this common mental disorder is the leading cause of disability and ill health worldwide. Depressive disorders are characterized by persistent sadness or loss of interest and pleasure, and a number of somatic and cognitive symptoms. They create a debilitating burden, including poor quality of life, increased morbidity and

mortality, higher utilization of health services, and an increased risk for a future diagnosis of dementia (Kaup et al., 2016).

Older adults may be particularly vulnerable to the ill effects of depression. The term **late-life depression** (LLD) typically refers to depressive episodes occurring after the age of 60; it includes both the first occurrence of a depressive disorder in late life and aging individuals with an earlier onset of depression. While not a natural consequence of aging, age-associated physical health and neurobiological changes, stressors related to loss and role transitions, and curtailment of daily activities may increase vulnerability to depressive disorders (Fiske, Wetherell, & Gatz, 2009). Despite the significant adverse impact of depressive disorders, LLD often goes undetected and untreated (Unützer, 2007). This disparity may be attributed in part to the differing presentations of depression among older versus younger adults. Older adults may be less likely to report depressed mood (Fiske et al., 2009) or guilt (Gallagher et al., 2010), and instead present with cognitive complaints (even in the absence of dementia; Morimoto, Kanellopoulos, Manning, & Alexopoulos, 2015) or an emphasis on somatic symptoms, such as fatigue, lack of stamina, decreased appetite, problems with sleep, and physical aches and pain (Hegeman, de Waal, Comijs, Kok, & van der Mast, 2015). Even when depression is detected, it may not be treated (Morichi et al., 2015). This failure to treat is often attributable to the "fallacy of good reasons" and therapeutic nihilism: When seemingly reasonable explanations exist for why a patient is depressed (e.g., loss of spouse or friends, loss of health and functioning), the provider may recognize the condition but fail to initiate treatment.

The tremendous burden of depressive disorders warrants routine **screening** and targeted treatment of older adults with these conditions. This chapter provides an overview of LLD, reviews the most common assessment measures for LLD, and discusses best practices and challenges. The term *depression* in this chapter refers to unipolar depression, which may encompass clinical presentations that run the gamut from an episode of major depressive disorder to chronic depression and subsyndromal depression that causes functional impairment. We differentiate this condition from bipolar depression (also known as the depressive phase of bipolar affective disorder or "manic depression"), which requires different therapeutic approaches. **Assessment** of LLD is an important part of the health assessment and clinical examination of older adults.

▶ Depression

The fifth edition of the *Diagnostic and Statistical Manual of Mental Disorders* (*DSM-V*) includes several categories of depressive disorders that may occur in older adults: major depressive disorder (MDD), persistent depressive disorder (previously referred to as *dysthymia*), substance/medication-induced depressive disorder, depressive disorder due to another medical condition, other specified depressive disorder, and unspecified depressive disorder (American Psychiatric Association [APA], 2013). Although all of these disorders impart a serious burden to the patients who experience them, major depressive disorder is the most severe. To make this diagnosis, at least five of the nine depressive symptoms must be present most of the day, nearly every day, for at least 2 weeks; **TABLE 22-1** lists these diagnostic criteria.

Persistent depressive disorder is a related unipolar depressive condition, and is characterized by chronic depressive symptoms that last for at least 2 years. Although fewer symptoms are required for a diagnosis of persistent depressive disorder relative to MDD (three versus five), the chronicity of this condition imparts functional impact and health consequences that are just as worthy of assessment and treatment considerations (Meeks, Vahia, Lavretsky, Kulkarni, & Jeste, 2011). Minor (subsyndromal) depression is classified in the *DSM-V* as "other specified depressive disorder" and refers to a depressive episode with a number of symptoms or duration insufficient to meet criteria for MDD. While the diagnosis of minor depression signifies the patient has fewer symptoms than in MDD, minor depression is more prevalent than MDD in older adults, and carries a considerable disease burden (Meeks et al., 2011).

▶ Assessment of Late-Life Depressive Disorders

Older adults with depression are likely to present to primary care and may report somatic symptoms

TABLE 22-1 *DSM-V* Diagnostic Criteria for Major Depressive Disorder	
Five (or more) of the following symptoms have been present most of the day, nearly every day, during the same 2-week period and represent a change from previous functioning; at least one of the symptoms is either (1) depressed mood or (2) loss of interest or pleasure. These symptoms cause clinically significant distress or impair important areas of functioning.	
Depressed mood	Fatigue or loss of energy
Anhedonia (markedly diminished interest or pleasure in all, or almost all, activities)	Feelings of worthlessness or excessive or inappropriate guilt
Insomnia or hypersomnia	Diminished ability to think or concentrate
Psychomotor agitation or retardation	Recurrent thoughts of death, or recurrent suicidal ideation or a suicide attempt
Significant weight loss (when not dieting) or weight gain, or decrease or increase in appetite	

Source: Data from American Psychiatric Association, 2013.

such as insomnia, fatigue, chronic pain, and complaints of fair or poor health (Fiske et al., 2009; Jackson, O'Malley, & Kroenke, 1998; Wuthrich, Johnco, & Wetherell, 2015). Older adults also present in a variety of other settings, including home health care, social services agencies, churches, community-based services and program, and medical and mental health specialist practices. Given the prevalence and functional impact of mood symptoms among older adults, a thorough geriatric assessment must include screening for depression. The U.S. Preventive Services Task Force recommends routine depression screening in the general adult population, with further evaluation when warranted (Siu et al., 2016). In contrast, case-finding is a more selective approach, in which only patients who are suspected of having depression are assessed (e.g., those with risk factors, such as chronic illness, chronic pain, or recent loss and associated grief and bereavement). Such a targeted approach may reveal more cases of depression than general screening, but it may also miss many more patients than would be identified through routine surveillance.

Routine depression screening may be conducted in person at a clinic or agency appointment, such as annual primary care visits. In addition, it can be reliably conducted over the telephone (Pinto-Meza, Serrano-Blanco, Peñarrubia, Blanco, & Haro, 2005) or online (Areán, Hallgren, et al., 2016). Recently, assessment conducted over the Internet or via applications on mobile devices has garnered considerable interest in the field; however, this modality offers both benefits (e.g., reduced access barriers) and challenges (e.g., issues of data sparsity and patient engagement; privacy and data security concerns) (Areán, Hoa Ly, & Andersson, 2016). Regardless of which assessment modality is used, providers should make a clinical judgment about whether the patient put forth his or her best performance. For example, when using telephone, webcam, or other remote assessment, the clinician should note whether the remote testing environment appeared free of distractions, whether any significant technological problems were noted, and whether the person appeared engaged in and understood the task.

Assessment of LLD has evolved substantially over the last two decades, and a number of new assessment tools have been introduced. Typically, two types of assessment measures are used to determine the presence of a depressive disorder: screening instruments (commonly using self-report measures) and clinical interviews (both structured and semi-structured). The purpose of depression assessment using one of these two approaches is four-fold: (1) screening for the elevated symptomatology, which may suggest presence of a depressive disorder; (2) precise diagnosis, including differential diagnosis and rating of severity and history of the disorder; (3) establishing a baseline level of symptoms, from which to guide treatment; and (4) assessing treatment response and tailoring clinical decision making ("measurement-based care" and "treatment-to-target") (Fortney et al., 2017). Determining the presence of a depressive disorder requires clinical skill as well as time and effort. Thus, the most efficient approach is a two-pronged method, beginning with screening using a validated self-report measure, and if that screening is positive, performing a clinical interview to confirm or rule out the diagnosis of depression. The most common screening assessment measures for depression are now considered a routine part of a comprehensive geriatric assessment, and the gold-standard assessment includes both a standardized scale and a good clinical assessment.

Patient Health Questionnaire

Perhaps the most commonly used depression screening instrument in routine clinical practice is the nine-item Patient Health Questionnaire (PHQ-9; **FIGURE 22-1**) (Spitzer, Williams, Kroenke, Hornyak, & McMurray, 2000). This status is due in part to this questionnaire's brevity, ease of use, and strong psychometric properties in primary care settings, including its accuracy in detecting the presence of a depressive disorder: It has 88% sensitivity and 88% specificity using a cut score of 10 or greater (Kroenke, Spitzer, & Williams, 2001). The data for this assessment tool are often collected via self-report, perhaps filled out by a patient while waiting for an annual primary care visit. The respondent endorses the presence and frequency

of the nine *DSM-V* symptoms of depression over the last 2 weeks, based on a range of 0 (*not at all*) to 3 (*nearly every day*). Out of a possible total score of 27, PHQ-9 scores of 5, 10, 15, and 20 correspond to mild, moderate, moderately severe, and severe depression, respectively (Kroenke et al., 2001). An additional follow-up question assesses the degree to which the depressive symptoms have interfered with the person's daily functioning.

Several factors of the PHQ-9 increase its utility as a screening tool. First, the PHQ-9 is in the public domain and easily accessible for clinical use. Second, in addition to the original English version, a validated Spanish translation and translations in a number of other languages are available. Third, the nine items of the PHQ-9 correspond to the nine core depressive symptoms in *DSM-V*, so this tool can assist a clinician with making a diagnosis of MDD or with tracking specific *DSM-V* symptoms of depression during a course of treatment. Fourth, a variant of the PHQ-9, called the PHQ-2 or the two-question screen, is available as an ultra-brief screener (Arroll, Khin, & Kerse, 2003). This instrument is composed of the first two questions of the PHQ-9: "During the last month, have you been bothered by . . . (1) feeling down, depressed, or hopeless? and (2) having little interest or pleasure in doing things?" These items correspond to the two cardinal symptoms of depressive disorders—dysphoria and anhedonia, respectively. Respondents may use the same 0–3 rating scales as used with the PHQ-9, or provide a dichotomous response (yes/no). A single "yes" response, or a score of 3 or greater (possible range: 0–6) detects MDD with a 61% to 83% sensitivity and 92% specificity in adult primary care settings (Arroll et al., 2010; Kroenke, Spitzer, & Williams, 2003). Some practices begin by screening all patients with the PHQ-2, then follow up with the PHQ-9 for only those patients who screen positive on the first two items.

The PHQ-9 can also be used to monitor treatment response in a standardized way through repeated assessment at follow-up visits. Many

PATIENT HEALTH QUESTIONNAIRE (PHQ-9)

NAME:_____   DATE:_____

Over the last *2 weeks,* how often have you been
bothered by any of the following problems?
(use "✓" to indicate your answer)

	Not at all	Several days	More than half the days	Nearly every day
1. Little interest or pleasure in doing things	0	1	2	3
2. Feeling down, depressed, or hopeless	0	1	2	3
3. Trouble falling or staying asleep, or sleeping too much	0	1	2	3
4. Feeling tired or having little energy	0	1	2	3
5. Poor appetite or overeating	0	1	2	3
6. Feeling bad about yourself—or that you are a failure or have let yourself or your family down	0	1	2	3
7. Trouble concentrating on things, such as reading the newspaper or watching television	0	1	2	3
8. Moving or speaking so slowly that other people could have noticed. Or the opposite — being so figety or restless that you have been moving around a lot more than usual	0	1	2	3
9. Thoughts that you would be better off dead, or of hurting yourself	0	1	2	3

add columns _____ + _____ + _____

(Healthcare professional: For interpretation of TOTAL,   TOTAL: _____
please refer to accompanying scoring card).

10. If you checked off *any problems,* how *difficult*
    have these problems made it for you to do
    your work, take care of things at home, or get
    along with other people?

    Not difficult at all _____
    Somewhat difficult _____
    Very difficult _____
    Extremely difficult _____

FIGURE 22-1 Patient Health Questionnaire.   *(continues)*

PHQ-9 Patient Depression Questionnaire

For initial diagnosis:

1. Patient completes PHQ-9 Quick Depression Assessment.
2. If there are at least 4 ✓s in the shaded section (including Questions #1 and #2), consider a depressive disorder. Add score to determine severity.

Consider Major Depressive Disorder

- if there are at least 5 ✓s in the shaded section (one of which corresponds to Question #1 or #2)

Consider Other Depressive Disorder

- if there are 2-4 ✓s in the shaded section (one of which corresponds to Question #1 or #2)

Note: Since the questionnaire relies on patient self-report, all responses should be verified by the clinician, and a definitive diagnosis is made on clinical grounds taking into account how well the patient understood the questionnaire, as well as other relevant information from the patient.
Diagnoses of Major Depressive Disorder or Other Depressive Disorder also require impairment of social, occupational, or other important areas of functioning (Question #10) and ruling out normal bereavement, a history of a Manic Episode (Bipolar Disorder), and a physical disorder, medication, or other drug as the biological cause of the depressive symptoms.

To monitor severity over time for newly diagnosed patients or patients in current treatment for depression:

1. Patients may complete questionnaires at baseline and at regular intervals (eg, every 2 weeks) at home and bring them in at their next appointment for scoring or they may complete the questionnaire during each scheduled appointment.
2. Add up ✓s by column. For every ✓: Several days = 1 More than half the days = 2 Nearly every day = 3
3. Add together column scores to get a TOTAL score.
4. Refer to the accompanying **PHQ-9 Scoring Box** to interpret the TOTAL score.
5. Results may be included in patient files to assist you in setting up a treatment goal, determining degree of response, as well as guiding treatment intervention.

Scoring: add up all checked boxes on PHQ-9

For every ✓ Not at all = 0; Several days = 1;
More than half the days = 2; Nearly every day = 3

Interpretation of Total Score

Total Score	Depression Severity
1-4	Minimal depression
5-9	Mild depression
10-14	Moderate depression
15-19	Moderately severe depression
20-27	Severe depression

Developed by Drs. Robert L. Spitzer, Janet B.W. Williams, Kurt Kroenke and colleagues, with an educational grant from Pfizer Inc. No permission required to reproduce, translate, display or distribute.

A2662B 10-04-2005

FIGURE 22-1 Continued

studies have validated utility of the PHQ-9 for screening and treatment monitoring with older adults in various settings, including primary care (Phelan et al., 2010) and community-based aging services (Richardson, Tu, & Conwell, 2008), concluding that it is comparable or superior to other measures. Nevertheless, the PHQ-9 may not perform as well for older adults with cognitive impairment (Boyle et al., 2011).

Beck Depression Inventory

Aaron T. Beck, the father of cognitive therapy, created the Beck Depression Inventory (Beck, Erbaugh, Ward, Mock, & Mendelsohn, 1961), a 21-item instrument designed to assess the presence and severity of depressive symptoms. With the advent of revised diagnostic criteria for MDD, a revised second edition of the inventory was released as the Beck Depression Inventory II (BDI-II; Beck et al., 1996); it remains in use today. The major changes between versions were modification of selected symptoms and a lengthening of time frame, to reflect *DSM* guidelines of assessing symptoms over the preceding 2 weeks. As with its predecessor, each of the 21 items on the BDI-II lists four statements that represent increasing severity of a symptom of depression, with each answer scored on a scale of 0 to 3. A summary score is calculated, ranging from 0 to 63, with higher total scores reflecting more severe depressive symptoms. The standardized cutoffs of 0–13, 14–19, 20–28, and 29–63 reflect minimal, mild, moderate, and severe depression, respectively. The proprietary software also includes an interpretative report that rates an individual patient's scores relative to a normative sample.

A seven-item adaptation of the BDI, the Beck Depressive Inventory for Primary Care (BDI-PC; Beck, Guth, Steer, & Ball, 1997), was developed to ascertain MDD among medical patients. Using the same rating scale as the BDI-II, each item is rated on a 4-point scale, for a maximum summary score of 21. When a cutoff score of 4 points is used among primary care patients, the BDI-PC identifies MDD with 97% sensitivity and 99% specificity (Steer, Cavalieri, Leonard, & Beck, 1999). This instrument has since been renamed the BDI-FastScreen for Medical Patients.

Although originally developed for use by a trained administrator, contemporary use of the BDI-II allows for self-reporting. However, whereas the PHQ-9 is relatively brief, the BDI-II takes approximately 5 to 10 minutes to administer, and the complex response format is not as simple as other popular self-report measures. Critics of the BDI-II argue that the reliance on multiple somatic items may artificially elevate depressive severity in medically ill older adults; however, studies examining the psychometric properties of the BDI-II in community-dwelling older adults suggest adequate support for use in geriatric assessment (Segal, Coolidge, Cahill, & O'Riley, 2008). The BDI measures are copyrighted, and a fee is required for each copy of the scale used. As of this writing, 25 BDI-II or 50 BDI-FastScreen record forms cost $58.85. Given that there are easy-to-use alternative measures available in the public domain with equivalent psychometric properties, the BDI-II has limitations for routine screening. Nonetheless, it remains commonly used in clinical practice, particularly in psychiatric settings.

Geriatric Depression Scale

Other screening instruments have been explicitly developed for assessment of depression in geriatric populations. The Geriatric Depression Scale (GDS) is one such self-report instrument. Originally developed with 30 items (Yesavage et al., 1983), the GDS has since been shortened to briefer versions (Dath et al., 1994; Parmelee, Lawton, & Katz, 1989; Sheikh & Yesavage, 1986; van Marwijk et al., 1995). One of the most commonly used short version forms is the 15-item version (GDS-15; items 1–4, 7–9, 10, 12, 14, 15, 17, and 21–23), for which more than five depressive responses suggest further assessment; this version has a sensitivity of 72% and specificity of 78% for diagnosing MDD (Marc, Raue, & Bruce, 2008). An even briefer 5-item version (GDS-5; items 1, 4, 10, 12, and 17) facilitates ease of administration; if the patient gives two depressive responses to these five items, further assessment is considered to be warranted (Hoyl et al., 1999). All versions of the GDS employ a simple dichotomous yes/no response format, with certain items being reverse scored.

Strengths of the GDS in geriatric depression assessment include its specific development for this population, along with its focus on the cognitive and behavioral symptoms of depression. Since somatic symptoms of depression might be conflated with symptoms of chronic disease, the GDS generally excludes somatic items to prevent spuriously elevated depression scores, thereby avoiding false-positive detection of depression among medically ill older adults. The GDS has demonstrated reliability and validity for detecting depression among older primary care patients (Friedman, Heisel, & Delavan, 2005) as well as nursing home residents (Lesher, 1986).

One limitation of the GDS is its decreased accuracy among cognitively impaired older adults (Burke, Houston, & Boust, 1989; Debruyne et al., 2009). Although the GDS is likely appropriate in more mildly impaired individuals (Midden & Mast, 2017), an informant report such as the Cornell Scale for Depression in Dementia (**BOX 22-1**) is preferable when assessing more impaired individuals.

BOX 22-1 Mood Assessment Scale

1. Are you basically satisfied with your life?
2. Have you dropped many of your activities and interests?
3. Do you feel that your life is empty?
4. Do you often get bored?
5. Are you hopeful about the future?
6. Are you bothered by thoughts you can't get out of your head?
7. Are you in good spirits most of the time?
8. Are you afraid that something bad is going to happen to you?
9. Do you feel happy most of the time?
10. Do you often feel helpless?
11. Do you often get restless and fidgety?
12. Do you prefer to stay at home, rather than going out and doing new things?
13. Do you frequently worry about the future?
14. Do you feel you have more problems with memory than most?
15. Do you think it is wonderful to be alive now?
16. Do you often feel downhearted and blue?
17. Do you feel pretty worthless the way you are now?
18. Do you worry a lot about the past?
19. Do you find life very exciting?
20. Is it hard for you to get started on new projects?
21. Do you feel full of energy?
22. Do you feel that your situation is hopeless?
23. Do you think that most people are better off than you are?
24. Do you frequently get upset over little things?
25. Do you frequently feel like crying?
26. Do you have trouble concentrating?
27. Do you enjoy getting up in the morning?
28. Do you prefer to avoid social gatherings?

29. Is it easy for you to make decisions?
30. Is your mind as clear as it used to be?

This is the original scoring for the scale: One point for each of these answers.

1.	no	6.	yes	11.	yes	16.	yes	21.	no	26.	yes
2.	yes	7.	no	12.	yes	17.	yes	22.	yes	27.	no
3.	yes	8.	yes	13.	yes	18.	yes	23.	yes	28.	yes
4.	yes	9.	no	14.	yes	19.	no	24.	yes	29.	no
5.	no	10.	yes	15.	no	20.	yes	25.	yes	30.	no

Cutoff: normal, 0–9; mild depression, 10–19; severe depression, 20–30.

Source: Courtesy of Yesavage, J.A., & Brink, T.L. (n.d.). Geriatric Depression Scale. Retrieved from https://web.stanford.edu/~yesavage/GDS.html

Other Measures

There exist a multitude of other measures for identifying clinical levels of depression, including the Zung Self-Rating Depression Scale (Zung, 1972), the General Health Questionnaire (GHQ; Goldberg, 1972), the Hospital Anxiety and Depression Scale (HADS; Zigmond & Snaith, 1983), the Montgomery Asberg Depression Rating Scale (MADRS-S; Montgomery & Asberg, 1979), and the Center for Epidemiological Studies Depression Scale (CES-D; Radloff, 1977). The CES-D is one of the instruments most commonly used in community samples for epidemiologic surveillance. For patients with dementia, the Cornell Scale for Depression in Dementia (Alexopoulos, Abrams, Young, & Shamoian, 1988) is an alternative to relying on self-report; this 19-item measure incorporates both clinician-provided and informant-based information to evaluate depressive symptoms in cognitively impaired patients.

None of the measures mentioned in this section is sufficient to establish a definitive diagnosis of a depressive disorder. Instead, a diagnosis must be confirmed by a structured or semi-structured diagnostic interview or a clinical assessment that confirms the impact of symptoms identified on a patient's ability to function, considers alternative explanations for presenting symptom patterns (such as medications or medical conditions), and considers alternative mental disorders such as dementia or bipolar affective disorder.

▶ Challenges and Best Practices in Assessment

Diagnostic Considerations

Clinicians should be aware of possible complications when assessing LLD. Many older adults have complex medical histories and health status, which may include overlapping symptoms between depression and physical health conditions (e.g., fatigue, sleep disturbances, appetite and weight changes) (APA, 2013). Furthermore, effects of prescription or nonprescription medications may overlap with, overshadow, cause, or worsen symptoms of depression (Areán & Reynolds, 2005). Given that depressed older adults may preferentially endorse somatic and cognitive concerns, relative to classic affective symptoms of depression (e.g., depressed mood or anhedonia), cases of LLD may be missed by clinicians, particularly among frail or medically complex older adults. Depression should be considered in all older adults who present with somatic or cognitive complaints that seem out of proportion to what is expected given their medical status; in older adults who report persistent affective or ruminative symptoms in the context of their medical comorbidity; and in those who have difficulty engaging effectively in health care or other services offered. Providers in primary care settings are apt to see numerous patients with multiple and persistent physical symptoms; in such patients, depression assessment and psychoeducation about the interplay of psychosocial stressors and somatic symptoms can be useful (Croicu, Chwastiak, & Katon, 2014). **TABLE 22-2** lists medical conditions and medications associated with depressive disorders.

Cohort effects may further complicate geriatric depression assessment. Although this may change with the aging of the baby boomer generation, both research findings and our clinical experience is that the current cohorts of older adults, particularly the "oldest old" (ages 80 and greater) are less likely to see themselves as depressed and more likely to perceive themselves as irritable, apathetic, or succumbing to "normal" aging (Sirey et al., 2001). Such ageism and therapeutic nihilism on behalf of the patient, as well as families, caregivers, and even clinicians, can further complicate diagnosis and treatment engagement.

TABLE 22-2 Medical Conditions and Medications Associated with Depressive Disorders

Medical Conditions

Neurologic disorders: stroke, Alzheimer's disease, Huntington's disease, Parkinson's disease, multiple sclerosis, traumatic brain injury

Coronary artery disease: hypertension, myocardial infarction, coronary artery bypass surgery, congestive heart failure

Metabolic disturbances: hypothyroidism or hyperthyroidism, Cushing's disease, diabetes mellitus

Other conditions: chronic obstructive pulmonary disease, rheumatoid arthritis, deafness, chronic pain, sexual dysfunction, renal dialysis

Medications

Antiviral agents
Cardiovascular agents (primarily antihypertensive medications)
Retinoic acid derivatives
Psychotropic medications (including antidepressants and antipsychotics)
Anticonvulsants
Antimigraine agents
Hormonal agents (including oral contraceptives)
Smoking cessation agents
Immunologic agents

Source: Data from American Psychiatric Association, 2013.

▶ Suicide

Specific consideration in the context of assessing depression should be given to the assessment of suicidality. Although older adults as a group evidence lower rates of MDD than younger cohorts (Kessler et al., 2003), older adults—particularly older white men—are among the highest-risk groups for completed suicide. The most recent U.S. data available at the time of this writing indicated a suicide rate of 16.6 per 100,000 people aged 65 and older, which is more than 20% greater than the national average (McIntosh, 2017). Depression and hopelessness are important risk factors in suicide among older adults; other notable risks include prior suicide attempts, the presence of comorbid physical illnesses (especially life-limiting conditions), social isolation, discord in the family or other important relationships, alcohol or prescription drug misuse, and impulsivity (Conwell, Van Orden, & Caine, 2011). Recent loss may increase the risk for suicide by increasing perceived burdensomeness and thwarting social connection, particularly among those persons with difficulty adapting to these changes. Such loss may include functional decline and loss of independence (e.g., mobility, vision), changes to the individual's social role (e.g., retirement, revocation of driving privileges), anticipatory grief due to a physical illness or other life-limiting condition, or death and bereavement (Van Orden et al., 2010).

Although depression alone does not account for all cases of suicide, the vast majority of older adults who complete suicide have a diagnosable psychiatric condition, most commonly MDD (Conwell et al., 2011). Moreover, research shows that most individuals who attempt or complete suicide sought care from their primary care provider (PCP) within 3 months of their suicidal act (De Leo, Draper, Snowdon, & Kölves, 2013; Mills, Watts, Huh, Boar, & Kemp, 2013). Thus, suicide is among the most devastating consequences of depression and other psychiatric illnesses, and potentially represents a missed opportunity for assessment and treatment. Although an assessment of suicide is crucial to the assessment of

LLD, we urge clinicians to assess suicidal ideation among nondepressed individuals as part of every comprehensive examination.

Notably, older adults are less likely to endorse suicide relative to their similarly depressed younger adults (Balsis & Cully, 2008). Given that older adults are more likely to complete suicide than their younger counterparts, this finding may represent a systematic under-reporting of suicidality, which behooves clinicians to use a broader range of evaluations to thoroughly assess suicide risk in older individuals. Suicidality comprises a spectrum ranging from passive thoughts of death (e.g., "It would just be easier to not wake up") to more specific and active thoughts, including planning, rehearsing, and preparing the means one would use to complete a suicidal act. These various levels of intensity require different assessment, response, and ongoing management.

While a comprehensive review of suicide assessment is beyond the scope of this chapter, we offer a few resources. The ninth item of the PHQ-9 depression screener (discussed earlier in this chapter) asks about the presence and frequency of "thoughts that you would be better off dead, or of hurting yourself in some way." Alternatively, a clinician can first assess for passive suicide ideation ("In the past couple of weeks, have things gotten so bad that you've had thoughts that life is not worth living, or that you'd be better off dead?") and follow up affirmative responses by assessing for active ideation ("Have you had any thoughts about hurting yourself or thoughts of suicide in the past couple of weeks?") (Raue et al., 2006; Raue, Ghesquiere, & Bruce, 2014). Any positive response to these inquiries warrants further assessment, including evaluation of intent, specific means and plan, previous attempts, and imminence of such action. The P4 suicidality screener (Dube, Kurt, Bair, Theobald, & Williams, 2010) offers structured screening questions to assess the four "Ps" of suicide risk: *p*ast attempts, *p*lan, *p*robability (how likely the person is to act on suicidal thoughts), and *p*reventive (or protective) factors against acting on suicidal thoughts (**FIGURE 22-2**).

P4 Suicidality Screener *

Have you had thoughts of actually hurting yourself?

NO YES

Four Screening Questions ← YES

1. **Have you ever attempted to harm yourself in the past?**

   NO **YES**

2. **Have you thought about how you might actually hurt yourself?**

   NO **YES** → [How? ________________]

3. **There's a big difference between having a thought and acting on a thought. How likely do you think it is that you will act on these thoughts about hurting yourself or ending your life some time over the next month?"**

   a. Not at all likely _____
   b. Somewhat likely _____
   c. Very likely _____

4. **Is there anything that would prevent or keep you from harming yourself?**

   NO **YES** → [What? ________________]

Risk Category	Shaded ("Risk") Response	
	Items 1 and 2	**Items 3 and 4**
Minimal	Neither is shaded	Neither is shaded
Lower	At least one item is shaded	Neither is shaded
Higher		At least one item is shaded

Reprinted with permission from: Dube P, Kroenke K, Bair MJ, Theobald D, Williams LS. The p4 screener: evaluation of a brief measure for assessing potential suicide risk in 2 randomized effectiveness trials of primary care and oncology patients. Prim Care Companion J Clin Psychiatry. 2010;12(6):PCC. 10m00978. Copyright 2018, Physicians Postgraduate Press. Reprinted by permission.

FIGURE 22-2 Suicide Screener.

http://gerocentral.org/wp-content/uploads/2013/04/P4-Suicide-Risk-Screener.pdf
Physicians Postgraduate Press. Reprinted by permission.

* P4 is a mnemonic for the 4 screening questions:
> → *past* history, *plan*, *probability*, *preventive* factors

---

Optional Clarifying Questions (if it is unclear if patient has a plan) *shaded response = risk*

1. Do you live alone?   (No ___   Yes ___)

2. Have you thought about taking an overdose of medication, driving your car off the road, using a gun, or doing something else serious like this?   (No ___   Yes ___ → What is it? _____)

3. Do you own a gun?   (No ___   Yes ___)

4. Have you been stockpiling (saving up) medication?   (No ___   Yes ___)

5. Do you feel hopeless about the future?   (No ___   A little ___   Somewhat ___   Very ___)

6. Do you feel you can resist your impulses to harm yourself?   (No ___   Yes ___)

7. Right now, how strong is your wish to die?   (No wish _____   Weak _____   Strong _____)

Reprinted with permission from: Dube P, Kroenke K, Bair MJ, Theobald D, Williams LS. The p4 screener: evaluation of a brief measure for assessing potential suicide risk in 2 randomized effectiveness trials of primary care and oncology patients. Prim Care Companion J Clin Psychiatry. 2010;12(6):PCC. 10m00978. Copyright 2018, Physicians Postgraduate Press. Reprinted by permission.

FIGURE 22-2 Continued

A thorough assessment of suicide (or other risk of harm, such as homicidal ideation) needs to be completed by a qualified mental health professional, to include appropriate referrals for acute stabilization and/or treatment. We refer readers to reviews by Raue and colleagues (Raue et al., 2006; Raue et al., 2014) and practice recommendations by Diggle-Fox (2016), and encourage continuing education in comprehensive risk of harm and suicide assessment.

▶ Differential Diagnosis

Depression is often comorbid with other psychiatric and medical conditions. One of the most important differential diagnoses to establish in this regard is the exclusion of bipolar affective disorder (previously called "manic depression"). Although the new onset of bipolar disorder in older adults is rare, a number of older adults who present with symptoms of depression may have had a prior episode of mania or hypomania. Use of standard depression treatments (e.g., antidepressant medications) may be ineffective with such patients, or it could increase the risk of a mixed or manic episode in patients at risk. Before making a diagnosis of unipolar depression, clinicians should enquire about prior episodes of mania or hypomania or earlier treatment for bipolar disorder or manic depression.

The complex interaction between depressive disorder and chronic medical illness was comprehensively articulated by Katon (2003) and considered earlier in this chapter. Moreover, depressive disorders are often comorbid with anxiety across the lifespan (Kessler et al., 2015). Recent epidemiologic findings suggest that even subsyndromal depressive conditions among adults age 55 years and older are associated with elevated risk of anxiety and personality disorders (Laborde-Lahoz et al., 2015). These comorbid mental health conditions may complicate assessment, diagnosis, and treatment of depression; thus, differential diagnosis is crucial.

While a thorough review of this subject is beyond the scope of this chapter, the importance of a good differential diagnosis of depression, dementia, and delirium (the "3 Ds" of geriatric psychiatry; Downing, Caprio, & Lyness, 2013) cannot be emphasized enough. Although these three conditions may overlap, each warrants a unique clinical work-up and treatment course; when unrecognized and untreated, each may complicate treatment and lead to poor health outcomes including premature death. Clinicians should consider disease onset, course, presentation, and information from a trusted informant in conjunction with a thorough medical evaluation.

Depression tends to have a gradual onset (perhaps over weeks or months) and a fluctuating and often recurring course. Poor concentration is the most common cognitive deficit or complaint. In contrast, dementia (particularly of the Alzheimer's type) tends to have an insidious onset and a gradual, progressive course, often spanning many years. With this condition, the most common cognitive symptom is in the domain of short-term memory, which will eventually result in functional impact and loss of independence in daily activities. Brief cognitive tests can help identify possible dementia and determine the need for further evaluation. The third "D," delirium, typically constitutes a more acutely presenting case of "brain failure," a medical emergency in older adults that may be particularly relevant in the setting of medical illness or the toxic effects of medications or other substances. It is characterized by a sudden change in mentation—specifically, an acute confusional state that manifests with poor attention, agitation, fluctuating consciousness, and disorganized thought. Differential diagnosis of these conditions is complicated by findings that depression may be a prodrome of dementia (Mirza et al., 2016), and that delirium is not only more prevalent among patients with dementia, but also may increase the risk of incident dementia (Davis et al., 2012; Gross et al., 2012).

▶ Recommendations for Practice

The assessments tools reviewed in this chapter include a few of the most popular instruments used in the assessment of LLD. Several attributes of an instrument should be considered when selecting a measure, particularly for use in population screening—namely, whether the instrument is easily administered, cost-effective (in terms of both expense of the measure and provider time), sensitive and specific for a particular patient population, and accepted by the patient.

We suggest routine screening of depression in any setting that routinely serves older adults, including primary care, aging service agencies, and specialty medical and mental health settings (including rehabilitative, medical inpatients, and long-term care). Staff should be trained in the importance of depression screening and its introduction to patients, the importance of standardized assessment, and ways to address concerns about confidentiality. The most notable risk of routine screening is false-positive diagnoses, which may subsequently expose the patient to potential harms in terms of anxiety or unnecessary treatment and associated costs and adverse effects. The potential of false-positive detection from screening measures further underscores the need to confirm elevated symptom reporting with a clinical assessment. While this will incur opportunity costs of provider time for follow-up assessment, it is necessary to ensure an accurate differential diagnosis and to develop an appropriate treatment plan.

A comprehensive assessment is pivotal to inform accurate detection and appropriate treatment of LLD and related conditions. A general health examination, including laboratory measures of overall health status (e.g., comprehensive metabolic panel, vitamin B_{12}, thyroid-stimulating hormone, complete blood count, serologic tests for syphilis and human immunodeficiency virus [HIV]), will inform the differential diagnosis and guide optimal treatment. Similarly, clinicians are encouraged to review prescription and nonprescription medications for all older adults, but particularly in regard to the differential diagnosis and pharmacologic treatment of LLD. We recognize there is often limited time in a clinic visit; with older adults who have multiple chronic, acute, or otherwise complex health conditions, attention to psychological problems may be considered a lower priority. When possible, working with an interdisciplinary healthcare team can optimize assessment and treatment from a biopsychosocial perspective that considers physical, psychological, and social contributors to depression and related conditions.

Finally, regardless of the assessment approach, treatment and follow-up are essential to successful care of the older adult with depression. While screening is important and useful for recognizing depression, it is necessary but not sufficient for improving clinical outcomes (Gilbody, Sheldon, & House, 2008).

Given that the overwhelming majority of depressed older adults initially present to primary care, rather than seek specialty mental health care, mental health treatment embedded in such settings is garnering increased attention from providers and policymakers. Older adults typically have established relationships with primary care providers, such that the stigma associated with mental health treatment is reduced in the primary care setting.

The IMPACT trial demonstrated that depressed older adults can be more successfully treated in primary care with a collaborative care approach than with care as usual (Unützer et al., 2002). This team-based model of care adds a care manager (e.g., counselor, clinical social worker) and psychiatric consultant to the existing patient–provider dyad. The care manager assists the PCP with a biopsychosocial assessment and psychoeducation; offers brief, evidence-based psychotherapy as the primary therapy or as an adjunct to pharmacotherapy prescribed by the primary care provider; measures and monitors treatment outcomes to ensure ineffective or partially effective treatments are changed proactively; and coaches patients in developing a relapse prevention plan. Psychiatric consultants offer systematic consultation on the entire panel of patients in active treatment, focusing on those patients who are not improving as expected. More than twice as many patients experienced significant improvement in depression with this population-focused, treat-to-target approach as compared with usual primary care, even when usual care included co-located behavioral health providers care (Unützer et al., 2002). IMPACT-treated patients also experienced significantly less physical pain, better social and physical functioning, and better overall quality of life as compared to usual-care–treated patients, even in the context of multiple comorbid physical conditions (Harpole et al., 2005). The collaborative care approach was found to be more effective than usual care for patients with and without prior depression treatment, and for patients from ethnic minority groups (Areán et al., 2005) and low socioeconomic status (Areán, Gum, Tang, & Unützer, 2007).

▶ Summary

Accurate assessment of LLD can help identify a common and disabling problem among older adults—a problem for which a wide range of effective treatments exist, ranging from psychotherapies to medications and other somatic treatments (Qaseem, Barry, & Kansagara, 2016; Renn & Areán, 2017). When they do undiagnosed, patients with depression often suffer from years of functional impairment that robs them of the ability to enjoy their later years. Successful assessment must address comorbid conditions and its results used to drive effective treatment and close follow-up. With the exponential increase in the older adult population, and the subsequent demands on primary and specialty care, social services agencies, and other geriatric settings, it is imperative that clinicians become proficient in the assessment and treatment (or referral to treatment) for LLD.

References

Alexopoulos, G. S., Abrams, R. C., Young, R. C., & Shamoian, C. A. (1988). Cornell Scale for Depression in Dementia. *Biological Psychiatry, 233,* 271–284.

American Psychiatric Association. (2013). *Diagnostic and statistical manual of mental disorders: DSM-V* (5th ed.). Washington, DC: American Psychiatric Publishing.

Areán, P. A., Ayalon, L., Hunkeler, E., Lin, E. H., Tang, L., Harpole, L., ... Unützer, J. (2005). Improving depression care for older, minority patients in primary care. *Medical Care, 43*(4), 381–390.

Areán, P. A., Gum, A. M., Tang, L. Q., & Unützer, J. (2007). Service use and outcomes among elderly persons with low incomes being treated for depression. *Psychiatric Services, 588,* 1057–1064.

Areán, P. A., Hallgren, K. A., Jordan, J. T., Gazzaley, A., Atkins, D. C., Heagerty, P. J., & Anguera, J. A. (2016). The use and effectiveness of mobile apps for depression: Results from a fully remote clinical trial. *Journal of Medical Internet Research, 18*(12), e330.

Areán, P. A., Hoa Ly, K., & Andersson, G. (2016). Mobile technology for mental health assessment. *Dialogues in Clinical Neuroscience, 182,* 163–169.

Areán, P. A., & Reynolds, C. F. (2005). The impact of psychosocial factors on late-life depression. *Biological Psychiatry, 584,* 277–282.

Arroll, B., Goodyear-Smith, F., Crengle, S., Gunn, J., Kerse, N., Fishman, T., ... Hatcher, S. (2010). Validation of PHQ-2 and PHQ-9 to screen for major depression in the primary care population. *Annals of Family Medicine, 84,* 348–353.

Arroll, B., Khin, N., & Kerse, N. (2003). Screening for depression in primary care with two verbally asked questions: Cross sectional study. *BMJ, 327*(7424), 1144–1146.

Balsis, S., & Cully, J. A. (2008). Comparing depression diagnostic symptoms across younger and older adults. *Aging and Mental Health, 126,* 800–806.

Beck, A. T., Erbaugh, J., Ward, C. H., Mock, J., & Mendelsohn, M. (1961). An inventory for measuring depression. *Archives of General Psychiatry, 46,* 561.

Beck, A. T., Guth, D., Steer, R. A., & Ball, R. (1997). Screening for major depression disorders in medical inpatients

with the Beck Depression Inventory for Primary Care. *Behavioral Research, 358,* 785–91.

Beck, A. T., Steer, R. A., Ball, R., & Ranieri, W. F. (1996). Comparison of Beck Depression Inventories-IA and-II in psychiatric outpatients. *Journal of Personality Assessment, 67*(3), 588–597.

Boyle, L. L., Richardson, T. M., He, H., Xia, Y., Tu, X., Boustani, M., & Conwell, Y. (2011). How do the PHQ-2, the PHQ-9 perform in aging services clients with cognitive impairment? *International Journal of Geriatric Psychiatry, 269,* 952–960.

Burke, W. J., Houston, M. J., & Boust, S. J. (1989). Use of the Geriatric Depression Scale in dementia of the Alzheimer type. *Journal of the American Geriatrics Society, 379,* 856–860.

Conwell, Y., Van Orden, K., & Caine, E. D. (2011). Suicide in older adults. *Psychiatric Clinics of North America, 342,* 451–468, ix.

Croicu, C., Chwastiak, L., & Katon, W. (2014). Approach to the patient with multiple somatic symptoms. *Medical Clinics of North America, 985,* 1079–1095.

D'Ath, P., Katona, P., Mullan, E., Evans, S., & Katona, C. (1994). Screening, detection and management of depression in elderly primary care attenders. I: The acceptability and performance of the 15 item Geriatric Depression Scale (GDS15) and the development of short versions. *Family Practice, 11*(3), 260–266.

Davis, D. H., Muniz Terrera, G., Keage, H., Rahkonen, T., Oinas, M., Matthews, F. E., . . . Brayne, C. (2012). Delirium is a strong risk factor for dementia in the oldest-old: A population-based cohort study. *Brain, 135*(Pt 9), 2809–2816.

Debruyne, H., Van Buggenhout, M., Le Bastard, N., Aries, M., Audenaert, K., De Deyn, P. P., & Engelborghs, S. (2009). Is the Geriatric Depression Scale a reliable screening tool for depressive symptoms in elderly patients with cognitive impairment? *International Journal of Geriatric Psychiatry, 246,* 556–562.

De Leo, D., Draper, B. M., Snowdon, J., & Kölves, K. (2013). Contacts with health professionals before suicide: Missed opportunities for prevention? *Comprehensive Psychiatry, 547,* 1117–1123.

Diggle-Fox, B. S. (2016). Assessing suicide risk in older adults. *Nurse Practitioner, 4110,* 28–35.

Downing, L. J., Caprio, T. V., & Lyness, J. M. (2013). Geriatric psychiatry review: Differential diagnosis and treatment of the 3 D's—delirium, dementia, and depression. *Current Psychiatry Reports, 156,* 365.

Dube, P., Kurt, K., Bair, M. J., Theobald, D., & Williams, L. S. (2010). The P4 screener: Evaluation of a brief measure for assessing potential suicide risk in 2 randomized effectiveness trials of primary care and oncology patients. *Primary Care Companion to the Journal of Clinical Psychiatry, 126.*

Fiske, A., Wetherell, J. L., & Gatz, M. (2009). Depression in older adults. *Annual Review of Clinical Psychology, 5,* 363–389.

Fortney, J. C., Unützer, J., Wrenn, G., Pyne, J. M., Smith, G. R., Schoenbaum, M., & Harbin, H. T. (2017). A tipping point for measurement-based care. *Psychiatric Services, 682,* 179–188.

Friedman, B., Heisel, M. J., & Delavan, R. L. (2005). Psychometric properties of the 15-item Geriatric Depression Scale in functionally impaired, cognitively intact, community-dwelling elderly primary care patients. *Journal of the American Geriatrics Society, 539,* 1570–1576.

Gallagher, D., Mhaolain, A. N., Greene, E., Walsh, C., Denihan, A., Bruce, I., . . . Lawlor, B. A. (2010). Late life depression: A comparison of risk factors and symptoms according to age of onset in community dwelling older adults. *International Journal of Geriatric Psychiatry, 2510,* 981–987.

Gilbody, S., Sheldon, T., & House, A. (2008). Screening and case-finding instruments for depression: A meta-analysis. *Canadian Medical Association Journal, 1788,* 997–1003.

Goldberg, D. P. (1972). *The detection of psychiatric illness by questionnaire: A technique for the identification and assessment of non-psychotic psychiatric illness.* London, United Kingdom, Oxford University Press.

Gross, A. L., Jones, R. N., Habtemariam, D. A., Fong, T. G., Tommet, D., Quach, I., . . . Inouye, S. K. (2012). Delirium and long-term cognitive trajectory among persons with dementia. *Archives of Internal Medicine, 172*(17), 1324–1331.

Harpole, L. H., Williams, J. W. Jr., Olsen, M. K., Stechuchak, K. M., Oddone, E., Callahan, C. M., . . . Unützer, J. (2005). Improving depression outcomes in older adults with comorbid medical illness. *General Hospital Psychiatry, 271,* 4–12.

Hegeman, J. M., de Waal, M. W., Comijs, H. C., Kok, R. M., & van der Mast, R. C. (2015). Depression in later life: A more somatic presentation? *Journal of Affective Disorders, 170,* 196–202.

Hoyl, M. T., Alessi, C. A., Harker, J. O., Josephson, K. R., Pietruszka, F. M., Koelfgen, M., . . . Rubenstein, L. Z. (1999). Development and testing of a five-item version of the Geriatric Depression Scale. *Journal of the American Geriatrics Society, 477,* 873–878.

Jackson, J. L., O'Malley, P. G., & Kroenke, K. (1998). Clinical predictors of mental disorders among medical outpatients: Validation of the "S4" model. *Psychosomatics, 395,* 431–436.

Katon, W. J. (2003). Clinical and health services relationships between major depression, depressive symptoms, and general medical illness. *Biological Psychiatry, 543,* 216–226.

Kaup, A. R., Byers, A. L., Falvey, C., Simonsick, E. M., Satterfield, S., Ayonayon, H. N., . . . Yaffe, K. (2016). Trajectories of depressive symptoms in older adults and risk of dementia. *JAMA Psychiatry, 735,* 525–531.

Kessler, R. C., Berglund, P., Demler, O., Jin, R., Koretz, D., Merikangas, K. R., . . . Wang, P. S. (2003). The epidemiology of major depressive disorder: Results from the National Comorbidity Survey Replication (NCS-R). *Journal of the American Medical Association, 289*(23), 3095–3105.

Kessler, R. C., Sampson, N. A., Berglund, P., Gruber, M. J., Al-Hamzawi, A., Andrade, L., . . . Wilcox, M. A. (2015). Anxious and non-anxious major depressive disorder in the World Health Organization World Mental Health Surveys. *Epidemiology and Psychiatric Sciences, 243,* 210–226.

Kroenke, K., Spitzer, R. L., & Williams, J. B. (2001). The PHQ-9: Validity of a brief depression severity measure. *Journal of General Internal Medicine, 169,* 606–613.

Kroenke, K., Spitzer, R. L., & Williams, J. B. (2003). The Patient Health Questionnaire-2: Validity of a two-item depression screener. *Medical Care, 4111,* 1284–1292.

Laborde-Lahoz, P., El-Gabalawy, R., Kinley, J., Kirwin, P. D., Sareen, J., & Pietrzak, R. H. (2015). Subsyndromal depression among older adults in the USA: Prevalence, comorbidity, and risk for new-onset psychiatric disorders in late life. *International Journal of Geriatric Psychiatry, 307,* 677–685.

Lesher, E. (1986). Validation of the Geriatric Depression Scale among nursing home residents. *Clinical Gerontologist, 44,* 21–28.

Marc, L. G., Raue, P. J., & Bruce, M. L. (2008). Screening performance of the 15-item Geriatric Depression Scale in a diverse elderly home care population. *American Journal of Geriatric Psychiatry, 1611,* 914–921.

McIntosh, J. (2017). USA state suicide rates and rankings for the nation, elderly, and young, 2015. American Association of Suicidology. Retrieved from http://www.suicidology.org/Portals/14/docs/Resources/FactSheets/2015/2015StatesTOY-corrected.pdf?ver=2017-01-09-215406-197

Meeks, T. W., Vahia, I. V., Lavretsky, H., Kulkarni, G., & Jeste, D. V. (2011). A tune in "A minor" can "B major": A review of epidemiology, illness course, and public health implications of subthreshold depression in older adults. *Journal of Affective Disorders, 129*(1–3):126–142.

Midden, A. J., & Mast, B. T. (2017). Differential item functioning analysis of items on the Geriatric Depression Scale-15 based on the presence or absence of cognitive impairment. *Aging and Mental Health,* 1–7.

Mills, P. D., Watts, B. V., Huh, T. J., Boar, S., & Kemp, J. (2013). Helping elderly patients to avoid suicide: A review of case reports from a National Veterans Affairs database. *Journal of Nervous and Mental Disease, 2011,* 12–16.

Mirza, S. S., Wolters, F. J., Swanson, S. A., Koudstaal, P. J., Hofman, A., Tiemeier, H., & Ikram, M. A. (2016). 10-year trajectories of depressive symptoms and risk of dementia: A population-based study. *The Lancet Psychiatry, 3*(7), 628–635.

Montgomery, S. A., & Asberg, M. (1979). A new depression scale designed to be sensitive to change. *British Journal of Psychiatry, 134,* 382–389.

Morichi, V., Dell'Aquila, G., Trotta, F., Belluigi, A., Lattanzio, F., & Cherubini, A. (2015). Diagnosing and treating depression in older and oldest old. *Current Pharmaceutical Design, 21*(13), 1690–1698.

Morimoto, S. S., Kanellopoulos, D., Manning, K. J., & Alexopoulos, G. S. (2015). Diagnosis and treatment of depression and cognitive impairment in late life. *Annals of the New York Academy of Sciences, 1345,* 36–46.

Parmelee, P., Lawton, M., & Katz, I. (1989). Psychometric properties of the Geriatric Depression Scale among the institutionalized aged. *Psychological Assessment, 14,* 331–338.

Phelan, E., Williams, B., Meeker, K., Bonn, K., Frederick, J., LoGerfo, J., & Snowden, M. (2010). A study of the diagnostic accuracy of the PHQ-9 in primary care elderly. *BMC Family Practice, 11,* 63.

Pinto-Meza, A., Serrano-Blanco, A., Peñarrubia, M. T., Blanco, E., & Haro, J. M. (2005). Assessing depression in primary care with the PHQ-9: Can it be carried out over the telephone? *Journal of General Internal Medicine, 208,* 738–742.

Qaseem, A., Barry, M. J., & Kansagara, D. (2016). Nonpharmacologic versus pharmacologic treatment of adult patients with major depressive disorder: A clinical practice guideline from the American College of Physicians. *Annals of Internal Medicine, 164,* 350–359.

Radloff, L. S. (1977). The CES-D Scale: A self-report depression scale for research in the general population. *Applied Psychological Measurement, 13,* 385–401.

Raue, P. J., Brown, E. L., Meyers, B. S., Schulberg, H. C., & Bruce, M. L. (2006). Does every allusion to possible suicide require the same response? A structured method for assessing and managing risk. *Journal of Family Practice, 55*(7), 605–613.

Raue, P. J., Ghesquiere, A. R., & Bruce, M. L. (2014). Suicide risk in primary care: Identification and management in older adults. *Current Psychiatry Reports,* 169.

Renn, B. N., & Areán, P. A. (2017). Psychosocial treatment options for major depressive disorder in older adults. *Current Treatment Options in Psychiatry, 4,* 1–12.

Richardson, T. M., Tu, X., & Conwell, Y. (2008). Psychometric properties of the Patient Heath Questionnaire (PHQ-2/9) among aging services clients. *American Journal of Geriatric Psychiatry, 163,* A62-A.

Segal, D. L., Coolidge, F. L., Cahill, B. S., & O'Riley, A. A. (2008). Psychometric properties of the Beck Depression Inventory-II (BDI-II) among community-dwelling older adults. *Behavioral Modification, 321,* 3–20.

Sheikh, J. I., & Yesavage, J. A. (1986). Geriatric Depression Scale (GDS): Recent evidence and development of a shorter version. *Clinical Gerontologist, 5,* 165–173.

Sirey, J. A., Bruce, M. L., Alexopoulos, G. S., Perlick, D. A., Raue, P., Friedman, S. J., & Meyers, B. S. (2001). Perceived stigma as a predictor of treatment discontinuation in young and older outpatients with depression. *American Journal of Psychiatry, 1583,* 479–481.

Siu, A. L., Bibbins-Domingo, K., Grossman, D. C., Baumann, L. C., Davidson, K. W., Ebell, M., ... Krist, A. H. (2016). Screening for depression in adults: US Preventive Services Task Force recommendation statement. *Journal of the American Medical Association, 315*(4), 380–387.

Spitzer, R. L., Williams, J. B., Kroenke, K., Hornyak, R., & McMurray, J. (2000). Validity and utility of the PRIME-MD patient health questionnaire in assessment of 3000 obstetric-gynecologic patients: The PRIME-MD Patient Health Questionnaire Obstetrics-Gynecology Study. *American Journal of Obstetrics and Gynecology, 1833,* 759–769.

Steer, R. A., Cavalieri, T. A., Leonard, D. M., & Beck, A. T. (1999). Use of the Beck Depression Inventory for Primary Care to screen for major depression disorders. *General Hospital Psychiatry, 212,* 106–111.

Unützer, J. (2007). Late-life depression. *New England Journal of Medicine, 357*(22), 2269–2276.

Unützer, J., Katon, W., Callahan, C. M., Williams, J. W. Jr., Hunkeler, E., Harpole, L., . . . Langston, C. (2002). Collaborative care management of late-life depression in the primary care setting: A randomized controlled trial. *Journal of the American Medical Association, 288*(22), 2836–2845.

van Marwijk, H. W., Wallace, P., de Bock, G. H., Hermans, J., Kaptein, A. A., & Mulder, J. D. (1995). Evaluation of the feasibility, reliability and diagnostic value of shortened versions of the Geriatric Depression Scale. *British Journal of General Practice, 45*(393), 195–199.

Van Orden, K. A., Witte, T. K., Cukrowicz, K. C., Braithwaite, S. R., Selby, E. A., & Joiner, T. E. Jr. (2010). The interpersonal theory of suicide. *Psychological Review, 1172,* 575–600.

World Health Organization. (2017). Depression: Let's talk. Retrieved from http://www.who.int/mental_health /management/depression/en/

Wuthrich, V. M., Johnco, C. J., & Wetherell, J. L. (2015). Differences in anxiety and depression symptoms: Comparison between older and younger clinical samples. *International Psychogeriatrics, 279,* 1523–1532.

Yesavage, J. A., Brink, T. L., Rose, T. L., Lum, O., Huang, V., Adey, M., & Leirer, V. O. (1983). Development and validation of a Geriatric Depression Screening scale: A preliminary report. *Journal of Psychiatric Research, 171,* 37–49.

Zigmond, A. S., & Snaith, R. P. (1983). The Hospital Anxiety and Depression Scale. *Acta Psychiatrica Scandinavica, 676,* 361–370.

Zung, W. W. (1972). The Depression Status Inventory: An adjunct to the Self-Rating Depression Scale. *Journal of Clinical Psychology, 284,* 539–543.

CHAPTER 23

Recognizing Mistreatment in Older Adults

Anthony Rosen, Alyssa Elman, and Terry Fulmer

CHAPTER OBJECTIVES

1. Elder mistreatment (EM) is a common phenomenon that has serious medical and social consequences, but it is dramatically under-recognized by clinicians and often not reported to authorities.
2. EM includes physical abuse, sexual abuse, neglect, abandonment, psychological abuse, and financial exploitation.
3. Clinical assessment should include observation of patient–caregiver interactions, clinical interview of the patient alone, and head-to-toe physical exam. When available, laboratory and imaging tests may be helpful. Implementing formal screening protocols may be valuable.
4. When concerned about EM, clinicians should document their findings in detail and report their suspicions to the appropriate authorities.

KEY TERMS

Abandonment
Elder mistreatment (EM)
Financial exploitation

Neglect
Physical abuse
Psychological abuse

Sexual abuse

▶ Introduction

Elder mistreatment (EM) is defined as action or negligence against an older adult that causes harm or risk of harm in a relationship with an expectation of trust or when an older adult is targeted based on age or disability. This mistreatment may include **physical abuse, sexual abuse, neglect, abandonment, psychological abuse**, and **financial exploitation** (TABLE 23-1)

TABLE 23-1	Types of Elder Mistreatment with Examples
Type	**Examples**
Physical abuse	■ Slapping, hitting, kicking, pushing, pulling hair ■ Use of physical restraints, force-feeding ■ Burning, use of household objects as weapons, use of firearms and knives
Sexual abuse	■ Sexual assault or battery, such as rape, sodomy, coerced nudity, and sexually explicit photographing ■ Unwanted touching, verbal sexual advances ■ Indecent exposure
Neglect	■ Withholding of food, water, clothing, shelter, medications ■ Failure to ensure the older adult's personal hygiene or to provide physical aids, including walker, cane, glasses, hearing aids, or dentures ■ Failure to ensure the older adult's personal safety and/or appropriate medical follow-up
Psychological abuse	■ Verbal berating, harassment, or intimidation ■ Threats of punishment or deprivation ■ Treating the older person like an infant ■ Isolating the older person from others
Financial exploitation	■ Stealing money or belongings ■ Cashing an older adult's checks without permission and/or forging his or her signature ■ Coercing an older adult into signing contracts, changing a will, or assigning durable power of attorney against his or her wishes or when the older adult does not possess the mental capacity to do so

Data from National Center on Elder Abuse. Types of abuse. Retrieved from https://ncea.acl.gov/faq/abusetypes.html

(Acierno et al., 2010; Connolly, Brandl, & Breckman, n.d.; Lachs & Pillemer, 2004; Lifespan of Greater Rochester, Weill Cornell Medical Center of Cornell University, & New York City Department for the Aging, 2011; National Research Council, 2003). Commonly, victims suffer from multiple types of EM concurrently (Acierno et al., 2010; Connolly et al., n.d.; Lachs & Pillemer, 2004; Lifespan of Greater Rochester et al., 2011; National Research Council, 2003). Recognizing EM can be challenging, but maintaining a high level of suspicion and evaluating for mistreatment is a critical part of geriatric assessment.

▶ Scope and Consequences of EM

EM is widespread, with an estimated 5% to 10% of community-dwelling older adults being victimized each year (Acierno et al., 2010; Connolly et al., n.d.; Lachs & Pillemer, 2004, 2015; Lifespan of Greater Rochester et al., 2011; National Research Council, 2003). Older adults in skilled nursing facilities are at even greater risk for EM by other residents (Albert, McCaig, & Ashman, 2013; Brownell, Wang, Smith, Stephens, & Hsia, 2014) or staff members (Ortmann, Fechner,

Bajanowski, & Brinkmann, 2001; Schiamberg et al., 2012). Research has demonstrated that psychological abuse, financial exploitation, and neglect are the more common types of EM, whereas physical abuse and sexual abuse occur more infrequently (Acierno et al., 2010; Amstadter et al., 2011; Laumann, Leitsch, & Waite, 2008).

EM can have serious medical and social consequences, including dementia (Dyer, Pavlik, Murphy, & Hyman, 2000), depression (Dyer et al., 2000), and much higher mortality (Dong et al., 2011; Lachs & Pillemer, 2015; Lachs, Williams, O'Brien, Pillemer, & Charlson, 1998). Older adults suffering from EM are more likely to present to the emergency department (Dong & Simon, 2013a; Lachs et al., 1997), be hospitalized (Dong & Simon, 2013c), and be placed in a nursing home (Dong & Simon, 2013b; Lachs, Williams, O'Brien, & Pillemer, 2002). The direct costs to society of this phenomenon are estimated to be many billions of dollars annually (Connolly et al., n.d.; Mouton et al., 2004).

EM is seldom identified, with as few as 1 in 24 cases of abuse reported to authorities (Lifespan of Greater Rochester et al., 2011). This failure in identification likely contributes to the high morbidity and mortality associated with EM (Murphy, Waa, Jaffer, Sauter, & Chan, 2013). Improving recognition is critical, as EM is expected to become more prevalent as the older adult population, especially the group older than age 85, continues to grow (American College of Emergency Physicians, 2013; Roskos & Wilber, 2006; Wilber et al., 2006).

▶ EM Risk and Vulnerability

Conceptual frameworks have been found to be useful to improve understanding of the causes of EM and for constructing approaches to assessment. One such approach is the risk and vulnerability model developed by Rose and Killien (1983), which has successfully applied to EM (Frost & Willette, 1994; Fulmer et al., 2005a) and

used to guide assessment approaches (Fulmer, Guadagno, & Bolton, 2004) (**FIGURE 23-1**). *Risk* refers to hazards or stressors in the external environment relevant to the older person that can contribute to the likelihood of mistreatment, such as having a caregiver who is emotionally unstable; *vulnerability* refers to characteristics within an older person, such as decreased cognitive status, that may influence the likelihood of mistreatment. Such a framework helps guide clinical thinking when approaching the EM assessment. Research in elder neglect has found that risks including functional status, history of trauma, and personality of the caregiver are contributing factors to such abuse (Fulmer et al., 2005a). Vulnerabilities include the older adult's personality, cognitive status, depression, functional capacity, social support, and childhood trauma (Fulmer et al., 2005a).

Other theories have been proposed to improve understanding of underlying causes of EM and to inform assessment and intervention (Jones, Holstege, & Holstege, 1997). Each of these adds valuable new insights into how to best shape an EM assessment.

▶ EM Assessment

Assessment for EM can be challenging in busy clinical settings, including emergency departments (Fulmer et al., 2005b). Nevertheless, these sites are an appropriate place for screening (Fulmer et al., 2005b; Fulmer et al., 2012; Rosen, Hargarten, Flomenbaum, & Platts-Mills, 2016). Many cases have only subtle indicators, and perpetrators and even victims often try to prevent detection of the abuse. The clinical encounter is an important potential opportunity to recognize EM (Fulmer, 2015), as evaluation by a healthcare provider may be the only time a mistreated older adult leaves the home (Rosen, Hargarten, et al., 2016). When possible, all geriatric patients should receive formal screening. Clinicians should use risk factors, elements of the medical history, and physical signs to aid their assessment.

CONSTRUCTS

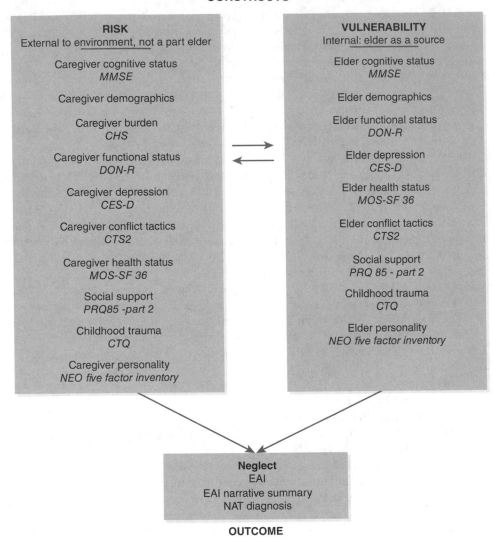

FIGURE 23-1 A risk vulnerability model of elder mistreatment.

Data from Vandeweerd, C., Paveza, G., Walsh, M., & Corvin, J.A. (2013). Physical mistreatment in persons with Alzheimer's disease. *Journal of Aging Research*, Article ID 920324, 2–10.

Observing Patient–Caregiver Interactions

When assessing geriatric patients, it is essential to closely observe interactions between the older adult and any family or paid caregivers present. These interactions may contain red flags suggesting that EM may be occurring. The clinician should note whether the older adult appears fearful of or hostile toward the caregiver. Another concerning indicator is if the caregiver interrupts the patient or does not allow him or her to answer questions, or if the older adult appears to look at the caregiver before responding to questions for approval or confirmation. Additionally, if the caregiver appears overwhelmed or burdened by, frustrated with, or angry at the older adult, the clinician's suspicions should be raised (Fulmer, 1990). A caregiver who appears unengaged and inattentive to the older adult's care should also be regarded as a worrisome sign. In clinical settings where other staff, including clerks, technologists, and receptionists, work, these staff should be encouraged to watch for concerning interactions between older adults and caregivers and to report them to clinicians (Rosen, Hargarten, et al., 2016).

Clinical Interview

It is imperative that older adults are assessed for EM without family or other caregivers present. If caregivers are resistant to allowing the patient to be evaluated alone, this reluctance should raise concern for EM. If a language barrier exists, professional translation services should be utilized. Use of family members, caregivers, or friends as interpreters should be avoided, regardless of whether they are suspected to be perpetrators. The clinician should assure the patient of privacy and confidentiality during the assessment. Many victims will be reluctant to divulge EM because of shame, guilt, and fear of reprisal.

The EM assessment should investigate the patient's functional status, cognition, and care needs, as well as the safety of the home environment (Lachs & Fulmer, 1993). The clinician should inquire about quality of life and explore whether an older adult feels isolated or depressed (Fulmer, Rodgers, & Pelger, 2014). The clinician should then ask questions about whether the older adult has experienced specific types of EM as well. Potential questions are included in **FIGURE 23-2**.

A separate interview with the caregiver/potential perpetrator may be helpful in clarifying the presence of EM (Lachs & Fulmer, 1993). Clinicians should avoid being critical or accusatory but approach the interview as an opportunity to learn more about the patient. The assessment should focus on the caregiver's knowledge and involvement in the patient's care. Also, the clinician should empathetically explore whether the caregiver feels overwhelmed and identify other responsibilities and recent changes in his or her life. It is important to note the presence of risk factors and symptoms of abuse and neglect, while also understanding the context in which it is occurring, so as to conduct an appropriate assessment (Fulmer et al., 2003).

Physical Examination

A complete head-to-toe physical examination of the older adult is a critical part of the EM assessment, as it may include signs suspicious for physical abuse, sexual abuse, or neglect (Chang, Wong, Endo, & Norman, 2013; Collins, 2006; Foreman, Theis, & Anderson, 1993; Gibbs, 2014; Palmer, Brodell, & Mostow, 2013; Speck et al., 2014; Wallace & Fulmer, 2003) (**TABLE 23-2**). When assessing an injury, it is essential to evaluate whether the physical findings are consistent with the reported mechanism. For example, it would be suspicious for an older adult to sustain four upper rib fractures from rolling off a bed two feet above the floor. A sexual assault forensic examination, typically performed by a forensically trained nurse, should be considered if the clinician has a concern for sexual abuse.

Laboratory and Imaging Studies

In clinical settings where available, laboratory and imaging studies may contribute to the assessment of EM. Laboratory tests evaluating for anemia, dehydration, malnutrition, hypothermia/hyperthermia, and rhabdomyolysis, though not diagnostic of EM, may support the clinician's suspicion (LoFaso & Rosen, 2014). Levels of medications and other drugs may also be helpful, particularly as part of a forensic investigation (LoFaso & Rosen, 2014). Inappropriately low levels of prescribed medications may suggest that a caregiver has been intentionally or unintentionally not providing an older adult with those pills (LoFaso & Rosen, 2014). A particular concern is diversion of narcotic pain medications (LoFaso & Rosen, 2014). High medication levels may indicate intentional or unintentional overdose. The detection of toxins or drugs that have not been prescribed may suggest poisoning (LoFaso & Rosen, 2014).

In the last 6 months:

*Please explore any positive responses in more detail.

PHYSICAL ABUSE	Has anyone tried to harm you? Have you been hit, slapped, pushed, grabbed, strangled, or kicked? Are there guns or other weapons in your home? Does anyone close to you have access to guns or other weapons?

SEXUAL ABUSE	Has anyone touched you in ways or places you did not want to be touched?

NEGLECT/ FUNCTIONAL STATUS	Have you relied on people for any of the following: bathing, dressing, shopping, banking, or meals?
	    If yes, have you had someone who helps you with this?
	    If yes, how often do you receive help? Is this help enough?
	    Have they done a good job? Are they reliable?
	    What happens if no one is available to help?
	Has anyone prevented you from getting food, clothes, medication, glasses, hearing aids, medical care, or anything else you need to stay healthy?

PSYCHOLOGICAL ABUSE	Has anyone close to you called you names, put you down, or yelled at you?
	    Has anyone close to you ever threatened to punish you or put you in an institution?
	    Have you felt sad or lonely at home?
	    Have you felt afraid of anyone close to you?
	    Do you distrust anyone close to you?
	    Does anyone close to you drink or use drugs?

FINANCIAL EXPLOITATION	Has anyone tried to force you to sign papers against your will, or that you did not understand? Has anyone pressured you to give them money or property? Has anyone taken money or things that belong to you without asking? Does anyone close to you rely on you for housing and/or financial support?

FIGURE 23-2 Questions to assess for elder mistreatment.

Data from Yaffe, M., Wolfson, C., Lithwick, M., & Weiss, D. (2008). Development and validation of a tool to improve physician identification of elder abuse: the elder abuse suspicion index (EASI). *Journal of Elder Abuse and Neglect, 20*(3), 276–300; Giraldo-Rodriguez, L., & Rosas-Carrasco, O. (2013). Development and psychometric properties of the geriatric mistreatment scale. *Geriatrics & Gerontology International, 13*(2), 466–474; Schofield, M. J., & Mishra, G. D. (2003). Validity of self-report screening scale for elder abuse: Women's Health Australia Study. *The Gerontologist, 43*(1), 110–120.

Although no imaging findings have been described that definitively identify EM, potentially suggestive findings exist (Murphy et al., 2013; Rosen, Bloemen, Harpe, et al., 2016; Wong et al., 2017). In particular, co-occurring old and new fractures, high-energy fractures despite assertion of a low-energy mechanism, and distal ulnar diaphyseal fractures should raise concern (Rosen, Bloemen, Harpe, et al., 2016; Wong et al., 2017).

When the possibility of EM, particularly physical abuse, is present, the clinician should communicate his or her suspicion to the radiologist and ask that professional to focus on whether the imaging findings are consistent with the purported mechanism. Additional screening imaging tests may be considered, including maxillofacial computed tomography (CT) scan and chest X-ray, to evaluate for acute and chronic fractures.

TABLE 23-2 Physical Signs Suspicious for Potential Elder Mistreatment

Physical Abuse

- Bruising in atypical locations (not over bony prominences; on lateral arms, back, face, ears, or neck)
- Patterned injuries (bite marks or injury consistent with the shape of a belt buckle, fingertip, or other object)
- Wrist or ankle lesions or scars (suggesting inappropriate restraint)
- Burns (particularly a stocking/glove pattern, suggesting forced immersion, or a cigarette pattern)
- Multiple fractures or bruises of different ages
- Traumatic alopecia or scalp hematomas
- Subconjunctival, vitreous, or retinal ophthalmic hemorrhages
- Intraoral soft-tissue injuries

Sexual Abuse

- Genital, rectal, or oral trauma (including erythema, bruising, lacerations)
- Evidence of sexually transmitted disease

Neglect

- Cachexia/malnutrition
- Dehydration
- Pressure sores/decubitus ulcers
- Poor body hygiene, unchanged diaper
- Dirty, severely worn clothing
- Elongated toenails
- Poor oral hygiene

Adapted from Chang et al., 2013; Collins, 2006; Foreman et al., 1993; Gibbs, 2014; Palmer et al., 2013; Speck et al., 2014; Wallace & Fulmer, 2003.

▶ Documentation

Comprehensive, accurate documentation is a critical element of EM clinical assessment. When documenting, the clinician should be mindful that the medical chart may be used in the future for investigation and prosecution, and the quality of the documentation can significantly impact whether justice and protection can be achieved for a victimized older adult (Coulourides et al., 2017). The patient's responses to questions in the interview should be documented in detail, using the patient's own words if possible. Social history information should be documented as well, including functional status, the caregiver's relationship to the patient, and living arrangements. The physical examination should be documented comprehensively, including the general appearance of the patient on arrival. In addition, the description should identify signs of potential neglect, including dirty clothing, poor dental hygiene, and untrimmed nails. For all injuries, documentation should include size, location, stage of healing, and whether consistent with the reported mechanism.

When documenting physical findings, clinicians should consider using a body diagram/traumagram, which is available as part of many electronic medical records, to increase accuracy. Whenever possible, clinicians should photograph physical findings and add these photographs to the medical chart, as these images may be useful forensically. A protocol for photographing injuries in the acute medical care setting has been recently published (Bloemen et al., 2016).

▶ Reporting to the Authorities

Reporting concerns about EM to the authorities is essential to ensure the safety of a vulnerable older adult. In most U.S. states, clinicians are mandatory reporters of suspected EM. Adult Protective Services (APS) are the county- or state-based agencies responsible for receiving and investigating these reports. In some states, clinicians are also required to report to law enforcement, who should always be contacted if a clinician believes an older adult is in immediate danger. For older adults who live in nursing homes, concerns should be reported to the state's long-term care ombudsman; the National Long-Term Care Ombudsman Resource Center has a website that can help the provider identify this contact (http://theconsumervoice.org/get_help).

▶ Tools for Formal Screening

The American Medical Association has recommended that healthcare providers routinely screen all geriatric patients for EM during healthcare assessments (American College of Emergency Physicians, 2013; American Medical Association, 1992). Several effective screening tools are described in the literature (Fulmer, 2002; Fulmer, Guadagno, Bitondo Dyer, & Connolly, 2004; National Center on Elder Abuse [NCEA], 2018), some of which have been validated in various clinical settings. Additional tools are currently in development. For a screening tool to be useful, it must be accurate, easy and efficient to use, and useful in a variety of clinical settings.

The Elder Assessment Instrument (EAI; **EXHIBIT 23-1**) is useful across varied clinical settings (Fulmer, 2008), including the emergency department; is easy to administer; and offers an efficient method for organizing observations relevant to a mistreatment judgment (Fulmer & Cahill, 1984; Fulmer, Paveza, Abraham, & Fairchild, 2000; Fulmer et al., 2005b; Fulmer, Street, & Carr, 1984). The Elder

---

EXHIBIT 23-1 Elder Assessment Instrument

Instructions: There is no "score" for this instrument. A patient should be referred to social services if the following exists: (1) if there is any positive evidence without sufficient clinical explanation, (2) whenever there is a subjective complaint by the older adult of elder mistreatment, or (3) whenever the clinician deems there is evidence of abuse, neglect, exploitation, or abandonment.
Purpose: To be used as a comprehensive approach for screening suspected elder abuse victims in all clinical settings.

1. General Assessment	Very Good	Good	Poor	Very Poor	Unable to Assess
a. Clothing					
b. Hygiene					
c. Nutrition					
d. Skin integrity					

Additional comments:

2. Possible Abuse Indicators	No Evidence	Possible Evidence	Probable Evidence	Definite Evidence	Unable to Assess
a. Bruising					
b. Lacerations					
c. Fractures					
d. Various stages of healing of any bruises or fractures					
e. Evidence of sexual abuse					
f. Statement by older adult related to abuse					

Additional comments:

3. Possible Neglect Indicators	No Evidence	Possible Evidence	Probable Evidence	Definite Evidence	Unable to Assess
a. Contractures					
b. Decubiti					
c. Dehydration					
d. Diarrhea					
e. Depression					
f. Impaction					
g. Malnutrition					

(continues)

EXHIBIT 23-1 Elder Assessment Instrument   *(continued)*

h.	Urine burns				
i.	Poor hygiene				
j.	Failure to respond to warning of obvious disease				
k.	Inappropriate medications (over/under)				
l.	Repetitive hospital admissions due to probable failure of healthcare surveillance				
m.	Statement by older adult related to neglect				
Additional comments:					

4. Possible Exploitation Indicators	**No Evidence**	**Possible Evidence**	**Probable Evidence**	**Definite Evidence**	**Unable to Assess**
a. Misuse of money					
b. Evidence					
c. Reports of demands for goods in exchange for services					
d. Inability to account for money/property					
e. Statement by older adult related to exploitation					
Additional comments:					

5. Possible Abandonment Indicators	No Evidence	Possible Evidence	Probable Evidence	Definite Evidence	Unable to Assess
a. Evidence that a caretaker has withdrawn care precipitously without making alternative arrangements					
b. Evidence that older adult is left alone in an unsafe environment for extended periods of time without adequate support					
c. Statement by older adult related to abandonment					
Additional comments:					

Summary	No Evidence	Possible Evidence	Probable Evidence	Definite Evidence	Unable to Assess
Evidence of abuse					
Evidence of neglect					
Evidence of exploitation					
Evidence of abandonment					
Additional comments:					

Comments: _____

Reproduced from Fulmer, T. (2003). Elder abuse and neglect assessment. *Journal of Gerontological Nursing, 29*(6), 4–5. Reproduced with permission of SLACK Incorporated.

Abuse Suspicion Index (EASI; **BOX 23-1**) is a short screening instrument validated for cognitively intact patients in family practice and ambulatory care settings, with a sensitivity of 0.47 and a specificity of 0.75 (Yaffe, Wolfson, Lithwick, & Weiss, 2008). It includes six questions and takes less than two minutes to conduct (Yaffe et al., 2008).

BOX 23-1 Clinical Screening for Elder Mistreatment: Elder Abuse Suspicion Index (EASI)

Questions 1 through 5 are answered by the patient. Question 6 is answered by the physician.

1. Have you relied on people for any of the following: bathing, dressing, shopping, banking, or meals?
2. Has anyone prevented you from getting food, clothes, medication, glasses, hearing aids, or medical care or from being with people you wanted to be with?
3. Have you been upset because someone talked to you in a way that made you feel shamed or threatened?
4. Has anyone tried to force you to sign papers or to use your money against your will?
5. Has anyone made you afraid, touched you in ways that you did not want, or hurt you physically?
6. Doctor: Elder abuse may be associated with findings such as poor eye contact, withdrawn nature, malnourishment, hygiene issues, cuts, bruises, inappropriate clothing, or medication compliance issues. Did you notice any of these today or in the last 12 months?

The patient can answer "yes," "no," or "unsure." A response of "yes" on one or more of questions 2 through 6 should prompt concern for abuse or neglect.

Reproduced from Yaffe, M. J., Wolfson, C., Lithwick, M., & Weiss, D. (2008). Development and validation of a tool to improve physician identification of elder abuse: The Elder Abuse Suspicion Index (EASI). *Journal of Elder Abuse and Neglect, 20*, 276–300. Reprinted by permission of the publisher, Taylor & Francis Ltd, http://www.tandfonline.com.

▶ Practice Challenges

EM assessment can be challenging for clinicians. Many older adults suffer from dementing illness, making it difficult to obtain a reliable medical history. A clinician should still interview older adults who are cognitively impaired, as recent studies have shown that individuals with dementia can often reliably report how an injury occurred (Wiglesworth et al., 2009; Ziminski, Wiglesworth, Austin, Phillips, & Mosqueda, 2013). In instances where the patient cannot provide history, collateral information should be obtained from other sources, such as other family members, neighbors, or the primary care provider.

Another challenge in EM assessment is the difficulty in distinguishing between EM and accidental trauma or illness. This task is made more challenging by the normal physiologic changes that occur with aging and older adults' frequent use of medications that affect bruising (Collins, 2006; Collins & Presnell, 2007; Collins & Sellars, 2005; Murphy et al., 2013; Rosenblatt, Cho, & Durance, 1996). Although only limited research exists to assist clinicians, recent studies have shown that physical abuse–related injuries are most frequently observed on the head, neck, and upper extremities (Murphy et al., 2013; Rosen, Hargarten, et al., 2016). In one study, abuse victims had bruises that were more often large (greater than 5 cm) and found on the face, lateral right arm, or posterior torso (Wiglesworth et al., 2009). Preliminary results from another study suggest that injuries to the left periorbital area, neck, and ulnar forearm may be much more common with abuse than with an accident (Wong et al., 2016). Future research to further inform EM assessment is ongoing.

BOX 23-2 Key Elements of the Clinical Assessment for Elder Mistreatment

- Observe patient–caregiver interactions.
- Interview the patient alone and provide assurance of privacy and confidentiality.
- Perform a head-to-toe physical examination, focusing on signs suggestive of physical abuse, sexual abuse, or neglect.
- Comprehensively document all findings from the assessment and consider taking photographs of any injuries or physical findings.
- Report any concerns to the appropriate authorities.

▶ Approach for Readers

Key elements of the clinical assessment for EM are highlighted in **BOX 23-2**. Ultimately, the most valuable tool for a clinician in assessing for EM is maintaining a high index of suspicion for this common, serious, but frequently missed phenomenon.

▶ Summary

Although abuse of older adults is common and has serious consequences, EM is both under-recognized and under-reported. The clinical encounter is an important opportunity to identify EM, and clinicians should routinely assess for it. A standardized approach and formal screening protocols may be helpful. The assessment should be comprehensively documented, and any concerns should be reported to the appropriate authorities. Identifying EM has the potential to dramatically impact the health and quality of life of the most vulnerable older adults.

References

Acierno, R., Hernandez, M. A., Amstadter, A. B., Resnick, H. S., Steve, K., Muzzy, W., . . . Kilpatrick, D. G. (2010). Prevalence and correlates of emotional, physical, sexual, and financial abuse and potential neglect in the United States: the National Elder Mistreatment Study. *American Journal of Public Health, 100*, 292–297.

Albert, M., McCaig, L. F., & Ashman, J. J. (2013). Emergency department visits by persons aged 65 and over: United States, 2009–2010. *NCHS Data Brief*, 1–8.

American College of Emergency Physicians. (2013). *Domestic family violence*. Retrieved from https://www.acep.org /Clinical---Practice-Management/Domestic-Family-Violence/

American Medical Association. (1992). *Diagnostic and treatment guidelines on elder abuse and neglect*. Chicago, IL: Author.

Amstadter, A. B., Zajac, K., Strachan, M., Hernandez, M. A., Kilpatrick, D. G., & Acierno, R. (2011). Prevalence and correlates of elder mistreatment in South Carolina: The South Carolina elder mistreatment study. *Journal of Interpersonal Violence, 26*, 2947–2972.

Bloemen, E. M., Rosen, T., Schiroo, C., Justina, A., Clark, S., Mulcare, M. R., . . . Hargarten, S. (2016). Photographing injuries in the acute care setting: Development and evaluation of a standardized protocol for research, forensics, and clinical practice. *Academic Emergency Medicine, 23*, 653–659.

Brownell, J., Wang, J., Smith, A., Stephens, C., & Hsia, R. Y. (2014). Trends in emergency department visits for ambulatory care sensitive conditions by elderly nursing home residents, 2001 to 2010. *JAMA Internal Medicine, 174*, 156–158.

Chang, A. L., Wong, J. W., Endo, J. O., & Norman, R. A. (2013). Geriatric dermatology: Part II. Risk factors and cutaneous signs of elder mistreatment for the dermatologist. *Journal of the American Academy of Dermatology, 68*, 533, e1–e10; quiz 43–44.

Collins, K. A. (2006). Elder maltreatment: A review. *Archives of Pathology & Laboratory Medicine, 130*, 1290–1296.

Collins, K. A., & Presnell, S. E. (2007). Elder neglect and the pathophysiology of aging. *American Journal of Forensic Medicine and Pathology, 28*, 157–162.

Collins, K. A., & Sellars, K. (2005). Vertebral artery laceration mimicking elder abuse. *American Journal of Forensic Medicine and Pathology, 26*, 150–154.

Connolly, M.T., Brandl, B., & Breckman, R. (n.d.). *The elder justice roadmap: A stakeholder initiative to respond to an emerging health, justice, financial, and social crisis*. Retrieved from https://www.justice.gov/file/852856/download

Coulourides, A., Kogan, A. N., Rosen, T., Homeier, D., Chennapan, K., & Mosqueda, L. (2017). Developing a tool to improve documentation of physical findings in injured older adults by health care providers: Insights from experts in multiple disciplines [Abstract]. *Journal of the American Geriatrics Society, 65*, S1–S289.

Dong, X., & Simon, M. A. (2013a). Association between elder abuse and use of ED: Findings from the Chicago Health and Aging Project. *American Journal of Emergency Medicine, 31*, 693–698.

Dong, X., & Simon, M. A. (2013b). Association between reported elder abuse and rates of admission to skilled nursing facilities: Findings from a longitudinal population-based cohort study. *Gerontology, 59,* 464–472.

Dong, X., & Simon, M. A. (2013c). Elder abuse as a risk factor for hospitalization in older persons. *JAMA Internal Medicine, 173,* 911–917.

Dong, X. Q., Simon, M. A., Beck, T. T., Farran, C., McCann, J. J., Mendes De Leon, C. F., . . . Evans, D. A. (2011). Elder abuse and mortality: The role of psychological and social wellbeing. *Gerontology, 57,* 549–558.

Dyer, C. B., Pavlik, V. N., Murphy, K. P., & Hyman, D. J. (2000). The high prevalence of depression and dementia in elder abuse or neglect. *Journal of the American Geriatrics Society, 48,* 205–208.

Foreman, M. D., Theis, S. L., & Anderson, M. A. (1993). Adverse events in the hospitalized elderly. *Clinical Nursing Research, 2,* 360–370.

Frost, M. H., & Willette, K. (1994). Risk for abuse/neglect: Documentation of assessment data and diagnoses. *Journal of Gerontological Nursing, 20,* 37–45.

Fulmer, T. T. (1990). The debate over dependency as a relevant predisposing factor in elder abuse and neglect. *Journal of Elder Abuse & Neglect, 2,* 51–72.

Fulmer, T. (2002). Elder mistreatment. *Annual Review of Nursing Research, 20,* 369–395.

Fulmer, T. (2003). Elder abuse and neglect assessment. *Journal of Gerontological Nursing, 29*(6), 4–5.

Fulmer, T. (2008). How to try this: Screening of mistreatment for older adults. *American Journal of Nursing, 108,* 52–59.

Fulmer, T. (2015). Nurses and the Elder Justice Act. *American Journal of Nursing, 115,* 11.

Fulmer, T. T., & Cahill, V. M. (1984). Assessing elder abuse: A study. *Journal of Gerontological Nursing, 10,* 16–20.

Fulmer, T., Firpo, A., Guadagno, L., Easter, T. M., Kahan, F., & Paris, B. (2003). Themes from a grounded theory analysis of elder neglect assessment by experts. *Gerontologist, 43,* 745–752.

Fulmer, T., Guadagno, L., Bitondo Dyer, C., & Connolly, M. T. (2004). Progress in elder abuse screening and assessment instruments. *Journal of the American Geriatrics Society, 52,* 297–304.

Fulmer, T., Guadagno, L., & Bolton, M. M. (2004). Elder mistreatment in women. *Journal of Obstetric, Gynecologic, and Neonatal Nursing, 33,* 657–663.

Fulmer, T., Paveza, G., Abraham, I., & Fairchild, S. (2000). Elder neglect assessment in the emergency department. *Journal of Emergency Nursing, 26,* 436–443.

Fulmer, T., Paveza, G., VandeWeerd, C., Fairchild, S., Guadagno, L., Bolton-Blatt, M., . . . Norman, R. (2005a). Dyadic vulnerability and risk profiling for elder neglect. *Gerontologist, 45,* 525–534.

Fulmer, T., Paveza, G., VandeWeerd, C., Guadagno, L., Fairchild, S., Norman, R., . . . Bolton-Blatt, M. (2005b). Neglect assessment in urban emergency departments and confirmation by an expert clinical team. *Journals*

of Gerontology, Series A: Biological Sciences and Medical Sciences, 60, 1002–1006.

Fulmer, T., Rodgers, R. F., & Pelger, A. (2014). Verbal mistreatment of the elderly. *Journal of Elder Abuse and Neglect, 26,* 351–364.

Fulmer, T., Strauss, S., Russell, S. L., Singh, G., Blankenship, J., Vemula, R., . . . Sutin, D. (2012). Screening for elder mistreatment in dental and medical clinics. *Gerontology, 29,* 96–105.

Fulmer, T., Street, S., & Carr, K. (1984). Abuse of the elderly: Screening and detection. *Journal of Emergency Nursing, 10,* 131–140.

Gibbs, L. M. (2014). Understanding the medical markers of elder abuse and neglect: Physical examination findings. *Clinics in Geriatric Medicine, 30,* 687–712.

Jones, J. S., Holstege, C., & Holstege, H. (1997). Elder abuse and neglect: Understanding the causes and potential risk factors. *American Journal of Emergency Medicine, 15,* 579–583.

Lachs, M. S., & Fulmer, T. (1993). Recognizing elder abuse and neglect. *Clinics in Geriatric Medicine, 9,* 665–681.

Lachs, M. S., & Pillemer, K. (2004). Elder abuse. *Lancet, 364,* 1263–1272.

Lachs, M. S., & Pillemer, K. A. (2015). Elder abuse. *New England Journal of Medicine, 373,* 1947–1856.

Lachs, M. S., Williams, C. S., O'Brien, S., Hurst, L., Kossack, A., Siegal, A., . . . Tinetti, M. E. (1997). ED use by older victims of family violence. *Annals of Emergency Medicine, 30,* 448–454.

Lachs, M. S., Williams, C. S., O'Brien, S., & Pillemer, K. A. (2002). Adult protective service use and nursing home placement. *Gerontologist, 42,* 734–739.

Lachs, M. S., Williams, C. S., O'Brien, S., Pillemer, K. A., & Charlson, M. E. (1998). The mortality of elder mistreatment. *Journal of the American Medical Association, 280,* 428–432.

Laumann, E. O., Leitsch, S. A., & Waite, L. J. (2008). Elder mistreatment in the United States: Prevalence estimates from a nationally representative study. *Journals of Gerontology, Series B: Psychological Sciences and Social Sciences, 63,* S248–S254.

Lifespan of Greater Rochester, Weill Cornell Medical Center of Cornell University, & New York City Department for the Aging. (2011, May). *Under the radar: New York State elder abuse prevalence study: Self-reported prevalence and documented case surveys.* Retrieved from http://ocfs.ny.gov/main/reports/Under%20the%20Radar%2005%2012%2011%20final%20report.pdf

LoFaso, V. M., & Rosen, T. (2014) Medical and laboratory indicators of elder abuse and neglect. *Clinics in Geriatric Medicine, 30,* 713–728.

Mouton, C. P., Rodabough, R. J., Rovi, S. L., Hunt, J. L., Talamantes, M. A., Brzyski, R. G., . . . Burge, S. K. (2004). Prevalence and 3-year incidence of abuse among postmenopausal women. *American Journal of Public Health, 94,* 605–612.

Murphy, K., Waa, S., Jaffer, H., Sauter, A., & Chan, A. (2013). A literature review of findings in physical elder abuse. *Canadian Association of Radiologists Journal, 64*, 10–14.

National Center on Elder Abuse (NCEA). (2018). *Frequently asked questions: Types of abuse*. Retrieved from https://ncea.acl.gov/faq/abusetypes.html

National Research Council. (2003). *Elder mistreatment: Abuse, neglect and exploitation in an aging America*. Washington, DC: National Academies Press.

Ortmann, C., Fechner, G., Bajanowski, T., & Brinkmann, B. (2001). Fatal neglect of the elderly. *International Journal of Legal Medicine, 114*, 191–193.

Palmer, M., Brodell, R. T., & Mostow, E. N. (2013). Elder abuse: Dermatologic clues and critical solutions. *Journal of the American Academy of Dermatology, 68*, e37–e42.

Rose, M. H., & Killien, M. (1983). Risk and vulnerability: A case for differentiation. *Advances in Nursing Science, 5*, 60–73.

Rosen, T., Bloemen, E. M., Harpe, J., Sanchez, A. M., Mennitt, K. W., McCarthy, T. J., . . . Lachs, M. S. (2016). Radiologists' training, experience, and attitudes about elder abuse detection. *American Journal of Roentgenology, 207*, 1210–1214.

Rosen, T., Bloemen, E. M., LoFaso, V. M., Clark, S., Flomenbaum, N. E., & Lachs, M. S. (2016). Emergency department presentations for injuries in older adults independently known to be victims of elder abuse. *Journal of Emergency Medicine 50*(3), 518–526.

Rosen, T., Hargarten, S., Flomenbaum, N. E., & Platts-Mills, T. F. (2016). Identifying elder abuse in the emergency department: Toward a multidisciplinary team-based approach. *Annals of Emergency Medicine, 68*, 378–382.

Rosenblatt, D. E., Cho, K. H., & Durance, P. W. (1996). Reporting mistreatment of older adults: The role of physicians. *Journal of the American Geriatrics Society, 44*, 65–70.

Roskos, E. R., & Wilber, S. T. (2006). 210: The effect of future demographic changes on emergency medicine. *Annals of Emergency Medicine, 48*, 65.

Schiamberg, L. B., Oehmke, J., Zhang, Z., Barboza, G. E., Griffore, R. J., Von Heydrich, L., . . . Mastin, T. (2012). Physical abuse of older adults in nursing homes: A random sample survey of adults with an elderly family member in a nursing home. *Journal of Elder Abuse & Neglect, 24*, 65–83.

Speck, P. M., Hartig, M. T., Likes, W., Bowdre, T., Carney, A. Y., Ekroos, R. A., . . . Faugno, D. K. (2014). Case series of sexual assault in older persons. *Clinics in Geriatric Medicine, 30*, 779–806.

Wallace, M., & Fulmer, T. (2003). Fulmer SPICES: An overall assessment tool of older adults. *Alabama Nurse, 30*, 26.

Wilber, S. T., Gerson, L. W., Terrell, K. M., Carpenter, C. R., Shah, M. N., Heard, K., . . . Hwang, U. (2006). Geriatric emergency medicine and the 2006 Institute of Medicine reports from the Committee on the Future of Emergency Care in the U.S. Health System. *Academic Emergency Medicine, 13*, 1345–1351.

Wiglesworth, A., Austin, R., Corona, M., Schneider, D., Liao, S., Gibbs, L., . . . Mosqueda, L. (2009). Bruising as a marker of physical elder abuse. *Journal of the American Geriatrics Society, 57*, 1191–1196.

Wong, N. Z., Rosen, T., Sanchez, A. M., Bloemen, E. M., Mennitt, K. W., Hentel, K., . . . Lachs, M. S. (2017). Imaging findings in elder abuse: A role for radiologists in detection. *Canadian Association of Radiologists Journal, 68*, 16–20.

Wong, N. Z., Sanchez, A. M., Bloemen, E. M., Mennitt, K. W., Hentel, K., Nicola, R.,... Lachs, M. (2016). Imaging findings in two cases of elder abuse: A role for radiologists in detection [Abstract]. *Journal of the American Geriatrics Society, 64*, S1–S311.

Yaffe, M. J., Wolfson, C., Lithwick, M., & Weiss, D. (2008). Development and validation of a tool to improve physician identification of elder abuse: The Elder Abuse Suspicion Index (EASI). *Journal of Elder Abuse and Neglect, 20*, 276–300.

Ziminski, C. E., Wiglesworth, A., Austin, R., Phillips, L. R., & Mosqueda, L. (2013). Injury patterns and causal mechanisms of bruising in physical elder abuse. *Journal of Forensic Nursing, 9*, 84–91, quiz E1–E2.

CHAPTER 24

Functional Assessment of Older Adults

Sherry A. Greenberg and Donna McCabe

CHAPTER OBJECTIVES

1. Describe the components of a functional assessment.
2. Describe use of valid, reliable tools to assess function in older adults.
3. Understand how functional assessment may be conducted in healthcare settings.
4. Identify factors and conditions that affect function in older adults.

KEY TERMS

Activities of daily living
Function

Functional assessment

Older adults

▶ Introduction

Functional assessment is a vital component of a comprehensive geriatric assessment. A person's level of **function** is affected by his or her overall state of health, yet is beyond a specific disease or health condition. Reflecting the broad scope of factors affecting function, **functional assessment** includes physical, psychological, socioeconomic, and environmental components. An emphasis is placed on knowing the individual's baseline status and making comparisons to that status. The focus on preservation of function relative to this baseline requires that declines be noticed as early as possible if they are to be improved or slowed in progression. Lack of systematic assessment using evidence-based tools and reliance on assumptions or patient self-report can limit the data obtained and lead to missed opportunities for preventing functional decline. Particularly concerning is the high risk for progressive loss of function among older adults with a preexisting need for assistance in **activities of daily living** (Graf, 2008, 2012; Resnick, 2016).

Physical functioning in some degree is a requirement for many facets of day-to-day life. For **older adults**, it may dictate their ability to live alone, where they are able to live, and what degree of assistance is required regardless of setting. In some sense, functional ability may be synonymous with overall good health. Older adults, in fact, often define the degree of their health in terms of their overall functioning—that is, their ability to do "what they do" on a daily basis (Boltz, Capezuti, Shabbat, & Hall, 2010).

Functional well-being, which comprises the maintenance of baseline optimal functioning, is a public health concern. *Healthy People 2020* (2017) has set forth a goal of reducing the proportion of older adults with moderate to severe functional limitations by 10%, from 29.3% in 2007 to 26.4% in 2020. Older adults living with or developing functional decline place a tremendous burden on government healthcare funding (Guralnik, Alecxih, Branch, & Wiener, 2002). Hence, it is healthcare providers' responsibility to assess function regularly and intervene quickly, as needed.

▶ Assessment and Best Practices

The basic elements of functional assessment are recommended to be completed at regular intervals to allow comparisons over time, quick identification of declines, and early intervention. Functional assessment should be completed formally at least yearly and informally during every encounter with an older adult. A functional assessment can be basic or comprehensive in nature. A complete functional assessment includes a thorough functional history and knowledge of the person's baseline functional status. The clinician must integrate functional assessment into the entire comprehensive exam that evaluates

the characteristics of the home environment, the role of caregivers, the existence of pain, and other elements that may affect function.

Caregivers, friends, and neighbors may provide information about a person's baseline functional status, as needed. The clinician should make direct observations of functional status whenever possible, however, as the client's or a family member's verbal report may not always be accurate. Document all findings. Do not assume that what is told is always the case, as functional status may change over time.

Functional assessment should be performed in all healthcare settings in which older adults are encountered. In the home setting, it is important to assess the older adult's ability to function in the home and surrounding environment at every home visit. Assess for safety issues, lighting, throw rugs, waxed floors, cooking items within reaching distance, condition of stairs and railings, wide doorways, raised toilet seats, handicap accessibility, and grab bars and/or a seat in the shower or bathtub.

In the primary care office, start assessing function upon a person's entrance into the office. Observe how the person walks; if an assistive device is used; if the person is holding onto the wall, objects, or other people for balance; and if the person needs assistance to change into an examination gown for the office physical examination.

In the acute care setting, assess the older adult's functional status and compare it to the baseline status. Assess level of activity and self-sufficiency. Family members and visiting friends may provide assistance in obtaining information about a person's baseline functional status. Although the primary focus during an acute care stay is assessment and management of the admitting health condition, there is increasing awareness of the importance of addressing the functional status needs of older adults, especially to prevent negative outcomes (Boltz, Resnick, & Galik, 2016; Resnick, Galik, Wells, Boltz, & Holtzman, 2015). In the post-acute care setting, assess the older adult's functional status upon admission, quarterly, and upon significant change in clinical status. The identification of functional decline is a major problem during transitions in health care, particularly upon entering and discharge from acute care setting. It is crucial to obtain a baseline history as a basis for making comparisons over time (Hoogerduijn et al., 2012).

Basic aspects of the health history and physical examination related to function of older adults include vision, hearing, oral health, nutrition, elimination, social support, cognition, and upper and lower extremity mobility. Aspects of visual function include assessment of eyes, extraocular movements, and visual fields; vision screening with glasses and/or contact lenses with a Snellen chart or book, if needed; and knowledge of the last ophthalmologist exam. Hearing function includes assessment for and removal of any cerumen, need for hearing aids and/or their battery function, and a whisper test to assess actual hearing of a soft voice. The condition of the mouth, oral mucosa, teeth, dentures, and tongue are important, as they relate to oral–systemic health. Note any difficulty chewing, eating, or swallowing. Ask about the last dental appointment or arrange for one, as needed.

In terms of nutrition, ask about ease of access to food and stores; dexterity to open cans, bottles, and packages; and ability to prepare meals and cook safely. In terms of mobility, assess upper and lower extremity function by determining range of motion and strength. Inquire about pain and any treatments used, as pain can affect overall function, mobility, and willingness to participate in physical and social activities.

In addition, assess ethnic, spiritual, and cultural factors that may affect any aspect of function or well-being. Ask about the person's social support system and participation in community activities, such as in a neighborhood senior center.

Interprofessional team members may assist in the comprehensive assessment of function for older adults. These team members include nurses, primary care providers, social workers, dietitians, dentists, podiatrists, and clergy members; physical, occupational, speech, and recreation therapists; and paid and nonpaid caregivers.

▶ Assessment Tools

The most common assessments for physical function examine the person's ability to perform activities of daily living (ADLs) and instrumental activities of daily living (IADLs) (Graf, 2008, 2012; Resnick, 2016). The Katz Index of Independence in Activities of Daily Living and the Lawton Instrumental Activities of Daily Living Scale (Lawton & Brody, 1969) are tools that are frequently used to assess the most common components of functional ability to live independently.

The Katz Index, which is used to assess for problems in performing ADLs, ranks adequacy of performance in the six functions of bathing, dressing, toileting, transferring, continence, and feeding (**BOX 24-1**). The individual receives a score of "yes" or "no" regarding independence in each of the six functions. A score of 6 indicates full function, 4 indicates moderate impairment, and 2 or less indicates severe functional impairment (Katz, 1983; Shelkey & Wallace, 2012).

The Lawton IADL Scale is used to assess independent living skills. It ranks adequacy in performance of eight complex activities: ability to use the telephone, shopping, food preparation, housekeeping, laundry, mode of transportation, responsibility for own medications, and ability to handle finances (**BOX 24-2**). People are scored according to their highest level of functioning in that category. The summary score ranges from 0 (low function, dependent) to 8 (high function, independent) (Graf, 2008, 2012; Lawton & Brody, 1969).

Many other tools may be used to develop a more detailed assessment of overall function and different facets of function other than just the physical domain. The Advanced Activities of Daily Living (AADL) tool is one such comprehensive assessment of overall functioning, whose results are highly dependent on cognitive abilities (Reuben & Solomon, 1989). The comprehensive nature of an AADL assessment provides data that indicate how the person is functioning in the environment on social, occupational, and more advanced levels such as hobbies and working. Cultural

BOX 24-1 Katz Index of Independence in Activities of Daily Living

Activities Points (1 or 0)	Independence: (1 Point) **No** supervision, direction, or personal assistance	Dependence: (0 Points) **With** supervision, direction, personal assistance, or total care
Bathing Points: _____	(1 Point) Bathes self completely or needs help in bathing only a single part of the body such as the back, genital area, or disabled extremity.	(0 Points) Needs help with bathing more than one part of the body, getting in or out of the tub or shower. Requires total bathing.
Dressing Points: _____	(1 Point) Gets clothes from closets and drawers and puts on clothes and outer garments complete with fasteners. May have help tying shoes.	(0 Points) Needs help with dressing self or needs to be completely dressed.
Toileting Points: _____	(1 Point) Goes to toilet, gets on and off, arranges clothes, cleans genital area without help.	(0 Points) Needs help transferring to the toilet, cleaning self, or uses bedpan or commode.
Transferring Points: _____	(1 Point) Moves in and out of bed or chair unassisted. Mechanical transferring aides are acceptable.	(0 Points) Needs help in moving from bed to chair or requires a complete transfer.
Continence Points: _____	(1 Point) Exercises complete self-control over urination and defecation.	(0 Points) Is partially or totally incontinent of bowel or bladder.
Feeding Points: _____	(1 Point) Gets food from plate into mouth without help. Preparation of food may be done by another person.	(0 Points) Needs partial or total help with feeding or requires parenteral feeding.

Total points = _____ 6 = High (patient independent) 0 = Low (patient very dependent)

Reproduced from Katz, S., Down, T.D., Cash, H.R., & Grotz, R.C. (1970). Progress in the development of the index of ADL. The Gerontologist, 1970, 10(1), 20-30, by permission of Oxford University Press.

BOX 24-2 Lawton Instrumental Activities of Daily Living Scale

A.   Ability to Use Telephone
   1.   Operates telephone on own initiative; looks up and dials numbers   1
   2.   Dials a few well-known numbers   1
   3.   Answers telephone, but does not dial   1
   4.   Does not use telephone at all   0
B.   Shopping
   1.   Takes care of all shopping needs independently   1
   2.   Shops independently for small purchases   0
   3.   Needs to be accompanied on any shopping trip   0
   4.   Completely unable to shop   0
C.   Food Preparation
   1.   Plans, prepares, and serves adequate meals independently   1
   2.   Prepares adequate meals if supplied with ingredients   0
   3.   Heats and serves prepared meals of prepares meals, but does not
      maintain adequate diet   0
   4.   Needs to have meals prepared and served   0
D.   Housekeeping
   1.   Maintains house alone with occasional assistance (heavy work)   1
   2.   Performs light daily tasks such as dishwashing, bed making   1
   3.   Performs light daily tasks, but cannot maintain acceptable level of cleanliness   1
   4.   Needs help with all home maintenance tasks   1
   5.   Does not participate in any housekeeping tasks   0
E.   Laundry
   1.   Does personal laundry completely   1
   2.   Launders small items, rinses socks, stockings, and so on   1
   3.   All laundry must be done by others   0
F.   Mode of Transportation
   1.   Travels independently on public transportation or drives own car   1
   2.   Arranges own travel via taxi, but does not otherwise use public transportation   1
   3.   Travels on public transportation when assisted or accompanied by another
   4.   Travel limited to taxi or automobile with assistance of another   0
   5.   Does not travel at all   0
G.   Responsibility for Own Medications
   1.   Is responsible for taking medication in correct dosages at correct time   1
   2.   Takes responsibility if medication is prepared in advance in separate dosages   0
   3.   Is not capable of dispensing own medication   0
H.   Ability to Handle Finances
   1.   Manages financial matters independently (budgets, writes checks, pays
      rent and bills, goes to bank); collects and keeps track of income   1
   2.   Manages day-to-day purchases, but needs help with banking, major
      purchases, and other tasks   1
   3.   Incapable of handling money   0

Scoring: For each category, circle the item description that most closely resembles the client's highest functional level (either 0 or 1).

Reproduced from Lawton, M.P., & Brody, E.M. (1969). Assessment of older people: Self-maintaining and instrumental activities of daily living. The Gerontologist, 9(3), 179–186, by permission of Oxford University Press.

and gender differences as well as socioeconomic factors may influence AADL performance (Dias, de Andrade, de Oliveira Duarte, Santos, & Lebrao, 2015). Recent research has shown that the number of AADLs performed is important in the maintenance of cognitive capacity, and that a smaller number of AADLs performed may predict cognitive decline (Dias et al., 2015).

Older adults with Alzheimer's dementia usually need assistance with advanced activities of daily living, which are unique needs based on activity preferences and routines (Takechi, Kokuryu, Kubota, & Yamada, 2012). Family caregivers are often the ones providing this support. Thus, assessment of caregiver needs is important to provide the individualized guidance and resources needed in general and in the community. Additionally, assessment of caregiver burden is needed to provide access to respite care and/or caregiver support groups as needed.

The Timed "Up and Go" (TUG) test is a short, reliable, and valid test for quantifying functional mobility. The individual may be observed by the healthcare practitioner during this kind of mobility testing, thereby providing a more accurate assessment compared to more subjective self-report functional assessment tools, which are potentially less reliable. As a descriptive tool, the TUG test provides valuable information about balance, gait speed, and functional ability. It measures the number of seconds taken by a person to stand up from a standard armchair, walk 3 meters, turn around, walk back to the chair, and sit down wearing usual footwear (Podsiadlo & Richardson, 1991). The length of time it takes to complete the TUG test provides information on fall risk: The longer it takes to complete it, the higher the risk of falls. Those individuals who complete the TUG test in less than 10 seconds are considered freely mobile; those who complete it in 10 to 19 seconds are mostly independent in mobility; those who complete it in 20 to 29 seconds have variable mobility; and those who complete it in greater than 29 seconds have impaired mobility (Podsiadlo & Richardson, 1991).

The PULSES Profile is a tool that measures functional performance in mobility and self-care, medical status, and psychosocial factors. The acronym stands for Physical condition, Upper limb function, Lower limb function, Sensory components, Excretory function, and Support factors (Granger, Sherwood, & Greer, 1977; Moskowitz, 1985). Each aspect should be assessed thoroughly.

Medications, including prescribed and over-the-counter drugs, laxatives, vitamins, and herbal remedies, should be assessed on each visit or every encounter in an institutional setting. Older adults at increased risk for adverse drug effects include those older than 85 years, those with low body weight or low body mass index, those with six or more concurrent chronic illnesses, those with impaired renal function, those who experienced a prior adverse drug event, and those with cognitive impairment (Resnick, 2016). Polypharmacy and medication use, misuse, or nonadherence can affect an older adult's functional status. The American Geriatrics Society (AGS) 2015 Updated Beers Criteria are designed to help reduce older adults' drug-related problems, including, but not limited to, exposure to potentially inappropriate medications, drug–disease interactions, and medications that warrant extra caution in the older adult population. The AGS Beers Criteria resources may aid the clinician in discerning how medication-related issues may affect an older adult's overall function (AGS, 2015; Greenberg, 2016).

Basic assessments of daily function do not evaluate cognitive function, although most of the elements require a certain level of cognitive ability to be carried out. The Montreal Cognitive Assessment (MoCA) is a brief assessment tool for mild cognitive impairment. It assesses the domains of attention and concentration, executive function, memory, language, visuo-constructional skills, conceptual thinking, calculations, and orientation. In general, the total possible score is 30 points, with a score of 26 or more being considered normal (Nasreddine et al., 2005). For more information about the MoCA, see the main website for this tool (http://www.mocatest.org).

The Functional Assessment Staging Test (FAST scale) is a valid measure of the course of dementia; it identifies seven stages that delineate the course of dementia based on a person's function (Reisberg, 1988):

- Stage 1: Normal adult with no cognitive deficits.
- Stage 2: Normal older adult.
- Stage 3: Early dementia/mild cognitive impairment (may last 7 years).
- Stage 4: Mild dementia (may last 2 years).
- Stage 5: Moderate dementia (may last 1.5 years).
- Stage 6 (a–e): Moderately severe dementia.
- Stage 7 (a–f): Severe dementia.

Beginning at Stage 4, people show difficulty with IADLs, such as paying bills, cooking, cleaning, and traveling outside of walking distance. In Stage 5, there may be difficulty selecting proper clothes. Stage 6 has five substages:

- Stage 6a: There is difficulty putting on clothes.
- Stage 6b: The person with dementia needs help bathing.
- Stage 6c: The person needs help toileting.
- Stage 6d: The person may have urinary incontinence.
- Stage 6e: The person may have bowel incontinence.

At Stage 7 on, there are greater deficits. Stage 7 has six substages:

- Stage 7a: The person can likely only speak five or six words during the day.
- Stage 7b: The person may only be able to speak one word clearly.
- Stage 7c: The person can no longer walk.
- Stage 7d: The person can no longer sit up.
- Stage 7e: The person can no longer smile.
- Stage 7f: The person can no longer hold up the head.

In Alzheimer's dementia, stages are not skipped. Thus, a significant variation from the staging suggests another etiology of dementia (Reisberg, 1988). It is important to note that for an older adult with later-stage Alzheimer's disease, difficulty with IADLs needing higher-level executive function, such as managing finances, will occur prior to difficulty with basic ADLs.

In addition to assessing cognitive function, assessment of mood is crucial. Feelings of low mood or depression may affect an individual's willingness to function, go out, and participate in daily functional and recreational activities. The Patient Health Questionnaire (PHQ) 2 and 9 are both publicly available instruments that are used in various electronic health records. Notably, the PHQ is used in the Centers for Medicare and Medicaid Services' home health agency Outcome and Assessment Information Set (OASIS-C2) as a screening tool for depression for all adults. The PHQ asks people to rate how often over the last two weeks they have been bothered by various problems.

While many instruments are available to measure depression, the Geriatric Depression Scale (GDS) has been tested and used extensively with the older adult population (Yesavage et al., 1983). The GDS—Long Form is a brief, 30-item questionnaire in which participants are asked to respond by answering "yes" or "no" in reference to how they felt over the past week. The GDS—Short Form, consisting of 15 questions, was developed in 1986 (Sheikh & Yesavage, 1986). Further assessment for depression is needed for a GDS—Long Form score greater than 10 or a GDS—Short Form score greater than 5. Consider referral to a nurse, primary care provider, social worker, or geropsychiatrist for further assessment as needed (Greenberg, 2012). The Geriatric Depression Scale is in the public domain; this scale and related information may be reviewed at http://www.stanford.edu/~yesavage/ACRC.html and https://web.stanford.edu/~yesavage/GDS.html.

▶ Functional Assessment: Case Exemplar

A change in function may be the first sign of an acute condition. This case involves a 78-year-old female who presents with a chief complaint of right hip pain. The pain began two weeks ago, without any trauma preceding its onset. Lately, the pain has become more severe. Tylenol has not helped. The pain has interfered with her weekly dancing routine and she now needs to walk with a cane. She has no significant past medical history, takes no medications, and rarely sees any healthcare providers. A complete physical examination is negative for any significant findings. Family members and friends thought the pain might be due to arthritis. Because the change in function and pain were so sudden, the clinician recommended an X-ray of the right hip. The X-ray showed a mass by the hip, which led to a medical work-up and follow-up. As this case suggests, acute changes in function should be taken seriously and assessed thoroughly.

▶ Summary

Functional assessment is complex and is crucial to the comprehensive care of older adults in all care settings. Components of the functional assessment may be completed by different members of the healthcare team. The physical therapist, who is often regarded as the expert in managing and intervening with limitations of movement and function, can be an important team member once functional decline has occurred. All interprofessional team members can participate in the multiple aspects of the functional assessment. It is the primary provider's responsibility to ensure that subjective and objective functional assessment data are collected and synthesized in conjunction with a comprehensive assessment. With the interprofessional team assessment approach, the individual's support team is motivated to maintain the client's function, optimize it, and quickly identify any decline in function. Social support systems are unique to each person, but healthcare providers should enlist friends, family, and formal or informal caregivers to take part in promoting clients' functional health. Every clinician, family member, and caregiver should remind older adults to stay active, keep the mind and body moving, and promote independence.

References

American Geriatrics Society (AGS) Beers Criteria Update Expert Panel. (2015). American Geriatrics Society 2015 Updated Beers Criteria for Potentially Inappropriate Medication Use in Older Adults. *Journal of the American Geriatrics Society, 63*(11), 2227–2246. doi:10.1111/jgs.13702

Boltz, M., Capezuti, E., Shabbat, N., & Hall, K. (2010). Going home better not worse: Older adults' views on physical function during hospitalization. *International Journal of Nursing Practice, 16*(4), 381–388.

Boltz, M., Resnick, B., & Galik, E. (2016). Preventing functional decline in the acute care setting. In B. Resnick (Ed.), *Geriatric nursing review syllabus: A core curriculum in advanced practice geriatric nursing* (5th ed., pp. 197–209). New York, NY: American Geriatrics Society.

Dias, E. F., de Andrade, F. B., de Oliveira Duarte, Y. A., Santos, J. L. F., & Lebrao, M. L. (2015). Advanced activities of daily living and the incidence of cognitive impairment in the elderly: SABE study. *Cad. Saude Publica, 31*(8), 1–13. doi.org/10.1590/0102-311X00125014

Graf, C. (2008). The Lawton Instrumental Activities of Daily Living Scale. *American Journal of Nursing, 108*(4), 52–62.

Graf, C. (2012). The Lawton Instrumental Activities of Daily Living (IADL) Scale. *Try This: Best Practices in Nursing Care to Older Adults, 23.* Retrieved from https://consultgeri .org/try-this/general-assessment/issue-23.pdf

Granger, C. V., Sherwood, C. C., & Greer, D. S. (1977). Functional status measures in a comprehensive stroke care program. *Archives of Physical Medicine and Rehabilitation, 58,* 555–561.

Greenberg, S. A. (2012). The Geriatric Depression Scale (GDS). *Try This: Best Practices in Nursing Care to Older Adults, 4.* Retrieved from https://consultgeri.org/try-this /general-assessment/issue-4.pdf

Greenberg, S. A. (2016). *Try This:* Issue 16: AGS 2015 Updated Beers Criteria for Potentially Inappropriate Medication Use in Older Adults. Hartford Institute for Geriatric Nursing. Retrieved from https://consultgeri .org/try-this/general-assessment/16beers2016-r2.pdf

Guralnik, J. M., Alecxih, L., Branch, L. G., & Wiener, J. M. (2002). Medical and long-term care costs when older persons become more dependent. *American Journal of Public Health, 92*(8), 1244–1245.

Healthy People 2020. (2017, December 6). U.S. Department of Health and Human Services, Office of Disease Prevention and Health Promotion. Retrieved from https://www.healthypeople.gov/2020/topics-objectives /topic/older-adults/objectives

Hoogerduijn, J. G., Buurman, B. M., Korevaar, J. C., Grobbee, D. E., de Rooij, S. E., & Schuurmans, M. J. (2012). The prediction of functional decline in older hospitalised patients. *Age and Ageing, 41*(3), 381–387.

Katz, S. (1983). Assessing self-maintenance: Activities of daily living, mobility and instrumental activities of daily living. *Journal of the American Geriatrics Society, 31*(12), 721–726.

Lawton, M. P., & Brody, E. M. (1969). Assessment of older people: Self-maintaining and instrumental activities of daily living. *The Gerontologist, 9*(3), 179–186.

Moskowitz, E. (1985). PULSES Profile in retrospect. *Archives of Physical Medicine and Rehabilitation, 66*, 647–648.

Nasreddine, Z. S., Phillips, N. A., Bédirian, V., Charbonneau, S., Whitehead, V., Collin, I.,... Chertkow, H. (2005). The Montreal Cognitive Assessment, MoCA: A brief screening tool for mild cognitive impairment. *Journal of the American Geriatrics Society, 53*, 695–699.

Podsiadlo, D., & Richardson, S. (1991). The Timed "Up & Go": A test of basic functional mobility for frail elderly persons. *Journal of the American Geriatrics Society, 39*(2), 142–148.

Reisberg, B. (1988). Functional Assessment Staging (FAST). *Psychopharmacology, 24*(4), 653–659.

Resnick, B. (Ed.). (2016). *Geriatric Nursing Review Syllabus (GNRS)* (5th ed.). New York, NY: American Geriatrics Society.

Resnick, B., Galik, E., Wells, C., Boltz, M., & Holtzman, C. (2015). Optimizing function and physical activity post trauma: Overcoming system and patient challenges. *International Journal of Orthopaedic and Trauma Nursing, 19*(4), 194206.

Reuben, D. B., & Solomon, D. H. (1989). Assessment in geriatrics. *Journal of the American Geriatrics Society, 37*(6), 570–572.

Sheikh, J. I., & Yesavage, J.A. (1986). Geriatric Depression Scale (GDS): Recent evidence and development of a shorter version. In T. L. Brink (Ed.), *Clinical gerontology: A guide to assessment and intervention* (pp. 165–173). New York, NY: Haworth Press.

Shelkey, M., & Wallace, M. (2012). Katz Index of Independence in Activities of Daily Living (ADL). *Try This: Best Practices in Nursing Care to Older Adults, 2.* Retrieved from https://consultgeri.org/try-this/general-assessment/issue-2.pdf

Takechi, H., Kokuryu, A., Kubota, T., & Yamada, H. (2012). Relative preservation of advanced activities in daily living among patients with mild-to-moderate dementia in the community and overview of support provided by family caregivers. *International Journal of Alzheimer's Disease,* 1–7. doi.org/10.1155/2012/418289

Yesavage, J. A., Brink, T. L., Rose, T. L., Lum, O., Huang, V., Adey, M. B., & Leirer, V. O. (1983). Development and validation of a geriatric depression screening scale: A preliminary report. *Journal of Psychiatric Research, 17*, 37–49.

CHAPTER 25

Physical Assessment

Vanessa M. Rodriguez and Rosanne M. Leipzig

CHAPTER OBJECTIVES

1. Describe the general approach to the physical assessment of older adults by system.
2. Appreciate the unique aspects of the physical examination of older adults.
3. Identify potential challenges that healthcare providers may encounter while performing a physical assessment of the older adult.

KEY TERMS

Assessment	Geriatric
Elderly	Physical examination

▶ Introduction

A good understanding of the unique aspects of taking a history and performing a physical **assessment** of a **geriatric** patient helps to support healthy aging, and also allows the detection of issues that may cause an older adult to decline. While geriatric patients experience a series of changes that are part of the normal aging process, this vulnerable population also has a propensity to develop syndromes, such as delirium and incontinence, for which the clinician must have a high index of suspicion.

Additionally, older adults may have more severe illness or unanticipated complications due to homeostenosis, the inability to compensate in the presence of stressors due to the decline of physiologic reserve in several systems (Cassel, 2003).

The **physical examination** starts with observation. In every healthcare setting (e.g., long-term care, ambulatory care center, hospital), healthcare providers and staff can begin to construct an initial impression of older patients as soon as they meet them. For example, an older adult walks into an ambulatory center and interacts with the front desk personnel, medical assistants, and nurses even before entering the room to meet with the provider.

Frequently, the precise sequence and timing of the examination must be modified when assessing an older person because of impaired hearing, sight, comprehension, or mobility. A study by Lo, Ryder, and Shorr (2005) of approximately 4000 adults age 45 years and older, evaluating how age could influence the duration of the ambulatory visit, found that despite the fact that those patients age 75 years and older had more medical conditions and were at higher risk for drug-related problems than younger patients, the duration of physician visits was similar across the age groups. Older adults with multiple medical issues presenting with several complaints will often benefit from a comprehensive evaluation completed over two or more visits rather than during an exhaustive initial encounter. In addition to the history and physical assessment, the assessment of other domains such as mobility and functional assessment will likely need further exploration that should not be done rapidly. For further details about the functional assessment of the older adult, refer to the *Functional Assessment: Activities of Daily Living and Instrumental Activities of Daily Living Assessment* chapter.

What makes the examination of older persons different is not the content of the examination, but rather the approach, which should be age- and person-appropriate and avoid undue discomfort, embarrassment, or stress. This approach should take into account whether the older adult has impaired special senses or diminished mobility and must allow for slower response times. The successful clinician must respectfully allow concerns that the person thinks are most important to be expressed. Caregivers and family may have concerns that need to be addressed within this context as well.

This chapter organizes the physical examination according to organ systems so as to provide a logical structure for the reader. In practice, in older people, the presenting symptom is often atypical or nonspecific—a signal that something is amiss somewhere but not necessarily in

the suspected organ system. Older adults can present very differently from younger people with similar medical problems, and findings in this age cohort can often be subtle or undifferentiated (Kurrle, Cameron, & Geeves, 2015). It is imperative to have a basic understanding of all the domains that characterize the general approach to the older adult, especially those that have special needs or considerations such as dementia. *The geriatric physical assessment differs from a typical medical evaluation in three ways: It includes nonmedical domains; it emphasizes functional capacity and quality of life; and it incorporates a multidisciplinary team approach that often includes a physician, nurses, nutritionist, social worker, and physical and occupational therapists.* This type of assessment often yields a more complete and relevant list of medical problems, functional impairments, and psychosocial issues (Landefeld, 2003). The main goal of performing such a thorough assessment is to detect or prevent disability and to increase safety. For those patients who already have some form of disability, knowing how to conduct a thoughtful history and physical examination may guide healthcare providers to develop a patient-centered plan that could reduce further disability and improve the patient's quality of life.

▸ Approach to the Geriatric Patient

Regardless of the setting, the clinician should utilize techniques that will aid in conducting an effective and culturally sensitive history and physical assessment. Ideally healthcare providers should anticipate barriers that could arise during the assessment, and have a plan to address them.

Because older persons frequently have impaired communication skills as a result of aging, illness, or lack of health literacy, the examiner must pay special attention to communication issues during the history taking and physical examination. For many older adults, English may be a second language; consequently, the examiner must keep in mind that the person may have difficulty in providing or understanding information during the interview. Of note, patients with dementia often lose fluency in a second language. A hearing problem may not be evident and can result in misunderstanding if not recognized. Someone who is hearing impaired may respond to questions inappropriately, resulting in misdiagnoses, especially of cognitive impairment. If the individual uses a hearing aid, the volume of both the hearing aid and the examiner's voice may need to be adjusted. When you are filling the role of examiner, make sure you have the patient's attention, that your mouth is visible, and that you speak clearly and slowly. If one of the patient's ears has better hearing, position yourself closer to that ear. In addition, it is a good practice to confirm that the listener heard you by asking that individual to repeat back what was heard, in the person's own words.

In most cultures (but not all), eye contact, a handshake, the use of last name, and appropriate physical contact are the rudiments of good communication with all persons, but particularly for older adults. Eye contact is important to establish a relationship. Prolonged eye contact can seem like staring, however, and in some cultures eye contact is considered inappropriate. Addressing the individual by the last name is a sign of respect in all cultures. Many older persons also appreciate a touch on the hand or shoulder. When done in a sincere and caring manner, a touch may reduce some of the anxiety associated with a trip to the clinician's office or during a home visit.

The environment of the encounter must be comfortable, with a minimum of noise, distractions, interruptions, and appropriate room temperature. It is important to speak to the older adult directly, rather than through others who may have accompanied him or her to the visit. For all but the most cognitively impaired patients, the clinician should talk to the caregiver only with the permission of the individual. The family members may appreciate some time alone with the practitioner to express their concerns without feeling embarrassed by the older person's presence. A natural time for this to occur is while the person undresses in preparation for the physical examination. Provide the patient and family with a brief explanation and description of what is to be accomplished during the visit. If there are multiple issues and concerns, let them know that several sessions may be required to address all concerns.

During the first visits, the provider should find out who the patient is, how that person spends his or her time, what is most important to the patient, and what is of greatest concern to the patient at this time. Some older adults may still be working or be active in their communities. Giving them a few minutes to open up and feel acknowledged as an individual can make a great difference in the tenor of the patient–provider relationship.

Practitioners rarely address the areas of religious or spiritual beliefs, which are often thought to be taboo. However, in completing the history, practitioners might ask the older person the following questions (avoiding a coercive or intrusive tone): What role does religion play in your life? Are you a member of a faith community? Do you participate actively with this community? Spirituality is discussed in more detail in the *Spiritual Assessment as a Key Component of Comprehensive Geriatric Care* chapter. Asking questions that pertain to meaning and purpose, as well as spiritual and religious issues, can open up a dialogue that will benefit the patient and enhance his or her relationship with the clinician.

▶ History Taking

Taking a history from an older adult can be anxiety provoking for healthcare providers whose time is limited. Having patients or their family members complete a health questionnaire prior to the first visit can allow the patient and family to assemble the requested medical information, such as current medications and doses, surgeries and hospitalizations, other healthcare providers and contact information, health maintenance, and family history, and activities of daily living (ADLs) and instrumental activities of daily living (IADLs), and to complete a review of systems. The time the clinician then spends with them can confirm this history and allow for probing further as needed. It will also give the clinician time to better understand what is most concerning for the patient and family, and decrease the likelihood that additional problems will be uncovered on their way out the door. Even if not completed in its totality, this history can provide some valuable information, and the staff can encourage its completion while the patient is waiting to see the provider.

Some older persons may be reluctant to share certain information in front of their family members, particularly things that might cause the family to question their living arrangements or autonomy, such as whether they have fallen, are incontinent, having difficulty bathing, or are sexually active. Asking the family to leave during the physical examination gives the clinician the opportunity to ask the patient these questions and to obtain information on sensitive concerns related to caregiver abuse and neglect. Some older adults are lonely or overly talkative, sharing at length numerous irrelevant incidents that happened long ago. Without showing disinterest or disrespect, the interviewer must strive to refocus the person on the issues at hand.

It is generally a good idea to use open-ended questions to obtain information. However, older adults often have difficulty with word finding, and their free recall is worse than when given cues or a choice. For this reason, it is sometimes helpful to supply a choice of words to help describe the problem. This is particularly true for patients with dementia. For example, "Describe your chest pain" is an open-ended question; "Was the pain sharp, stabbing, dull, or crushing?" may help the older individual be more precise in the description.

TABLE 25-1 outlines content for a review of systems related to geriatric syndromes. As mentioned earlier, this review can be completed before the initial encounter.

For older adults with multiple chronic conditions and functional limitations, it is important that the provider ask specific questions about when problems started and if they resolved at any point. When multiple concerns or serious symptoms are present, a good starting point is often "When was the last time you felt really well?"—this question enables the clinician to gauge the severity of the problems and their effect on function.

Be specific when asking about pain. The 2011 National Health and Aging Trends Study on prevalence and impact of pain among older adults found that older adults endorsed multiple sites of pain, and pain was strongly associated with decreased physical function (Patel, Guralnik, Dansie, & Turk, 2013). The question "What is your pain level on a scale from 0 to 10?" is unanswerable to someone with multiple sites of pain. Typically, a thorough investigation of the etiologies of pain, using a multimodal approach, is required in such a case. (See the *Pain Assessment* chapter for more information.)

Special attention should be paid to patients with dementia, as they may have a limited ability to communicate their needs and sources of discomfort. Remember that patients with dementia can be accurate when reporting what is going on at the moment, but less so when describing about something over time.

▶ Sexual Health Assessment

The sexual health of older adults is an important component of the overall health assessment. Unfortunately, this area may inadvertently be omitted because of stereotypic beliefs regarding aging and sexuality. Although certain physiologic functions related to sexuality change with aging, healthy sex lives among older adults are the norm. Libido and sexual response may be inhibited, however, when individuals are ill or on medications that may blunt sexual arousal response.

TABLE 25-1 Geriatric Review of Systems

General	<ul><li>Weight loss/gain</li><li>Fatigue</li><li>Weakness</li><li>Fever</li><li>Chills</li><li>Loss of appetite</li><li>Snores</li><li>Night sweats</li><li>Swollen lymph nodes</li><li>Pain</li></ul>	Gastrointestinal	<ul><li>Abdominal pain</li><li>Constipation</li><li>Diarrhea</li><li>Blood in stools</li><li>Excessive gas/bloating</li><li>Painful swallowing</li><li>Trouble swallowing</li><li>Nausea</li><li>Vomiting</li><li>Heartburn</li></ul>
Eyes	<ul><li>Visual loss</li><li>Blurry vision</li><li>Double vision</li><li>Eye pain</li><li>Itchy/burning eyes</li></ul>	Genitourinary	<ul><li>Leakage of urine</li><li>Frequent nighttime urination</li><li>Urinary frequency</li><li>Urination urgency</li><li>Painful urination</li><li>Blood in urine</li><li>Problems with erection</li><li>Vaginal itching/dryness</li><li>Spotting/discharge</li><li>Painful intercourse</li></ul>
Ears	<ul><li>Hearing loss</li><li>Ear discharge</li><li>Ear pain</li><li>Room spinning sensation</li><li>Loss of balance</li><li>Ringing in the ears</li></ul>	Breast	<ul><li>Nipple discharge</li><li>Pain</li><li>Breast mass</li></ul>
Nose/Throat	<ul><li>Bloody nose</li><li>Congestion</li><li>Smell changes</li><li>Runny nose</li><li>Sore throat</li><li>Hoarseness</li></ul>	Musculoskeletal	<ul><li>Falls</li><li>Fear of falling</li><li>Neck pain</li><li>Painful gait</li><li>Back pain</li><li>Joint pain or swelling</li><li>Muscle pain</li><li>Stiffness</li></ul>
Oral	<ul><li>Dry mouth</li><li>Bleeding gums</li><li>Mouth pain</li><li>Tongue problems</li><li>Taste changes</li><li>Jaw pain</li><li>Dentures (if yes, ask about fit, pain)</li></ul>	Skin	<ul><li>Itching</li><li>Rash</li><li>Easy bruising</li><li>Mass or swelling</li></ul>

TABLE 25-1 Geriatric Review of Systems			*(continued)*
Respiratory	■ Cough ■ Shortness of breath ■ Wheezing ■ Productive sputum ■ Blood in sputum	Endocrine	■ Hot flashes ■ Heat/cold intolerance ■ Excessive thirst
Cardiovas-cular	■ Chest pain ■ Palpitations ■ Swelling of the legs ■ Shortness of breath with exertion ■ Sleeping with many pillows for better breathing ■ Wakes up due to difficulty breathing ■ Painful varicose veins	Neurologic	■ Memory loss ■ Dizziness or lightheadedness ■ Headaches ■ Fainting ■ Loss of consciousness ■ Numbness or tingling of hands or feet ■ Tremors ■ Seizures ■ Sudden weakness of arm or legs ■ Speech problems ■ Leg cramps
Psychiatric	■ Depression ■ Anxiety ■ Sleep problems ■ Irritability ■ Visual hallucinations ■ Hear voices ■ Suicidal ideations ■ Homicidal ideations ■ Abusive relationship ■ Alcoholism ■ Substance abuse problems	Other	

In conducting a sexual health history, it is important to review systematically the individual's regular patterns of sexual activity, expectations related to sex, and any changes in capacity or enjoyment, and to elicit the client's goals for a healthy sex life. Once the clinician understands these goals, he or she can recommend appropriate treatment and/or actions such as counseling, adjunct therapy, or physical aids to increase sexual capacity.

It is key that the clinician understand that sexuality in late life is a normal and positive experience of aging. Clinicians need to assess their own level of comfort in eliciting a sexual history from the older adult, because any discomfort on their part is likely to inhibit the older adult's ability to discuss his or her sexual life frankly. Key components of a sexual history must include an understanding of what the older adult's normal sexual patterns and interests have been over the course of his or her life and whether any changes have transpired that now affect sexual capacity and performance.

During the course of the overall health assessment, the clinician should elicit any sexual concerns or chief complaints from the patient. Most important, the clinician must determine whether the individual's sexual activities are meeting his or her expectations and whether that person perceives there to be any sexual difficulties. In some cases, it might be useful to interview the older adult's partner, as his or her responses may be different. Finally, homosexuality; unsafe intercourse resulting in sexually transmitted disease, including HIV infection; and sexual trauma from rape and other types of sexual assault are all issues that should not be overlooked due to stereotypes held about older people.

▶ Physical Assessment

For older adults, the examination should require as few changes in position as possible. Observe the patient, including behavior, dress and grooming, and any particular strong smells, such as urine, that could signal difficulty with self-care or neglect. Is the patient wearing eyeglasses or hearing aids, using an assistive device, or wearing a medical information bracelet or a fall alert device? Is the patient cachectic or obese? Evaluate the patient's demeanor and level of alertness, and adjust the interaction accordingly to create a space of safety and respect for the patient. A change in alertness may be a sign of a serious medical issue such as delirium, but could also be evidence of a mental health problem or dementia. Note the pace, fluency, and clarity of speech.

With the patient seated, the head, eyes, ears, nose, throat, neck, heart, lungs, joints, and neurologic examinations follow in turn. The patient is then positioned supine for examination of the lower extremities, abdomen, peripheral pulses, breasts, genitalia, and inguinal regions. The patient should then turn to the lateral decubitus position for rectal examination. Finally, have the patient stand so that postural blood pressure and pulse changes can be detected. Balance and gait can be tested at the beginning or end of the exam.

▶ Components of the Examination

Vital Signs

The blood pressure (BP) measurement of any patient, but particularly the older adult, should be done carefully. Before measuring BP, the provider should ask about pain and any contraindications to the use of an extremity, such as lymphedema, infections, rash, or vascular access as in patients undergoing dialysis. The balloon of the blood pressure cuff should encircle about two-thirds of the arm's circumference. If the person is obese, a wide cuff is used because a smaller cuff may overestimate the blood pressure. The blood pressure should be measured in both arms at least once. Differences between arms may be due to asymmetrical atherosclerotic involvement.

Before measuring BP in an older person, an Osler maneuver can be performed to determine whether the reading may be spuriously high due to stiff peripheral arteries. This maneuver is performed by palpating the radial or brachial artery, inflating the blood pressure cuff above systolic pressure, and determining whether the pulseless artery is palpable. If so, the true intra-arterial blood pressure reading may be lower than the blood pressure obtained by auscultation. In one study, persons whose arteries remained palpable (Osler positive) when the cuff was inflated above systolic pressure had a blood pressure reading taken by auscultatory methods that was 20% higher than the intra-arterial measured pressure (Messerli, Ventura, & Amodeo, 1985). Some subjects had a diastolic cuff reading of 120 or 100 mm Hg while a simultaneous intra-arterial pressure was 80 mm Hg. Such persons have pseudo-hypertension, which might cause them to be erroneously diagnosed as hypertensive. The cuff should be inflated to at least 200 mm Hg, and the examiner should continue to listen until a pressure of 50 to assure that there is no auscultatory gap, where the sounds disappear only to reappear again at a lower pressure. Korotkoff sounds are identified by listening with the bell of the stethoscope pressed lightly over the brachial artery. The pressure at which the sounds are first heard is the systolic pressure. The sounds may become muffled before they disappear, but the point at which the sounds are no longer heard is the diastolic pressure. If the auscultatory gap is not recognized, the diastolic pressure may be erroneously recorded as higher than its true value, or the systolic pressure may be erroneously recorded as lower than its true value.

Isolated systolic hypertension (ISH) is defined as a blood pressure of greater than 160 mm Hg systolic, while the diastolic blood pressure remains less than 90 mm Hg. This condition mostly occurs in older patients. Data from the Framingham Heart Study and the National Health and Nutrition Examination Survey (NHANES) have shown that the systolic pressure rises and the diastolic pressure falls after age 60 years in both normotensive and untreated hypertensive subjects (Franklin et al., 1997) and that ISH accounts for 60% to 80% of cases of hypertension in the elderly (Franklin, Jacobs, Wong, Gilbert, & Lapuerta, 2001; Kannel, 1996).

The target blood pressure for older adults remains in dispute (James et al., 2014; Wright et al., 2015). Differing results were found two major trials (ACCORD and SPRINT) that had a target systolic blood pressure goal of 120 mm Hg and included high-risk patients (Group, 2010; Wright et al., 2015). A recent systematic review by Weiss et al. (2017) that considered the benefits and harms of intensive blood pressure treatment in older adults did not find substantial and strong evidence to suggest that lowering blood pressure to less than the current BP target (less than 150/90 mm Hg) significantly reduces mortality, stroke, or cardiac events. There remains concern that aggressive treatment of hypertension could be associated with greater medication burden and higher risk for

adverse effects, such as hypotension and syncope. The appropriate BP goals are particularly unclear for more frail older adults, such as those who are institutionalized or with multimorbidity, as they are underrepresented in most trials.

If the patient reports dizziness, or if diuretics, antihypertensives, or other medications associated with postural hypotension are to be started, blood pressure and pulse should be measured in both the lying and standing positions. Postural hypotension is defined as a drop in systolic blood pressure of 20 mm Hg or more, a drop in diastolic blood pressure of 10 mm Hg or more, or an increase in heart rate increase of 20 beats/min or more, within 3 minutes of standing. In an older adult, it is appropriate to use a two-position approach to measure BP: First measure the blood pressure and pulse after the patient rests supine for 5 minutes, and then remeasure them within 3 minutes after the patient stands up (Bickley & Szilagyi, 2016). In healthy **elderly** individuals, postural hypotension occurs infrequently and is usually asymptomatic (Mader, Josephson, & Rubenstein, 1987; Myers, Kearns, Kennedy, & Fisher, 1978). In older persons who are frail, postural hypotension can be a symptomatic disorder associated with increased falls and syncope (Tinetti et al., 2014). The fall in blood pressure on standing can be exaggerated if the blood volume is low or if the reflex orthostatic mechanisms are impaired because of age or medications. Even mild volume depletion secondary to use of diuretics can result in marked postural hypotension in older adults, although no such change occurs in younger subjects (Shannon, Wei, Rosa, Epstein, & Rowe, 1986).

Feeling the pulse and measuring the heart rate can identify bradycardia, tachycardia, or an irregular pulse, all of which could signify a serious medical issue or the side effect of a medication (e.g., cholinesterase inhibitors, albuterol). The radial artery is convenient for determining the heart rate. When the pulse is irregular, it is further characterized as regularly irregular or irregularly irregular. A regularly irregular pulse may indicate consistently dropped beats, as in a second-degree atrioventricular (A-V) block, or added beats, such as occurs with premature ventricular contractions. An irregularly irregular pattern often represents atrial fibrillation but can also be caused by very frequent premature ventricular or atrial contractions. Atrial fibrillation, particularly when accompanied by mitral stenosis or an enlarged left atrium, is a significant risk factor for stroke. Abnormal rates or rhythms should be followed up with an electrocardiogram.

Observing and measuring the respiratory rate, depth, and effort can help identify an uncontrolled chronic medical condition (e.g., heart failure, pain), an acute illness, or even a mental health disease such as anxiety. The respirations should be observed—for use of accessory muscles of respiration and for retraction in the supraclavicular fossae—and counted. The usual respiratory rate in adults is approximately 12 to 18 breaths per minute.

Measuring baseline temperature is particularly important in older adults. The definitions of a fever in frail older adults (e.g., residents in long-term care facilities) are all considerably lower than those used to define fever in the general adult population (High et al., 2009; Norman, 2000), including a single oral temperature greater than 37.8°C (100°F), persistent oral or tympanic membrane temperature of 37.2°C (99.0°F) or greater, rectal temperature of 37.5°C (99.5°F) or greater, or a rise in temperature of 1.1°C (2°F) or more above baseline temperature (High et al., 2009). Fever, as it is usually defined in adults, is the cardinal feature of infection, but is absent in 30% to 50% of frail, older adults, even in the setting of serious infections such as pneumonia or endocarditis (Henschke, 1993; Musgrave & Verghese, 1990), which explains why it is so important to take a baseline reading and use the definitions given previously.

Height, Weight, and Nutrition

Older persons are at increased risk of malnutrition because of inappropriate food intake, social isolation, disability, and chronic medical conditions and medications (Nutrition Screening Initiative, 1991). Good nutritional status is critical for adequate functioning, energy, and a sense of well-being. Malnourished people are at greater risk of infections, delay in recovery from illness, complications from procedures, and mortality.

The four components of the nutritional assessment can be remembered by the mnemonic ABCD:

- **A**nthropometric measurement such as height and weight
- **B**iochemical parameters such as serum albumin and hemoglobin
- **C**linical assessment (medical history, physical examination, and other domains discussed in this text)
- **D**ietary history, such as the content and adequacy of the diet and the use of nutritional supplements

Careful attention to these components is critical, as they could indicate an underlying medical issue, the progression of a medical condition (e.g., dementia), a loss of appetite due to medications, no access to meals, or poor oral health.

The body mass index (BMI) is measure of body fat based on height and weight. It is calculated by dividing the weight of the person in kilograms by the square of that person's height in meters. Multiple free online calculators are available to determine BMI, such as that from the National Heart, Lung, and Blood Institute (2006). Clinical guidelines developed by the National Heart, Lung, and Blood Institute in cooperation with the National Institute of Diabetes and Digestive and Kidney Diseases, and in concert with many other professional organizations, have defined overweight as a BMI between 25 and 29.9 and obesity as a BMI of 30 or higher (NHLBI Obesity Education Initiative Expert Panel, 1998). For older adults, however, a healthy BMI is higher—in the range of 22 of 27 (Joanna Briggs Institute, 2017). The BMI may also be inaccurate in older adults due to weight increase from edema or loss of height from osteoporotic vertebral collapses (Nazarko, 2002).

...nd weight should ideally be reeval-
...the same circumstances—for exam-
...vithout shoes or with the same shoes.
...ıces guidelines published by the Joann
Briggs ... ıstitute (2017) recommend that height be measured with the person standing straight, without shoes, heels together, and looking straight ahead. Three methods are detailed in the report for measuring height in those who are unable to stand: knee height by caliper, "fingertip to fingertip," and the demi-span measurement. The last two methods may be difficult to complete in patients who are confined to bed, have upper limb disabilities, or have chest and back deformities, such as kyphosis or scoliosis. The type of scale used (standing, chair, or bed) depends on the physical condition of the person. If weight is being recorded daily, it should be measured at the same time of the day using the same scale.

Skin

Skin assessment can reveal new growths, pressure ulcers, and suggest elder abuse. The assessment can occur during the examination of other areas of the body and when the patient is disrobed. Older adults have less subcutaneous fat and fewer sweat and sebaceous glands, which consequently leads to thinner, drier skin that bruises and bleeds more easily. With age, skin elasticity is lost, and skin turgor is routinely diminished, even in patients who are adequately hydrated. Wrinkling and creasing occur, resulting in "crow's feet" at the corners of the eyes and lines on the forehead. Common new findings that occur in aging include the development of hyperpigmented macular lesions called solar lentigenes (popularly known as age, sun, or liver spots). Skin tags are fleshy soft growths, typically with a pedicle, and are benign unless irritated by clothing or jewelry. Other important lesions in older adults include seborrheic keratoses, skin cancers, dermatitis, and infections such as zoster.

Signs of elder abuse, which may include skin-related signs such as burns or bruises, may be missed by professionals due to lack of awareness and inadequate training on detecting abuse. The elderly may be reluctant to report abuse themselves because of fear of retaliation, lack of physical and/or cognitive ability to report, or reluctance to get the abuser in trouble. Elder abuse is fully covered in the *Recognizing Mistreatment in Older Adults* chapter.

The skin should be assessed for pressure ulcers, particularly in frail older adults or those with limited mobility. Pressure ulcers are staged as follows:

- Stage 1: The skin is intact and may be warm or tender. In lighter-skinned people, the area is reddened and does not blanch (lose color with finger pressure); in darker-skinned people, the area is not red but has a different color than the surrounding area.
- Stage 2: The skin is broken, and the area is tender and painful.
- Stage 3: The ulcer extends into the subcutaneous tissue.
- Stage 4: Muscle and bone can be seen.

Pressure ulcers covered by an eschar or sloughing are of concern for a deep tissue injury since the depth of injury is unknown. Pressure ulcers and skin tears result in pain, disfigurement, decreased quality of life, increased healthcare costs, longer hospitalizations, and increased morbidity (Bergquist, 2003; Brillhart, 2005). A pressure ulcer can develop over a short period of time (e.g., as a result of several hours of lying in place). Constant vigilance is required to prevent the development of pressure ulcers in institutionalized or hospitalized older adults (Brandeis, Morris, Nash, & Lipsitz, 1990). Recurrent or extensive decubiti in older adults might signal abuse or neglect.

Hair and Nails

Changes in the color and distribution of hair occur with normal aging. Hair color becomes gray or whitened. Progressive thinning of all body hair, including hair of the axillae and pubis, occurs with age. The growth of facial hair in older women can sometimes be quite distressing, but measures to reduce the problem, such as depilatory agents, can be recommended. A lack of hair on the lower extremities may indicate diminished peripheral circulation but is often a normal finding in older adults.

The nails of older adults are frequently afflicted by onychomycosis, a chronic fungal condition of the nail. Increased risk of onychomycosis is associated with multiple factors, including male sex, old age, smoking, underlying medical diseases (e.g., peripheral arterial disease, diabetes, and immunodeficiency), and predisposing genetic factors (de Berker, 2009; Gupta & Ricci, 2006; Gupta et al., 2000; Surjushe et al., 2007). The thickened, brittle, and crumbling nail is difficult to treat and is a common problem for neglected persons living alone.

Head

Many healthcare providers prefer to conduct their physical examination from head to toe, working their way down the body. The head is best examined with the patient sitting. The head and skull should be examined for evidence of trauma, especially in cases of delirium or sudden changes in level of consciousness. Frontal bossing or an increase in hat size are changes in the skull that are characteristic of Paget's disease.

Palpate the temporal arteries for tenderness. Temporal arteritis (or giant cell arteritis) is a condition in which the temporal arteries become tender and may lose their pulsations, and can result in blindness. Symmetrical pain and weakness of shoulders and hips (polymyalgia rheumatic) can accompany temporal arteritis.

Eyes

Age-related changes in the eyes include darkening of the skin around the orbits, crow's feet, smaller pupils, slower pupillary light reflex, decreased tearing, and decreased adaptation to the dark. The older person, perhaps because of diminished pupil size and increased thickness and opacity of the lens, needs more illumination to compensate than a younger person. Provision of excellent lighting in waiting and examination rooms is essential.

The structures surrounding the eye itself are inspected first. Xanthomas are fat deposits sometimes seen in the skin near the eyes and may be associated with elevated levels of blood lipids. Loss of the lateral third of the eyebrows, although a classic sign of hypothyroidism, may be a normal finding in some older persons. On each eyelid, the examiner will find a central, relatively rigid tarsal plate that, in advancing age, may become lax, leading to ectropion (eversion of the lids), thereby exposing the eyes to drying and infection. The margin of the lid may roll backward toward the eye as well, so that eyelashes brush against the cornea, causing entropion.

Evaluate the eyes for discharge, ocular redness, conjunctival color, extraocular movements, bleeding, and protrusion, as they all may be indicative of an underlying or uncontrolled medical condition. The pupils may react more sluggishly to light but should be equal in size. The extraocular muscles are checked for full range of motion: up and down, left and right. Check visual acuity for reading and distance using a Snellen chart, with and without glasses. This can be followed by peripheral vision testing using a confrontation test. The person giving this test sits facing the patient, approximately 3 feet away. The patient covers one eye while the tester covers the contralateral eye. The tester holds his or her arms straight out to the sides while putting up a certain number fingers. The patient looks straight ahead to the tester's nose, and is asked to state the number of fingers the tester is holding up.

Some eye disorders are especially common in older adults. Macular degeneration is a major cause of visual disability in older persons. The macula—the region of the retina with the sharpest acuity—is affected in this condition. Visual acuity is decreased, but peripheral vision is preserved. Special studies by an ophthalmologist may be required to make the diagnosis of senile macular degeneration. Many disorders may cause asymmetry of the pupils, including central nervous system lesions and diabetes; drugs can have this effect as well.

In glaucoma, the intraocular pressure is elevated, and contraction of the visual field results in a loss of peripheral vision. Glaucoma is a silent disease that ideally should be diagnosed before a significant loss of visual fields occurs; an ophthalmologist can screen for it.

Blurred vision and poor night vision may be due to cataracts. A cataract may be best visualized by focusing on the lens with a bright light or an ophthalmoscope: The cataract appears as an opaque or a black area against the orange reflection from the retina. The precise significance of the cataract depends on how much it interferes with the person's vision, function, and work. Cataract is the most common eye disease and the leading cause of reversible blindness (Huan, 2010; Robman & Taylor, 2005). After cataract removal, the pupil is irregular.

Ears

Observation and the otoscope are used to examine the ears. Common changes seen with age include increased ear lobe length, hair growth in the canal, and accumulation of cerumen. Painless nodules on the pinnae of the ears could be basal cell carcinomas, rheumatoid nodules, or even gouty tophi.

The normal tympanic membrane is gray or pink, with a light reflex produced by its cone shape. The malleus—the first of the three small bones in the inner ear—can be seen indenting this membrane, pointing posteriorly. The tympanic membrane may be thickened in the older person (tympanosclerosis), possibly as a result of scarring from prior infections. Effusions occur in relationship to eustachian tube dysfunction, as in allergy or upper respiratory tract infections.

Hearing assessment is critical in older adults. The U.S. Preventive Services Task Force (USPSTF) found that the whispered voice test and single-question screening ("Do you have difficulty with your hearing?") seem to be nearly as accurate for detecting hearing loss as more detailed questionnaires or handheld audiometers (Moyer et al., 2012). The whispered voice test is performed by standing 2 feet behind the seated patient so that the individual cannot read the examiner's lips. The nontested ear should be occluded with a finger. The clinician should fully exhale before whispering to ensure a quiet voice, then whisper a combination of three numbers and letters, such as 2-A-3. The test is abnormal if after two repetitions of different combinations of letters and numbers, four out of the six total numbers and letters are incorrect. Families and patients may disagree on whether the patient has a hearing problem. In this case, negative findings on handheld audiometers can be particularly helpful in ruling out hearing loss greater than 40 dB.

Hearing loss may, for the sake of simplicity, be divided into conductive loss and sensorineural loss. Conductive hearing loss implies interference in the conduct of sound energy into the inner ear. It can be due to foreign bodies, cerumen, abnormalities of the tympanic membrane, otitis media or externa, or involvement of the ossicles with Paget's disease, rheumatoid arthritis, or otosclerosis (in which the stapes becomes fixed to the oval window of the cochlea) (Mader, 1984). Cerumen in the canal may be the primary or a contributing cause of hearing loss that is easily remedied. In the primary care setting, it can be easily visualized with an otoscope. If the hearing loss persists after cerumen removal, the patient should be referred to an ear/nose/throat (ENT) specialist for further evaluation. External otitis can be due to allergic reactions or irritation due to hearing aids. Malignant otitis externa is a *Pseudomonas* infection that involves the ear canal and presents as granulation tissue at the juncture of bone and cartilage.

Sensorineural hearing loss is due to disease that may occur anywhere from the organ of Corti in the inner ear to the brain. With aging, the hair cells in the basal turn of the organ of Corti are lost. These cells are sensitive to high frequencies, so their absence results in high-frequency hearing loss, or presbycusis. In presbycusis, consonants and sibilants become unintelligible (e.g., *f*, *s*, *th*, *ch*, and *sh*), impairing the ability to understand speech. Vowel sounds have a low frequency, so ability to understand them remains intact.

Often both conductive and sensorineural hearing losses are present simultaneously, and the precise nature of the defect requires sophisticated audiometric testing. The combination of hearing loss and cognitive impairment can lead to social isolation and paranoia, and may make mental status testing a real challenge. It has been concluded that hearing loss is independently associated with accelerated cognitive decline and incident cognitive impairment in community-dwelling older adults.

Nose

A bright light or an otoscope can be used to examine the nasal mucosa and the internal nasal architecture. Nasal patency is tested by occluding one nostril. The clinician should also palpate the paranasal sinuses for tenderness. Chronic nasal drainage resistant to therapy should be investigated because it can be a symptom of cancer in the sinuses.

The sense of smell decreases with age, which in turn affects the sense of taste. This factor can be significant for nutrition and safety. The smell of food cooking stimulates the appetite and can make eating enjoyable. Conversely, the inability to smell leaking natural gas creates a risk of serious accident.

Oral Cavity

Oral health is often overlooked by healthcare providers. Multiple factors are associated with poor oral health, such as being disabled, homebound, or institutionalized (Vargas, Kramarow, & Yellowitz, 2001). Dental care is not covered by regular Medicare, so older adults may not see a dentist regularly. Thus, healthcare providers should thoroughly examine the oral cavity, especially in patients with dysphagia, weight loss, cough, or oral pain, and in those who smoke. Older adults who use systemic steroids or inhalers may be predisposed to oral fungal infections or ulcers.

Examination of the mouth may reveal any of several aging-related changes. Cheilosis, or fissures at the angles of the mouth, may be a sign of poor nutrition and vitamin deficiency. Xerostomia (dry mouth), which can lead to mucositis, caries, cracked lips, and fissured tongue, is often an adverse effect of medications, particularly in those persons taking more than four daily prescription medications (Stein & Aalboe, 2015; Yellowitz & Schneiderman, 2014). Carcinomatous lesions may occur on the lips, which typically have high exposure to sunlight. The oral mucosa should be carefully inspected for lesions by using the tongue blade to move the buccal mucosa away from the teeth. Remove the dentures when inspecting the mouth surfaces for areas of irritation and for suspicious lesions. The upper and lower lips should also examined, including hidden surfaces.

Leukoplakia is a white patch or plaque on any of the mucous membranes of the mouth that may appear to be painted on the surface. These patches may be present for years and represent a premalignant condition. Such lesions should be biopsied for definitive diagnosis. Other lesions with a similar appearance include those caused by *Candida* (thrush) and lichen planus. Traumatic injury—in particular, from ill-fitting dentures—may damage the oral mucosa, producing erythematous tissue changes.

In addition to inspection, a moistened glove may be used to palpate the buccal cavity, including the lips and floor of the mouth, for areas of induration. Palpation is particularly important to evaluate complaints related to the oral region, to assess suspicious areas, and to evaluate persons at risk of oral cancer (e.g., those with a history of tobacco or alcohol use).

A lesion of the hard palate—albeit one with no particular clinical significance except that it be recognized as benign—is the torus palatinus. Any masses not in the midline, however, are suspect as neoplasms. A slowly growing asymptomatic lesion with a rough surface, irregular margin, and firm consistency should be biopsied, no matter how long it has been there.

The clinician should also examine the tongue. A sore, red inflamed tongue is associated with vitamin B_{12} or iron deficiency. Hairy or black tongue is a condition in which it looks as if the tongue is growing short hairs. This asymptomatic condition appears during treatment with antibiotics that inhibit normal bacteria and permit fungal overgrowth. The tongue may also be observed for fasciculations, which indicate lower motor neuron disease, and for abnormal movements such as tardive dyskinesia.

Tooth loss and the use of dentures are extremely common in older persons. Poorly fitting dentures may have far-reaching consequences, such as malnutrition, and can result in numerous problems, such as traumatic ulcers, denture stomatitis, and possibly even cancer. Any dental malocclusion, as well as abnormal speech sounds, such as slurred "s" sounds, clicks, or whistles, which signal improperly fitting dentures, should be recognized. The person may fail to realize that the dentures no longer fit properly. Older adults with dentures should be encouraged to visit the dentist every year or two so that dentures can be adjusted to account for changing mandibular bone structure.

Dental caries may appear as soft white, yellow, or brown areas on the tooth. When they are present, the person may complain of sensitivity to extremes of temperature.

Periodontal disease—a major cause of tooth loss—involves inflammation and destruction of the supporting structures of the teeth (Gordon & Jahnigen, 1986). When examining the oral cavity, bad breath, red or swollen gums, tender or bleeding gums, painful chewing, loose teeth, sensitive teeth, gums that have pulled away from the teeth, any change in the way the teeth fit together when the patient bites, and any change in the fit of partial dentures may be evidence of periodontal disease (National Institute of Dental and Craniofacial Research, 2003). Foul breath odor is common with dental infections, retention of food particles in the teeth or dentures, or chronic periodontal disease.

Neck

The neck presents several important structures for examination: the lymph nodes, the trachea, the thyroid gland, the carotid arteries, and jugular veins. During the physical examination, the clinician should palpate the posterior and anterior cervical lymph node chains as well as the supraclavicular area. Virchow's node—that is, enlargement of the lymph node in the left supraclavicular fossa—is a classic sign of metastatic gastrointestinal carcinoma. Check the trachea for lateral deviation and a look for jugular venous distention, which could be a sign of heart failure. Prominent pulsations above the clavicle may represent kinking of a carotid artery or prominence of the innominate artery.

The carotids should be gently palpated. The pulses should be symmetrical. A bounding or collapsing pulse, in which the upstroke of the pulse wave is very sharp and the downstroke falls rapidly, may be noted in a person with essential hypertension, thyrotoxicosis, aortic regurgitation, or an extreme emotional state. Listen to the carotids using the bell of the stethoscope. Bruits, which signify turbulent blood flow (and not necessarily hemodynamically significant narrowing), may be a clue to atherosclerosis and could be an important finding in an individual with a history of syncope, stroke, or transient ischemic attack. In asymptomatic persons, bruits are probably more indicative of coronary artery disease than of cerebrovascular disease, at least in older men (Sauvé, Laupacis, Østbye, Feagan, & Sackett, 1993).

Attempt to palpate the thyroid gland for enlargement from both in front and in back of the person, even though this gland is generally not easily palpated. If the gland is enlarged, it must be determined whether the gland is diffusely enlarged (goiter) or exhibits discrete nodularity. Sometimes a bruit may be heard over vascular thyroid lesions, and occasionally a thrill is felt. Thyroid disease in older adults is notorious for its subtle presentation. For example, hypothyroidism may manifest solely as depression or mental deterioration. The symptoms of hypothyroidism are easily misinterpreted by the older adult or the physician, and include dry skin, constipation, sleepiness, lethargy, cold intolerance, and fatigue. Hyperthyroidism or thyrotoxicosis may present with weight loss or atrial fibrillation instead of the signs and symptoms usually found in younger persons, such as exophthalmos, restlessness, hyperactivity, and tachycardia.

Heart and Lungs

An estimated 85.6 million American adults have one or more types of cardiovascular disease. Of these individuals, 43.7 million are estimated to be 60 years or older (American Heart Association, 2016). The typical presentation of heart disease in older persons may differ from that in younger adults. Angina pectoris may present as dyspnea, palpitations, or syncope on exertion, rather than as chest pain (Konstam, 1994). Myocardial infarction should be considered in the differential diagnosis of older patients who present with transient ischemic attack, stroke, or an episode of confusion. Even when the pain is typical, an older person may ascribe it to other causes—for example, attributing jaw pain to arthritis or epigastric pain to hiatal hernia or ulcer. Heart disease may also be associated with nonspecific fatigue or weakness in older adults.

The heart and lungs should be examined while the patient is still seated. The clinician places the palm over the apex of the patient's heart to palpate the point of maximal impulse (PMI), also known as the apex pulsation. Normally the PMI covers an area the size of a half-dollar in the midclavicular line. If the PMI is not easily palpated, the patient should be asked to lean forward or to move into a left lateral decubitus position. When the heart is hypertrophied as a result of hypertension, the PMI is small and vigorous. Dilated ventricles, as from mitral regurgitation, cause the PMI to shift lateral to the midclavicular line. The heart size generally

remains unchanged in healthy older persons (Potter, Elahi, Tobin, & Andres, 1982).

Auscultate the heart starting at the apex by using the diaphragm of the stethoscope, inch across to the left lower sternal border, then to the left second intercostal space, and then cross to the right and down the right sternal border. Palpation of the carotid pulse with simultaneous auscultation of the heart is helpful in timing murmurs or other sounds emanating from the heart. The first and second heart sounds are assessed first. Because the first heart sound is produced by the closure of the mitral and tricuspid valves, it sounds louder than the second heart sound over the apex of the heart and the right lower sternal border (the mitral and tricuspid areas, respectively). The third and fourth heart sounds (S_3 and S_4) are low in pitch and best heard at the apex with the bell of the stethoscope. The S_4 sound is normal in older adults; it is due to the arterial stiffening that accompanies aging. The S_3 sound (also known as ventricular gallop) is abnormal, signifying high left ventricular filling pressures and an abrupt deceleration inflow across the mitral valve at the end of the rapid filling phase of diastole (Kono, Rosman, Alam, Stein, & Sabbah, 1993; Shah et al., 2008). An S_3 sound could occur secondary to heart failure, decreased myocardial contractility, ventricular volume overload from aortic and mitral regurgitation, and left-to-right shunts.

Next, listen for murmurs and for silence in systole and diastole. High-pitched clicks and many murmurs will best be heard using the diaphragm of the stethoscope. Lower-pitched sounds such as gallops and diastolic rumbles arising from the mitral and tricuspid valves will best be heard with the bell of the stethoscope. Diastolic murmurs are always significant and may be caused by mitral stenosis or by aortic or pulmonic regurgitation. Mitral stenosis may be silent in older adults.

Systolic murmurs are very common in persons older than age 65 years. Functional flow murmurs from a dilated aortic annulus are short, early systolic murmurs heard at the cardiac base. The second heart sound is normally split, and the carotid upstrokes are normal. The murmur of aortic stenosis is a systolic ejection (diamond-shaped murmur) at the base classically accompanied by diminished carotid upstrokes, sustained apical impulse, and a fourth heart sound. Some of these findings may not be present in the older person. Tips for differentiating aortic stenosis from aortic sclerosis (a common benign murmur in older adults) are as follows:

1. Check the carotid upstroke compared with the PMI. A delayed upstroke suggests aortic stenosis (pulsus parvus et tardus).
2. Check for radiation to the right carotid artery and right clavicle. Aortic stenosis can radiate to either, whereas aortic sclerosis does not (Williams, 2012).
3. Listen carefully to S_2. A diminished S_2 sound suggests aortic stenosis, as does a paradoxically split S_2.
4. Check the pulse pressure. If it is less than 40 mm Hg, the systolic murmur is likely aortic stenosis, since aortic sclerosis does not affect the pulse pressure.

Holosystolic murmurs that are maximal at the apex and radiate into the left axilla are usually mitral regurgitation (Wei & Gersh, 1987). Some cardiac murmurs are also better heard when the patient is lying down.

After the cardiac examination, the clinician should examine the patient's lungs by auscultation and percussion. During auscultation, when asking the person to take a few deep breaths, be alert for signs of hyperventilation, such as dizziness, to avoid inducing syncope. Normally, only so-called vesicular breath sounds are heard over the chest. Bronchial or tubular breath sounds can be heard over the trachea. Such sounds heard over the peripheral lung fields are suggestive of consolidation.

Rales are sounds produced by the movement of fluid or exudate in the airways and suggest heart failure or pneumonia. Nevertheless, basilar rales may be heard in older adults without heart failure, particularly in those who are aged, debilitated, or bedridden. These sounds are often due to atelectasis in people who are habitually shallow breathers, and will disappear after the person takes a few deep breaths and coughs. It is significant if rales are still present after the patient adequately performs these maneuvers. Moist rales or rhonchi are gurgling sounds arising from larger bronchi. Wheezes indicate bronchospasm and may accompany heart failure.

To identify a consolidation or effusion, the clinician should percuss the lungs for areas of dullness. Both consolidations (e.g., pneumonia) and effusions yield dullness or flatness on percussion. They can be differentiated by listening to breath sounds and performing tactile fremitus. Bronchial breath sounds are heard over a consolidation, whereas an effusion is associated with a relative absence of sound.

To assess for tactile fremitus, the clinician places the ulnar surfaces of both hands to either side of the person's chest, and asks the patient to say "ninety-nine." Fremitus will be increased over consolidation and decreased over an effusion.

In chronic obstructive pulmonary disease, the lungs are often hyperresonant, meaning the pitch on percussion is higher than that over the normal lung. When examining patients with chronic obstructive pulmonary disease (COPD) who use inhalers, the clinician should consider observing the patient using the inhaler to verify the technique. Although not a direct component of the physical examination, poor technique can help explain why a patient is not improving with treatment or is having recurrent respiratory exacerbations.

Musculoskeletal System

While examining the lungs, the clinician should identify the presence of any kyphosis or scoliosis. Severe kyphosis can interfere with breathing and cardiovascular function. Tenderness over the spinous processes may suggest a vertebral fracture.

Careful evaluation of the joints will identify deformities, contractures, injuries, joint infections, and evidence suggestive of arthritis. Ask the patient to move the joints in all directions (active range of motion); if the active range of motion is limited, the clinician should move the joints to determine what is limiting the patient's movement (passive range of motion). Limitation of external rotation of the hip can be an early sign of osteoarthritic involvement. Contractures are due to muscle spasticity from inadequate joint motion and are prevalent in patients with advanced dementia or other neurologic illnesses. They can result in pain, increased fall risk, and decreased functional ability (Wagner & Clevenger, 2010).

The location of the swelling and deformity of the hand joints can help determine the type of arthritis. Osteoarthritis is common in older adults, and especially affects the distal interphalangeal joints of the hands as well as the knees and hips. Bony overgrowths at the distal interphalangeal joint are called Heberden's nodes. Rheumatoid arthritis in the hands tends to affect the proximal interphalangeal and metacarpophalangeal (MCP) joints. The joint swelling seen in rheumatoid joints is not bone, but rather synovia and soft tissue swelling that can be felt along the dorsal surface of the involved joint. Progression of the disease produces ulnar deviation in the hands at the MCP joints, as well as a tendency for joints to sublux. Gout will often present with hand arthritis rather than the classic great toe metatarsophalangeal (MTP) inflammation in older adults.

Common musculoskeletal disorders in older adults may result in falls as well as gait and balance conditions. Polymyalgia rheumatica is the most common inflammatory rheumatic disease in the elderly. It is characterized by abrupt-onset pain and stiffness of the shoulder and pelvic girdle muscles (Patil & Dasgupta, 2013) and requires a high index of suspicion. Lumbar spinal stenosis can cause pain and limit walking. Absence of pain when seated and improvement of symptoms when bending forward are the most useful individual findings.

Diagnosis requires an appropriate clinical picture and radiographic findings (Suri, Rainville, Kalichman, & Katz, 2010).

Clubbing of the fingers may indicate an underlying chronic disorder resulting in hypoxia. A normal nail, when viewed from the side, forms an angle with the skin of the nail bed. Clubbing results when the angle is greater than normal and the finger has a "rounded" appearance. Clubbing is seen in chronic lung disorders, carcinoma of the lung, and other disorders associated with chronic hypoxia.

To examine the lower extremities, the patient should be asked to lie down. It is important to make the older person as comfortable as possible for this part of the examination. A pillow can be used or the head of the examining table can be elevated slightly to support the head and upper back; a perfectly flat position is uncomfortable for some older adults. Use sheets appropriately for warmth and modesty.

With the patient supine, check the peripheral pulses in the feet. Palpate the femoral arteries in the groin and auscultate them for bruits. Bruits heard in the femoral arteries are evidence of diffuse atherosclerotic disease. While examining the area of the groin, the physician can check for lymph node swelling. Examine the skin of the lower extremity for lesions and breakdown as discussed earlier. Examine the legs for evidence of arterial insufficiency—namely, laterally placed ulcers, loss of the skin appendages, and delayed capillary refill when the toenails are pressed and released. Venous insufficiency may manifest as pigmented, medially placed ulcers. Examine the feet for changes in the joints as well as for clubbing. Frequently, the examination of the foot reveals evidence of diabetes, neglect, or peripheral vascular disease.

Abdomen

Inspect the abdomen, noting any distention or scars from previous surgery. Listen to the abdomen before proceeding with palpation to avoid inducing peristaltic activity. Pay attention to changes in facial expression during the examination, especially when examining patients with limited ability to communicate, such as those with dementia. The clinician should consider distracting anxious patients when attempting to identify areas of discomfort. Note that older adults with peritoneal irritation are less likely to manifest abdominal wall rigidity compared to younger persons.

Partial bowel obstruction produces rushing sounds; when obstruction is complete, the sounds may become tinkling or very high pitched. Ileus produced by obstruction or from other causes, such as pneumonia or appendicitis, may result in absence of bowel sounds. Conversely, a silent abdominal mass may be the only sign of a gastrointestinal carcinoma.

Tortuosity or aneurysm of the abdominal aorta may be felt as a pulsatile mass in the abdomen. An abdominal aortic aneurysm may have both lateral and anteroposterior pulsation, which distinguishes it from a mass in front of the aorta, which merely transmits the pulsations to the examining hand. In thin persons, the aortic pulsation may be felt normally and may be quite alarming to the unsuspecting examiner. An abdominal ultrasound is a noninvasive way to evaluate the person for the possibility of an aneurysm. A leaking aneurysm and mesenteric ischemia are major, serious considerations in the differential diagnosis of abdominal pain in older adults.

Constipation may produce a mass of feces that can easily be palpated and mistaken for a tumor. A rectal examination is invaluable in the evaluation of constipation.

In addition to palpating and percussing the liver to estimate its size, the clinician should palpate the mid-lower abdomen to check for bladder distention. Such a finding may be important in the evaluation of incontinence or as a sign of urinary retention, which could occur secondary to constipation or be due to prostatic hypertrophy in males. Urinary retention may also be the cause of otherwise unexplainable confusion.

Breasts

Palpate and examine the breasts. Ideally, this examination is done both while the patient is sitting and again while the patient is supine during the abdominal examination. The clinician should search for nipple retraction, skin changes, and masses, which because of loss of connective tissue and adipose are often more easily appreciated in the older woman. Nipples that are retracted secondary to age-related changes can be everted with gentle pressure around the nipple. Inability to evert the nipple with gentle pressure suggests that the retraction is due to an underlying growth. Palpate the nipples so as to express any discharge present. Examine all four quadrants of both breasts, including the axillary tail, and carefully inspect them for any asymmetry. The skin under large, pendulous breasts should be examined for maceration due to perspiration.

Male breasts are not exempt from disease and must also be examined. Gynecomastia (breast enlargement) in an older male can result from a variety of causes, including bronchiogenic carcinoma, obesity, thyroid disease, testicular tumors, drugs (e.g., spironolactone), liver cirrhosis, and other types of cancer.

Genitourinary System and Rectal Examination

Examine the genitalia in conjunction with the rectal examination. This part of the examination may be deferred, but should never be neglected.

Examine the male genitalia for sores, discharge, and testicular masses. The glans of the penis in an uncircumcised man is checked by retracting the foreskin. The prostate is palpated during the rectal examination. The prostate is frequently enlarged in older men and normally feels soft and non-nodular; patients should be referred to a urologist for evaluation of a palpated nodule. The two lobes of the prostate can usually be distinguished by the median furrow between them. Because lobes of the prostate not palpable by the examining finger may enlarge centrally and cause obstruction, a normal-sized gland on physical examination does not rule out urinary obstruction from prostatic enlargement. Do not neglect the evaluation of the prostate in the work-up of back pain.

Inspect the female genitalia for lesions of the skin. If urinary incontinence is a problem, perform a bimanual and a speculum pelvic examination. Older women may not want to bring urinary incontinence to the attention of their doctor, preferring instead to make adjustments on their own, such as decreasing fluid intake and using absorbent napkins, so be sure to inquire about this condition. Note any cystocele, rectocele, or uterine prolapse that may occur as the pelvic musculature becomes lax with age. Attempt to examine for leakage of urine. To perform a stress test, observe for urine loss with coughing or the Valsalva maneuver while the patient is either in the lithotomy position or standing, if tolerated (Holroyd-Leduc, Tannenbaum, Thorpe, & Straus, 2008). Instantaneous urine leakage on coughing or during a Valsalva maneuver is a positive test and is consistent with stress incontinence. Leakage after these events suggests urge incontinence. After menopause, the estrogen-responsive tissues of the genitalia and the lower urinary tract atrophy, which then leads to dryness of the vagina, shrinkage of the vagina and its surrounding structures, altered bacterial resistance, and weakened uterine ligaments. Urinary incontinence and infections may result.

Postmenopausal changes in the vagina cause itching, burning, and dyspareunia (painful intercourse)—symptoms that often older women may be reluctant to spontaneously disclose. The context of the pelvic examination, however, is a natural one in which to broach such subjects in a straightforward and supportive manner. Vaginal atrophy may also be associated with bleeding, and could be a sign of underlying uterine carcinoma. Additionally, palpable ovaries are never normal in an older woman. In terms of education and screening for cervical cancer, the U.S. Preventive Services Task Force recommends against screening women older than 65 years who had adequate prior screening and are not otherwise at high risk for cervical cancer. In addition, the USPSTF recommends against screening in women who have had a hysterectomy with removal of the cervix and who do not have history of a high-grade precancerous lesion or cervical cancer (Moyer, 2012).

Rectal examination may be performed after the patient is helped into the lateral decubitus position; alternatively, the patient may be asked to bend over the examination table. Explain to the patient what to expect and when. The anus is inspected for tears, irritation, and external hemorrhoids, and the tone of the anal sphincter, which may diminish with age, is noted. A gloved finger is used to make a sweep of the entire rectum, being sure to take in its entire circumference. The patient is asked to strain to bring down any lesions just outside the reach of the examining finger. A stool sample to test for occult blood is obtained, and healthcare providers should discuss with patients what the plan would be if the test is positive. Some patients may prefer to forgo further diagnostic evaluations, or a work-up may not be in alignment with their goals.

In addition to pelvic examination in women and prostate examination in men, the clinician should perform neurologic testing for perineal sensation and sacral reflexes, examine the abdomen for a grossly distended bladder, and look for leaking of urine as previously described. Fecal incontinence is a serious problem among institutionalized older adults and is a significant risk factor for formation of decubiti.

Nervous System

The neurologic examination is performed with the patient initially in a sitting position. It has six components: intellectual function, the cranial nerves, motor examination, sensory examination, reflexes, and cerebellar examination. The mental status examination is discussed at length in the *Cognitive/Mentation Assessment* chapter and the mobility assessment in the chapter of that name. Age-related changes in the nervous system include decreased vibratory sensation (especially in the legs), depression of the Achilles tendon reflex, some decreased ability to look upward, and mild swaying on the Romberg test (Halter et al., 2009). To assess the patient's position sense (proprioception), the patient is asked to identify the direction in which the toes or fingers are displaced by the examiner. Older persons asked to stand with their feet together and eyes closed (Romberg test) may have some difficulty with this task because of impaired proprioception, decreased strength, and more reliance of balance on visual input. This test is useful for the evaluation of patients with disequilibrium or gait abnormalities.

To evaluate sensation, the clinician determines the person's ability to feel a soft cotton-tipped applicator, sharp pinprick, and vibrating tuning fork. Such an examination is often quite subjective, and sometimes deficits are not reproducible. Impaired mental status or aphasia may make sensory examination more difficult, prone to error, or even impossible to perform. More complex sensory integration is examined by asking the patient to identify common objects placed in his or her hands, such as a coin, comb, or paper clip (stereognosis).

Motor tone is frequently increased in older persons. Passive movement of the person's limb by the examiner may commonly demonstrate involuntary rigidity, which should not be mistaken for lack of cooperation. Strength may be decreased as well as muscle mass, especially in the small muscles of the hands.

Essential tremors may involve the head as well as the hands, improve after alcohol use, and worsen with stress or fatigue. This form of tremor is usually seen during action, such as when eating, writing, or holding a posture. Parkinsonian tremors, in contrast, most often occur at rest, when the body part is relaxed.

Another aspect of the nervous system evaluation is testing of the strength of the extremities. If the patient has difficulty rising from a chair (hip muscles) or combing his or her hair

(shoulder girdle), the weakness is proximal; if the patient has difficulty standing on his or her toes (gastrocnemius/soleus) or doing fine work with the hands (intrinsics), the muscle weakness is distal (Saguil, 2005). Although many myopathies are associated with proximal weakness (e.g., polymyositis), a small number are associated predominantly with distal weakness (e.g., inclusion body myositis in adults older than age 50).

Gait and Balance

Falling is an example of a geriatric syndrome with multiple contributing causes and serious consequences; it requires careful delineation of the circumstances of the fall and a thorough search for underlying physical illness. The risk of falling increases with advancing age, and simple diagnostic evaluation may identify persons at increased risk (Nevitt, Cummings, Kidd, & Black, 1989; Rogers, Rogers, Takeshima, & Islam, 2003; Studenski et al., 1994; Tinetti, Speechley, & Ginter, 1988). The clinician should observe the patient sitting and rising from a chair, walking and turning around, and bending down to pick up an object off the floor (Tinetti & Speechley, 1989). Does the individual rise from a chair in a single movement? Is he or she steady in walking and turning without grasping for support while using smooth continuous movement? Does the person seem sure of himself or herself when bending? Observe, if possible, the patient climbing and descending a flight of stairs (Tinetti, 1986). A relatively quick screen is the 8-foot up-and-go test. In this test, the patient begins in a seated position and is then instructed to stand, walk 8 feet forward (a spot on the floor may be indicated), turn, return to the chair, and sit. The patient is asked to do this as quickly as safety allows. This task assesses speed, agility, and dynamic balance (Rikli & Jones, 1999).

Balance should also be tested in a standard way. In the three-stage balance test, the patient stands with the feet next to each other (side by side), then slides one foot forward so that its heel is next to the arch of the other foot (semi-tandem), and finally puts the heel of one foot touching the toe of the other (full tandem). The patient should assume each of the three poses for 10 seconds each. Patients who cannot do each of these poses are at a higher risk of falls and may respond to physical therapy. The *Mobility Assessment* chapter has more information on this aspect of the physical examination.

▶ Practice Challenges

The physical examination of the older person is not markedly different from the physical examination of any adult, but is distinguished by the focus on factors contributing to functional loss, the frequent barriers to communication present in older adults (such as impaired special senses), the likelihood of multiple comorbidities, the increased risk of developing a geriatric syndrome, and differences in what is considered abnormal. Such an examination complements the functional, social, economic, and values assessment. For the older adult, evaluation of these other domains is often the key to the solution of the multifaceted problems of living presented by older adults to the primary care practitioner and others who care for older persons.

While this chapter serves as a guide, each encounter with an older adult may vary widely from these guidelines. A reliable caregiver is not always available, and the resources to gather the data required for informed decision making may be lacking. For example, the information accompanying patients who are transferred to a hospital from a nursing home or the outpatient setting may be incomplete and has been shown to vary in quality, with gaps often including medication regimen and prescription histories (Tamblyn et al., 2014). It may be difficult to get the patient into the best position for the different parts of the physical examination. Special equipment may be needed, for example, to weigh or measure the patient, or to maximize the individual's hearing. Finally, given scheduling practices, a comprehensive examination may need to be spread over several visits.

▶ Summary

The physical assessment of older patients is both an art and a science. It requires that practitioners become skilled at evaluating functional domains as well as organ systems, and that they be able to differentiate normal from not normal, and sick from not sick, in the context of older adults. The physical assessment serves many purposes, including diagnosis of symptomatic, asymptomatic, and atypically presenting disease. It also provides the data that allow clinicians to stratify patients as robust, vulnerable, or frail—information they can then use to help the patient and family prioritize prevention and treatment and discuss their goals for life and care. This type of holistic, patient-centered approach can be mastered with training, but requires the ability to make correct diagnoses and to estimate prognosis, both of which depend on the clinician's physical assessment skills.

References

American Heart Association. (2016). Older Americans & Cardiovascular Diseases. [Fact Sheet]. Retrieved from https://www.heart.org/idc/groups/heart-public /@wcm/@sop/@smd/documents/downloadable /ucm_483970.pdf

Bergquist, S. (2003). Pressure ulcer prediction in older adults receiving home health care: Implications for use with the OASIS. *Advances in Skin & Wound Care, 16*(3), 132–139.

Bickley, L., & Szilagyi, P. G. (2016). *Bates' guide to physical examination and history-taking.* Philadelphia, PA: Lippincott Williams & Wilkins.

Brandeis, G. H., Morris, J. N., Nash, D. J., & Lipsitz, L. A. (1990). The epidemiology and natural history of pressure ulcers in elderly nursing home residents. *Journal of the American Medical Association, 264*(22), 2905–2909.

Brillhart, B. (2005). Pressure sore and skin tear prevention and treatment during a 10-month program. *Rehabilitation Nursing, 30*(3), 85–91.

Cassel, C. K. (2003). *Geriatric medicine: An evidence-based approach.* New York, NY: Springer Science & Business Media.

de Berker, D. (2009). Clinical practice: Fungal nail disease. *New England Journal of Medicine, 360*(20), 2108–2116. doi: 10.1056/NEJMcp0804878

Franklin, S. S., Gustin, W., Wong, N. D., Larson, M. G., Weber, M. A., Kannel, W. B., & Levy, D. (1997). Hemodynamic patterns of age-related changes in blood pressure. *Circulation, 96*(1), 308–315.

Franklin, S. S., Jacobs, M. J., Wong, N. D., Gilbert, J. L., & Lapuerta, P. (2001). Predominance of isolated systolic hypertension among middle-aged and elderly US hypertensives. *Hypertension, 37*(3), 869–874.

Gordon, S. R., & Jahnigen, D. W. (1986). Oral assessment of the dentulous elderly patient. *Journal of American Geriatrics Society, 34*(4), 276–281.

Group, A. S. (2010). Effects of intensive blood-pressure control in type 2 diabetes mellitus. *New England Journal of Medicine, 2010*(362), 1575-1585.

Gupta, A. K., & Ricci, M. J. (2006). Diagnosing onychomycosis. *Dermatology Clinics, 24*(3), 365–369. doi: 10.1016/j.det.2006.03.008

Gupta, A. K., Taborda, P., Taborda, V., Gilmour, J., Rachlis, A., Salit, I., ... Summerbell, R. C. (2000). Epidemiology and prevalence of onychomycosis in HIV-positive individuals. *International Journal of Dermatology, 39*(10), 746–753.

Halter, J., Ouslander, J., Tinetti, M., Studenski, S., High, K., & Asthana, S. (2009). *Hazzard's geriatric medicine and gerontology.* New York, NY: McGraw-Hill Prof Med/Tech.

Henschke, P. J. (1993). Infections in the elderly. *Medical Journal of Australia, 158*(12), 830–834.

High, K. P., Bradley, S. F., Gravenstein, S., Mehr, D. R., Quagliarello, V. J., Richards, C., & Yoshikawa, T. T. (2009). Clinical practice guideline for the evaluation of fever and infection in older adult residents of long-term care facilities: 2008 update by the Infectious Diseases Society of America. *Clinical Infectious Diseases, 48*(2), 149–171.

Holroyd-Leduc, J. M., Tannenbaum, C., Thorpe, K. E., & Straus, S. E. (2008). What type of urinary incontinence does this woman have? *Journal of the American Medical Association, 299*(12), 1446–1456.

Huan, S. L. (2010). Risk factors of cataract formation. *International Journal of Ophthalmology, 10*(6), 1128–1130.

James, P. A., Oparil, S., Carter, B. L., Cushman, W. C., Dennison-Himmelfarb, C., Handler, J., ... Ortiz, E. (2014). 2014 evidence-based guideline for the management of high blood pressure in adults: Report from the panel members appointed to the Eighth Joint National Committee (JNC 8). *Journal of the American Medical Association, 311*(5), 507–520. doi: 10.1001/jama.2013.284427

Joanna Briggs Institute. (2017). Recommended Practice. *Observations: Weight and Height (older adult).* Ovid Joanna Briggs Institute EBP. (JBI2344).

Kannel, W. B. (1996). Blood pressure as a cardiovascular risk factor: Prevention and treatment. *Journal of the American Medical Association, 275*(20), 1571–1576.

Kono, T., Rosman, H., Alam, M., Stein, P. D., & Sabbah, H. N. (1993). Hemodynamic correlates of the third heart sound during the evolution of chronic heart failure. *Journal of the American College of Cardiology, 21*(2), 419–423.

Konstam, M. A. (1994). Heart failure: Evaluation and care of patients with left-ventricular systolic dysfunction. *Journal of Cardiac Failure, 1*(2), 183–187.

Kurrle, S., Cameron, I., & Geeves, R. (2015). A quick ward assessment of older patients by junior doctors. *BMJ, 350*, h607.

Landefeld, C. S. (2003). Improving health care for older persons. *Annals of Internal Medicine, 139*(5 Pt 2), 421–424.

Lo, A., Ryder, K., & Shorr, R. I. (2005). Relationship between patient age and duration of physician visit in ambulatory setting: Does one size fit all? *Journal of American Geriatrics Society, 53*(7), 1162–1167. doi: 10.1111/j.1532-5415.2005.53367.x

Mader, S. (1984). Hearing impairment in elderly persons. *Journal of American Geriatrics Society, 32*, 548–553.

Mader, S. L., Josephson, K. R., & Rubenstein, L. Z. (1987). Low prevalence of postural hypotension among community-dwelling elderly. *Journal of the American Medical Association, 258*(11), 1511–1514.

Messerli, F. H., Ventura, H. O., & Amodeo, C. (1985). Osler's maneuver and pseudohypertension. *New England Journal of Medicine, 312*(24), 1548–1551.

Moyer, V. A. (2012). Screening for cervical cancer: US Preventive Services Task Force recommendation statement. *Annals of Internal Medicine, 156*(12), 880–891.

Moyer, V. A. (2012). Screening for hearing loss in older adults: US Preventive Services Task Force recommendation statement. *Annals of Internal Medicine, 157*(9), 655–661.

Musgrave, T., & Verghese, A. (1990). Clinical features of pneumonia in the elderly. *Seminars in Respiratory Infections, 5*(4), 269–275.

Myers, M. G., Kearns, P. M., Kennedy, D., & Fisher, R. (1978). Postural hypotension and diuretic therapy in the elderly. *Canadian Medical Association Journal, 119*(6), 581.

National Heart, Lung, and Blood Institute. (2006). Calculate your body mass index. Retrieved from https://www.nhlbi.nih.gov/health/educational/lose_wt/BMI/bmi-m.htm

National Institute of Dental and Craniofacial Research. (2003, September). *Periodontal (gum) disease: Causes, symptoms, and treatments.* Retrieved from https://www.nidcr.nih.gov/OralHealth/Topics/GumDiseases/PeriodontalGumDisease.htm?_ga=1.182919663.878490602.1415283936

Nazarko, L. (2009). *Nursing in care homes.* John Wiley & Sons.

Nevitt, M. C., Cummings, S. R., Kidd, S., & Black, D. (1989). Risk factors for recurrent nonsyncopal falls: A prospective study. *Journal of the American Medical Association, 261*(18), 2663–2668.

NHLBI Obesity Education Initiative Expert Panel on the Identification, Evaluation, and Treatment of Obesity in Adults. (1998). *Clinical guidelines on the identification, evaluation, and treatment of overweight and obesity in adults: The evidence report.* Bethesda, MD: National Heart, Blood, and Lung Institute. Retrieved from https://www.ncbi.nlm.nih.gov/books/NBK1996/

Norman, D. C. (2000). Fever in the elderly. *Clinical Infectious Diseases, 31*(1), 148–151.

Nutrition Screening Initiative. (1991). *Report of nutrition screening 1: Toward a common view.* Washington, DC: Author.

Patel, K. V., Guralnik, J. M., Dansie, E. J., & Turk, D. C. (2013). Prevalence and impact of pain among older adults in the United States: Findings from the 2011 National Health and Aging Trends Study. *Pain, 154*(12), 2649–2657.

Patil, P., & Dasgupta, B. (2013). Polymyalgia rheumatica in older adults. *Aging and Health, 9*(5), 483–495.

Potter, J. F., Elahi, D., Tobin, J. D., & Andres, R. (1982). Effect of aging on the cardiothoracic ratio of men. *Journal of the American Geriatrics Society, 30*(6), 404–409.

Rikli, R. E., & Jones, C. J. (1999). Development and validation of a functional fitness test for community-residing older adults. *Journal of Aging and Physical Activity, 7*(2), 129–161.

Robman, L., & Taylor, H. (2005). External factors in the development of cataract. *Eye, 19*(10), 1074–1082.

Rogers, M. E., Rogers, N. L., Takeshima, N., & Islam, M. M. (2003). Methods to assess and improve the physical parameters associated with fall risk in older adults. *Preventive Medicine, 36*(3), 255–264.

Saguil, A. (2005). Evaluation of the patient with muscle weakness. *American Family Physician, 71*(7), 1327–1336.

Sauvé, J.-S., Laupacis, A., Østbye, T., Feagan, B., & Sackett, D. L. (1993). Does this patient have a clinically important carotid bruit? *Journal of the American Medical Association, 270*(23), 2843–2845.

Shah, S. J., Marcus, G. M., Gerber, I. L., McKeown, B. H., Vessey, J. C., Jordan, M. V., . . . Michaels, A. D. (2008). Physiology of the third heart sound: Novel insights from tissue Doppler imaging. *Journal of the American Society of Echocardiography, 21*(4), 394–400.

Shannon, R. P., Wei, J. Y., Rosa, R. M., Epstein, F. H., & Rowe, J. W. (1986). The effect of age and sodium depletion on cardiovascular response to orthostasis. *Hypertension, 8*(5), 438–443.

Stein, P., & Aalboe, J. (2015). Dental care in the frail older adult: Special considerations and recommendations. *Journal of the California Dental Association, 43*(7), 363–368.

Studenski, S., Duncan, P. W., Chandler, J., Samsa, G., Prescott, B., Hogue, C., & Bearon, L. B. (1994). Predicting falls: The role of mobility and nonphysical factors. *Journal of the American Geriatrics Society, 42*(3), 297–302.

Suri, P., Rainville, J., Kalichman, L., & Katz, J. N. (2010). Does this older adult with lower extremity pain have the clinical syndrome of lumbar spinal stenosis? *Journal of the American Medical Association, 304*(23), 2628–2636.

Surjushe, A., Kamath, R., Oberai, C., Saple, D., Thakre, M., Dharmshale, S., & Gohil, A. (2007). A clinical and mycological study of onychomycosis in HIV infection. *Indian Journal of Dermatology, Venereology, and Leprology, 73*(6), 397–401.

Tamblyn, R., Poissant, L., Huang, A., Winslade, N., Rochefort, C. M., Moraga, T., & Doran, P. (2014). Estimating the information gap between emergency department records of community medication compared to on-line access to the community-based pharmacy records. *Journal of the American Medical Informatics Association, 21*(3), 391–398. doi: 10.1136/amiajnl-2013-001704

Tinetti, M. E. (1986). Performance-oriented assessment of mobility problems in elderly patients. *Journal of American Geriatrics Society, 34*(2), 119–126.

Tinetti, M. E., Han, L., Lee, D. S., McAvay, G. J., Peduzzi, P., Gross, C. P., . . . & Lin, H. (2014). Antihypertensive medications and serious fall injuries in a nationally representative sample of older adults. *JAMA Internal Medicine, 174*(4), 588–595.

Tinetti, M. E., & Speechley, M. (1989). Prevention of falls among the elderly. *New England Journal of Medicine, 320*(16), 1055–1059.

Tinetti, M. E., Speechley, M., & Ginter, S. F. (1988). Risk factors for falls among elderly persons living in the community. *New England Journal of Medicine, 319*(26), 1701–1707.

Vargas, C. M., Kramarow, E. A., & Yellowitz, J. A. (2001). The oral health of older Americans. *Aging Trends, 3,* 1–8.

Wagner, L. M., & Clevenger, C. (2010). Contractures in nursing home residents. *Journal of the American Medical Directors Association, 11*(2), 94–99.

Wei, J. Y., & Gersh, B. J. (1987). Heart disease in the elderly. *Current Problems in Cardiology, 12*(1), 7–65.

Weiss, J., Freeman, M., Low, A., Fu, R., Kerfoot, A., Paynter, R., . . . Kansagara, D. (2017). Benefits and harms of intensive blood pressure treatment in adults aged 60 years or older: A systematic review and meta-analysis. *Annals of Internal Medicine, 166*(6), 419–429.

Williams, M. (2012, January 18). *Cardiac auscultation in the older adult.* Retrieved from http://www.medscape.com/viewarticle/756829_10

Wright, J. T. Jr., Williamson, J. D., Whelton, P. K., Snyder, J. K., Sink, K. M., Rocco, M. V., . . . Ambrosius, W. T. (2015). A randomized trial of intensive versus standard blood-pressure control. *New England Journal of Medicine, 373*(22), 2103–2116. doi: 10.1056/NEJMoa1511939

Yellowitz, J. A., & Schneiderman, M. T. (2014). Elder's oral health crisis. *Journal of Evidence Based Dental Practice, 14,* 191–200.

CHAPTER 26

Pain Assessment

Keela Herr and Staja Q. Booker

CHAPTER OBJECTIVES

1. Describe the importance and impact of unrecognized and undertreated pain in older adults.
2. Provide best practice recommendations for assessment of pain in older adults, with and without cognitive impairment.

KEY TERMS

Acute pain
Central pain

Mixed and undetermined pain
Neuropathic pain

Peripheral nociceptive pain
Persistent or chronic pain

▶ Introduction

With an increasing older adult population globally, the issue of pain has taken on new importance, demanding timely and thorough assessment approaches. A number of provider, political, and payment/regulatory issues affect quality pain care practice, including the role and approach to assessment. Several guidelines have been developed in the United States, the United Kingdom, and elsewhere that describe the "why, how, and when" of pain assessment, but lack of strong evidence in some areas to guide practice hinders providers' consistent implementation of guidelines. Moreover, national policy constraints, regulations, and licensing requirements can limit older adults' access to opioids and other non-drug treatments. In such cases, older adults may feel less inclined to report pain if they believe that adequate treatment will not be provided.

Assessment is the foundation to developing a clear, collaborative, and effective pain treatment plan. This chapter provides practical approaches for pain assessment in older adults, including an evidence-based hierarchical approach for assessing pain in older adults. For a comprehensive review of pain assessment and treatment, clinical practice guidelines on acute and persistent pain are available (Arnstein & Herr, 2015; Cornelius, Herr, Gordon, & Kretzer, 2016).

▸ Importance of Pain Assessment

Demographics and Prevalence of Pain

One of the key elements in improving assessment of pain is to recognize the important role that unrecognized and undertreated pain has in determining quality of life and function in older adults. The prevalence of bothersome pain within the past month has been reported to be as high as 53% of non-institutionalized older adults in the United States, or approximately 18.7 million people (Patel, Guralnik, Dansie, & Turk, 2013). Although acute and chronic non-cancer-related pains are among the most common complaints of older adults, care of pain in older adults is often overlooked in efforts to manage more "pressing" chronic conditions, such as diabetes, hypertension, and kidney dysfunction. Women and individuals with obesity, musculoskeletal conditions, or depressive symptoms are at higher risk for pain (Patel et al., 2013).

Effects of Pain on Older Adults' Health

While the impact of acute pain on short- and long-term outcomes in older adults is less studied and understood, certainly persistent pain negatively affects all aspects of older adults' lives, impairing everything from social interactions, sleep, and nutritional status, to mood and cognitive function. Pain has a profound effect on comfort level, functional ability, and quality of life. According to Hunt et al. (2015), 43% of older adults with dementia report pain that limits function or contributes to their inability to perform activities of daily living. Specifically, high-impact pain is defined as moderate to severe pain lasting 3 months or longer that interferes with daily life activities and limits participation in key social roles. The majority of older persons with pain have multiple sites of pain that impact physical and psychosocial function and pose serious threats to quality of life. Pain not well managed from conditions such as osteoarthritis, chronic back pain, and vertebral fractures and herniation can lead to activity avoidance, falls, and social isolation. Relevant goals from *Healthy People 2020* that apply to older adults are to (1) decrease the prevalence of adults having high-impact chronic pain and (2) reduce the mean level of joint pain among adults with doctor-diagnosed arthritis (*Healthy People 2020*, 2014). These goals underscore the importance of assessing for pain during each clinical encounter and determining a mutual agreed-upon goal for comfort, function, and mood.

The pain experience in older adults is different from that in other adult groups, partly due to age-related differences in physiological and psychological mechanisms, communication, pain perception, beliefs and attitudes toward pain, coping, and social support. Although it has long been postulated that older adults do not experience pain with the same intensity as younger adults because of age-related changes in the nervous system, differences in pain threshold and tolerance increase risk for under-recognition and undertreatment. Additionally, a growing body of evidence indicates that altered pain perception strongly impacts frail individuals with dementia and may contribute to unjustified undertreatment of pain (DeFrin et al., 2015; Gibson & Lauterbacher, 2017). When pain goes unrecognized and is undertreated, it has significant consequences for health, often resulting in disability and frailty. In fact, physiological stressors–associated frailty decreases older adults' reserve to adapt or effectively inhibit additional nociceptive stressors such as pain, a phenomenon called "pain homeostenosis" (Lohman, Whiteman, Greenberg, & Bruce, 2017; Shega et al., 2012). Emerging evidence also suggests that persistent pain may be a contributing or co-occurring factor in the frailty phenotype (Lohman et al., 2017). Pain may add to the level of frailty and/or frailty may increase pain, leading to physical and cognitive function disabilities.

▶ Best Assessment Practices

Booker, Bartoszczyk, and Herr (2016) describe an approach to pain assessment and management in frail older adults. A comprehensive evaluation for the underlying cause of pain, pain characteristics, and impact on physical and psychosocial function and quality of life is key to developing an effective treatment approach. Multiple factors (e.g., anxiety, depression, beliefs, insomnia, fear avoidance, biomechanical issues), when combined with pain, can cause impairment or dysfunction and should be considered during the evaluation. History taking to identify underlying diseases known to be painful and determine the patient's analgesic history (e.g., effectiveness and adverse effects, current and previous prescription and over-the-counter drugs) provides important information that can guide treatment planning. Assessment of activities of daily living and instrumental activities of daily living is very helpful in delineating the impact of the person's pain on function.

A complete physical examination of the pain source and the musculoskeletal, peripheral vascular, and neurologic systems is important given the predominance of pain-related problems originating in these systems. The physical examination should also target potential pain contributors (e.g., leg length discrepancy, myofascial pain, sacroiliac joint syndrome). Laboratory and diagnostic tests should be used to establish etiologic diagnosis, but caution is warranted in interpreting their results: More than half of older patients with radiographic evidence of degenerative joint disease are pain-free, and imaging studies are often not necessary or useful.

When gathering information regarding the pain experience from the older adult, different approaches are often needed depending on the individual's level of cognitive ability. This section focuses on the interpersonal interaction between patient and provider. Specifically, a focused hierarchy is presented for older adults who can and cannot self-report, with this hierarchy integrating components of the pain characteristics, functional assessment, and psychosocial assessment. Providers' interpersonal assessment approach can be complemented by emerging mobile and other technologies (Docking, 2016).

Self-Reporting Individuals

The best method for assessment currently remains self-report. That is, the older adult verbalizes the occurrence of pain and rates pain using standardized pain tools. A patient's self-report is the most reliable evidence of pain intensity and impact of function. Only the patient truly knows the severity of the pain that he or she is experiencing, and providers continue to underestimate pain based on their personal judgment. The role of the provider, then, is to actualize accurate pain assessment by asking about pain, accepting the patient's report and taking it seriously, and taking action when pain is reported. Based on research, best practices, and previous guidelines, the authors of this chapter have developed and advocate for a stepwise approach to guide assessment (**TABLE 26-1**).

In case exemplar 1, several best practices were apparent. First, self-report using a validated pain intensity tool was elicited, and the provider also inquired about the effect of pain on the patient's everyday functional ability. This questioning prompted the patient to readily offer additional information related to pain locations, symptoms, and medications used. Also, a focused assessment was followed up with a more comprehensive physical examination and diagnostic tests. After diagnosis, the provider appropriately assessed and incorporated the patient's comfort–function goal into the plan of care. The only issue with this scenario is the lack of a standardized tool for assessment of pain interference and mood.

TABLE 26-1 Hierarchy of Pain Assessment for Self-Reporting Older Adults

Step 1: Determine the patient's ability to reliably self-report pain and attempt to obtain self-report.

Step 2: Determine presence/absence of pain by asking older adult if he or she is experiencing pain, hurt, aches, or discomfort "right now/at this moment" *and* "with activities/movement." Also ask about location and radiation, duration, frequency or pattern, and precipitating and ameliorating factors to help determine the cause.

Step 3: Measure self-reported pain intensity using a valid, reliable, and preferred pain scale, such as the Faces Pain Rating Scale—Revised (FPS-r), Iowa Pain Thermometer (IPT) and Verbal Descriptor Scale (VDS), or Numeric Rating Scale (NRS). The VDS, with or without a thermometer, is preferred by the majority of older adults, although there are individual differences.

Step 4: Assess the impact of pain on function to determine pain tolerability, such as by using the Brief Pain Inventory (BPI) or the PEG (a Veterans Administration–developed three-item version of the BPI) (Krebs et al., 2009).

Step 5: Assess interference of pain with sleep and emotional stability. Strong associations between sleep, pain, and depression support emphasis on good sleep hygiene (Eslami, Zimmerman, Grewal, Katz, & Lipton, 2016).

Step 6: Develop a multimodal plan of pain care with realistic goals for comfort, function, and mood, **making sure each step is documented**. Use of a pain diary by patients can help assess the relationship between pain and activity and provides a record of pain intensity during various activities, as well as effect of analgesics and other treatments.

Reproduced and modified with permission from copyright holders: Booker, S., & Herr, K. University of Iowa, College of Nursing. © 2015.

🔍 CASE EXEMPLAR 1

Mrs. H, a 78-year-old widow, sees you for the first time because "no one has been able to help me with my pain." She has hypertension and diet-controlled diabetes, but her principal concern is ongoing pain. She says that the pain is "all over" and has been present for weeks. You identify a pain intensity scale that Mrs. H understands (Iowa Pain Thermometer–Revised [IPT-R]) and ask her to rate her current pain on one of the scales. She rates her "pain now" as 8/10 on the IPT-R.

After a focused exam, which reveals nothing alarming or emergent, you ask Mrs. H how the pain interferes with her usual activities. She reveals that she has difficulty moving in the morning and completing her morning activities of daily living, but this condition improves somewhat later in the day. Without prompting, she further states that the pain is primarily in her upper arms, back, and neck. Over-the-counter acetaminophen had some effect, but did not eliminate the pain. She also notes some "feverishness" and fatigue.

Armed with this new information, you direct your exam to the appropriate areas, finding limited active and passive range of motion of the shoulders, but no findings of arthritis. The erythrocyte sedimentation rate is 95 and confirms the diagnosis of polymyalgia rheumatica. When you ask Mrs. H about her primary goal for comfort and function, she states that she wants to be able to work in her garden. Mrs. H's symptoms improve dramatically within a few days after she agrees to take a low dose of prednisone and perform alternating application of cold and heat.

Non-Self-Reporting Individuals

Inability to report may stem from cognitive impairment, intellectual disabilities, or aphasic conditions. Although evaluation of pain in older adults with cognitive impairments and intellectual disabilities may be difficult, there is no evidence that cognitive impairment "masks" the pain. However, behaviors such as agitation and confusion may be misinterpreted as dementia-related behaviors rather than as distress and discomfort from pain. Many older adults without severe dementia are able to self-report pain

(Lukas, Barber, Johnson, & Gibson, 2013). Direct attempts to obtain self-reports from older adults with dementia are therefore a critical component of pain assessment, given that no psychosocial and behavioral indicators can be substituted for such a self-report, but rather complement pain assessment (Breland et al., 2015). Thus, using a validated behavioral observational tool is a key component of the hierarchy of pain assessment for patients who are unable to self-report their pain; this hierarchy is described in **TABLE 26-2**.

🔍 *CASE EXEMPLAR 2*

Mr. A.J. is an 83-year-old retired farmer with osteoarthritis in his shoulders, hip, and lower back pain; he currently resides in a local long-term care facility. He is unable to care for himself, and the nurses' aides must dress and feed him. Mr. A.J. was diagnosed with moderate dementia. Some days he is able to verbalize his needs and says "Pain, pain all over"; on other days he cannot make such a self-report.

This morning, as Mr. A.J. was being dressed, he moaned and resisted the aides when putting on his shirt. The aides stretched his arms out and he hollered loudly. The nurse entered the room and suggested that Mr. A.J. was agitated because he is "demented." The nurse dismissed Mr. A.J.'s behavior and did not assess for pain by using a pain tool such as Pain Assessment in Advanced Dementia (PAINAD). Although he has an "as needed" (prn) order for acetaminophen and hydrocodone, she gave him a low-dose of lorazepam and noted in the patient chart the behaviors observed and medication administered.

Later, it was noted that Mr. A.J. did not eat much breakfast and resisted range-of-motion exercises. He did not moan or cry out for the remainder of the day, but appeared despondent. By that point, Mr. A.J.'s pain had not been addressed for 8 hours.

In case exemplar 2, given the patient's history of osteoarthritis, many opportunities for use of best practices and assuring quality pain care were missed, such as attempting self-report of pain, assessing for other reasons for behavior, using a validated pain observation tool, and attempting

an analgesic trial. While the nurse did enter the room and observe the patient, document behaviors and medication administration, and attempt a range-of-motion intervention, all these actions were arbitrary and not guided by a best practice framework to determine cause of behaviors.

TABLE 26-2 Hierarchy of Pain Assessment for Non-Self-Reporting Older Adults

Step 1: Determine the patient's ability to reliably self-report pain and attempt to obtain self-report. Note whether the patient has a diagnosis of cognitive impairment or dementia. If the patient is able to self-report, continue with steps 2–6 in Table 26-1. If the patient is unable to self-report, continue with steps 2–6 below.

Step 2: Search for possible causes/sources of pain. Ensure basic comfort measures have been met and etiologies that may be painful have been treated.

Step 3: Observe for potential pain behaviors using a reliable and valid pain-behavior observation tool, such as Pain Assessment in Advanced Dementia (PAINAD), or Pain Assessment Checklist for Seniors with Limited Ability to Communicate-II (PACSLAC-II), during key physical activities (e.g., transfers, ambulation, repositioning) noting changes in behavior between rest and movement.

Step 4: Incorporate proxy reporting. Examples of information that professional and personal caregivers may provide include changes in function or usual activities, such as altered gait or falls, agitation, resistance to care, impaired sleep, or escalated pacing.

Step 5: Initiate an analgesic trial to evaluate whether pain is the cause of behaviors when other causes have been ruled out and the patient is not responding to nondrug interventions. A guide to be adjusted based on comorbidities and contraindications follows (Reuben et al., 2017):

- Try acetaminophen first (if no hepatic dysfunction). Order a scheduled dose, rather than "as needed" dosing. Acetaminophen is often effective in improving behaviors and/or function.
  - If there is no response to acetaminophen and localized inflammatory pain is suspected, try topical nonsteroidal anti-inflammatory drugs (NSAIDs).
  - If there is no response, try oral morphine sulfate (5 mg every 12 hours, up to a maximum dose of 10 mg every 12 hours) or buprenorphine transdermal patch (5 mcg/hour, up to maximum mcg/hr).
- If there is no response to acetaminophen and neuropathic pain is suspected, try pregabalin 25 mg/day, up to a maximum dose of 300 mg/day.

Carefully monitor the response to analgesics with each change as the agent and dose are titrated to achieve pain relief yet avoid undesirable adverse effects.

Step 6: If the analgesic trial confirms pain, **develop a balanced, multimodal plan of pain care while evaluating treatment options' risks and benefits and documenting in medical record and advance directives**. Measurable and realistic goals for comfort, function, mood, and behavioral improvement should be established.

Reproduced and modified with permission from copyright holders: Booker, S., & Herr, K. University of Iowa, College of Nursing. © 2015.

▶ Practice Challenges: Barriers and Facilitators

Multiple patient and provider attitudinal and communication barriers might interfere with the assessment and successful treatment of pain in older adults. Some older individuals will deny having pain but admit to experiencing discomfort or aching. Other older adults may fear the cause of pain or the diagnostic tests, and be unwilling to report pain. Other barriers may include lack of providers' time or interest, and some providers may fail to assess pain and instead normalize pain as an aspect of aging. Developing collaborative and trusting relationships between patient and provider will encourage patients to readily offer report of pain. Assessment of pain in the older adult can be challenging, but best practices can inform and guide quality pain assessment. **TABLE 26-3** describes the various types of pain that providers should consider during the pain assessment.

Gaps in provider knowledge about pain, in general and across disciplines, suggest a strong need for improvements in healthcare provider education regarding best practices for assessment and management of pain (Fishman et al., 2013). An interprofessional panel of experts reached consensus on core pain competencies that all healthcare providers and healthcare students should be competent to perform, including addressing the needs of vulnerable populations such as older adults (Fishman et al., 2013). Making evidence-based assessment a culture of practice at institutions is also essential to facilitate greater attention to its importance among healthcare staff.

TABLE 26-3 Types of Pain

Acute pain	Typically has a distinct onset with evident pathology (e.g., a new injury from a recent fall, skin tear, inflammation, postsurgical) and may be caused by exacerbation of a chronic problem (e.g., a vertebral fracture in a person with osteoporosis). Short duration and self-limiting.
Persistent or chronic pain	Does not respond to usual treatments within expected amount of time; often associated with functional and psychological impairment; may occur in the absence of any past injury or body damage. Chronic pain occurs on at least half of the days for 6 months or more (National Pain Strategy, 2016), and is referred to as persistent pain after this point. Persistent or chronic pain may result from conditions such as osteoarthritis, rheumatoid arthritis, chronic back pain, myalgias, other rheumatologic conditions, or cancer.
Peripheral nociceptive pain	Caused by mechanical deformation mediated by stretch receptors (e.g., pain related to the bowel is either visceral obstruction or renal colic; described as "colicky," "cramping," and "squeezing"; poorly localized and referred). Somatic pain is caused by tissue injury mediated by pain receptors (e.g., pain related to a fracture or joint pain from osteoarthritis; described as "aching," "stabbing," and "throbbing"; well localized). Most often, the degree of pain is proportional to the degree of tissue injury. Nociceptive pain usually responds to traditional medications and nondrug treatments.
Nociplastic pain	Pain that arises from altered nociception despite no clear evidence of actual or threatened tissue damage causing the activation of peripheral nociceptors or evidence for disease or lesion of the somatosensory system causing the pain.

(continues)

TABLE 26-3 Types of Pain		*(continued)*
Neuropathic pain	Involves disease or injury to either the central or peripheral nervous system. Neuropathic pain is often described as "burning," "pricking," or "shooting" and is often associated with sensory disturbances such as allodynia (i.e., a painful response to a nonpainful stimulus) or paresthesia (i.e., abnormal sensation such as tingling or numbness). Examples include phantom limb pain, postherpetic neuralgia, and diabetic neuropathy. The pain may continue without ongoing tissue damage. This type of pain may not respond to the usual analgesic therapies, but may respond to adjuvant treatments such as tricyclic antidepressants and anticonvulsants.	
Central pain	A special case of neuropathic pain that is caused by damage to pain transmission pathways of the spinothalamic tract or the thalamus itself. Post-stroke syndrome is one such type of central pain.	
Mixed and undetermined pain	Associated with no identifiable pathologic processes and mechanisms; may be widespread and out of proportion to identifiable organic pathology, such as recurrent headaches or fibromyalgia. Treatment is often difficult and usually requires a combination of medications and nondrug therapies, including cognitive-behavioral therapy.	

▶ Summary

With the current and future demographic shifts in the U.S. population, increased recognition of the problem of pain in older adults calls for more research to identify and test new assessment techniques and tools in a variety of settings. The geriatric practitioner can improve skills in this area by keeping in mind the principles of assessment discussed in this chapter. Initiating quality pain assessment and treatment in and between prehospital, acute, long-term, hospice, and ambulatory care settings is a worthwhile effort with the potential to have a considerable positive effect on the quality of life of older adults.

References

Arnstein, P. A., & Herr, K. (2015). *Persistent pain in older adults: Evidence-based practice guideline.* Iowa City, IA: University of Iowa, Csomay Center for Gerontological Excellence. Retrieved from http://www.iowanursingguidelines.com/category-s/124.htm?searching=Y&sort=7&cat=124&show=6&page=4

Booker, S. S., Bartoszczyk, D. A., & Herr, K. A. (2016). Managing pain in frail elders. *American Nurse Today, 11*(4), 1–9. Retrieved from https://americannursetoday.com/managing-pain-frail-elders/

Breland, J. Y., Barrera, T. L., Snow, A. L., Sansgiry, S., Stanley, M. A., Wilson, N., . . . Kunik, M. E. (2015). Correlates of pain intensity in community-dwelling individuals with mild to moderate dementia. *American Journal of Alzheimer's Disease & Other Dementias, 30*(3), 320–325. doi: 10.1177/1533317514545827

Cornelius, R., Herr, K., Gordon, D., & Kretzer, K. (2016). *Acute pain management in older adults: Evidence-based practice guideline.* Iowa City, IA: University of Iowa, Csomay Center for Gerontological Excellence. Retrieved from http://www.iowanursingguidelines.com/category-s/124.htm

DeFrin, R., Amanzio, M., de Tommaso, M., Dimova, V., Filipovic, S., Finn, D. P., . . . Kunz, M. (2015). Experimental pain processing in individuals with cognitive impairment: Current state of the science. *Pain, 156*(8),1396–1408. doi: 10.1097/j.pain.0000000000000195

Docking, R. E. (2016). Role of emerging technologies in geriatric pain management. *Clinics in Geriatric Medicine, 32*(4), 787–795. http://dx.doi.org/10.1016/j.cger.2016.06.011

Eslami, V., Zimmerman, M. E., Grewal, T., Katz, M., & Lipton, R. B. (2016). Pain grade and sleep disturbance in older adults: Evaluation the role of pain, and stress for depressed and non-depressed individuals. *International Journal of Geriatric Psychiatry, 31*(5), 450–457. doi: 10.1002/gps.4349

Fishman, S. M., Young, H. M., Arwood, E. L., Chou, R., Herr, K., Murinson, B. B., . . . Strassels, S. A. (2013). Core competencies for pain management: Results of an interprofessional consensus summit. *Pain Medicine, 14*, 971–981.

Gibson, S., & Lauterbacher, S. (2017). Pain perception and report in persons with dementia. In S. Lauterbacher & S. Gibson (Eds.), *Pain in dementia* (pp. 31–42). Philadelphia, PA: Wolters Kluwer.

Healthy People 2020. (2014). Arthritis, osteoporosis, and chronic back conditions. Retrieved from https://www.healthypeople.gov/2020/topics-objectives/topic/Arthritis-Osteoporosis-and-Chronic-Back-Conditions/objectives

Hunt, L. J., Covinsky, K. E., Yaffe, K., Stephens, C. E., Miao, Y., Boscardin, W. J., & Smith, A. K. (2015). Pain in community-dwelling older adults with dementia: Results from the National Health and Aging Trends Study. *Journal of the American Geriatric Society, 63*(8), 1503–1511. doi: 10.1111/jgs

Krebs, E. E., Lorenz, K. A., Bair, M. J., Damush, T. M., Wu, J., Sutherland, J. M., . . . Kroenke, K. (2009). Development and initial validation of the PEG, a three-item scale assessing pain intensity and interference. *Journal of General Internal Medicine, 24*(6), 733–738. http://dx.doi.org/10.1007/s11606-009-0981-1

Lohman, M. C., Whiteman, K. L., Greenberg, R. L., & Bruce, M. L. (2017). Incorporating persistent pain in phenotypic frailty measurement and prediction of adverse health outcomes. *Journals of Gerontology. Series A, Biological Sciences and Medical Sciences, 72*(2), 216–222. doi: 10.1093/gerona/glw212

Lukas, A., Barber, J. B., Johnson, P., & Gibson, S. J. (2013). Observer-rated pain assessment instruments improve both the detection of pain and the evaluation of pain intensity in people with dementia. *European Journal of Pain, 17*(10), 1558–1568. doi: 10.1002/j.1532-2149.2013.00336.x

National Pain Strategy. (2016). Interagency Pain Research Coordinating Committee. Retrieved from https://iprcc.nih.gov/National_Pain_Strategy/NPS_Main.htm

Patel, K. V., Guralnik, J. M., Dansie, E. J., & Turk, D.C. (2013). Prevalence and impact of pain among older adults in the United States: Findings from the 2011 National Health and Aging Trends Study. *Pain, 154*(12), 2649–2657. doi: 10.1016/j.pain.2013.07.029

Reuben, D. B., Herr, K. A., Pacala, J. T., Pollock, B. G., Potter, J. F., & Semla, T. P. (Eds.). (2017). *Geriatrics at your fingertips.* (19th ed.) New York, NY: American Geriatrics Society.

Shega, J. W., Dale, W., Andrew, M., Paice, J., Rockwood, K., & Weiner, D. (2012). Persistent pain and frailty: A case for homeostenosis. *Journal of the American Geriatrics Society, 60*, 113–117. doi: 10.1111/j.1532-5415.2011.03769.x

CHAPTER 27

Caregiver Assessment

Rhonda J. V. Montgomery, Sandy Atkins, and W. June Simmons

CHAPTER OBJECTIVES

1. Explain the importance of caregivers to the health and well-being of older adults.
2. Describe the tools used to assess caregiver needs, burden, and qualification for services.

KEY TERMS

Caregiver   Burden

▶ Introduction

The vast majority of long-term services and supports for community-dwelling older adults in the United States are provided by family and other informal/unpaid **caregivers**—a contribution amounting to more than $450 billion per year (AARP Public Policy Institute, 2011). Approximately two-thirds of older adults with functional impairments living at home receive all of their care from family members—usually daughters and spouses (Doty, 2010). The spouses are likely to be as old as the care recipient and the daughters tend to be in their 50s or 60s—and both of these groups of caregivers are likely to have their own health and economic challenges. Caregiver assessment and interventions are crucial for the well-being of both the caregiver and the person being cared for. The caregiver can be the most effective partner to healthcare providers in their efforts to prolong independence, health, and quality of life for frail and disabled older adults.

▶ Why Caregiver Assessment Is Important: Demographics and Prevalence

For many, if not most, older adults with complex chronic conditions and functional impairment, the presence and help of a family caregiver is essential to enable the patient to reside at home. The family caregiver is arguably the most important member of a care team. The support that family members provide goes well beyond management of medications and assistance with activities of daily living (ADLs) and mobility. As caregivers, family members provide emotional support for patients and assume the roles of home care workers, nurses, money managers, advocates, drivers, shoppers, and schedulers. They are also communicators with medical personnel, translating medical information and expectations to patients and representing the needs and values of the patients to providers. The presence of a family caregiver has been shown to prevent unnecessary or inappropriate physician and emergency room visits and readmission to hospitals (Bass, Clark, Looman, McCarthy, & Eckert, 2003). There is also strong evidence that family caregivers can prevent or delay out-of-home placement (Lavelle, Mancuso, Huber, & Felver, 2014; Mittelman, Haley, Clay, & Roth, 2006).

Unfortunately, the benefits that family caregivers afford patients come at the cost of increased stress, interference with family and work obligations, and negative impacts on the caregivers' own physical and mental health. Caregivers consistently report poorer subjective health status than non-caregivers (Berglund, Lytsy, & Westerling, 2015; Pinquart & Sorenson, 2003) and commonly experience sleep disturbance, fatigue, pain, loss of physical strength, loss of appetite, and weight loss (Stenberg, Ruland, & Miaakowski, 2010). Numerous studies have shown caregivers to have higher rates, compared to their non-caregiver peers, of depression and chronic conditions including hypertension, high cholesterol, chronic obstructive pulmonary disease (COPD), and heart disease (Beach, Schulz, Yee, & Jackson, 2000; Capistrant, Moon, Berkman, & Glymour, 2012; Ho, Collins, Davis, & Doty, 2005; Ji, Zoller, Sundquist, & Sundquist, 2012; Schulz et al., 2009; Vitaliano, Zhang, & Scanlan, 2003). Alone or cumulatively, these negative outcomes for caregivers often impede the quality of patient care and, ultimately, lead to out-of-home placement of the patient.

Given the significant influence that family caregivers have on the quality of patient care and patient outcomes, and the potential negative impact of caregiving on the health and well-being of both the patient and the caregiver, it is clear that provision of effective support for caregivers is a strategic investment. Yet only recently healthcare providers have begun to include caregiver assessments as a routine part of patient care protocols, largely in response to growing advocacy efforts (Feinberg & Levine, 2015).

▶ Best Practices

Just as good patient care begins with a good assessment, so effective support for family caregivers begins with a good assessment and an understanding of the purpose for the assessment. Because health providers are primarily focused on the needs of the patient, it is not uncommon for them to limit their view of family caregivers, seeing them as merely sources of assistance and of information about the patient's condition. Consequently, when caregiver assessment has been included in patient care protocols, the focus has often been limited to evaluating the caregiver's skills and physical ability to provide the type and level of care needed by the patient. Until recently little, if any, attention was given to the physical and emotional **burden** that caregivers experience and the identification of resources to support their efforts.

A good caregiver assessment will incorporate questions and measures that are both *necessary and sufficient* to (1) identify the caregiver's knowledge and understanding of the patient's needs and (2) assess the well-being and needs of the caregiver. The following domains are suggested for inclusion in a caregiver assessment that addresses both of these purposes:

- Relationship of caregiver to patient
- Types and extent of care tasks
- Other obligations (e.g., family or work obligations)
- Availability of financial and social supports
- The accuracy of the caregiver's knowledge about the patient's condition
- Care tasks and responsibilities
- Physical health
- Depression
- Stress/anxiety/emotional burden
- Strain/quality of the relationship between the caregiver and the patient/relationship burden
- Caregiver's perception regarding the difficulty of the care tasks and responsibilities/workload burden

If the assessor working with the caregiver does not have access to patient information, it is also important to include questions about patient diagnoses and functional levels (e.g., ADL and instrumental activities of daily living [IADL] measures, cognitive status).

When an assessment tool is well constructed, it will include reliable, valid, and normed measures and will be easy to use. Psychometrically sound measures enable the provider to reliably assess the caregiver's current condition, monitor changes, and document success or failure of interventions. A trained staff member with good clinical skills should be able to conduct the assessment in less than an hour in a manner that enables caregivers to easily and willingly share critical information. Most important, the information gained through such an assessment should guide the creation of a care plan for the caregiver and help inform the patient's care plan.

Caregiver assessment cannot be a stand-alone service. Effective caregiver interventions incorporate an assessment of caregivers' needs and preferences, and then tailor interventions accordingly (National Academies of Sciences, 2016). A well-designed assessment is not useful if it does not lead to a care plan that effectively supports the caregiver. To be useful, a caregiver assessment must provide trained professionals with the information necessary to diagnose caregivers' needs and create care plans linked to supports and re sources tailored to those needs. The assessment must also provide a mechanism for ascertaining the success of the care plan and monitoring for changes as the patient's condition worsens.

Although no single assessment tool or process has been widely adopted by healthcare or long-term care providers, a wide array of caregiver assessment measures are available at the Family Caregiver Alliance (2012) website. Additionally, the Rosalyn Carter Institute for Caregiving maintains a database of caregiver interventions on its website (www.rosalynncarter.org/caregiver _intervention_database/), many of which include caregiver assessment tools.

Generally, assessment tools developed for studies of specific caregiver interventions have one or more limitations that make them inappropriate for adoption into routine practice without modification to fit each health and human services setting (Gitlin, Marx, Stanley, & Hodgson, 2015; Nichols, Martindale-Adams, Burns, Zuber, & Graney, 2016). First, many of the available assessments were created specifically for use with caregivers of dementia patients (e.g., Bass et al., 2013; Czaja et al., 2009; Mittelman et al., 2006). Second, assessments designed for multicomponent interventions tend to focus on triaging caregivers based on the limited set of resources that are part of the intervention (e.g., Czaja et al., 2009). Third, assessments developed for intervention studies tend to be too long, because they incorporate questions to determine eligibility for the study and to identify factors affecting outcomes.

▶ Where to Start

Two caregiver assessments have been designed, tested, and used to support the broader population of caregivers. Both assessment processes have been reviewed as part of the Administration of Community Living (ACL, 2017) Aging and Disability Evidence-Based Programs and Practices (ADEPP) program and are included as evidence-based programs on the ACL website (https://www.acl.gov/programs/strengthening -aging-and-disability-networks/aging-and -disability-evidence-based-programs). The BRI Care Consultation intervention (www.benrose .org/bricareconsultation/) is a coaching program that includes an assessment and consultation process conducted via telephone. The Tailored Caregiver Assessment and Referral (TCARE) system (Montgomery, Kwak, Kosloski, & O'Connell Valuch, 2011; see also www.tailored care.com) was specifically designed to assess caregivers' needs and link them with a full array of services available within an organization and the larger community. The TCARE system is based on extensive research and field use and includes an assessment tool, software with embedded decision algorithms that guide the development of care plans tailored to caregivers' specific needs, and a process for ongoing monitoring of caregivers' needs.

Regardless of the instrument used, the rationale for conducting a family caregiver assessment is that the needs of family caregivers are diverse and change over time, and must be addressed to protect the health and spirit of caregivers. Services and supports need to be tailored to the identified needs (Brodaty, Green, & Koschera, 2003).

▶ Practice Challenges

Organizations must overcome two major challenges to implement an effective caregiver assessment process. The first challenge is to convey to the leadership and practice teams the central role that family caregivers play in patient care and patient decision making. The second challenge is to allocate sufficient resources to implement an effective process and services.

All too often, healthcare providers fail to recognize family caregivers as essential care partners and fail to adequately support practitioners by giving them the time and tools needed to assess and address caregivers' needs. For the most part, caregiver assessment and support services are viewed as unfunded "add-on" benefits for which there is no source of third-party payment. Efficient creation of successful care plans for caregivers requires both an established process and sufficient staff time. In the absence of training and an established process, professionals working with families must rely solely on their own skills to interpret and integrate extensive and complex information about the caregiver and the patient. As a result, the creation of a care plan can consume too much staff time and result in care plans that are restricted to the limited range of services with which a care manager is familiar. Caregiver assessment will remain limited in scope and inadequate unless a provider organization recognizes family caregivers as care partners who, with adequate support, can help improve the quality of patient care and the organization's bottom line.

▶ Summary

At the practice level, implementation of a caregiver assessment program requires some level of training for professionals to become informed about the diversity and changing nature of the caregiving experience and the challenges that families and friends can face when they assume the caregiver role. Professionals serving as caregiver specialists also need to be knowledgeable about the availability of resources within organization to support caregivers and have ready access to detailed information about additional resources available in the community.

It is also important to help the caregiver understand the value of assessment and for the assessment to occur at a time and place that is convenient for family members and professionals (Levine, Halper, Rutberg, & Gould, 2013). While in-home visits are often seen as the best option, the time and resources required for such visits may be prohibitive. Often the best time to conduct caregiver assessment is when the caregiver accompanies a patient for a physician visit or a medical procedure that entails waiting on the part of the caregiver. Regardless of location, it is best to avoid conducting a caregiver assessment in the presence of the patient. Because the primary focus of family caregivers is the needs of the patient, it is critical to first assure the caregiver that the needs of the patient will be addressed. Only then will caregivers be open to help with addressing their own needs.

References

AARP Public Policy Institute. (2011). *Valuing the invaluable: 2011 update, the economic value of family caregiving.* Washington, DC: Author.

Administration on Community Living (ACL). (2017, April 30). Aging and disability evidence-based programs and practices. Retrieved from https://www.acl.gov /programs/strengthening-aging-and-disability-networks /aging-and-disability-evidence-based-programs/

Bass, D. M., Clark, P. A., Looman, W. J., McCarthy, C. A., & Eckert, S. (2003). The Cleveland Alzheimer's managed care demonstration: Outcomes after 12 months of implementation. *Gerontologist, 43*(1), 73–85.

Bass, D. M., Judge, K. S., Lynn Snow, A., Wilson, N. L., Morgan, R., Looman, W. J., . . . Kunik, M. E. (2013). Caregiver outcomes of Partners in Dementia Care: Effect of a care coordination program for veterans with dementia and their family members and friends. *Journal of the American Geriatrics Society, 61*(8), 1377–1386.

Beach, S. R., Schulz, R., Yee, J. L., & Jackson, S. (2000). Negative and positive health effects of caring for a disabled spouse: Longitudinal findings from the Caregiver Health Effects Study. *Psychology and Aging, 15*(2), 259–271.

Berglund, E., Lytsy, P., & Westerling, R. (2015). Health and wellbeing in informal caregivers and noncaregivers: A comparative cross-sectional study of the Swedish general population. *Health and Quality of Life Outcomes, 13*(1), 1–11.

Brodaty, H., Green, A., & Koschera, A. (2003). Meta-analysis of psychosocial interventions for caregivers of people with dementia. *Journal of the American Geriatrics Society, 51*(5), 657–664.

Capistrant, B. D., Moon, J. R., Berkman, L. F., & Glymour, M. M. (2012). Current and long-term spousal caregiving and onset of cardiovascular disease. *Journal of Epidemiology and Community Health, 66*(10), 951–956.

Czaja, S. J., Gitlin, L. N., Schulz, R., Zhang, S., Burgio, L. D., Stevens, A. B., . . . Gallagher-Thompson, D. (2009). Development of the Risk Appraisal Measure: A brief screen to identify risk areas and guide interventions for dementia caregivers. *Journal of the American Geriatrics Society, 57*(6), 1064–1072.

Doty, P. (2010). The evolving balance of formal and informal, institutional and non-institutional long-term care for older Americans: A thirty-year perspective. *Public Policy & Aging Report, 20*(1), 3–9.

Family Caregiver Alliance. (2012, December). *Selected caregiver assessment measures: A resource inventory for practitioners* (2nd ed.). Retrieved from https:// www.caregiver.org/sites/caregiver.org/files/pdfs /SelCGAssmtMeas_ResInv_FINAL_12.10.12.pdf

Feinberg, L. F., & Levine, C. (2015). Family caregiving: Looking to the future. *Generations, 39*(4), 11–20.

Gitlin, L. N., Marx, K., Stanley, I. H., & Hodgson, N. (2015). Translating evidence-based dementia caregiving interventions into practice: State-of-the-science and next steps. *Gerontologist, 55*(2), 210–226.

Ho, A., Collins, S. R., Davis, K., & Doty, M. M. (2005). A look at working-age caregivers' roles, health concerns, and need for support. *Issue Brief (Commonwealth Fund), 854*, 1–12.

Ji, J., Zoller, B., Sundquist, K., & Sundquist, J. (2012). Increased risks of coronary heart disease and stroke among spousal caregivers of cancer patients. *Circulation, 125*(14), 1742–1747.

Lavelle, B., Mancuso, D., Huber, A., & Felver, B. E. M. (2014). *Expanding the eligibility for family caregiver support program in SFY: Updated findings.* Olympia, WA: Department of Social and Health Services, Research and Data Analysis Division.

Levine, C., Halper, D., Rutberg, J., & Gould, D. A. (2013). Engaging family caregivers as partners in transitions. TC–QuIC: A Quality Improvement Collaborative. Retrieved from https://www.uhfnyc.org/assets/1111

Mittelman, M. S., Haley, W. E., Clay, O. J., & Roth, D. L. (2006). Improving caregiver well-being delays nursing home placement of patients with Alzheimer's disease. *Neurology, 67*(9), 1592–1599.

Montgomery, R. J. V., Kwak, J., Kosloski, K., & O'Connell Valuch, K. (2011). Effects of the TCARE⁻ intervention on caregiver burden and depressive symptoms: Preliminary findings from a randomized controlled study. *Journals of Gerontology, Series B: Psychological Sciences and Social Sciences, 66*(5), 640–647. doi: 10.1093 /geronb/gbr088

National Academies of Sciences. (2016). *Families caring for an aging America.* Washington, DC: The National Academies Press. doi: 10.17226/23606

Nichols, L. O., Martindale-Adams, J., Burns, R., Zuber, J., & Graney, M. J. (2016). REACH VA: Moving from translation to system implementation. *Gerontologist, 56*(1), 135–144.

Pinquart, M., & Sorensen, S. (2003). Differences between caregivers and noncaregivers in psychological health and physical health: A meta-analysis. *Psychology and Aging, 18*(2), 250–267. doi: 10.1037/0882-7974.18.2.250

Schulz, R., Beach, S. R., Hebert, R. S., Martire, L. M., Monin, J. K., Tompkins, C. A., & Albert, S. M. (2009). Spousal suffering and partner's depression and cardiovascular disease: The Cardiovascular Health Study. *American Journal of Geriatric Psychiatry, 17*(3), 246–254.

Stenberg, U., Ruland, C. M., & Miaakowski, C. (2010). Review of the literature on the effects of caring for a patient with cancer. *Journal of Psycho-Oncology, 19*(10), 1099–1611.

Vitaliano, P. P., Zhang, J., & Scanlan, J. M. (2003). Is caregiving hazardous to one's physical health? A meta-analysis. *Psychological Bulletin, 129*(6), 946–972. doi: 10.1037/0033-2909.129.6.946

CHAPTER 28

Spiritual Assessment as a Key Component of Comprehensive Geriatric Care

Betty Ferrell and Anne Reb

CHAPTER OBJECTIVES

1. Define the concept of spirituality and describe the importance of spirituality in geriatric assessment and care.
2. Identify spiritual assessment tools for use in geriatric care.
3. Recognize how spiritual assessment can direct spiritual interventions.
4. Apply the principles of spiritual assessment to a case example.

KEY WORDS

Geriatric care	Spirituality
Spiritual assessment	

▶ Introduction

Spirituality is a key aspect of quality of life that frequently becomes more important as individuals age or experience serious illness. Spirituality is often thought of as synonymous with religion, yet current consensus definitions have provided an expanded view of this concept. In 2009, a national consensus conference of more than 50 interdisciplinary experts defined spirituality as "The aspect of humanity that refers to the way individuals seek and express meaning and purpose and the way they experience their connectedness to the moment, to self, to others, to nature and to the significant or sacred" (Puchalski et al., 2009, p. 887).

The definition of spirituality takes on important meaning as older individuals reflect on their lives, their legacy, a lifetime of relationships, and decades of sometimes changing religious affiliations. Participation in religious practices and services has positive effects on mental health and provides a source of social and emotional support for many older adults (McFarland, 2010). Participation in formal religion tends to decline when health and mobility issues arise, although individual spiritual practices such as prayer, reading the Bible, and meditating are prevalent in adults age 65 and older (Maddox, 2013; Pew Research Center, 2014). Despite the decline in formal religious affiliation, 65% of American adults age 65 and older believe religion is "very important" and another 20% rate it as "somewhat important" (Pew Research Center, 2014). Compared with younger adults, older adults are more likely to view religion, and more broadly spirituality, as important (Nelson-Becker, 2018). Individuals with terminal illnesses often value spirituality as a key contributor to quality of life and as a resource to help them to cope with their illness (Taylor, 2015).

▶ Spirituality and Health Outcomes

Research supports a relationship between spirituality and improved health outcomes such as recovery from illness, finding meaning, and quality of life (Puchalski, 2015). Spirituality is often associated with other geriatric outcomes such as depression, distress, and anxiety (Jim et al., 2015; Salsman et al., 2015; Sherman et al., 2015). Higher levels of spirituality predict better mental and physical health (Hodge, 2015). In *Spirituality, Religion, and Aging*, social work scholar Holly Nelson-Becker (2018) reviews definitions of spirituality related to aging. Kathleen

Fischer (1998) defines spirituality as not just one compartment of life, but rather as the deepest dimension of life. Individuals' spiritual awareness typically increases as they face the end of life, and researchers have found that attention to patients' and family members' spirituality at this critical point in time is vitally important (Taylor, 2015).

Healthcare professionals are tasked with examining the state of their patients' spiritual health, so as to render care that supports the best possible quality of life. Spiritual well-being "concerns our inner life and our relationship with the outside world ... the environment, others, and with ourselves, but the focus is on maintaining or regaining healthy balance" (Nelson-Becker, 2018, p. 42).

Spiritual suffering or distress is the opposite of spiritual well-being. Suffering individuals experience distress as they grapple with existential questions related to the meaning they have achieved—or failed to achieve—in life (Nelson-Becker, 2018). Major life changes, loss, grief, loss of faith, and concerns with meaning and purpose in life can all cause individuals to experience spiritual distress. Conversely, spiritual issues can cause or influence physical and psychological symptoms such as depression, anxiety, and pain (Puchalski, 2015). Spiritual care or promoting spiritual health is intended to relieve spiritual distress and to bring about spiritual healing (Nelson-Becker, 2018).

Spiritual care begins with a screening or spiritual history. Healthcare practitioners of all disciplines should have basic knowledge and skill in **spiritual assessment** as a component of whole-person, comprehensive care.

▶ Spiritual Assessment

Spiritual assessments are used to reveal spiritual needs, spiritual distress, and spiritual resources (Ferrell, Borneman, & Reb, in press). Spiritual needs include a wide array of issues, such as a relationship with a higher power, needs for forgiveness, regrets, and meaning or purpose in life.

Spiritual resources may include a patient's faith community, or friends and family who serve as sources of support.

Spiritual assessments are performed in two stages. The first stage involves a brief, initial screening, which is then followed by a second, more in-depth assessment or spiritual history to determine whether spiritual needs exist (Ferrell et al., in press). The initial screening can reveal the person's religious or spiritual orientation and whether further in-depth assessment is needed (Puchalski et al., 2009). Spiritual assessments should occur at the initiation of care and continue throughout the period of clinical care, as patients or clients may grow more comfortable with their clinicians and begin to reveal their concerns or problems related to this realm (Nelson-Becker, 2018). Also, spiritual assessments should be performed whenever a patient's health status changes (Puchalski, 2015). For example, a patient may decline a referral to chaplaincy, but if a life-threatening disease is diagnosed, the patient or family may then perceive that chaplaincy would be helpful.

Clinicians providing **geriatric care** are challenged to identity efficient assessment tools given the imperative to measure multiple domains of geriatric care. These domains include function, psychosocial issues, social support, quality of life, and symptoms associated with chronic illness. Notably, an ever-increasing body of evidence suggests that spirituality is also an important dimension of care (Brady, Peterman, Fitchett, Mo, & Cella, 1999; Steinhauser et al., 2000). The National Comprehensive Cancer Network's (2016a) Distress Management guidelines define spiritual distress and symptoms and provide recommendations for provision of spiritual care including chaplaincy care (Puchalski, 2015).

Initial spiritual screening can be done by nurses, social workers, physicians, or chaplains on a medical team to identify those patients most in need of spiritual care. Chaplains are the spiritual care specialists who conduct a more detailed spiritual assessment and can advise clinicians on how to help with patients' spiritual issues. They can also coordinate involvement of clergy and parish nurses, if appropriate (Puchalski, 2015). Unfortunately, chaplains are often too few in number given the overwhelming demands of busy inpatient and outpatient care settings. It is not uncommon for hospitals to have only one chaplain for several hundred beds in the inpatient setting, and no chaplaincy in the outpatient setting. Given this reality, it is important for all clinicians to possess the basic skills to assess spiritual needs so as to identify those patients most in need of spiritual support. The findings from the spiritual assessment, including spiritual beliefs and values, should be incorporated into the care plan (Puchalski, 2015).

▶ Spiritual Screening Tools

Numerous instruments exist to measure spirituality, although most have been designed for research use rather than clinical application. Several papers have evaluated spiritual assessment tools (Koenig, 2011; Koenig, King, & Carson, 2012; Lucchetti, Bassi, & Lucchetti, 2013; Monod et al., 2011; Selman, Harding, Gysels, Speck, & Higginson, 2011; Selman, Siegert, et al., 2011). A recent paper by Steinhauser and colleagues (2017) provides a state-of-the-science review of spirituality research in palliative care, including exploration of spirituality, outcomes, and measures. Nelson-Becker (2018) recommends that an initial screening pose the following reflective questions:

- What helps you to experience a deep sense of meaning, purpose, hope, or guidance for values in your life?
- Is spirituality, religion, or faith important in your life? If so, please give examples. If not, please explain why they are not important, or if you prefer, we do not need to discuss this.
- If important to you, what terms for referring to spirituality, religion, or faith do you prefer?
- Would you like to incorporate "spirituality, religion, or faith" (or "meaning, life satisfaction" if patient prefers these terms) in our work together? Please explain.

Various other brief assessment tools that may be useful in geriatric assessment can be found in **TABLE 28-1**. Dr. Christina Puchalski and colleagues developed the FICA Spiritual History Tool, which is probably the most widely cited spiritual assessment instrument (Puchalski, 2010; Puchalski & Romer, 2000). The domains assessed with this tool include (1) faith, belief, and what gives meaning in one's life; (2) importance of faith or spiritual practices in one's life and how these values influence coping and healthcare decision making; (3) participation in a spiritual or religious community or other support groups; and (4) interventions to address spiritual needs. The FICA Spiritual History Tool is designed to elicit a patient's spiritual history—specifically,

those elements that a clinician would need to know in a clinical setting—and has been validated in patients with cancer (Borneman, Ferrell, & Puchalski, 2010).

Another widely used mnemonic assessment tool is HOPE (Anandarajah & Hight, 2001). The HOPE assessment format is an especially easy one for healthcare professionals to remember and to use. In this tool, H denotes the sources of hope, meaning, comfort, strength, peace, love, and connection; O is for organized religion; P represents personal spirituality and practices; and E is for effects on medical care and end-of-life issues. The HOPE tool addresses terminal event planning, provides for ongoing spiritual care, and has been purported to have fewer religious

TABLE 28-1 Spiritual Assessment Tools	
Tool	**Description**
FICA (Puchalski & Romer, 2000)	Open-ended questions assess: ■ **F:** Faith/spirituality ■ **I:** Importance of spirituality ■ **C:** Faith community ■ **A:** Patient preference for addressing spirituality in health care
"Are you at peace" (Steinhauser et al., 2006)	Single item measure developed by Steinhauser
SPIRIT (Maugans, 1996)	Assesses: ■ **S:** Spiritual belief system ■ **P:** Personal spirituality ■ **I:** Integration with a spiritual community ■ **R:** Ritualized practices and restrictions ■ **I:** Implications for medical care ■ **T:** Terminal event planning
FACIT (Peterman, Fitchett, Brady, Hernandez, & Cella, 2002)	12-item instrument; ordinal scale measures dimensions of religious and existential/spiritual well-being
HOPE (Anandarajah & Hight, 2001)	Measures sources of: ■ **H:** Hope ■ **O:** Organized religion ■ **P:** Personal spiritual practices ■ **E:** Effects on medical care and/or issues

overtones compared to some other brief screening tools (Blaber, Jones, & Willis, 2015).

Another spiritual assessment tool is titled SPIRIT (Maugans, 1996). This mnemonic tool assesses the patient's formal religious affiliation and personal belief practices, sources of support, daily spiritual rituals and restrictions, and implications for medical and end-of- life care.

The Functional Assessment of Chronic Illness Therapy—Spiritual Well-being (FACIT-Sp-12) is a short 12-item instrument that has been used in health-related research (Peterman et al., 2002). It includes subscales measuring faith, meaning, and peace and is a widely used measure in patients with cancer (Munoz, Salsman, Stein, & Cella, 2015).

The Spiritual Distress Assessment Tool (SDAT) is a relatively new spiritual distress tool that has been tested with older hospitalized adults (Monod et al., 2010). In studies using this instrument, 65% of older hospitalized patients reported some distress, with 22% reporting serious spiritual distress on at least one item (Monod, Martin, Spencer, Rochat, & Bula, 2012). Patients and clinicians have found SDAT to be a valuable assessment tool that assesses five areas of spiritual need, termed *unmet needs*: (1) need for life balance, (2) need for connection, (3) values acknowledgment, (4) need to maintain control, and (5) need to maintain identity. The patient's needs are assessed with regard to each category, including the extent to which these needs have not been met (Nelson-Becker, 2018).

▶ Practice Challenges in Performing a Spiritual Assessment

Even with the right assessment tool, initiating a spiritual assessment may not be an easy task. Older patients may be reluctant to raise spiritual topics; moreover, if these topics are introduced by the nurse, patients may be hesitant to engage in a discussion about them. By definition, spiritual needs are personal, often complex issues, and the patient may not be comfortable enough initially to discuss them. Religion may have caused the patient pain or suffering in the past—a possibility that should be kept in mind (Nelson-Becker, 2018). However, research supports that most patients want their healthcare providers to address their religious and spiritual concerns, and a significant subset report that their spiritual needs are not adequately met (Blaber et al., 2015; Peteet & Balboni, 2013). In a study addressing spiritual issues across the bone marrow transplant trajectory, patients reported a desire for their healthcare team to discuss spiritual issues especially at critical junctures such as diagnosis, post-transplant, and survivorship (Sinclair et al., 2015). Patients appreciated providers who listened carefully for spiritual concerns, engaged in a meaning-based conversation, and used a "non-agenda" approach.

Once spiritual needs are identified, clinicians may feel unprepared or uncomfortable addressing the issues that arise. When spiritual themes arise, the clinician can follow up with open-ended questions and listen reflectively to understand the patient's concerns. Compassionate listening to the patient's and family's story may reveal spiritual issues such as anger, feeling abandoned by God, lack of meaning, despair, and forgiveness needs (Puchalski, 2015). The clinician can initiate a referral to a chaplain or pastoral counselor if religious and spiritual symptoms are identified (Denlinger et al., 2016). Referrals can also be made to a social worker or mental health professional depending on the symptoms and the patient's preferences. According to Taylor (2015), it is important that nurses explore how their own spiritual beliefs may affect their interaction with their patients. She counsels that nurses develop their own "spiritual self-awareness" so that they will be prepared to assist a patient in addressing spiritual needs. For example, nurses can ask themselves similar questions they anticipate asking their patients (Taylor, 2015).

The clinician must decide on a case-by-case basis whether a structured instrument would be helpful in assessing a patient's spiritual needs or whether a general clinical assessment would be more useful. Some spiritual experiences do not lend themselves to measurement (Nelson-Becker, 2018). For example, spiritual themes may arise in the context of listening to patients' stories about their diagnosis or exploring their most important concerns. Incorporating the cultural context in discussions about spirituality is also important (Puchalski, Vitillo, Hull, & Reller, 2014). For example, spiritual genograms may be useful when working with Muslims, as they incorporate the patients' relationships with family members into the assessment process (Hodge, 2015).

Time and practice constraints may also influence which assessment approach is taken. Use of brief spiritual screening tools should be incorporated in palliative care and other settings, as they are accessible to everyday care providers and promote holistic patient-centered care (Blaber et al., 2015). For inpatients, a spiritual screening should be included in the psychosocial section of the intake assessment (Puchalski, 2010). In outpatient settings, a diagnosis of a life-threatening illness, cancer recurrence, symptoms such as unrelieved pain, or a psychosocial issue may prompt an inquiry into the patient's fears, concerns, and coping resources that may be linked to spiritual or existential issues. Incorporating screening instruments as part of usual care may facilitate exploration of spiritual issues and concerns.

Despite the practice constraints and/or difficulties in performing a spiritual assessment, healthcare professionals should remember that spiritual assessment is the first step in identifying a patient's spiritual needs, which can then lead to appropriate spiritual care. Rendering spiritual care and helping to restore or ensure a patient's spiritual well-being are integral to effective palliative care. Since an assessment can and should be performed not just once, but on an ongoing basis, the nurse should gather spiritual needs data as they are revealed in the everyday encounters (Taylor, 2015).

▶ Which Tool to Use?

As described earlier, many instruments are available for clinical assessment and research purposes to assess spirituality and many factors should be considered. Based on the authors' experiences over many years, we offer the following general advice.

For clinical assessment, the FICA tool developed by Puchalski, a geriatrician and national leader in spirituality, offers a simple approach and provides clinicians with the language to best communicate with patients about spirituality. The tool and extensive information about it is available on the George Washington Institute for Spirituality and Health website (https://smhs.gwu.edu/gwish/).

For research purposes or for a more comprehensive assessment of spirituality providing quantitative scoring, we recommend the FACIT-Sp-12 tool (www.FACIT.org). This simple 12-item tool offers the benefit of assessing dimensions of spirituality including faith, meaning, and peace.

ASSESSMENT EXEMPLAR

Mr. Pedro Garcia is a 78-year-old man who has been seen in a community medicine clinic for the past 20 years. He has been well managed for multiple chronic illnesses including hypertension, diabetes, and arthritis. For the past 12 years, Mr. Garcia cared for his wife, Emelia, during a difficult course of Alzheimer's disease. Emelia was placed in a long-term care facility one year ago and died six months later.

Today, Mr. Garcia was being seen in the oncology clinic and received the results of recent tests, which revealed a diagnosis of Stage IV colon cancer. Mr. Garcia says he is not surprised, as he has had symptoms for the past two years but was just too busy caring for Emelia to focus on his own health.

The oncology nurse practitioner sees Mr. Garcia after the oncologist shares the diagnostic information. The nurse practitioner conducts a comprehensive assessment to assist in identifying treatment options. The assessment includes aspects of Mr. Garcia's medication history and cognition. The nurse practitioner tells Mr. Garcia that the oncology clinic also seeks to provide spiritual support to patients facing a serious diagnosis of colon cancer. She uses the FICA assessment tool to gather information about Mr. Garcia's faith, religion, spiritual community, and resources. Mr. Garcia shares that he "was Catholic" but has not attended mass in two years and has struggled to keep his faith after seeing all the suffering Emelia endured.

The nurse, sensing Mr. Garcia's distress, also asks the spiritual assessment question, "Are you at peace?" (Steinhauser et al., 2006). Mr. Garcia says that he feels he has been "a good man" but notes that he is estranged from his son, who could not understand why he had to place Emelia in long-term care. The nurse asks Mr. Garcia if he would like to be introduced to the clinic chaplain at his next clinic visit, and he agrees. She also shares the spiritual assessment and the other comprehensive assessment information with the oncology team in their weekly review of new patients.

Case Commentary

The case of Mr. Garcia illustrates the importance of spiritual assessment as a component of comprehensive patient assessment. By using the FICA tool to guide the spiritual assessment as well as the single-item "at peace" measure, the nurse has gained important information about the patient's spirituality, encompassing aspects of religion, life meaning, distress, and relationships. The assessment findings will be shared with the interdisciplinary team, so that clinicians can provide spiritual support to Mr. Garcia.

▶ Summary

As with other aspects of geriatric assessment, spirituality assessment is performed to identify needs and possible strategies for care. Spiritual assessment can be useful in identifying areas of distress—for example, spiritual longing, broken relationships, need for forgiveness, religious or spiritual struggles, and need for chaplaincy to provide rituals, religious/spiritual coping, and support. If spiritual distress is identified, treatment or care plans can include referral to chaplains and other spiritual care providers for spiritual counseling. If patients experience guilt or hopelessness with depressive symptoms, they should also be referred to a mental health professional for further assessment (National Comprehensive Cancer Network, 2016a). Care plans may include spiritual goals, mind–body interventions, spiritual practices, journaling, and other contemplative interventions (Puchalski, 2015). **BOX 28-1** lists resources for additional information regarding spirituality in health care.

BOX 28-1 Key Resources for Clinicians

- George Washington University Institute for Spirituality in Health: https://smhs.gwu.edu/gwish/
- City of Hope Pain/Palliative Care Resource Center: http://prc.coh.org (See Spirituality Section)
- Puchalski, C., & Ferrell, B. (2010). *Making health care whole*. West Conshohocken, PA: Templeton Press.
- Cobb, M., Puchalski, C. M., & Rumbold, B. (Eds.). (2012). *Oxford textbook of spirituality in healthcare*. New York, NY: Oxford University Press.

Recently, life review interventions such as Dignity Therapy have been tested to assist seriously ill patients in reviewing their lives, addressing meaning and legacy (Chochinov et al., 2011; Steinhauser, Alexander, Byock, George, & Tulsky, 2009). Mindfulness practices have been shown to benefit older adults and may be an inclusive spiritual approach for baby boomers who identify with a more secular view of spirituality (Stevens, 2016). Mindfulness practices such as meditation, yoga, qigong, guided imagery, and relaxation therapies incorporate physical, mental, social, and existential dimensions. Mindfulness training can enhance psychological resilience and foster the search for meaning and other psychosocial tasks relevant during this phase of life (Nilsson, 2014). Many of these practices are accessible even to those with significant physical limitations.

Spirituality is a key component of quality of life, and older people may have even greater spirituality-related concerns as they face chronic or serious illness. Spiritual assessment is an interdisciplinary commitment and is critical to quality geriatric care.

References

Anandarajah, G., & Hight, E. (2001). Spirituality and medical practice: Using the HOPE questions as a practical tool for spiritual assessment. *American Family Physician, 63*(1), 81–89.

Blaber, M., Jones, J., & Willis, D. (2015). Spiritual care: Which is the best assessment tool for palliative settings? *International Journal of Palliative Nursing, 21*(9), 430–438. doi: 10.12968/ijpn.2015.21.9.430

Borneman, T., Ferrell, B., & Puchalski, C. M. (2010). Evaluation of the FICA tool for spiritual assessment. *Journal of Pain and Symptom Management, 40*(2), 163–173. doi: 10.1016/j.jpainsymman.2009.12.019

Brady, M. J., Peterman, A. H., Fitchett, G., Mo, M., & Cella, D. (1999). A case for including spirituality in quality of life measurement in oncology. *Psychooncology, 8*(5), 417–428.

Chochinov, H. M., Kristjanson, L. J., Breitbart, W., McClement, S., Hack, T. F., Hassard, T., & Harlos, M. (2011). Effect of dignity therapy on distress and end-of-life experience in terminally ill patients: A randomised controlled trial. *Lancet Oncology, 12*(8), 753–762. doi: 10.1016/s1470-2045(11)70153-x

Denlinger, C. S., Ligibel, J. A., Are, M., Baker, K. S., Broderick, G., Demark-Wahnefried, W., ... Ku, G. H. (2016). NCCN guidelines insights: Survivorship, version 1.2016. *Journal of the National Comprehensive Cancer Network, 14*(6), 715–724.

Ferrell, B., Borneman, T., & Reb, A. (In press). Spirituality and cancer survivorship. In P. J. Haylock & C. Curtiss (Eds.), *Cancer survivorship: Transdisciplinary, patient-centered approaches to the seasons of survival.* Pittsburgh, PA: Oncology Nursing Society.

Fischer, K. (1998). *Winter grace: Spirituality and aging.* Nashville, TN: Upper Room.

Hodge, D. R. (2015). Administering a two-stage spiritual assessment in healthcare settings: A necessary component of ethical and effective care. *Journal of Nursing Management, 23*(1), 27–38. doi: 10.1111/jonm.12078

Jim, H. S., Pustejovsky, J. E., Park, C. L., Danhauer, S. C., Sherman, A. C., Fitchett, G., ... Salsman, J. M. (2015). Religion, spirituality, and physical health in cancer patients: A meta-analysis. *Cancer, 121*(21), 3760–3768. doi: 10.1002/cncr.29353

Koenig, H. (2011). *Spirituality and health research: Methods, measurement, statistics, and resources.* West Conshohocken, PA: Templeton Press.

Koenig, H. G., King, D., & Carson, V. B. (2012). *Handbook of religion and health* (2nd ed.). New York, NY: Oxford University Press.

Lucchetti, G., Bassi, R. M., & Lucchetti, A. L. (2013). Taking spiritual history in clinical practice: A systematic review of instruments. *Explore (NY), 9*(3), 159–170. doi: 10.1016/j.explore.2013.02.004

Maddox, G. L. (2013). *The encyclopedia of aging: A comprehensive resource in gerontology and geriatrics.* New York, NY: Springer.

Maugans, T. A. (1996). The SPIRITual history. *Archives of Family Medicine, 5*(1), 11–16.

McFarland, M. J. (2010). Religion and mental health among older adults: Do the effects of religious involvement vary by gender? *Journals of Gerontology, Series BL Psychological Sciences and Social Sciences, 65*(5), 621–630. doi: 10.1093/geronb/gbp112

Monod, S., Brennan, M., Rochat, E., Martin, E., Rochat, S., & Bula, C. J. (2011). Instruments measuring spirituality in clinical research: A systematic review. *Journal of General Internal Medicine, 26*(11), 1345–1357. doi: 10.1007/s11606-011-1769-7

Monod, S., Martin, E., Spencer, B., Rochat, E., & Bula, C. (2012). Validation of the Spiritual Distress Assessment Tool in older hospitalized patients. *BMC Geriatrics, 12,* 13. doi: 10.1186/1471-2318-12-13

Monod, S., Rochat, E., Bula, C. J., Jobin, G., Martin, E., & Spencer, B. (2010). The Spiritual Distress Assessment Tool: An instrument to assess spiritual distress in hospitalised elderly persons. *BMC Geriatrics, 10,* 88. doi: 10.1186/1471-2318-10-88

Munoz, A. R., Salsman, J. M., Stein, K. D., & Cella, D. (2015). Reference values of the Functional Assessment of Chronic Illness Therapy—Spiritual Well-Being: a report from the American Cancer Society's studies of cancer survivors. *Cancer, 121*(11), 1838–1844. doi: 10.1002/cncr.29286

National Comprehensive Cancer Network. (2016a). Distress management (version 2.2016). Retrieved from https://www.nccn.org/professionals/physician_gls/f_guidelines.asp#supportive

Nelson-Becker, H. (2018). *Spirituality, religion, and aging.* Thousand Oaks, CA: Sage.

Nilsson, H. (2014). A four-dimensional model of mindfulness and its implications for health. *Psychology of Religion and Spirituality, 6*(2), 162–174.

Peteet, J. R., & Balboni, M. J. (2013). Spirituality and religion in oncology. *CA: Cancer Journal for Clinicians, 63*(4), 280–289. doi: 10.3322/caac.21187

Peterman, A. H., Fitchett, G., Brady, M. J., Hernandez, L., & Cella, D. (2002). Measuring spiritual well-being in people with cancer: The Functional Assessment of Chronic Illness Therapy—Spiritual Well-being Scale (FACIT-Sp). *Annals of Behavioral Medicine, 24*(1), 49–58.

Pew Research Center. (2014). Religious Landscape Study: Religious composition of adults ages 65 and older. Retrieved from http://www.pewforum.org/religious-landscape-study/age-distribution/65/

Puchalski, C. (2010). Formal and informal spiritual assessment. *Asian Pacific Journal of Cancer Prevention, 11*(Suppl. 1), 51–57.

Puchalski, C. (2015). Spirituality in geriatric palliative care. *Clinics in Geriatric Medicine, 31*(2), 245–252. doi: 10.1016/j.cger.2015.01.011

Puchalski, C., Ferrell, B., Virani, R., Otis-Green, S., Baird, P., Bull, J., … Sulmasy, D. (2009). Improving the quality of spiritual care as a dimension of palliative care: The report of the Consensus Conference. *Journal of Palliative Medicine, 12*(10), 885–904. doi: 10.1089/jpm.2009.0142

Puchalski, C., & Romer, A. L. (2000). Taking a spiritual history allows clinicians to understand patients more fully. *Journal of Palliative Medicine, 3*(1), 129–137. doi: 10.1089/jpm.2000.3.129

Puchalski, C., Vitillo, R., Hull, S. K., & Reller, N. (2014). Improving the spiritual dimension of whole person care: Reaching national and international consensus. *Journal of Palliative Medicine, 17*(6), 642–656. doi: 10.1089/jpm.2014.9427

Salsman, J. M., Pustejovsky, J. E., Jim, H. S., Munoz, A. R., Merluzzi, T. V., George, L., … Fitchett, G. (2015). A meta-analytic approach to examining the correlation between religion/spirituality and mental health in cancer. *Cancer, 121*(21), 3769–3778. doi: 10.1002/cncr.29350

Selman, L., Harding, R., Gysels, M., Speck, P., & Higginson, I. J. (2011). The measurement of spirituality in palliative care and the content of tools validated cross-culturally: A systematic review. *Journal of Pain and Symptom Management, 41*(4), 728–753. doi: 10.1016/j.jpainsymman.2010.06.023

Selman, L., Siegert, R., Harding, R., Gysels, M., Speck, P., & Higginson, I. J. (2011). A psychometric evaluation of measures of spirituality validated in culturally diverse palliative care populations. *Journal of Pain and Symptom Management, 42*(4), 604–622. doi: 10.1016/j.jpainsymman.2011.01.015

Sherman, A. C., Merluzzi, T. V., Pustejovsky, J. E., Park, C. L., George, L., Fitchett, G., … Salsman, J. M. (2015). A meta-analytic review of religious or spiritual involvement and social health among cancer patients. *Cancer, 121*(21), 3779–3788. doi: 10.1002/cncr.29352

Sinclair, S., McConnell, S., Raffin Bouchal, S., Ager, N., Booker, R., Enns, B., & Fung, T. (2015). Patient and healthcare perspectives on the importance and efficacy of addressing spiritual issues within an interdisciplinary bone marrow transplant clinic: A qualitative study. *BMJ Open, 5*(11), e009392. doi: 10.1136/bmjopen-2015-009392

Steinhauser, K. E., Alexander, S. C., Byock, I. R., George, L. K., & Tulsky, J. A. (2009). Seriously ill patients' discussions of preparation and life completion: An intervention to assist with transition at the end of life. *Palliative and Supportive Care, 7*(4), 393–404. doi: 10.1017/s147895150999040x

Steinhauser, K. E., Fitchett, G., Handzo, G. F., Johnson, K. S., Koenig, H. G., Pargament, K. I., … Balboni, T. A. (2017). State of the science of spirituality and palliative care research part I: Definitions, measurement, and outcomes. *Journal of Pain and Symptom Management, 54*(3), 428–440.

Steinhauser, K. E., Christakis, N. A., Clipp, E. C., McNeilly, M., McIntyre, L., & Tulsky, J. A. (2000). Factors considered important at the end of life by patients, family, physicians, and other care providers. *Journal of the American Medical Association, 284*(19), 2476–2482.

Steinhauser, K. E., Voils, C. I., Clipp, E. C., Bosworth, H. B., Christakis, N. A., & Tulsky, J. A. (2006). "Are you at peace?": One item to probe spiritual concerns at the end of life. *Archives of Internal Medicine, 166*(1), 101–105. doi: 10.1001/archinte.166.1.101

Stevens, B. A. (2016). Mindfulness: A positive spirituality for ageing? *Australasian Journal on Ageing, 35*(3), 156–158. doi: 10.1111/ajag.12346

Taylor, E. J. (2015). Spiritual assessment. In B. Ferrell, N. Coyle, & J. A. Paice (Eds.), *Oxford textbook of palliative nursing* (4th ed., pp. 531–545). New York, NY: Oxford University Press.

CHAPTER 29

Substance Use Assessment

Paul Sacco

CHAPTER OBJECTIVES

1. Understand the current prevalence of drinking and other drug use among older adults and projections regarding use and abuse of drugs in the future.
2. Become familiar with substances typically used by older adults as well as risk factors for use and abuse among older adults.
3. Understand unique risks of alcohol and other drug use among older adults compared with younger populations.
4. Learn fundamental tenets of substance use assessment including screening and assessment tools preferred for older adult patients.

KEY TERMS

At-risk drinking
Cannabis
Prescription drug misuse

Screening, Brief Intervention, and Referral for Treatment (SBIRT)

▶ Introduction

For many of older adults, alcohol use is a part of normal aging. Approximately 45% of older adults aged 65 and older report past 12-month alcohol use (Moore et al., 2009). Smaller percentages of older adults (age 65-plus) use other substances, most commonly **cannabis** (1.4%) (Han, Sherman, et al., 2017), opioids (1%), and tranquilizers (0.2%) (Schepis & McCabe, 2016). For many older adults, alcohol and/or other drug use is simply a long-term habit that started earlier in life. In this sense, substance use may provide a sense of continuity for older adults (Burruss, Sacco, & Smith, 2015). For others, however, it may be a distinct change in behavior from earlier life stages; in retirement, alcohol and other drug use may increase because of more free time or because of the stresses associated with aging itself. These processes are likely complex in nature (Kuerbis & Sacco, 2012).

Whether older adults begin to use alcohol or other substances in early adulthood or later in life, they likely use substances for a variety of different but overlapping reasons, including socialization, enhancement, and coping motivations. Social motives refer to the role of alcohol, in particular, as a so-called social lubricant; enhancement motives are simply drinking for the immediate effects of alcohol. In addition to these reasons, older adults may drink as a means of coping with difficult emotions or life experiences (Gilson et al., 2013; Gilson, Bryant, & Judd, 2017). Other research has found that older adults may use alcohol or other drugs for medicinal purposes (Aira, Hartikainen, & Sulkava, 2008; Haug et al., 2017; Immonen, Valvanne, & Pitkälä, 2011).

As a foundation for screening and assessment, it is important to recognize that alcohol and other drug use is common among older adults and commonly seen during clinic visits. A recent multi-site study in primary care found that approximately 13.9% of patients in primary care had an alcohol use disorder and 14% had a drug use disorder (Wu et al., 2017). Although older age is associated with decreased risk of such disorders (Sacco, 2017), it is clear that substance use and substance use disorders are under-recognized in health care. In addition, it is important to note that older adults use alcohol and other drugs for many of the same reasons that younger people do.

A variety of terms are used to describe the spectrum of risk behavior in this population. Current use of alcohol or drugs typically means any use in the past year or past month, and at-risk use refers to exceeding the daily and/or weekly consumption guidelines for alcohol. The term *binge drinking* is synonymous with exceeding daily risk limits, and *heavy drinking* often refers to exceeding total limits. It is notable that drinking limits in guidelines for older adults age 65 and older are much lower than they are for younger groups. The limit for men younger than age 65 is no more than 14 standard drinks per week and no more than 4 drinks on a given occasion. The limit for older adults (men age 65 and older and women of all ages) is no more than 7 standard drinks per week and no more than 3 drinks on a given occasion (National Institute on Alcohol Abuse and Alcoholism, 2007). The term *problem use* describes alcohol and/or drug use that leads to at least one identified problem. The terms *alcohol use disorder* and *drug use disorder* denote an individual who meets the full *Diagnostic and Statistical Manual of Mental Disorders* (*DSM-V*) criteria for these conditions (American Psychiatric Association, 2013). They represent the most severe forms of alcohol- and drug-related problems, respectively, among older adults.

In many cases, older adults who are at risk due to substance use may share specific sociodemographic and health-related risk factors. Men display higher rates of at-risk drinking, alcohol-related disorders (American Psychiatric Association, 2013; Sacco, Bucholz, & Harrington, 2014), and drug use disorder (Wu & Blazer, 2011) compared to women (Blazer & Wu, 2009). Alcohol and drug use disorders are also more common among the youngest older adults, and less common among older seniors (Reynolds, Pietrzak, El-Gabalawy, Mackenzie, & Sareen, 2015). In terms of racial/ethnic differences, white race is positively associated with at-risk patterns of alcohol consumption (e.g., binge drinking and heavy drinking) (Merrick et al., 2008), while African American race may be associated with drug use (specifically cocaine) among older adults (Wu & Blazer, 2011). **At-risk drinking** among older adults may be associated with higher socioeconomic status (Blazer & Wu, 2009; Moos, Brennan, Schutte, & Moos, 2010). Conversely, drug use disorders are more common among individuals with lower levels of income and educational attainment (Wu & Blazer, 2011). Broadly speaking, alcohol (Sacco, Bucholz, & Spitznagel, 2009) and drug-related problems (Wu & Blazer, 2011) among older adults are associated with lower likelihood of being currently married.

Aside from sociodemographic correlates of at-risk drinking and drug use, older adults may present with a variety of comorbid mental health and substance-related conditions. Depression is associated with at-risk drinking (Choi & DiNitto, 2011; Han, Moore, Sherman, Keyes, & Palamar, 2017; Sacco et al., 2009) and drug use (Wu & Blazer, 2011) among older adults, and a variety of anxiety disorders (e.g., generalized anxiety disorder, post-traumatic stress disorder [PTSD], and panic disorders) are also comorbid with alcohol-related problems in older adult populations (Kuerbis, Chernick, & Gardner, 2016). Tobacco use (not reviewed in the current chapter) also commonly co-occurs with at-risk alcohol use (Han, Moore, et al., 2017; Sacco et al., 2009) and drug use (Han, Sherman, et al., 2017). Older adults who have one substance use disorder (e.g., alcohol) frequently use other substances as well, and trend data suggest that today's older adults presenting for treatment services are more commonly using drugs in addition to alcohol compared with previous generations (Arndt, Gunter, & Acion, 2005; Sacco, Kuerbis, Goge, & Bucholz, 2013; Substance Abuse and Mental Health Services Administration, 2011). Although mental health and substance abuse comorbidity are common, older adults who present with alcohol and other drug-related problems may be relatively healthy compared with their non-substance-using peers (Gavens, Goyder, Hock, Harris, & Meier, 2016; Han, Moore, et al., 2017; Holdsworth et al., 2017). Older adults may lose the capacity to use alcohol and other drugs as their health deteriorates, although individuals with drug use disorders often have multiple medical conditions, especially older men (Wu & Blazer, 2011).

Although research has identified risk factors for at-risk alcohol use, drug use, and substance use disorder, these variables are not deterministic in predicting who may suffer consequences related to use. Clinicians should assess all older adults for these issues, because the consequences of untreated problems can be serious. These effects reflect the type of drug used and may arise from acute exposure (e.g., effects of intoxication or medication interaction) or chronic use (e.g., alcoholic liver disease).

Alcohol is the most commonly used substance among older adults. Its acute effects include increased risk of falls, suicide, motor vehicle accidents secondary to intoxication (Sorock, Chen, Gonzalgo, & Baker, 2006), alcohol and drug interactions (Cousins et al., 2014), and insomnia (Kuerbis, Sacco, Blazer, & Moore, 2014). Although older adults are at lower risk for driving under the influence (Fell, Tippetts, & Voas, 2009), changes in metabolism in older adulthood (Meier & Seitz, 2008) may be specifically problematic for them. Laboratory research suggests that even with consumption of moderate amounts of alcohol, older adults experience greater impairment but are less aware of it (Sklar, Boissoneault, Fillmore, & Nixon, 2014; Sklar, Gilbertson, Boissoneault, Prather, & Nixon, 2012). Both chronic and acute alcohol use may lead to greater vulnerability to elder abuse among older drinkers as well (Johannesen & LoGiudice, 2013; Teaster & Brossoie, 2016). Potential chronic effects of alcohol use include alcohol-related liver disease (Ferreira & Weems, 2008) and increased risk for certain types of cancer (i.e., head and neck, liver, pancreas, and breast) (Savage, Finnell, & Choflet, 2016). Low-risk drinking, however, is associated with lower cardiovascular risk and mortality overall—reinforcing the idea that alcohol may have beneficial as well as detrimental effects on health, depending on dose and pattern of use (Ronksley, Brien, Turner, Mukamal, & Ghali, 2011; Smyth et al., 2015).

Compared to alcohol use, the consequences of nonmedical drug use are relatively understudied in older adults. Drugs such as benzodiazepines, opioids, and barbiturates have sedating effects that may lead to problems with falls and other types of accidents in older adults (Kuerbis et al., 2014). Cannabis use may increase risk for a heart attack in the period just after use, and it also affects short-term memory (Kuerbis et al., 2014). Given the current opioid crisis, intentional and unintentional overdoses among older adults are a major concern (West, Severtson, Green, & Dart, 2015). Research on older heroin users has identified a wide swathe of health comorbidities associated with intravenous drug use, including human immunodeficiency virus (HIV) and hepatitis C virus (HCV) infection (Rosen, Hunsaker, Albert, Cornelius, & Reynolds, 2011). The current lack of research in these areas is problematic, as it limits the information that providers can share with older adult patients. For alcohol, there is a clear guideline for safe use, but for other drugs such as cannabis, educating patients about safe use among older adults is more complicated. Less guidance is available for clinicians, even as states move toward full legalization and the prevalence of past-year cannabis use increases among older adults. Fortunately, the National Institutes of Health (2017) has recently created a funding opportunity for researchers to learn more about the causes and consequences of nonmedical drug use among older adults.

▶ Screening, Brief Intervention, and Referral for Treatment: A Best Practice

Rather than focusing broadly on options for assessment, this chapter puts forward a specific model for screening and assessment that is relatively simple, time efficient, flexible, and evidence based (Babor et al., 2007; Schonfeld et al., 2009; U.S. Department of Health and Human Services, 2014). **Screening, Brief Intervention, and Referral for Treatment (SBIRT)** is a model that was developed to guide primary care practices in assessment of substance use (Bradley et al., 2002). SBIRT uses a population-based public health approach to identify individuals at risk of unhealthy alcohol and other drug use through structured screening. Those who display increased risk based on screening receive a brief intervention to facilitate change in substance use behavior. For those who are identified as showing the highest risk (i.e., probable substance use disorder), the patient receives a referral to treatment. The value of SBIRT for geriatric healthcare providers is that the intervention nests well into an overall health assessment, rather than requiring a separate assessment. SBIRT has also been implemented widely in elder-specific contexts such as senior centers; it does not have to occur in a healthcare setting (Schonfeld et al., 2009).

▶ Screening

Before the assessment process begins, it is important to remember that alcohol and other drug problems remain highly stigmatized in society, and older adults share many of these attitudes. The challenge for the clinician is to avoid language that inadvertently reinforces the stigma associated with substance use disorders. For example, the clinician should avoid the use of the terms *addict* and *alcoholic*, as they are pejorative and conjure up images in patients that decrease the likelihood that they will provide valid answers to screening questions. As an alternative, the clinician can use person-first language such as *person with a drug-use disorder* rather than *drug addict*. In addition, all interventions with older adults, including SBIRT, should be built on a foundation of respect and a recognition of the individual's right to self-determination. These concepts are crucial to ethical practice but are also valuable components of effective intervention.

Structured brief screening instruments provide a starting point for obtaining valid information about alcohol and other drug use. Well-constructed screening tools prevent clinicians from asking vague questions about use or questions that invoke social desirability. For instance, if a provider states, "You don't have an alcohol problem, do you?" the likelihood that a patient will report alcohol use accurately is low. Similarly, screening questions discriminate very well between individuals who are at low risk and those who use alcohol or other drugs. The development of the screening instruments leads to a very small number of questions but questions that say a great deal about the person's specific risk. On a related note, the scores of screening measures can be used to compare a patient's drinking to overall norms for older adults based on quantity and frequency as well as overall score with respect to alcohol-related problems. This information can be used as a starting point for a supportive discussion with the older adult patient about his or her use of alcohol and its relationship to the patient's overall health and well-being (i.e., the brief intervention).

In preparing for screening, the clinician should ask permission to conduct the screening with the older adult and answer any questions he or she might have about the purpose of the screening. This is another reason why routine screening of all patients is valuable. If all patients are screened, then the process becomes normalized as part of routine care. Consequently, older adults will see alcohol assessment as a part of quality healthcare practice.

Alcohol Screening Instruments

Although multiple alcohol screening measures are available, the Alcohol Use Disorders Identification Test (AUDIT; Babor, Higgins-Biddle, Saunders, & Monteiro, 2001) and the Comorbidity Alcohol Risk Evaluation Tool (CARET; Barnes et al., 2010) are especially helpful when assessing older adults. The AUDIT screen gathers data on consumption patterns (i.e., quantity and frequency of drinking), alcohol-related problems (e.g., loss of control), and feedback from healthcare providers about drinking (see **BOX 29-1**). The CARET measure is elder-specific, including quantity and frequency of alcohol use but also potentially harmful medication interactions (e.g., benzodiazepines) and medical comorbidities (e.g., depression). The CAGE questions (Ewing, 1984), although commonly used in healthcare settings, are not recommended

for assessing elderly patients' alcohol use. This instrument does not assess recent use, and the CAGE questions focus on the most severe signs and symptoms of use, so they do not detect recent at-risk drinking among older adults (Adams, Barry, & Fleming, 1996).

Providers can nest AUDIT or CARET in a structured assessment interview or have the patient self-administer the questions. For the screening measure to be scored appropriately, all questions should be asked verbatim to the patient; research even suggests that self-administration may lead to greater disclosure by patients of their substance use (Hankin, Haley, Baugher, Colbert, & Houry, 2015).

Once complete, the AUDIT screen (Babor et al., 2001) provides an overall score for the respondent, a level of risk, and responses to each question. For CARET (Barnes et al., 2010), a similar set of risk categories is provided that are specific to older adults.

Drug Screening Instruments

Unlike for alcohol measures, there are few drug-screening instruments developed specifically for older adults. The National Institute on Drug Abuse (NIDA) Quick Screen is recommended (see **BOX 29-2**); it asks about use of prescription drugs nonmedically and illicit drugs during the past year (National Institute on Drug Abuse, 2011).

If the patient reports any use in the past year, then the clinician can use a modified version of the Alcohol, Smoking and Substance Involvement Screening Test (ASSIST; Humeniuk, Henry-Edwards, Ali, Poznyak, & Monteiro, 2010), a more in-depth screen for both drug and alcohol use. This instrument collects data on lifetime and recent use of drugs in different classes and provides a risk score by drug. Although the ASSIST is much longer than the AUDIT screen, fewer older adult patients will likely report past-year use. In the ASSIST, the patient is asked questions about specific drugs used, quantity of use, frequency, and consequences associated with use.

BOX 29-1 AUDIT Questionnaire

Please circle the answer that is correct for you.

1. How often do you have a drink containing alcohol?
   - Never
   - Monthly or less
   - 2–4 times a month
   - 2–3 times a week
   - 4 or more times a week
2. How many standard drinks containing alcohol do you have on a typical day when drinking?
   - 1 or 2
   - 3 or 4
   - 5 or 6
   - 7 to 9
   - 10 or more
3. How often do you have six or more drinks on one occasion?
   - Never
   - Less than monthly
   - Monthly
   - Weekly
   - Daily or almost daily
4. During the past year, how often have you found that you were not able to stop drinking once you had started?
   - Never
   - Less than monthly
   - Monthly
   - Weekly
   - Daily or almost daily
5. During the past year, how often have you failed to do what was normally expected of you because of drinking?
   - Never
   - Less than monthly
   - Monthly
   - Weekly
   - Daily or almost daily
6. During the past year, how often have you needed a drink in the morning to get yourself going after a heavy drinking session?
   - Never
   - Less than monthly
   - Monthly
   - Weekly
   - Daily or almost daily
7. During the past year, how often have you had a feeling of guilt or remorse after drinking?
   - Never
   - Less than monthly
   - Monthly
   - Weekly
   - Daily or almost daily

8. During the past year, have you been unable to remember what happened the night before because you had been drinking?
   - Never
   - Less than monthly
   - Monthly
   - Weekly
   - Daily or almost daily
9. Have you or someone else been injured as a result of your drinking?
   - No
   - Yes, but not in the past year
   - Yes, during the past year
10. Has a relative or friend, doctor or other health worker been concerned about your drinking or suggested you cut down?
    - No
    - Yes, but not in the past year
    - Yes, during the past year

Scoring the AUDIT

Scores for each question range from 0 to 4, with the first response for each question (e.g., never) scoring 0, the second (e.g., less than monthly) scoring 1, the third (e.g., monthly) scoring 2, the fourth (e.g., weekly) scoring 3, and the last response (e.g., daily or almost daily) scoring 4. For questions 9 and 10, which have only three responses, the scoring is 0, 2 and 4 (from top to bottom). A score of 8 or more is associated with harmful or hazardous drinking; a score of 13 or more in women, and 15 or more in men, is likely to indicate alcohol dependence.

Saunders J.B., Aasland O.G., Babor T.F., de la Fuente J.R. and Grant M. Development of the Alcohol Use Disorders Identification Test (AUDIT): WHO Collaborative Project on Early Detection of Persons with Harmful Alcohol Consumption II. Addiction 1993; 88:791–804. Retrieved from http://auditscreen.org. This is a WHO approved instrument.

BOX 29-2 NIDA Quick Screen

In the past year, how often have you used the following?

Prescription drugs for nonmedical reasons:
- Never
- Once or twice
- Monthly
- Weekly
- Daily or almost daily

Illegal drugs:
- Never
- Once or twice
- Monthly
- Weekly
- Daily or almost daily

Modified from National Institute on Drug Abuse. (2011). Screening for drug use in general medical settings: Resource guide. In National Institutes of Health (Ed.). Bethesda, Maryland: U.S. Department of Health and Human Services. Retrieved from https://www.drugabuse.gov/sites/default/files/resource_guide.pdf

▶ A Brief Discussion of Brief Intervention

Data from the alcohol and other drug screens give the practitioner information about next steps in the assessment process. If the older adult does not report high-risk alcohol or drug use, then the clinician can take the opportunity to educate the older adult about healthy drinking guidelines for older adults. In contrast, for individuals who display at-risk drinking or drug use, a clinician should offer a brief intervention. This intervention starts the same way as the screening, in that the provider asks permission to talk about the results of the screening. In cases where the patient declines, the intervention ends, but that is a rare event. The act of asking permission itself creates a tone of respectfulness and collaboration that is central to the SBIRT model.

If the older adult is agreeable, the clinician should share information about overall score, level of risk, and contributing factors for risks related to alcohol, prescription drugs, and illicit drugs. The clinician should then inform the individual about the risks associated with at-risk drinking, many of which were noted at the beginning of this chapter. In addition, a wealth of materials on drinking and substance use among older adults are available from the National Institute on Alcohol Abuse and Alcoholism (2007, 2015) and National Institute on Aging (2017) that are brief, clear, and easy to read. Rather than the clinician simply giving these materials to the client, this information should be shared as part of a conversation about health.

In the SBIRT intervention, the clinician begins a discussion with the client about his or her reactions about the information. Using the seminal motivational interviewing (MI) intervention model (Miller & Rollnick, 2013; Rollnick & Miller, 1995), the clinician facilitates a dialogue about at-risk use. Although SBIRT is not directly equivalent to MI (Miller & Rollnick, 2009), it borrows some basic techniques of the intervention that are helpful in decreasing defensiveness and encouraging behavior change among individuals whose drinking or drug use is unhealthy. The MI skills include open-ended questions, affirmations, reflections, and summarizations (OARS). Open-ended questions are simply questions that can be answered without a set list of responses. For instance, the clinician could ask, "Now that I have shared the results of the screening with you, what are your thoughts?" The patient then has the opportunity to respond in any number of ways. Affirmations are responses that support the client's efforts and positive health behaviors, such as self-care behaviors. Reflective listening is the process of communicating the clinician's understanding of the message shared by the older adult in a nonjudgmental and accurate manner; it involves rephrasing and restating the message sent by the individual. Summarizing is the process of integrating multiple strains of a conversation into a whole and then offering that information back to the older adult.

While in-depth review of these concepts is beyond the purview of this chapter, the clinician should avoid taking the expert role, threatening the older adult, or engaging in other behaviors that engender resistance. Instead, the clinician should listen for *change talk*—a term from the MI model that encompasses any statements from the client that reflect *his or her own perception* of the need or desire for change related to the use of alcohol or other drugs. The job of the clinician is to simply reflect change talk back to the client. Similarly, the provider should avoid arguing with and directly confronting the patient about his or her use. One difference between the MI model and the SBIRT model is that the clinician can advise the patient to make a behavior change, but advising should include listening to the patient's concerns about change and trying to understand alcohol and drug use from the patient's perspective.

Decisional Balance

One technique for achieving this end is decisional balance. Another MI technique, decisional balance is a simple but powerful means of helping the patient to think about potential consequences of the alcohol or drug use and the value of change. In decisional balance, the practitioner is asked to discuss the positive aspects of the client's use of alcohol or other substances; that is, the provider listens and reflects on the person's thoughts about what drives the behavior. The value of asking for positive aspects of use is that the older adult understands the behavior as volitional and will display less resistance to discussing the negative aspects. The clinician then asks about negative aspects of use and reflects on those with the patient. The idea is to help the older adult patient to think about how use of substances is affecting his or her health and overall functioning.

Readiness Ruler

The readiness ruler is another approach borrowed from MI. In this technique, patients are asked to rate themselves on their readiness to change on a scale from 1 to 10. The theoretical underpinning of this approach comes from the Transtheoretical Model of Change (Prochaska, DiClemente, & Norcross, 1992), which posits that individuals proceed through a multiple-stage change process including precontemplation, contemplation, preparation, action, and maintenance phases. The readiness ruler is a means of gauging where the older adult is in the change process and can facilitate motivation for change by the individual.

Using the rating scale, the clinician asks the client to rate himself or herself on a scale based on readiness to make a change in a focal behavior (e.g., alcohol consumption). For example, the patient might report being a "4." Rather than asking the client why he or she is not ready to change, the provider asks the client to discuss why he or she *did not identify as a lower number.* For example, the clinician might say, "Tell me why you are not a 2?" The immediate effect of this approach is to encourage change talk. The client will talk about reasons for change, and the job of the clinician is then to reflect back to the client what he or she is saying. SBIRT works when the client is talking about the value of making a change and thinking about his or her own way of going about it. The SBIRT model primarily engages the clinician as facilitator and consultant rather than as an expert.

After a brief discussion using these techniques, the clinician then pivots to asking about what the older adult would like to do going forward. It is valuable to listen to the patient and think with him or her about a range of options. Assuming an older adult has the capacity to make decisions independently, the clinician should work collaboratively. This may mean accepting a plan for change that is different from what the clinician might recommend. When using a harm reduction approach (Marlatt & Witkiewitz, 2002), an older adult may decide to get a taxi rather than drive under the influence or decide to decrease his or her drinking rather than abstain from drinking altogether. If an older adult expresses motivation to pursue treatment services, either formal or informal, this is an opportunity for the clinician to assist the person and help him or her through the process.

Referral for Treatment

In assessing older adults, it is valuable to recognize and communicate to the patient that outcomes for older adults in treatment are as good or even better than they are for younger groups (Kuerbis & Sacco, 2013). Unfortunately, too few older adults who need treatment obtain such services (Sacco et al., 2013). For all patients, clinicians should facilitate a "warm handoff" to treatment (Substance Abuse and Mental Health Services Administration, 2016). This involves identifying a provider and making an effort to connect the older adult to the provider while the patient is present. In settings where behavioral health services are co-located with healthcare providers, the clinician can even personally introduce the patient to the treatment provider.

▶ Practice Challenges

Assessment of alcohol and other substance abuse through SBIRT is a practical approach for assessment of substance use among older adults. Within busy practice settings, however, finding the time to complete an SBIRT intervention can be a challenge, especially for primary care providers. Team-based approaches to addressing substance use can be helpful in such cases. Screenings can be completed by providers in the waiting room and can be incorporated into mobile health devices. In integrated behavioral health settings, health educators or other health professionals can conduct SBIRT interventions. Provider stereotypes about older adults may influence whether they even ask the questions, and older adult stigma may limit disclosure by patients. Nevertheless, use of structured screening instruments and routine screening of 100% of older adult patients will limit these issues.

Even though treatment is effective for older adults, there are not enough addiction providers effectively trained to work with older adults and not enough geriatric specialists who have training in addressing substance use among patients (Jeste et al., 1999). Therefore, it is incumbent upon all practitioners to create an appropriate system of resources that draw upon what is available to ensure that this important screening takes place. For example, a social worker or nurse who has an interest in substance disorders but who does not have specific training can obtain needed education and serve as a local resource.

▶ Summary

Unlike many aspects of geriatric assessment, assessment of substance use is not complicated; rather, the primary obstacle for clinicians in identifying substance use in their patients is omission of such assessment. Only about one in six of Americans is asked by a healthcare provider about alcohol use (McKnight-Eily et al., 2014). Although older adults are a relatively low-risk group, routine screening can help to prevent

harm and address use when necessary, and older adults can benefit from a variety of intervention approaches.

References

Adams, W. L., Barry, K. L., & Fleming, M. F. (1996). Screening for problem drinking in older primary care patients. *Journal of the American Medical Association, 276*(24), 1964–1967.

Aira, M., Hartikainen, S., & Sulkava, R. (2008). Drinking alcohol for medicinal purposes by people aged over 75: A community-based interview study. *Family Practice, 25*(6), 445–449. doi: 10.1093/fampra/cmn065

American Psychiatric Association. (2013). *Diagnostic and statistical manual of mental disorders* (5th ed.). Arlington, VA: American Psychiatric Publishing.

Arndt, S., Gunter, T. D., & Acion, L. (2005). Older admissions to substance abuse treatment in 2001. *American Journal of Geriatric Psychiatry, 13*(5), 385–392. doi: 10.1097/00019442-200505000-00007

Babor, T. F., Higgins-Biddle, J., Saunders, J. B., & Monteiro, M. G. (2001). *The Alcohol Use Disorders Identification Test: Guidelines for use in primary care* (2nd ed.). Geneva, Switzerland: World Health Organization.

Babor, T. F., McRee, B. G., Kasselbaum, P., Grimaldi, P. L., Ahmed, K., & Bray, J. (2007). Screening, Brief Intervention, and Referral to Treatment (SBIRT): Toward a public health approach to the management of substance abuse. *Substance Abuse, 28*(3), 7–30. doi: 10.1300/J465v28n03_03

Barnes, A. J., Moore, A. A., Xu, H., Ang, A., Tallen, L., Mirkin, M., & Ettner, S. L. (2010). Prevalence and correlates of at-risk drinking among older adults: The Project SHARE study. *Journal of General Internal Medicine, 25*(8), 840–846. doi: 10.1007/s11606-010-1341-x

Blazer, D. G., & Wu, L. (2009). The epidemiology of at risk and binge drinking among middle-aged and elderly community adults: National Survey on Drug Use and Health. *American Journal of Psychiatry, 166*, 1162–1169.

Bradley, K. A., Epler, A. J., Bush, K. R., Sporleder, J. L., Dunn, C. W., Cochran, N. E., . . . Fihn, S. D. (2002). Alcohol-related discussions during general medicine appointments of male VA patients who screen positive for at-risk drinking. *Journal of General Internal Medicine, 17*(5), 315–326.

Burruss, K., Sacco, P., & Smith, C. A. (2015). Understanding older adults' attitudes and beliefs about drinking: Perspectives of residents in congregate living. *Ageing & Society, 35*(9), 1889–1904. doi: 10.1017/S0144686x14000671

Choi, N. G., & DiNitto, D. M. (2011). Heavy/binge drinking and depressive symptoms in older adults: Gender differences. *International Journal of Geriatric Psychiatry, 26*(8), 860–868. doi: 10.1002/gps.2616

Cousins, G., Galvin, R., Flood, M., Kennedy, M.-C., Motterlini, N., Henman, M., . . . Fahey, T. (2014). Potential for alcohol and drug interactions in older adults: Evidence from the Irish longitudinal study on ageing. *BMC Geriatrics, 14*(1), 57.

Ewing, J. A. (1984). Detecting alcoholism: The CAGE questionnaire. *Journal of the American Medical Association, 252*(14), 1905–1907. doi: 10.1001/jama.1984.03350140051025

Fell, J. C., Tippetts, A. S., & Voas, R. B. (2009). Fatal traffic crashes involving drinking drivers: What have we learned? *Annals of Advances in Automotive Medicine /Annual Scientific Conference, 53*, 63–76.

Ferreira, M. P., & Weems, M. K. S. (2008). Alcohol consumption by aging adults in the United States: Health benefits and detriments. *Journal of the American Dietetic Association, 108*(10), 1668–1676.

Gavens, L., Goyder, E., Hock, E., Harris, J., & Meier, P. (2016). Alcohol consumption after health deterioration in older adults: A mixed-methods study. *Public Health, 139*, 79–87. doi: 10.1016/j.puhe.2016.05.016

Gilson, K.-M., Bryant, C., Bei, B., Komiti, A., Jackson, H., & Judd, F. (2013). Validation of the Drinking Motives Questionnaire (DMQ) in older adults. *Addictive Behaviors, 38*(5), 2196–2202. doi: http://dx.doi.org/10.1016/j.addbeh.2013.01.021

Gilson, K.-M., Bryant, C., & Judd, F. (2017). Understanding older problem drinkers: The role of drinking to cope. *Addictive Behaviors, 64*, 101–106. doi: http://dx.doi.org/10.1016/j.addbeh.2016.08.032

Han, B. H., Moore, A. A., Sherman, S., Keyes, K. M., & Palamar, J. J. (2017). Demographic trends of binge alcohol use and alcohol use disorders among older adults in the United States, 2005–2014. *Drug and Alcohol Dependence, 170*, 198–207. doi: http://dx.doi.org/10.1016/j.drugalcdep.2016.11.003

Han, B. H., Sherman, S., Mauro, P. M., Martins, S. S., Rotenberg, J., & Palamar, J. J. (2017). Demographic trends among older cannabis users in the United States, 2006–13. *Addiction, 112*(3), 516–525. doi: 10.1111/add.13670

Hankin, A., Haley, L., Baugher, A., Colbert, K., & Houry, D. (2015). Kiosk versus in-person screening for alcohol and drug use in the emergency department: Patient preferences and disclosure. *Western Journal of Emergency Medicine, 16*(2), 220–228. doi: 10.5811/westjem.2015.1.24121

Haug, N. A., Padula, C. B., Sottile, J. E., Vandrey, R., Heinz, A. J., & Bonn-Miller, M. O. (2017). Cannabis use patterns and motives: A comparison of younger, middle-aged, and older medical cannabis dispensary patients. *Addictive Behaviors, 72*, 14–20. doi: https://doi.org/10.1016/j.addbeh.2017.03.006

Holdsworth, C., Frisher, M., Mendonca, M., De Oliveiria, C., Pikhart, H., & Shelton, N. (2017). Lifecourse transitions, gender and drinking in later life. *Ageing & Society, 37*(3), 462–494. doi: 10.1017/S0144686X15001178

Humeniuk, R., Henry-Edwards, S., Ali, R., Poznyak, V., & Monteiro, M. (2010). *The Alcohol, Smoking and Substance Involvement Screening Test (ASSIST): Manual for use in primary care.* Geneva, Switzerland: World Health Organization.

Immonen, S., Valvanne, J., & Pitkälä, K. H. (2011). Older adults' own reasoning for their alcohol consumption. *International Journal of Geriatric Psychiatry, 26*(11), 1169–1176. doi: 10.1002/gps.2657

Jeste, D. V., Alexopoulos, G. S., Bartels, S. J., Cummings, J. L., Gallo, J. J., Gottlieb, G. L., . . . Lebowitz, B. D. (1999). Consensus statement on the upcoming crisis in geriatric mental health. *Archives of General Psychiatry, 56*, 848–853.

Johannesen, M., & LoGiudice, D. (2013). Elder abuse: a systematic review of risk factors in community-dwelling elders. *Age and Ageing, 42*(3), 292–298. doi: 10.1093/ageing/afs195

Kuerbis, A., Chernick, R., & Gardner, D. S. (2016). Alcohol use and comorbid psychiatric and subsyndromal disorders among older adults. In A. Kuerbis, A. A. Moore, P. Sacco, & F. Zanjani (Eds.), *Alcohol and aging: Clinical and public health perspectives* (pp. 35–53). Cham, Switzerland: Springer International Publishing.

Kuerbis, A., & Sacco, P. (2012). The impact of retirement on the drinking patterns of older adults: A review. *Addictive Behaviors, 37*(5), 587–595. doi: 10.1016/j.addbeh.2012.01.022

Kuerbis, A., & Sacco, P. (2013). A review of existing treatments for substance abuse among the elderly and recommendations for future directions. *Substance Abuse: Research and Treatment, 7*, 13–37. doi: 10.4137/SART.S7865

Kuerbis, A., Sacco, P., Blazer, D., & Moore, A. A. (2014). Substance use disorders in older adults. *Clinics in Geriatric Medicine, 30*(3), 629–654.

Marlatt, G. A., & Witkiewitz, K. (2002). Harm reduction approaches to alcohol use. *Addictive Behaviors, 27*(6), 867–886. doi: http://dx.doi.org/10.1016/S0306-4603(02)00294-0

McKnight-Eily, L. R., Liu, Y., Brewer, R. D., Kanny, D., Lu, H., Denny, C. H., . . . Collins, J. (2014). Vital signs: Communication between health professionals and their patients about alcohol use—44 states and the District of Columbia, 2011. *Morbidity and Mortality Weekly Report, 63*(1), 16–22.

Meier, P., & Seitz, H. K. (2008). Age, alcohol metabolism and liver disease. *Current Opinion in Clinical Nutrition & Metabolic Care, 11*(1), 21–26.

Merrick, E. L., Horgan, C. M., Hodgkin, D., Garnick, D. W., Houghton, S. F., Panas, L., . . . Blow, F. C. (2008). Unhealthy drinking patterns in older adults: Prevalence and associated characteristics. *Journal of the American Geriatrics Society, 56*(2), 214–223.

Miller, W. R., & Rollnick, S. (2009). Ten things that motivational interviewing is not. *Behavioural and Cognitive Psychotherapy, 37*(02), 129–140.

Miller, W. R., & Rollnick, S. (2013). *Motivational interviewing: Helping people change.* New York, NY: Guilford.

Moore, A. A., Karno, M. P., Grella, C. E., Lin, J. C., Warda, U., Liao, D. H., & Hu, P. (2009). Alcohol, tobacco, and nonmedical drug use in older U.S. adults: Data from the

2001/02 National Epidemiologic Survey of Alcohol and Related Conditions. *Journal of the American Geriatrics Society, 57*(12), 2275–2281.

Moos, R. H., Brennan, P. L., Schutte, K. K., & Moos, B. S. (2010). Social and financial resources and high-risk alcohol consumption among older adults. *Alcoholism: Clinical and Experimental Research, 34*(4), 646–654. doi: 10.1111/j.1530-0277.2009.01133.x

National Institute on Aging. (2017). *Facts about aging and alcohol.* Retrieved from https://www.nia.nih.gov/health/facts-about-aging-and-alcohol

National Institute on Alcohol Abuse and Alcoholism. (2007). *Helping patients who drink too much: A clinician's guide.* NIH Publication No. 07-3769. Bethesda, MD: National Institutes of Health.

National Institute on Alcohol Abuse and Alcoholism. (2015). *Older adults and alcohol: You can get help.* NIH Publication No. 11-7350. Retrieved from https://pubs.niaaa.nih.gov/publications/olderAdults/olderAdults.htm

National Institute on Drug Abuse. (2011). *Screening for drug use in general medical settings: Resource guide.* National Institutes of Health (Ed.). Bethesda, MD: U.S. Department of Health and Human Services.

National Institutes of Health. (2017). *Marijuana, prescription opioid, or prescription benzodiazepine drug use among older adults.* Retrieved from https://grants.nih.gov/grants/guide/pa-files/PA-17-196.html

Prochaska, J. O., DiClemente, C. C., & Norcross, J. C. (1992). In search of how people change: Applications to addictive behaviors. *American Psychologist, 47*(9), 1102–1114. doi: 10.1037/0003-066X.47.9.1102

Reynolds, K., Pietrzak, R. H., El-Gabalawy, R., Mackenzie, C. S., & Sareen, J. (2015). Prevalence of psychiatric disorders in U.S. older adults: Findings from a nationally representative survey. *World Psychiatry, 14*(1), 74–81. doi: 10.1002/wps.20193

Rollnick, S., & Miller, W. R. (1995). What is motivational interviewing? *Behavioural and Cognitive Psychotherapy, 23*, 325–334.

Ronksley, P. E., Brien, S. E., Turner, B. J., Mukamal, K. J., & Ghali, W. A. (2011). Association of alcohol consumption with selected cardiovascular disease outcomes: A systematic review and meta-analysis. *BMJ, 342*, d671. doi: 10.1136/bmj.d671

Rosen, D., Hunsaker, A., Albert, S. M., Cornelius, J. R., & Reynolds, C. F. III (2011). Characteristics and consequences of heroin use among older adults in the United States: A review of the literature, treatment implications, and recommendations for further research. *Addictive Behaviors, 36*(4), 279–285. doi: http://dx.doi.org/10.1016/j.addbeh.2010.12.012

Sacco, P. (2017). Understanding alcohol consumption patterns among older adults: Continuity and change. In A. Kuerbis, A. Moore, P. Sacco, & F. Zanjani (Eds.), *Alcohol and aging: Clinical and public health perspectives* (pp. 19–34). Cham, Switzerland: Springer International Publishing.

Sacco, P., Bucholz, K. K., & Harrington, D. (2014). Gender differences in stressful life events, social support, perceived stress, and alcohol use among older adults: Results from a national survey. *Substance Use & Misuse, 49*(4), 456–465. doi: 10.3109/10826084.2013.846379

Sacco, P., Bucholz, K. K., & Spitznagel, E. L. (2009). Alcohol use among older adults in the National Epidemiologic Survey on Alcohol and Related Conditions: A latent class analysis. *Journal of Studies on Alcohol and Drugs, 70*(6), 829–838.

Sacco, P., Kuerbis, A., Goge, N., & Bucholz, K. K. (2013). Help seeking for drug and alcohol problems among adults age 50 and older: A comparison of the NLAES and NESARC surveys. *Drug and Alcohol Dependence, 131*(1–2), 157–161. doi: http://dx.doi.org/10.1016/j.drugalcdep.2012.10.008

Savage, C. L., Finnell, D. S., & Choflet, A. (2016). Cancer, alcohol, and aging. In A. Kuerbis, A. A. Moore, P. Sacco, & F. Zanjani (Eds.), *Alcohol and aging: Clinical and public health perspectives* (pp. 65–77). Cham, Switzerland: Springer International Publishing.

Schepis, T. S., & McCabe, S. E. (2016). Trends in older adult nonmedical prescription drug use prevalence: Results from the 2002–2003 and 2012–2013 National Survey on Drug Use and Health. *Addictive Behaviors, 60*, 219–222. doi: http://dx.doi.org/10.1016/j.addbeh.2016.04.020

Schonfeld, L., King-Kallimanis, B. L., Duchene, D. M., Etheridge, R. L., Herrera, J. R., Barry, K. L., & Lynn, N. (2009). Screening and brief intervention for substance misuse among older adults: The Florida BRITE Project. *American Journal of Public Health, 100*(1), 108–114. doi: 10.2105/ajph.2008.149534

Sklar, A. L., Boissoneault, J., Fillmore, M. T., & Nixon, S. (2014). Interactions between age and moderate alcohol effects on simulated driving performance. *Psychopharmacology, 231*(3), 557–566. doi: 10.1007/s00213-013-3269-4

Sklar, A. L., Gilbertson, R., Boissoneault, J., Prather, R., & Nixon, S. J. (2012). Differential effects of moderate alcohol consumption on performance among older and younger adults. *Alcoholism: Clinical and Experimental Research, 36*(12), 2150–2156. doi: 10.1111/j.1530-0277.2012.01833.x

Smyth, A., Teo, K. K., Rangarajan, S., O'Donnell, M., Zhang, X., Rana, P., . . . Yusuf, S. (2015). Alcohol consumption and cardiovascular disease, cancer, injury, admission to hospital, and mortality: A prospective cohort study. *Lancet, 386*(10007), 1945–1954. doi: 10.1016/S0140-6736(15)00235-4

Sorock, G. S., Chen, L. H., Gonzalgo, S. R., & Baker, S. P. (2006). Alcohol-drinking history and fatal injury in older adults. *Alcohol, 40*(3), 193–199.

Substance Abuse and Mental Health Services Administration, Center for Behavioral Health Statistics and Quality. (2011). *The TEDS report: Older adult admissions reporting alcohol as a substance of abuse: 1992 and 2009.* Rockville, MD: Author.

Substance Abuse and Mental Health Services Administration. (2016, January 7). *Screening, Brief Intervention, and Referral to Treatment (SBIRT)*. Retrieved from http://www.samhsa.gov/sbirt

Teaster, P. B., & Brossoie, N. (2016). The intersection of elder abuse and alcohol misuse. In A. Kuerbis, A. A. Moore, P. Sacco, & F. Zanjani (Eds.), *Alcohol and aging: Clinical and public health perspectives* (pp. 131–147). Cham, Switzerland: Springer International Publishing.

U.S. Department of Health and Human Services. (2014). *NREPP: SAMHSA's National Registry of Evidence-based Programs and Practices*. Retrieved from https://www.samhsa.gov/nrepp

West, N. A., Severtson, S. G., Green, J. L., & Dart, R. C. (2015). Trends in abuse and misuse of prescription opioids among older adults. *Drug and Alcohol Dependence, 149*(0), 117–121. doi: http://dx.doi.org/10.1016/j.drugalcdep.2015.01.027

Wu, L.-T., & Blazer, D. G. (2011). Illicit and nonmedical drug use among older adults: A review. *Journal of Aging & Health, 23*(3), 481–504. doi: 10.1177/0898264310386224

Wu, L.-T., McNeely, J., Subramaniam, G., Brady, K. T., Sharma, G., VanVeldhuisen, P., . . . Schwartz, R. P. (2017). *DSM-V* substance use disorders among adult primary care patients: Results from a multisite study. *Drug & Alcohol Dependence, 179*, 42–46. doi: 10.1016/j.drugalcdep.2017.05.048

CHAPTER 30

Medication Assessment in Older Adults

Carla Bouwmeester and John W. Devlin

CHAPTER OBJECTIVES

1. Recognize both the importance and the challenges of improving safe medication use in older adults.
2. Apply practice guidelines and validated assessment tools to evaluate the appropriateness of medication use in older adults.
3. Discuss deprescribing strategies to optimize medication outcomes in older adults.

KEY TERMS

Deprescribing   Medication reconciliation   Polypharmacy
Medication adherence

▶ Introduction

Medication assessment in the older adult is a complex process and should consider the psychological, physical, and cognitive aspects of the patient's life. When evaluating medication appropriateness, it is important to consider how each of these three domains contributes to overall patient functioning and well-being. The goal of medication assessment is to determine the most appropriate medication regimen based on the underlying medical condition, balance effectiveness with the risk for potential adverse effects, ensure medication accessibility, and consider the patient's healthcare preferences. To achieve these goals, healthcare providers should start with **medication reconciliation** and use general screening tools to gather information on current medication use and behaviors. If specific medication-associated problems are identified through this strategy, then a more focused assessment is warranted and individualized solutions should be developed.

▶ Importance of Polypharmacy

Older adults, as compared to those who are younger, are more likely to have multiple chronic conditions (multimorbidity) and take several medications—often prescribed by different healthcare providers. Multimorbidity is present in two-thirds of older (age greater than 65 years) and 80% of very old (age greater than 85 years) adults (Salive, 2013). The number of prescribed medications increases with both age and multimorbidity. It is estimated that more than 20% of U.S. community-dwelling older adults take more than 10 prescription medications (Hajjar et al., 2005). More than one-third of older adults take five or more medications, and when over-the-counter (OTC) medications are included, this prevalence increases to 67% (Qato, Wilder, Schumm, Gillet, & Alexander, 2016).

Polypharmacy, while often defined in many ways, most commonly refers to the use of multiple medications that may be unnecessary, ineffective, or not clinically indicated (Hamilton, Gallagher, Ryan, Byrne, & O'Mahony, 2011). Medication-related adverse effects associated with polypharmacy may also result in falls, cognitive decline, and increased healthcare utilization (Fried et al., 2014; Hamilton et al., 2011; Hill-Taylor et al., 2013). Drug-associated admissions to hospital are prevalent in older adults. Medication assessment is an important strategy to identify and reduce polypharmacy in older adults.

▶ Medication Assessment Tools

Medication reconciliation is a foundational component of medication assessment and is straightforward to perform. This process involves comparing all the medications a patient is taking to the prescription orders or a medication list(s) maintained by the healthcare provider(s). At a minimum, medication reconciliation should include the medication name, directions for use, and how the individual is currently taking the medication. The goal of medication reconciliation is to create an up-to-date and accurate list of medications that can be shared seamlessly from patient to provider regardless of the healthcare setting where the patient is receiving care.

The Joint Commission has developed a five-step process for medication reconciliation (**TABLE 30-1**) ("Using Medication Reconciliation to Prevent Errors," 2006). When this reconciliation process is used in older adults, step 1 should also include OTC medications, herbal therapies, and dietary supplements, and step 5 should incorporate communication with other healthcare providers where appropriate.

Ideally, medication reconciliation should occur at each encounter with a healthcare provider. This process is especially important during transitions of care from one healthcare setting to another (e.g., home to hospital, hospital to rehabilitation facility) so as to maintain accurate medication lists and prevent medication errors.

Determining the appropriateness of prescribed medication(s) through implicit or explicit criteria represents a more complex form of medication assessment. Several tools, such as the American Geriatric Society's (2015) Updated Beers Criteria for Potentially Inappropriate Medication Use in Older Adults (Beers Criteria), are available to guide this process. The Beers Criteria, which are based on a synthesis of published evidence and developed through consensus by a multidisciplinary group of geriatric experts, provide explicit guidelines for

TABLE 30-1 Medication Reconciliation Process

Step 1: Obtain a list of current medications that include prescription and over-the-counter medications, herbal therapies, and dietary supplements.

Step 2: Develop a list of medications that are currently prescribed by all healthcare providers.

Step 3: Compare the lists from step 1 and step 2.

Step 4: Make clinical decisions to continue, modify, or stop each medication based on the comparison from step 3.

Step 5: Communicate the recommendations and revised medication plan to the patient, caregiver(s) (where appropriate), and other healthcare providers.

Data from Joint Commission. (2006). Using medication reconciliation to prevent errors. *The Joint Commission Journal on Quality and Patient Safety, 32*, 230–232.

the appropriateness of medications that are commonly considered for use in older adults. Within these guidelines, medication classes and individual drugs are categorized as potentially inappropriate in older adults, potentially inappropriate based on specific drug–disease or drug–syndrome interactions, or appropriate but should be used with caution. The Beers Criteria also identify medications with the potential to cause serious drug–drug interactions, requiring dosing adjustments based on kidney function, and having strong anticholinergic properties (and thus increasing the risk for falls, urinary retention, and delirium).

In 2015, the American Geriatrics Society published a companion article to the Beers Criteria suggesting medication alternatives for drugs considered to be high-risk agents in the elderly or to pose a substantial risk for drug–disease interactions (Hanlon, Semla, & Schmader, 2015). Medication assessment using these criteria requires the clinician to consider patient-specific factors—a step generally not required when the Beers Criteria are explicitly applied. This extra evaluation step may result in a decision by the clinician that a medication listed on the Beers Criteria may, in fact, be appropriate for a patient based on a careful consideration

of clinical status, concomitant conditions, and current medications.

The Screening Tool of Older People's Prescriptions (STOPP) and Screening Tool to Alert to Right Treatment (START) criteria are additional examples of medication assessment tools utilizing explicit criteria (O'Mahony et al., 2015). The STOPP/START criteria were updated in 2015 to include 80 STOPP criteria for potentially inappropriate medications and 34 START criteria representing potential omissions of medication therapy (O'Mahony et al., 2015). While a consensus panel of healthcare practitioners from 13 European countries developed the updated criteria, these guidelines have since been evaluated in research and clinical settings around the world and found to be valid (Khodyakov et al., 2017). Benefits of using the STOPP/START criteria in combination with the Beers Criteria include keeping a focus on clinically relevant adverse drug reactions and potential prescribing omissions, neither of which are addressed in the Beers Criteria.

The Medication Appropriateness Index (MAI) is a medication assessment tool that provides implicit (versus explicit) criteria and, therefore, requires the clinician conducting the assessment to have some knowledge of pharmacology and clinical therapeutics. The MAI, which consists of 10 questions, rates the use of each medication as appropriate, marginally appropriate, or inappropriate (Hanlon et al., 1992; Hanlon & Schmader, 2013). Elements of the MAI are listed in **TABLE 30-2**, along with key clinical considerations that a healthcare provider should consider when conducting this medication assessment. Although the MAI was originally published in 1992 (Hanlon et al., 1992), it is updated regularly and is available upon request from the primary author.

Clinical research studies have demonstrated that the MAI has good inter-rater and intra-rater reliability, can predict both adverse and positive health outcomes, and is able to detect inappropriate prescribing more frequently than medication assessment tools using explicit criteria like the Beers Criteria (Hanlon & Schmader, 2013). Since the MAI criteria must be applied to each individual medication, the time spent conducting this assessment may be considerable in a patient prescribed a large number of medications.

TABLE 30-2 Medication Considerations Based on Elements of the Medication Appropriateness Index

Elements	Considerations
Indication for use	Medications without a known indication can be considered for discontinuation
Effectiveness	Determine effectiveness of the medication for the stated indication
Dosage	Confirm the correct dosage based on patient-specific factors (e.g., age, kidney function) and clinical indication
Correct directions	Directions for use should be consistent with clinical indication, dosage form, and duration of therapy
Practical directions	Medication directions should be practical for the patient and easy to implement
Drug–drug interactions	Identify any clinically relevant, potential drug–drug interactions and strategies to minimize the risk for adverse effects
Drug–disease interactions	Consider how medications may exacerbate other medical conditions
Duplication	Medications with overlapping indications and/or mechanisms of action may be considered for discontinuation
Duration	Determine the expected duration of therapy and time-to-benefit for each medication (i.e., is the time to anticipated medication benefit appropriate relative to the patient's life expectancy?)
Expense	Evaluate each medication for a lower-cost alternative and consider medication expenses based on patient-specific factors (e.g., insurance coverage, medication assistance programs, accessibility)

Data from Hanlon, J. T., Schmader, K. E., Samsa, G. P., Weinberger, M., Uttech, K. M., Lewis, I. K., . . . Feussner, J. R. (1992). A method for assessing drug therapy appropriateness. *Journal of Clinical Epidemiology, 45*, 1045–1051.

Medication **deprescribing** is another important implicit approach to medication assessment and can be a valuable strategy to reduce polypharmacy. Deprescribing refers to the systematic removal of inappropriate medications supervised by a healthcare professional (Reeve, Gnjidic, Long, & Hilmer, 2015). In addition to reviewing medications, it is important to consider patient preferences during deprescribing. Patients and their caregivers, when appropriate, should be included in all deprescribing decisions to ensure adherence to this intervention and maintain patient–healthcare provider trust (Scott et al., 2015).

A common approach to deprescribing is outlined in **TABLE 30-3**.

The goal of medication assessment is to reduce inappropriate polypharmacy and improve patient outcomes. The most direct and simplest form of assessment is medication reconciliation, whereas explicit and implicit criteria can be applied to perform a more patient-specific and comprehensive review. The most common medication assessment tools include the Beers Criteria, STOPP/START criteria, and the MAI; however, specialized assessment tools are available for specific circumstances. Based on the patient's risk profile and medication regimen,

TABLE 30-3 Stepwise Approach to Deprescribing

Key Step	Considerations
1. Determine which medications the patient is taking and how they are taking them.	■ Ensure the patient brings a complete list (or the actual vials) for prescription and over-the-counter medications (including vitamins and dietary supplements) ■ Ask the patient how he or she takes each medication to assess adherence
2. Consider the potential harm of each medication when determining deprescribing priority.	■ Consider the number of drugs, potential adverse effects, and use of "high-risk" drugs when determining medication risk ■ Evaluate for the presence of factors that increase risk of harm, such as cognition issues, substance abuse, nonadherence, and multimorbidity
3. Assess whether a medication should be discontinued.	■ Assess the medication's indication, current effectiveness, and observed or potential adverse effects ■ Determine whether a medication is being used to treat an adverse effect from another medication ■ Ask the patient about his or her expectations and preferences ■ Identify medications unlikely to provide benefit during the patient's remaining lifespan
4. Prioritize the medications for discontinuation.	■ Discontinuation prioritization should be based on: 1. Greatest harm and/or least benefit 2. Ease of discontinuation 3. Patient preference for discontinuation
5. Implement the deprescribing plan and monitor the patient for adverse effects associated with medication discontinuation.	■ Reach agreement on the plan with the patient ■ Discontinue medications one at a time ■ Taper medications that may have withdrawal effects ■ Document the plan and rationale for deprescribing

Data from Scott, I. A., Hilmer, S. N., Reeve, E., Potter, K., LeCouteur, D., Rigby, D., . . . Martin, J. H. (2015). Reducing inappropriate polypharmacy: The process of deprescribing. *JAMA Internal Medicine, 175*, 827–834.

there are tools to assess anticholinergic burden, sedative load, overall drug burden, and inappropriate medications at the end of life (Gnjidic, Tinetti, & Allore, 2017). Assessment tools can be chosen based on the healthcare provider's scope of practice and expertise, the time required to complete the assessment, and concordance with patient-specific risk factors.

▶ Challenges

Medication assessment is inherently limited by the quality and quantity of information available about the patient's medication regimen, medical conditions, and psychosocial variables (e.g., religious beliefs, economic status, housing, and health literacy). Accurate medication reconciliation is possible only if the patient or caregiver is able to supply information about each medication such as directions of use, frequency of dosing, and adherence. Medication assessment with explicit criteria also requires knowledge of the patient's medical conditions, medical history, and laboratory values. In addition, assessment tools with implicit criteria require application of the healthcare provider's clinical judgment to determine medication appropriateness.

Despite these limitations, accurate medication reconciliation during transitions of care remains a high priority as older adults navigate ever-more complex healthcare systems. In one study, medication reconciliation in older adults discharged from a Veterans Administration (VA) hospital detected that 44% were receiving at least one unnecessary medication (Hajjar et al., 2005). Strategies to improve medication reconciliation can be as straightforward as ensuring every older adult and his or her caregiver carries an accurate and up-to-date medication list. This medication list should be updated with each medication change and shared with the primary healthcare provider, all medical specialists, and the pharmacist.

Once an accurate medication list is established, practitioners must also consider the older adult's ability to access medications. The ability to pay for medications is directly related to **medication adherence** and may vary throughout the year based on Medicare Part D coverage or seasonal incomes. Medicare beneficiaries with Part D medication plans may fall within the coverage gap or "doughnut hole," such that they may be unable to afford all of their medications. Prescription drug plans offered through Medicare have different formularies, premiums, copayments, and network pharmacies. It is important for older adults to annually review their options through Medicare's plan finder (https://www.Medicare.gov); the results from this analysis will help identify the most beneficial plan. Medication costs may also be lessened through state Medicaid programs and manufacturers' prescription drug plans for low-income patients.

Additional factors related to medication accessibility include medication delivery and storage requirements. During the medication assessment process, healthcare providers should ascertain whether medications are received from a pharmacy on a regular basis. Many pharmacies offer door-to-door delivery services or mail-order options at reduced or no cost to customers as well as automatic refills of medications. If patients are enrolled in automatic refill programs, it is important to notify the pharmacy when the prescription directions change or the medication is discontinued to prevent polypharmacy and potential medication errors. Medication assessment should also include a review of any specific medication storage requirements (e.g., unopened insulin vials should be stored in the refrigerator) or shortened expiration dates once medication packaging is opened. All medications should be stored in a cool, dry place away from direct heat and humidity. Medications with the potential for abuse, such as opioids, benzodiazepines, or stimulants, should be stored in a locked box or cabinet to prevent unintentional overdose or diversion.

Adherence packaging is another factor to consider when performing a medication assessment. Medication pillboxes can be filled by older adults or their caregivers on a daily or weekly basis to increase adherence and prevent underdosing or overdosing. Pharmacies may also provide medications in blister packs in which each dose is individually packaged on a single card or multiple medications, intended to be taken at the same time, are packaged in a single "bubble." Technology can also be used to provide medication reminders through automated home dispensing machines, telephone or computer application alerts, or medication reminder programs (often available in assisted living facilities or other group living arrangements). Regardless of the method used to boost adherence, it is imperative for the patient and/or caregiver to communicate all medication changes to the person responsible for organizing the pillboxes, bubble packs, or medication reminders.

Medication assessment should also take into account how medications are being taken by a patient or administered by a caregiver. Incorrect administration technique may lead to reduced efficacy, increased adverse effects, and potential patient harm. Although patients receive administration instructions when a medication is first prescribed, these instructions should be reviewed at regular intervals until the technique is mastered. One study of older adults with chronic obstructive pulmonary disease (COPD) found inadequate inhaler technique to be associated with increased healthcare utilization, oral steroid and antibiotic use, and poorer disease control (Melani et al., 2011). The provision of inhaler technique training to older adults by pharmacists, even in the setting of cognitive impairment, improves their ability to properly use this medication delivery system (Bouwmeester, Kraft, & Bungay, 2015). In addition to inhalers, the ability of older adults to self-administer eyedrops, eardrops, nasal sprays, and transdermal patches should always be evaluated. Medication administration guides in patient-friendly language can be obtained from the pharmacy or on websites such as the American Society of Health-System Pharmacists' Safe Medication website (http://www.safemedication.com).

▶ Summary

Polypharmacy and inappropriate prescribing are all too prevalent in older adults. Medication assessment should be regularly completed in all older adults, particularly during care transitions, to determine medication regimen appropriateness, risk for adverse effects, and barriers to medication accessibility. Medication reconciliation, using the Joint Commission criteria, can be easily completed by nurses, physicians, and pharmacists, and is the foundation for medication assessment in older adults. A number of well-validated, explicit (e.g., Beers Criteria) and implicit (e.g., MAI) criteria tools are available to evaluate medication appropriateness and guide deprescribing efforts in the older adult population. The ability for older adults to self-administer their medications and afford them are also important considerations in the medication assessment process.

References

American Geriatrics Society 2015 Beers Criteria Update Expert Panel. (2015). American Geriatrics Society 2015 Updated Beers Criteria for Potentially Inappropriate Medication Use in Older Adults. *Journal of the American Geriatrics Society, 63,* 2227–2246.

Bouwmeester, C., Kraft, J., & Bungay, K. M. (2015). Optimizing inhaler use by pharmacist-provided education to community dwelling elderly. *Respiratory Medicine, 109,* 1363–1368.

Fried, T. R., O'Leary, J., Towle, V., Goldstein, M. K., Trentalange, M., Martin, D. K. (2014). Health outcomes associated with polypharmacy in community-dwelling older adults: a systematic review. *Journal of the American Geriatrics Society, 62,* 2261–2272.

Gnjidic, D., Tinetti, M., & Allore, H. G. (2017). Assessing medication burden and polypharmacy: Finding the perfect measure. *Expert Review of Clinical Pharmacology, 10,* 345–347.

Hajjar, E. R., Hanlon, J. T., Sloane, R. J., Lindblad, C. I., Pieper, C. F., Ruby, C. M., . . . Schmader, K. E. (2005). Unnecessary drug use in frail older people at hospital discharge. *Journal of the American Geriatrics Society, 53*(9), 1518–1523.

Hamilton, H., Gallagher, P., Ryan, C., Byrne, S., & O'Mahony, D. (2011). Potentially inappropriate medications defined by STOPP criteria and the risk of adverse drug events in older hospitalized patients. *Archives of Internal Medicine, 13,* 1013–1019.

Hanlon, J. T., & Schmader, K. E. (2013). The Medication Appropriateness Index at 20: Where it started, where it has been and where it may be going. *Drugs and Aging, 30,* 10.

Hanlon, J. T., Schmader, K. E., Samsa, G. P., Weinberger, M., Uttech, K. M., Lewis, I. K., . . . Feussner, J. R. (1992). A method for assessing drug therapy appropriateness. *Journal of Clinical Epidemiology, 45,* 1045–1051.

Hanlon, J. T., Semla, T. P., & Schmader, K. E. (2015). Alternative medications for medications in the use of high-risk medications in the elderly and potentially harmful drug–disease interactions in the elderly quality measures. *Journal of the American Geriatrics Society, 63,* e8–e18.

Hill-Taylor, B., Sketris, I., Hayden, J., Byrne, S., O'Sullivan, D., & Christie, R. (2013). Application of the STOPP/START criteria: A systematic review of the prevalence of potentially inappropriate prescribing in older adults, and evidence of clinical, humanistic and economic impact. *Journal of Clinical Pharmacy and Therapeutics, 38,* 360–372.

Khodyakov, D., Ochoa, A., Olivieri-Mui, B. L., Bouwmeester, C., Zarowitz, B. J., Patel, M., . . . Briesacher, B. (2017). Screening tool of older person's prescriptions/screening tools to alert doctors to right treatment medication criteria modified for U.S. nursing home setting. *Journal of the American Geriatrics Society, 65,* 586–591.

Melani, A. S., Bonavia, M., Cilenti, V., Cinti, C., Lodi, M., Martucci, P., . . . Neri, M. (2011). Inhaler mishandling remains common in real life and is associated with reduced disease control. *Respiratory Medicine, 105,* 930–938.

O'Mahony, D., O'Sullivan, D., Byrne, S., O'Connor, M. N., Ryan, C., & Gallagher, P. (2015). STOPP/START criteria for potentially inappropriate prescribing in older people: Version 2. *Age and Ageing, 44,* 213–218.

Qato, D. M., Wilder, J., Schumm, L. P., Gillet, V., & Alexander, G. C. (2016). Changes in prescription and over-the-counter medication and dietary supplement use among older adults in the United States, 2005 vs 2011. *JAMA Internal Medicine, 176,* 473–482.

Reeve, E., Gnjidic, D., Long, J., & Hilmer, S. (2015). A systematic review of the emerging definition of "deprescribing" with network analysis: Implications for future research and clinical practice. *British Journal of Clinical Pharmacology, 80,* 1254–1268.

Salive, M. E. (2013). Multimorbidity in older adults. *Epidemiology Reviews, 35,* 75–83.

Scott, I. A., Hilmer, S. N., Reeve, E., Potter, K., Le Couteur, D., Rigby, D., . . . Martin, J. H. (2015). Reducing inappropriate polypharmacy: The process of deprescribing. *JAMA Internal Medicine, 175,* 827–834.

Using medication reconciliation to prevent errors. (2006). *Joint Commission Journal on Quality and Patient Safety, 32,* 230–232.

CHAPTER 31

Mobility Assessment

Victoria Hornyak, David Wert, and Jennifer Brach

CHAPTER OBJECTIVES

1. Describe the prevalence and consequences of mobility limitations in older adults.
2. Recognize appropriate measures and tools to quantify and describe mobility.
3. Identify challenges to the assessment of mobility.

KEY TERMS

Assessment   Mobility   Walking

▶ Introduction

Walking is a chief component of **mobility**. In older adults, walking difficulty is a common and costly problem that is associated with loss of independence as well as higher rates of morbidity and mortality. **Assessment** of mobility should be part of the healthcare management of older persons, particularly for rehabilitation professionals for whom the goal of intervention is often to improve mobility. Such an assessment is critical to the management of the care of the older adult. Healthcare professionals need to (1) recognize who has a problem,

(2) determine when interventions are appropriate and often what those interventions should be, (3) determine whether the interventions were effective, (4) predict risk for future disability, and (5) plan for the public health needs of the older adult.

This chapter defines mobility and discusses its importance, provides a framework for selecting measures for the assessment of mobility, and presents some of the challenges associated with mobility assessment. The overall goal is to provide individuals caring for older persons with a guide that can be used in selecting measures of mobility.

Mobility: Definition and Epidemiology

Mobility is the ability to move one's body through space. It includes a range of activities, from turning in bed; transferring from lying to sitting, and from sitting to standing; and walking. This chapter focuses on walking, a fundamental mobility task for human life. Older adults who need supervision or assistance to walk, walk slowly, report difficulty walking, or are unsteady or have gait abnormalities can be classified as having walking difficulty.

The epidemiology of walking difficulty can be considered from the perspective of basic- or higher-level mobility. An example of basic mobility would be walking around inside the home. Examples of higher-level mobility include walking outside or walking longer distances such as a quarter or half mile. Basic walking problems are uncommon in community-dwelling older adults, but frequently occur in institutionalized older people. Among community-dwelling older adults, fewer than 10% are dependent when walking around inside; by comparison, among older adults who are institutionalized, approximately 80% are dependent when walking around inside. Walking difficulty—a less severe mobility problem than dependence—is a common problem in community-dwelling older adults. Almost half of all community-dwelling older adults report walking difficulty, defined as difficulty walking a quarter of a mile, and of those without such difficulty, approximately 22% will develop new difficulty over one year (Hoffman, Ciol, Huynh, & Chan, 2010).

Mobility difficulty is not always permanent or fixed. In fact, it is often transient, fluctuating over weeks, months, or years (Manini, 2013). Mobility disability increases dramatically with age, is more common in women than in men, and is more prevalent in nonwhites than in whites (Freedman et al., 2013; Hung, Ross, Boockvar, & Siu, 2011).

Mobility problems have serious consequences. Mobility difficulty in older adults contributes to loss of independence, higher rates of morbidity, and increased mortality (Cesari et al., 2005; Guralnik et al., 1994; Perera et al., 2016; Studenski et al., 2011). Mobility loss is also a sentinel predictor of other disabilities that restrict independent living (Fried, Bandeen-Roche, Chaves, & Johnson, 2000). Individuals with walking difficulty are also less likely to remain in the community, and are more likely to experience social isolation and decreased quality of life (Guralnik et al., 1994; Webber, Porter, & Menec, 2010). Compared to those without walking difficulty, older adults with walking difficulty are less physically active and spend a greater amount of time in sedentary activities, which in turn puts them at increased risk for a number of chronic diseases.

Walking difficulty is also a costly problem. In one study, compared to older adults without self-reported walking difficulty, those who developed mild walking difficulty over one year had higher healthcare costs (mean $1128 per person). When these data are extrapolated to the estimated 22% of older adults who develop walking difficulty annually, the cost to society is an additional $3.6 billion per year (Hoffman et al., 2010).

Given the prevalence of walking dependence and difficulty in older adults and the high associated healthcare costs, identification of those persons with walking problems is an important part of comprehensive geriatric assessment. Numerous mobility assessments exist, but no single measure can describe all levels of walking ability in a way that is meaningful to clinicians under all circumstances (Brach, Rosano, & Studenski, 2017). Therefore, rather than take a "one size fits all" approach to mobility assessment, a framework is offered here that takes three factors into consideration: (1) the clinical characteristics of the person to be assessed, (2) the corresponding construct of the measure and the relevant psychometric properties, and (3) the feasibility of the measure.

Measures of Mobility

TABLE 31-1 identifies several measures of mobility related to walking, as well as key normative

TABLE 31-1 Performance and Self-Report-Based Assessment Tools with Associated Values of Interest

Assessment Tool	Values of Interest
Performance-Based	
Gait speed	Normative values (Perry, 1992): 1.23–1.37 m/s ■ Indicators of function (Bowden, Balasubramanian, Behrman, & Kautz, 2008): ■ <0.4 m/s: Household ambulator ■ 0.4–0.8 m/s: Limited community ambulator ■ >0.8 m/s: Community ambulator Indicators of change: MCID (Perera, Mody, Woodman, & Studenski, 2006) ■ Small: 0.05 m/s ■ Substantial: 0.10 m/s

Timed Up and Go (TUG)	Normative values (Steffen, Hacker, & Mollinger, 2002) (seconds):
	■ 60–69 years:
	  • Male: 8
	  • Female: 8
	■ 70–79 years:
	  • Male: 9
	  • Female: 9
	■ 80–89 years:
	  • Male: 10
	  • Female: 11
	
	Indicators of function (Shumway-Cook, Brauer, & Woollacott, 2000): > 14 s = fall risk
	
	Indicators of change (Wright, Cook, Baxter, Dockerty, & Abbott, 2011): MCID = 0.8–1.4 s

Short Physical Performance Battery (SPPB)	Indicators of function: ■ 0–4: Greater risk of rehospitalization/death (Volpato et al., 2011) ■ <10: Predictive of mobility disability (Guralnik et al., 1994)/mortality (Pavasini et al., 2016) Indicator of change: MCID (Perera et al., 2006) ■ Small: 0.5 point ■ Substantial: 1.0 point

(continues)

TABLE 31-1 Performance and Self-Report-Based Assessment Tools with Associated Values of Interest *(continued)*

Assessment Tool	Values of Interest

6-Minute Walk Test	Normative values (Steffen et al., 2002) (meters):
	
	■ 60–69 years:
	  • Male: 572
	  • Female: 538
	
	■ 70–79 years:
	  • Male: 527
	  • Female: 471
	
	■ 80–89 years:
	  • Male: 417
	  • Female: 392
	
	Indicators of function (Harada, Chiu, & Stewart, 1999):
	>300 meters (community ambulator)
	
	Indicator of change: MCID (Perera et al., 2006)
	
	■ Small: 20 m
	■ Substantial: 50 m

Dynamic Gait Index (DGI)	Indicators of function: <19 = fall risk (Shumway-Cook & Baldwin, 1997; Wrisley & Kumar, 2010) Indicators of change: MCID (Pardasaney et al., 2012) = 1.90 points

Self-Report-Based

Activity Measure for Post-Acute Care (AM-PAC): "6 clicks"	Indicators of function: ■ 42.9 (Basic Mobility Score): Cut-point for D/C to home setting (Jette et al., 2014) ■ 39.4 (Daily Activity Score): Cut point for D/C to home setting (Jette et al., 2014) Indicators of change (Jette et al., 2014): ■ MCD90: 4.73 points (Basic Mobility) ■ MCD90: 5.49 points (Daily Activity)
Lifespace Questionnaire	Normative values (Peel et al., 2005; Stalvey, Owsley, Sloane, & Ball, 1999): ■ 65–74 years: 71.3 points ■ 75–84 years: 60.0 points ■ 85+ years: 45.8 points
Late-Life Function and Disability Instrument (LLFDI): Function	Indicators of change (Beauchamp, Schmidt, Pedersen, Bean, & Jette, 2014): MCID = 2.7 (Overall function)

Abbreviations: D/C: Discharge; MCID: Minimal Clinically Important Difference.

values associated with each measure. The measures are classified as self-report or performance based, and then further described according to the constructs they incorporate. Self-report measures are questionnaires that capture patients' perception of their mobility or a report of what they think they can do. In contrast, a performance-based measure requires the patient to perform the task and provides information on what the patient can actually do. Self-report and performance-based measures are often only moderately correlated at best, indicating that the measures provide slightly different, but complementary, information about a patient's mobility (Reuben, Valle, Hays, & Siu, 1995). If possible, to capture a more complete picture of a person's mobility, it is often suggested to administer both self-report and performance-based measures.

When choosing a measure, it is also important to consider the ease of administration and/or potential burden to the patient. For example, gait speed is a performance-based measure that is associated with mobility disability, fall risk, and mortality; it requires little training to measure correctly and takes just a few seconds to measure. Because it is easily measured over any known distance, gait speed can be assessed in nearly any setting (Fritz & Lusardi, 2009). In contrast, the Late-Life Function and Disability Instrument (LLFDI) is a self-reported 48-item questionnaire. It is typically administered by interview, takes approximately 15 minutes to complete, and requires some training to administer and to score (Haley et al., 2002; Jette et al., 2014). Table 31-1 shows additional measures and values of interest to the clinician who is assessing mobility.

▶ Clinical Characteristics

Several person-centered characteristics can influence the selection of mobility measures. Some active medical problems or diagnoses can impact walking in a very specific way—for example, a recent joint replacement or a diagnosis of Parkinson's disease. The gait of a person who

has recently undergone a total knee replacement will be heavily influenced by pain and lack of range of motion, while the gait of a person with Parkinson's disease will be primarily affected by impaired neuromuscular control, resulting in difficulty initiating gait or festination. Individuals may seek help for their mobility problems if those difficulties are getting in the way of daily activities, such as when walking through the grocery store becomes impossible due to the shortness of breath and fatigue of chronic obstructive pulmonary disease (COPD). A person may have a history of falls and subsequently limit his or her mobility outside the home due to fear of having another fall.

That being said, many walking problems represent a decline or dysfunction in the overall health of an older adult, especially as age advances (Studenski et al., 2011). Since walking requires the coordination of multiple body systems—neurologic, musculoskeletal, cardiovascular, and pulmonary—declines in walking ability can be a signal of systemic dysfunction (Ferrucci et al., 2000). For this reason, gait speed has been proposed as the "sixth vital sign" for older adults (Fritz & Lusardi, 2009).

▶ Intent of the Measure

After identifying the characteristics of the mobility problem, clinicians should consider what the clinical complaint represents in terms of mobility. For example, a person who has recently undergone a joint replacement may struggle with a slow, painful gait, and difficulty rising from a chair. Measures of mobility disability may be able to quantify the extent to which this individual is limited in her ability to participate in home and community activities. Considering her primary complaint of slow walking speed and concern about her future performance, measures of mobility disability including gait speed and the Short Physical Performance Battery (SPPB) may be most informative. **TABLE 31-2** describes this clinical scenario and others, with suggested measures of mobility and the associated rationales.

TABLE 31-2 Clinical Examples of Mobility Impairments and Suggested Measures

Clinical Example (Person-Specific Characteristics)	Intent of Mobility Assessment	Suggested Measures	Rationale
A 65-year-old male is reluctant to leave his home because of weakness, fatigue, and shortness of breath. He has a history of coronary artery disease (CAD) and chronic obstructive pulmonary disease (COPD).	Describe functional endurance and track performance over time	6-minute walk test Life Space Assessment	Measures of endurance: ■ Establishes maximum walking distance, which can be tracked over time ■ Defines the extent of his community boundaries given his impairments
A 75-year-old female is 6 weeks post total knee replacement. She still feels very slow and is having difficulty getting up from chairs. She attends a local health fair and wants to know how she is doing. She asks, "I am I always going to feel like this?"	Predict risk of future disability	Gait Speed SPPB	Measures of mobility disability: ■ Indicator of overall health; establishes comparison point for future rehabilitation; predicts mortality and disability ■ Combines walking speed, chair stands (lower-extremity strength), and static balance; a predictor of mobility disability
An 81-year-old male is hospitalized for 4 days with community-acquired pneumonia and feels weak and debilitated from the illness. The case managers are asking the healthcare team for discharge recommendations.	Describe mobility as it relates to the person's ability to return home	AMPAC "6-Clicks" Gait speed	Measures of basic mobility: ■ AMPAC "6-Click" cut-off scores indicate safe discharge to a home setting ■ Ranges of gait speeds have been established that categorize performance into those who are likely to be community ambulators, likely to be household ambulators, or likely to be institutionalized
An 89-year-old community-dwelling female consults a physical therapist due to a recent change in mobility. She reports difficulty walking outside and participating in social activities.	Evaluate mobility and monitor change with intervention	LLFDI DGI	Measures of higher functioning: ■ LLFDI is useful for higher-functioning people, since items range from basic to advanced activities such walking a mile or more and stair climbing ■ DGI consists of higher-level mobility tasks, which can uncover problems more likely to be encountered when walking in the community

▶ Challenges

While physical performance and self-report measures of mobility continue to be commonly used tools for clinical and research-related assessment of function and mobility in older adults, each of the two categories of assessment (physical performance and self-report) presents certain challenges that need to be recognized prior to specific measure selection and implementation.

The inherent nature of physical performance measures makes them less susceptible to "opinion" and "subjective influences," so that they can provide quantitative measures that can also discriminate small but important or preclinical differences (Brach et al., 2017). Despite this strength, physical performance measures may not always be the most appropriate category of mobility assessments to complete for a variety of reasons. Performance testing requires direct instruction and observation, necessitating the real-time presence of a clinician/researcher for completion of the assessment. In some instances, this approach may not be as cost-effective or as clinically efficient as self-report measures that do not require direct involvement of an assessor. Additionally, performance-based measures often require more time to complete, special training or certification prior to administering the assessment tool, access to a variety of equipment/testing items, and a larger area in which to perform the assessment (Brach et al., 2017; Guralnik, Branch, Cummings, & Curb, 1989; Kempen, Steverink, Ormel, & Deeg, 1996). Lastly, there is a lack of consensus in the literature as to whether mobility is best assessed and characterized using performance measures that do allow or do not allow the use of an assistive device (Chung, Demiris, & Thompson, 2015).

Self-report measures of mobility and function have high face validity, in that they directly reflect the opinion of the patient/client (Brach et al., 2017). Despite such measures providing the strong personal perceptions of the patient/client, self-report measures also come with a number of limitations and challenges. Research suggests that self-report measures are less accurate than performance-based measures because they are assessing "perception" rather than actual "performance" (Chung et al., 2015; Faber, Bosscher, & van Wieringen, 2006; Hoeymans, Feskens, vandenBos, & Kromhout, 1996; Wang, Yeh, & Hu, 2011); thus, they assess what individuals "think" they can do versus what they can *actually* do. Additionally, researchers have found that self-report measures are more strongly confounded by personality (cognitive/recall) and affective (depression) factors, as well as cultural, education, and language backgrounds (Bravell, Zarit, & Johansson, 2011; Kempen et al., 1996). Self-report measures have been shown to be less accurate, and have lower concordance with performance-based outcomes, for individuals with moderate to severe cognitive deficits (Kempen et al., 1996). Additionally, the greater the time period over which individuals are requested to recall mobility abilities, the greater the error in accurate recall (over-estimation or under-estimation) of abilities. Individuals with depression or low self-efficacy have also been shown to have more discordance between self-reported abilities and performance-based abilities, specifically showing tendencies in underestimating their ability compared to actual performance measures (Reuben et al., 1995). Likewise, individuals have been shown to overestimate or underestimate self-reported abilities based on their cultural upbringing. Moreover, some studies have shown that lower socioeconomic status can impact self-reported outcomes (underestimation of abilities) (Chung et al., 2015; Reuben et al., 1995).

In light of these limitations, the choice of assessment tool should be made based on the underlying purpose or intent of the assessment, the feasibility of using the instrument, and the clinical characteristics of the individual being assessed (Chung et al., 2015). That being said, the challenges reported here clearly demonstrate that physical performance and self-report measures of mobility/function do not provide equivalent information about a patient's functional status. Consequently, it has been overwhelmingly recommended that both types of assessments be completed, as they provide complementary information that allows for a more accurate account of mobility/function (Brach et al., 2017; Bravell et al., 2011; Farag et al., 2012; Kempen et al., 1996).

▶ Summary

Walking is a fundamental mobility task that is associated with the overall health and independence of older adults. Many tools are available that describe walking and related mobility tasks, each of which can be used to measure different aspects of mobility. It is important that clinicians be able to describe the clinical presentation of the client's mobility problem, consider the intent of the mobility assessment, and be knowledgeable about the construct and psychometric properties of a measure when choosing assessments. Clinicians can choose from self-reported measures or performance-based tests, or both, recognizing that each type of assessment yields slightly different information. Just as all walking problems are not created equal, so assessment of mobility should not be considered a "one size fits all" approach. Expert clinicians can take advantage of the nuances that each measurement offers and provide a personalized assessment of an individual's mobility that can be used to describe function, drive intervention, track progress, or predict risk.

References

Beauchamp, M. K., Schmidt, C. T., Pedersen, M. M., Bean, J. F., & Jette, A. M. (2014). Psychometric properties of the Late-Life Function and Disability Instrument: A systematic review. *BMC Geriatrics, 14*, 12.

Bowden, M., Balasubramanian, C., Behrman, A. L., & Kautz, S. (2008). Validation of speed-based classification system using quantitative measures of walking performance poststroke. *Neurorehabilitation & Neural Repair, 22*(6), 672–675.

Brach, J., Rosano, C., & Studenski, S. (2017). Mobility. In J. Halter, J. Ouslander, S. Studenski, K. High, S. Asthana, M. Supiano, & C. Ritchie (Eds.), *Hazzard's Geriatric Medicine and Gerontology* (1175–1790). China: McGraw-Hill Education. 1775–1790.

Bravell, M. E., Zarit, S. H., & Johansson, B. (2011). Self-reported activities of daily living and performance-based functional ability: A study of congruence among the oldest old. *European Journal of Ageing, 8*(3), 199–209.

Cesari, M., Kritchevsky, S. B., Penninx, B. W., Nicklas, B. J., Simonsick, E. M., Newman, A. B., . . . Pahor, M. (2005). Prognostic value of usual gait speed in well-functioning older people: Results from the Health, Aging and Body Composition Study. *Journal of the American Geriatrics Society, 53*(10), 1675–1680.

Chung, J., Demiris, G., & Thompson, H. J. (2015). Instruments to assess mobility limitation in community-dwelling older adults: A systematic review. *Journal of Aging and Physical Activity, 23*(2), 298–313.

Faber, M. J., Bosscher, R. J., & van Wieringen, P. C. W. (2006). Clinimetric properties of the Performance-Oriented Mobility Assessment. *Physical Therapy, 86*(7), 944–954.

Farag, I., Sherrington, C., Kamper, S. J., Ferreira M., Moseley, A. M., Lord, S. R., & Cameron, I. D. (2012). Measures of physical functioning after hip fracture: Construct validity and responsiveness of performance-based and self-reported measures. *Age and Ageing, 41*(5), 659–664.

Ferrucci, L., Bandinelli, S., Benvenuti, E., Di Iorio, A., Macchi, C., Harris, T. B., & Guralnik, J. M. (2000). Subsystems contributing to the decline in ability to walk: Bridging the gap between epidemiology and geriatric practice in the InCHIANTI study. *Journal of the American Geriatrics Society, 48*(12), 1618–1625.

Freedman, V., Spillman, B., Andreski, P. M., Cornman, J. C., Crimmins, E. M., Kramarow, E., . . . Waidmann, T. A. (2013). Trends in late-life activity limitations in the United States: An update from five national surveys. *Demography, 50*(2), 661–671.

Fried, L. P., Bandeen-Roche, K., Chaves, P. H. M., & Johnson, B. A. (2000). Preclinical mobility disability predicts incident mobility disability in older women. *Journals of Gerontology Series A: Biology, 55*(1), M43–M52.

Fritz, S., & Lusardi, M. (2009). White paper: Walking speed: The sixth vital sign. *Journal of Geriatric Physical Therapy, 32*(2), 2–5.

Guralnik, J., Branch, L., Cummings, S., & Curb, J. (1989). Physical performance measures in aging research. *Journal of Gerontology: Medical Sciences, 44*, M141–M146.

Guralnik, J. M., Simonsick, E. M., Ferrucci, L., Glynn, R. J., Berkman, L. F., Blazer, D. G., & Wallace, R. B. (1994). A short physical performance battery assessing lower extremity function: Association with self-reported disability and prediction of mortality and nursing home admission. *Journal of Gerontology, 49*(2), M85–M94.

Haley, S. M., Jette, A. M., Coster, W. J., Kooyoomjian, J. T., Levenson, S., Heeren, T., & Ashba, J. (2002). Late Life Function and Disability Instrument: II. Development and evaluation of the function component. *Journals of Gerontology Series A: Biological Sciences and Medical Sciences, 57*(4), M217–222.

Harada, N. D., Chiu, V., & Stewart, A. L. (1999). Mobility-related function in older adults: Assessment with a 6-minute walk test. *Archives of Physical Medicine & Rehabilitation, 80*(7), 837–841.

Hoeymans, N., Feskens, E. J. M., vandenBos, G. A. M., & Kromhout, D. (1996). Measuring functional status: Cross-sectional and longitudinal associations between performance and self-report (Zutphen Elderly Study 1990–1993). *Journal of Clinical Epidemiology, 49*(10), 1103–1110.

Hoffman, J. M., Ciol, M. A., Huynh, M., & Chan, L. (2010). Estimating transition probabilities in mobility and total costs for Medicare beneficiaries. *Archives of Physical Medicine and Rehabilitation, 91*(12), 1849–1855.

Hung, W. W., Ross, J. S., Boockvar, K. S., & Siu, A. L. (2011). Recent trends in chronic disease, impairment and disability among older adults in the United States. *BMC Geriatrics, 11*(1), 47.

Jette, D. U., Stilphen, M., Ranganathan, V. K., Passek, S. D., Frost, F. S., & Jette, A. M. (2014). AM-PAC "6-Clicks" functional assessment scores predict acute care hospital discharge destination. *Physical Therapy, 94*(9), 1252–1261.

Kempen, G. I., Steverink, N., Ormel, J., & Deeg, D. J. (1996). The assessment of ADL among frail elderly in an interview survey: Self-report versus performance-based tests and determinants of discrepancies. *Journals of Gerontology Series A: Psychological Sciences and Social Sciences, 51*(5), P254–P260.

Manini, T. M. (2013). Mobility decline in old age: A time to intervene. *Exercise and Sport Sciences Reviews, 41*(1), 2–2.

Pardasaney, P. K., Latham, N. K., Jette, A. M., Wagenaar, R. C., Ni, P., Slavin, M. D., & Bean, J. F. (2012). Sensitivity to change and responsiveness of four balance measures for community-dwelling older adults. *Physical Therapy, 92*(3), 388–397.

Pavasini, R., Guralnik, J., Brown, J. C., Di Bari, M., Cesari, M., Landi, F., & Campo, G. (2016). Short Physical Performance Battery and all-cause mortality: Systematic review and meta-analysis. *BMC Medicine, 14*, 215. https://doi.org/10.1186/s12916-016-0763-7

Peel, C., Baker, P. S., Roth, D. L., Brown, C. J., Bodner, E. V., & Allman, R. M. (2005). Assessing mobility in older adults: The UAB Study of Aging Life-Space Assessment. *Physical Therapy, 85*(10), 1008–1019.

Perera, S., Mody, S., Woodman, R., & Studenski, S. (2006). Meaningful change and responsiveness in common physical performance measures in older adults. *Journal of the American Geriatrics Society, 54*(5), 743–749.

Perera, S., Patel, K. V., Rosano, C., Rubin, S. M., Satterfield, S., Harris, T., & Studenski, S. A. (2016). Gait speed predicts incident disability: A pooled analysis. *Journals of Gerontology Series A: Biology, 71*(1), 63–71.

Perry, J. (1992). *Gait analysis: Normal and pathological function.* Thorofare, NJ: Slack.

Reuben, D. B., Valle, L. A., Hays, R. D., & Siu, A. L. (1995). Measuring physical function in community-dwelling older persons: A comparison of self-administered, interviewer-administered, and performance-based measures. *Journal of the American Geriatrics Society, 43*(1), 17–23.

Shumway-Cook, A., & Baldwin, M. (1997). Predicting the probability for falls in community-dwelling older adults. *Physical Therapy, 77*(8), 812–819.

Shumway-Cook, A., Brauer, S., & Woollacott, M. (2000). Predicting the probability for falls in community-dwelling older adults using the Timed Up & Go Test. *Physical Therapy, 80*(9), 896–903.

Stalvey, B. T., Owsley, C., Sloane, M. E., & Ball, K. (1999). The Life Space Questionnaire: A measure of the extent of mobility of older adults. *Journal of Applied Gerontology, 18*(4), 479–498.

Steffen, T. M., Hacker, T. A., & Mollinger, L. (2002). Age- and gender-related test performance in community-dwelling elderly people: Six-Minute Walk Test, Berg Balance Scale, Timed Up & Go Test, and gait speeds. *Physical Therapy, 82*(2), 128–137.

Studenski, S., Perera, S., Patel, K., Rosano, C., Faulkner, K., Inzitari, M., & Guralnik, J. (2011). Gait speed and survival in older adults. *Journal of the American Medical Association, 305*(1), 50–58.

Volpato, S., Cavalieri, M., Sioulis, F., Guerra, G., Maraldi, C., Zuliani, G., . . . Guralnik, J. (2011). Predictive value of the Short Physical Performance Battery following hospitalization in older patients. *Journals of Gerontology Series A: Biological Sciences and Medical Sciences, 66A*(1), 89–96.

Wang, C. Y., Yeh, C. J., & Hu, M. H. (2011). Mobility-related performance tests to predict mobility disability at 2-year follow-up in community-dwelling older adults. *Archives of Gerontology and Geriatrics, 52*(1), 1–4.

Webber, S. C., Porter, M. M., & Menec, V. H. (2010). Mobility in older adults: A comprehensive framework. *Gerontologist, 50*(4), 443–450.

Wright, A., Cook, C., Baxter, G., Dockerty, J., & Abbott, J. (2011). A comparison of 3 methodological approaches to defining major clinically important improvement of 4 performance measures in patients with hip osteoarthritis. *Journal of Orthopaedic & Sports Physical Therapy, 41*(5), 319–327.

Wrisley, D. M., & Kumar, N. A. (2010). Functional gait assessment: Concurrent, discriminative, and predictive validity in community-dwelling older adults. *Physical Therapy, 90*(5), 761–773.

CHAPTER 32

Nutritional Assessment as a Key Component of Comprehensive Geriatric Care

Mary Jane Koren

▶ Introduction

In Maslow's hierarchy of needs, the first, and most fundamental need is that the physiological demands for air, water, and food must be met if the human body is to function (CommonLit Staff, 2015). In the United States, except for obesity, clinicians often take access to food and nutritional status for granted. Yet, for older adults especially, assumptions of nutritional adequacy may well be misguided. Nutrition can be affected as a result of aging-related changes in several physiological functions, the increased likelihood of a variety of health-related issues, or the presence of complicating social or economic factors.

Before exploring nutritional assessment, it is necessary to first clarify terms. *Malnutrition* simply means "bad" (*mal*) nutrition and can be a result of either over- or under-consumption, or an imbalance of nutrients. Thus, *obesity*, which is readily apparent to even the casual observer, is a form of malnutrition in which a person gets far too many calories, which has negative consequences for health. For the purposes of this chapter, however, it is the other end of the nutritional spectrum that will be considered. *Under-nutrition* is a type of malnutrition in which a person may be either not eating enough food or not getting sufficient amounts of appropriately balanced quantities of protein, calories, or other essential nutrients required to maintain health. Detecting under-nutrition, which can have subtle signs or symptoms (Gariballa, 2000) or go unrecognized as the underlying cause of some other illness, requires that a comprehensive geriatric assessment include an assessment of nutritional status. Omitting this component of the geriatric assessment puts both the health and the well-being of the older adult at risk.

▸ Why Under-nutrition Is Common in Older Adults

Because of the way the human body ages (i.e., the physiologic changes associated with aging), older people are actually predisposed to become under-nourished. Assessing nutritional status, therefore, is an important component of comprehensive **geriatric care**.

For example, there is a natural phenomenon in which the desire for adequate quantities of food declines commensurate with the decline in physical activity seen in the very old. Sometimes referred to as the "anorexia of aging" (Landi et al., 2016), this condition means that older adults may not feel hungry at mealtimes, leading them to eat only a little bit or even to skip meals. Compounding that, the stomach loses elasticity, or becomes less compliant, as people age, so they may feel "full" faster. This sensation of satiation is further mediated by the release of such hormones as cholecystokinin, leptin, and dynorphin, which act both on the brain and on the gut.

The senses of smell and taste likewise diminish with age: Food loses its flavor, making meals less interesting and enjoyable, and causing older adults to tend to eat less. Oral problems, such as poor dentition or decreased saliva production, are common in old age, which can make eating uncomfortable. It has been estimated that dental problems alone may decrease food intake by as much as 100 kcal/day—not a lot for one day, perhaps, but cumulatively, over weeks and months, enough to cause an insidious and inexorable loss of weight (Merck & Co., 1995).

Swallowing problems (dysphagia) can also make mealtimes a source of stress, rather than enjoyment. People who have experienced difficulty swallowing may be reluctant to eat very much or be very selective about what they try to eat because of their fear of choking. In addition, older adults do not get as thirsty as young people, which, especially in hot weather or for people with congestive heart failure on diuretics, can cause dehydration with serious sequelae including dizziness, delirium, and falls (Alexander, 2000). In all these ways, the aging process itself sets the stage for energy-protein malnourishment and inanition.

Likewise, a host of medical problems and social issues may further compromise an older person's ability to maintain optimal nutrition. One of the most common causes of under-nutrition is depression. Research has shown that depressive symptoms are associated with insufficient food intake and nutritional deficiencies, especially in poor elderly people living at home (German et al., 2011), because of loss of appetite, diminished enjoyment of food, difficulty with food preparation, and consumption of a less varied diet (Sharkey et al., 2002). A vicious circle starts in which depression leads to poor intake, which worsens depressive feelings, and so on. It can be a hard circle to break, especially in homebound elderly individuals, who may become lonely, withdrawn, and apathetic. One study, for example, found that depressive symptoms, which were more common among women in the study, were linked with diminished mobility and social interaction (Perrino et al., 2011).

Another condition that is a major factor in under-nutrition in the elderly is dementia—a slowly progressive neurologic disease found in almost 50% of people older than the age of 85. Dementia is the fifth leading cause of death for persons older than 65 years (Hebert, Weuve, Scherr, & Evans, 2013). It tends to strike women with far greater frequency than it affects men, with two-thirds of the cases being women, whom census data show are also far more likely than men to be poor and live alone. Older adults with dementia may quite literally forget to eat and, even if they do remember, may be unable to figure out how to prepare even the most rudimentary of meals. In this all too common scenario, the probability of admission to a nursing home rises exponentially.

Depression and dementia are not the only illnesses that may lead to under-nutrition in older adults. Most older people have one or more chronic conditions, such as high blood pressure, arthritis, diabetes, heart disease, or chronic obstructive pulmonary disease (COPD). Among persons older than age 65, approximately 50% have two to four chronic conditions. Among those older than age 75, almost 20% have five or more chronic illnesses (AARP Public Policy Institute, 2009). The presence of multiple chronic conditions takes a huge toll on normal function. Even something as simple as not being able to stand comfortably or lift things can compromise a person's ability to shop, prepare a meal, and sometimes even eat. The presence and perceived effect of individual diseases and conditions on daily activities is an important component of what is termed the "the burden of disease"— and the more illnesses a person has, the heavier that "burden" becomes. When people do not feel well, appetite is often suppressed, which leads to insufficient energy (calorie)-protein intake and weight loss.

Unfortunately, treating people's illnesses may actually worsen their nutritional situation. National surveys show that more than 90% of older adults are taking prescription medications. According to the National Health and Nutrition Examination Survey, 64% of U.S. adults age 60 and older are taking three or more prescription drugs per month. Almost 40% are taking five or more prescription medications per month (Gu, Dillon, & Burt, 2010)—and that is the average! In a population with such a high burden of illness, the likelihood that people will be on multiple medications is all but certain. Some drugs, such as digitalis, a medication commonly prescribed for heart problems, directly suppress appetite. Approximately 36% of all modern antihypertensive and antihyperlipidemic medications cause changes in the senses of smell and taste (Doty, Philip, Reddy, & Kerr, 2003), which may in turn result in decreased food intake. Others, such as medications for arthritis or antibiotics, can cause gastric irritation. Finally, some drugs, such as Dilantin, some antacids, and tetracycline, can actually inhibit the uptake of nutrients from the intestinal tract.

Physical disability, frailty, and dementia, separately or in combination, mean that many older adults experience difficulty with shopping and meal preparation. For example, people who have "aged in place" either in rural or suburban areas may find themselves living miles from a grocery store and in an area where grocery delivery services may be unavailable. If and when they are no longer able to drive, they become dependent on the goodwill of neighbors, friends, or relatives to get out to shop for food or to have food brought in. Even in areas with reasonably good public transportation, buses and subways may be difficult for the frail and disabled to use, especially if they are trying to carry groceries or maneuver a small shopping cart. Furthermore, some frail older adults are afraid to venture beyond their apartments, fearing they may be targeted as "easy prey" for gangs or others in the neighborhood. As a consequence, many older adults default to a "tea and toast" diet, essentially devoid of nutritional benefit because they feel trapped in their own homes and cannot, or will not, risk a trip to the store for food.

Aside from clinically related issues, many other social factors may lead to **food insecurity**—that is, the state of having limited or uncertain availability of nutritionally adequate, safe foods (Carter, Dubois, Tremblay, & Taljaard, 2012). An example of unsafe food would be food that has been left too long in a refrigerator and become seriously moldy. Older adults with impaired eyesight or diminished sense of smell or taste may not notice when things "have gone off"—with potentially dire consequences. Sometimes older adults may have limited or uncertain ability to acquire acceptable foods in socially acceptable ways and eat pet food or get discarded food out of dumpsters (WBOC 16, 2013).

Among older adults in the United States, food insecurity increased by 25% after the recession that began after 2007. The poverty rate (i.e., living at or below the federally established poverty line of $11,800 in 2017) for women 65 and older at that time was 10.3%, 3.3 percentage points higher than the poverty rate for older men (7.0%) (Administration on Aging, 2010). Approximately 50% of those on Medicare live at or below 200% of the federal poverty level ($23,760 in 2017). Data from numerous studies have shown that poverty and hunger (an individual-level physiological condition that may result from food insecurity) go hand in hand in the elderly (Hall Bryan, 2005). In a 2011 survey by AARP's Public Policy Institute (Rix, 2011), one-fourth of those surveyed who were age 50 or older said they had already exhausted all their savings during the recession that began in 2008; more than one-third were having difficulty making ends meet and had to stop or cut back on saving for retirement.

Food insecurity is a problem that will only grow as more and more older adults must rely on Social Security as the major source of their retirement income. A 2016 study by AARP (Shelton, 2016), estimates that approximately 21% of people age 65 and older derive 90% or more of their family income from Social Security, which at the time averaged $1300/month or approximately $16,000/year. For an individual, this income level is just slightly above the federal poverty limit, which often puts older people in a position of having to choose between housing and related costs, medicine, or food.

▶ Health Outcomes from Under-nutrition

The **health consequences of under-nutrition** are numerous and may be profound—which explains why a nutritional assessment is an important element of a comprehensive geriatric assessment. (Culp & Cacchione, 2008). Whether the problem is not enough calories to maintain weight, insufficient protein to maintain muscles and other vital organs, or deficiencies of vitamins and micronutrients such as zinc, the outcome is the same: Unless older adults eat enough "good food," bad things can happen. For example, research has linked under-nutrition to the following health conditions:

- Weight loss. In at least two longitudinal studies, the findings suggested that weight loss in later life was predictive of mortality (Institute of Medicine, 2000).
- Skin problems, such as very dry skin or poor wound healing, especially of the skin tears that are such a common occurrence with the papery skin seen in the oldest old. These wounds leave people vulnerable to infections of the surrounding skin, soft tissues, and underlying bone.
- Sarcopenia. The decline of skeletal muscle tissue with age is one of the most important causes of functional decline and loss of independence in older adults. It causes loss of strength and function, which then predispose older adults to weakness and increased falls and may lead to hospitalization, nursing home placement, and even death (Fielding et al., 2011).

- Suppressed immune function. Such immuno-suppression renders people more susceptible to infections and less able to mount a defense against otherwise minor infections.
- Fatigue. This condition exacerbates depressive symptoms and saps any energy an individual might have to stay engaged with the community and wider social network.
- Increased frailty. The loss of physiologic reserve increases the risk of disability, which is a sort of precursor state to being dependent on another individual to compensate for functional deficits (Rockwood, Fox, Stolee, Robertson, & Beattie, 1994).
- Functional decline and impairment. When people have trouble managing their own personal care (e.g., bathing) and functions such as ambulation, they increase their risk of falls and gradual loss of the capacity to independently manage routine household tasks such as grocery shopping and meal preparation.
- Higher complication rates and more severe complications from underlying chronic conditions or acute comorbid illnesses, such as pneumonia, and longer lengths of stay when hospitalized.
- Depression, loneliness, and sometimes pseudodementia.
- Falls. Falls may arise from altered function brought about by any number of vitamin deficiencies (such as hypovitaminosis D or vitamin B_{12} deficiency) or from unrecognized dehydration.
- Delirium (Culp & Cacchione, 2008). Even when transient, delirium has been shown to have long-term sequelae.
- Anemia from deficiencies of vitamin B_6 (sideroblastic anemia), vitamin B_{12} (megaloblastic anemia), or iron (microcytic anemia). This type of condition leaves people feeling exhausted and can even worsen heart failure.

The sheer length of this list illustrates how poor nutrition can compromise virtually every system in the body. Moreover, while these negative health outcomes stemming from under-nutrition may be devastating to the individual, they also have enormous implications for health services utilization. For example, as mentioned earlier, many of the consequences of malnutrition produce effects that increase the risk of falls. According to the Centers for Disease Control and Prevention (CDC, 2016):

- One in three adults age 65 and older falls each year (Hausdorff, Rios, & Edelberg, 2001).
- Of those who fall, 20% to 30% suffer moderate to severe injuries that make it hard for them to get around or live independently and that increase their chances of early death (Alexander, Rivara, & Wolf, 1992).
- Older adults are hospitalized for fall-related injuries five times more often than they are hospitalized for injuries from other causes.

These statistics help explain rising healthcare expenditures. For example:

- In 2000, the total direct cost of all fall injuries for people 65 and older exceeded $19 billion: $0.2 billion for fatal falls, and $19 billion for nonfatal falls (Stevens, Corso, Finkelstein, & Miller, 2006).
- By 2020, the annual direct and indirect costs of fall mediated injuries are expected to reach $54.9 billion (in 2007 dollars) (Englander, Hodson, & Terregrossa, 1996).
- In a study of people age 72 and older, the average healthcare cost of a fall injury totaled $19,440, which included hospital, nursing home, emergency room, and home health care (Rizzo et al., 1998).

▶ Nutritional Assessment and Assessment Tools

While there are few rapid methods to screen the overall dietary intakes of older adults (Bailey et al., 2009), one or two screening tools have been developed that can be used as a first step to ascertain nutritional status or confirm suspicions that malnutrition may be present. The Mini-Nutritional Assessment—Short Form (MNA-SF) works well for such screening purposes. In its longer form, the full MNA still takes only 10 to 15 minutes to administer and can provide some limited additional information about the possible causes of malnutrition in persons identified as malnourished or at risk for malnutrition.

Nevertheless, none of these screening tools is a substitute for a complete assessment performed by a trained nutritional professional. Such an assessment includes four components:

- Evaluation of the person's anthropometrics (e.g., height, weight, skin-fold thickness, grip strength)
- Lab tests for different biochemical markers of nutritional status, such as total protein, vitamin B_{12}, and lipid levels
- Clinical factors or findings (the most obvious is weight loss)
- A thorough dietary history

Complete dietary histories can be time-consuming to complete because they query the individual about the frequencies and amounts of multiple categories of food and rely, to a great extent, on the patient's ability to recall intake accurately—an ability that can be compromised in someone with even mild dementia. A good example of a food frequency questionnaire (FFQ) is the Diet History Questionnaire (DHQ), developed by the U.S. Department of Agriculture. The DHQ is free and is available in several versions and in both paper and electronic formats to facilitate its use by researchers, clinicians, and teachers. At 36 pages in length, it is probably more than a patient's primary care practitioner wants to undertake routinely, but in patients at high risk for malnutrition or in complex cases its use can be extremely helpful in identifying underlying dietary patterns and spearheading a successful intervention. A somewhat shorter version, the brief self-administered DHQ (BDHQ), a 58-item fixed-portion-type questionnaire, is also available.

ASSESSMENT EXEMPLAR

Mr. D is a frail 87-year-old African American male with hypertension and fairly advanced COPD, probably from smoking (although he quit several years ago). A widower for the last 2 years, he lives on his Social Security benefits in a small, un-air-conditioned, third-floor walk-up rental apartment. His two adult children visit infrequently, and he has no other living relatives. On a recent visit, however, his daughter notices his clothes are baggy on him, he seems a little unsteady, and that there is not much food in the refrigerator. She also notices a couple of empty whiskey bottles in the trash. She tells her father to "make an appointment at that clinic you go to."

You are Mr. D's new primary care practitioner. Mr. D is not aware of whether he has lost weight but concedes his pants feel loose. When you ask, he tells you that he just does not feel very hungry, that "old age is getting to him" and that he misses his wife. He also complains that the stairs to his apartment "are too much" for him these days. His weight is down approximately 20 pounds from when he was last in the clinic 6 months ago. He takes hydrochlorothiazide, digoxin, and an inhaler (for his COPD).

Case Commentary

Attuned as you now are to the very real possibility that Mr. D is under-nourished, his history raises several red flags as to potential causes that should be investigated. You start with the full Mini-Nutritional Assessment. This instrument's findings, plus Mr. D's history and physical examination, give you important information about the patient's nutritional status that reflects his clinical condition (e.g., the unsteadiness may be partly from a vitamin B_{12} deficiency, especially if he is drinking a lot), his psychological state (he is probably depressed), and the care he is receiving (his medications may be affecting his appetite). You have also gained some important insights into the patient's social and economic situation—that is, Mr. D is living just above the federal poverty level, is socially isolated, may be dehydrated (i.e., he is on a diuretic and in an un-air-conditioned apartment), may be drinking too much, and cannot get in and out of his apartment easily to shop for food (although apparently the liquor store delivers!). All of these factors will have to be addressed for Mr. D's nutritional status to improve. The assessment findings should be shared with the entire interdisciplinary team, as the expertise of each member of the team will be needed to address Mr. D's problems. In addition to the clinical interventions, you realize that to really help Mr. D, the team will have reach out to and involve several community-based organizations, including the local area agency on aging to get him home-delivered meals; perhaps enroll him in a social day care program (and maybe even Alcoholics Anonymous); do an in-home falls assessment; and arrange for transportation to take Mr. D to church on Sundays.

▶ Summary

Having access to and partaking of adequate and appropriate food is a key component of physical health as well as quality of life. Older people may be at even higher risk of malnutrition as they become frail, face chronic or serious illness, or are constrained by poverty or any of the other social determinants of health. Clinicians must keep the possibility of under-nutrition or food insecurity in the forefront of their thinking as they care for their older adult patients, as many of their patients' signs and symptoms may stem from malnutrition rather than other disease processes. Likewise, assessment of food security and nutritional adequacy must be recognized as an interdisciplinary commitment and brought to the team for its thinking about how to remedy what are usually very complex issues. Including the evaluation of nutritional status within the comprehensive geriatric assessment is critical to the delivery of quality geriatric care.

References

AARP Public Policy Institute. (2009). *Beyond 50.09 chronic care: A call to action for health reform.* Retrieved from https://www.aarp.org/health/medicare-insurance/info-03-2009/beyond_50_hcr.html

Administration on Aging. (2010). *A profile of older Americans: 2010.* U.S. Department of Health and Human Services. Retrieved from https://aging.ca.gov/docs/DataAnd Statistics/Statistics/OtherStatistics/AoA2010profile.pdf

Alexander, B. H., Rivara, F. P., & Wolf, M. E. (1992). The cost and frequency of hospitalization for fall-related injuries in older adults. *American Journal of Public Health, 82*(7), 1020–1023.

Bailey, R. L., Miller, P. E., Mitchell, D. C., Hartman, T. J., Lawrence, F. R., Sempos, C. T., & Smiciklas-Wright, H. (2009). Dietary screening tool identifies nutritional risk in older adults. *American Journal of Clinical Nutrition, 90*(1), 177–183. doi: 10.3945/ajcn.2008.27268

Carter, M. A., Dubois, L., Tremblay, M. S., & Taljaard, M. (2012). Local social environmental factors are associated with household food insecurity in a longitudinal study of children. *BMC Public Health, 12*, 1038–1038. doi: 10.1186/1471-2458-12-1038

Centers for Disease Control and Prevention (CDC). (2016). *Costs of falls among older adults.* Retrieved from https://www.cdc.gov/homeandrecreationalsafety/falls/fall cost.html

CommonLit Staff. (2015). *Maslow's hierarchy of needs.* Retrieved from http://www.pearlandisd.org/cms/lib/TX01918186/Centricity/Domain/3004/Maslows%20 Hierarchy%20of%20Needs.pdf

Culp, K. R., & Cacchione, P. Z. (2008). Nutritional status and delirium in long-term care elders. *Applied Nursing Research, 21*(2), 66–74. doi: 10.1016/j.apnr.2006.09.002

Doty, R. L., Philip, S., Reddy, K., & Kerr, K. L. (2003). Influences of antihypertensive and antihyperlipidemic drugs on the senses of taste and smell: A review. *Journal of Hypertension, 21*(10), 1805–1813. doi: 10.1097/01 .hjh.0000084769.37215.16

Englander, F., Hodson, T. J., & Terregrossa, R. A. (1996). Economic dimensions of slip and fall injuries. *Journal of Forensic Science, 41*(5), 733–746.

Fielding, R. A., Vellas, B., Evans, W. J., Bhasin, S., Morley, J. E., Newman, A. B., . . . Zamboni, M. (2011). Sarcopenia: An undiagnosed condition in older adults. Current consensus definition: Prevalence, etiology, and consequences. International Working Group on Sarcopenia. *Journal of the American Medical Directors Association, 12*(4), 249–256. doi: 10.1016/j.jamda.2011.01.003

Fletcher, A. J., & Besdine, R. W. (2000). *The Merck manual of geriatrics.* M. H. Beers, & R. Berkow (Eds.). Whitehouse

Station, NJ: Merck Research Laboratories. Retrieved at https://www.merckmanuals.com/professional/geriatrics/falls-in-the-elderly/falls-in-the-elderly#v1136435

Gariballa, S. E. (2000). Nutritional support in elderly patients. *Journal of Nutrition, Health & Aging, 4*(1), 25.

German, L., Kahana, C., Rosenfeld, V., Zabrowsky, I., Wiezer, Z., Fraser, D., & Shahar, D. R. (2011). Depressive symptoms are associated with food insufficiency and nutritional deficiencies in poor community-dwelling elderly people. *Journal of Nutrition, Health, and Aging, 15*(1), 3–8.

Gu, Q., Dillon, C. F., & Burt, V. L. (2010). Prescription drug use continues to increase: U.S. prescription drug data for 2007–2008. *NCHS Data Brief, 42*, 1–8.

Hall Bryan, L. J. B. (2005). Food security among older adults in the United States. *Food Insecurity and Special Populations, 20*(4), 329–338.

Hausdorff, J. M., Rios, D. A., & Edelberg, H. K. (2001). Gait variability and fall risk in community-living older adults: A 1-year prospective study. *Archives of Physical Medicine and Rehabilitation, 82*(8), 1050–1056.

Hebert, L. E., Weuve, J., Scherr, P. A., & Evans, D. A. (2013). Alzheimer disease in the United States (2010–2050) estimated using the 2010 census. *Neurology, 80*(19), 1778–1783. doi: 10.1212/WNL.0b013e31828726f5

Institute of Medicine. (2000). *The role of nutrition in maintaining health in the nation's elderly: Evaluating coverage of nutrition services for the Medicare population.* Washington, DC: National Academies Press.

Landi, F., Calvani, R., Tosato, M., Martone, A. M., Ortolani, E., Savera, G., . . . Marzetti, E. (2016). Anorexia of aging: Risk factors, consequences, and potential treatments. *Nutrients, 8*(2), 69.

Perrino, T., Brown, S. C., Huang, S., Brown, C. H., Gómez, G. P., Pantin, H., & Szapocznik, J. (2011). Depressive symptoms, social support, and walking among Hispanic older adults. *Journal of Aging and Health, 23*(6). doi: 10.1177/0898264311404235

Rix, S. E. (2011). *Recovering from the Great Recession: Long struggle ahead for older Americans.* AARP Public Policy Institute. Retrieved from https://www.aarp.org/work/retirement-planning/info-05-2011/insight_50.html

Rizzo, J. A., Friedkin, R., Williams, C. S., Nabors, J., Acampora, D., & Tinetti, M. E. (1998). Health care utilization and costs in a Medicare population by fall status. *Medical Care, 36*(8), 1174–1188.

Rockwood, K., Fox, R. A., Stolee, P., Robertson, D., & Beattie, B. L. (1994). Frailty in elderly people: An evolving concept. *Canadian Medical Association Journal, 150*(4), 489–495.

Sharkey, J. R., Branch, L. G., Zohoori, N., Giuliani, C., Busby-Whitehead, J., & Haines, P. S. (2002). Inadequate nutrient intakes among homebound elderly and their correlation with individual characteristics and health-related factors. *American Journal of Clinical Nutrition, 76*(6), 1435–1445.

Shelton, A. (2016). Social Security: Who's Counting on It? AARP, March.

Stevens, J. A., Corso, P. S., Finkelstein, E. A., & Miller, T. R. (2006). The costs of fatal and non-fatal falls among older adults. *Injury Prevention, 12*(5), 290–295.

WBOC 16. (2013). Some seniors in Kent County strapped for cash, eat pet food to save money. Retrieved from http://www.wboc.com/story/23662934/some-seniors-in-kent-county-strapped-for-cash-eat-pet-food-to-save-money

William, B., Abrams, M. D., & Mark, B. M. D. (1995). The Merck Manual of Geriatrics.

CHAPTER 33

Transitions of Care

Megan Burke, Bruce Leff, and Alicia Arbaje

CHAPTER OBJECTIVES

1. Describe the importance and significance of care transitions in the current healthcare system.
2. Understand key factors that contribute to poor care transitions.
3. Describe several effective evidence-based models of care transitions, with a special focus on issues related to assessment of patients in the context of care transitions.

KEY TERMS

Care transition	Geriatric assessment	Hospital readmission

TRANSITIONS OF CARE INTRODUCTORY CASE

An 84-year-old man with mild cognitive impairment who lives alone is admitted to the cardiology floor after experiencing chest pain at home and being diagnosed with an NSTEMI (non-ST-elevation myocardial infarction) in the emergency department. His family declines cardiac catheterization and opts for medical management. Treatment is initiated with aspirin, a beta blocker, a statin, and an angiotensin-converting enzyme inhibitor. His chest pain resolves and his team plans for discharge back home.

▶ Introduction

A *care transition* refers to a patient's movement between one level of care, location, or set of providers to another within the healthcare system.

Transitions of care can occur across multiple settings and among multiple providers. Patients—especially adults age 65 years and older—are especially vulnerable to adverse events during care transitions. *Transitional care* refers to the set of actions designed to ensure the coordination and continuity of health care during care transitions (Coleman, 2003). One of the most common and complex transitions of care for older patients is the discharge from the inpatient hospital to the community.

After hospital discharge, almost 20% of Medicare-covered patients will be readmitted within 30 days and more than one-third will be readmitted in 90 days (Jencks, Williams, & Coleman, 2009). More than 20% of patients will experience a preventable adverse event—defined as an injury resulting from medical management rather than underlying disease processes—within 2 weeks of the discharge (Forster, Murff, Peterson, Gandhi, & Bates, 2003).

In this chapter, we describe key factors that contribute to poor care transitions. We also introduce several effective evidence-based models of care transitions, with a special focus on issues related to the assessment of patients in the context of care transitions.

▶ Key Factors That Contribute to Poor Care Transitions

Multiple factors contribute to the complexity of care transitions and adverse care transition–related outcomes. A review of these factors is useful to understand issues related to assessment in the context of care transitions.

Over the past two decades, hospital lengths of stay have decreased, patients have become sicker, and the majority of hospitalized patients have begun to be cared for by hospitalists, or practitioners who do not care for those patients outside of the hospital (Kuo, Sharma, Freeman, & Goodwin, 2009). Discharging, or transitioning, a patient out of the hospital involves assimilating and communicating a large amount of complex patient-related

information among multiple people with varying levels of clinical knowledge (e.g., patient, family members, primary care doctor, outpatient consultants, home care teams including coordinators, nurses, and rehabilitation therapists). Currently, there is no single accepted standardized approach used to ensure high-quality care transitions.

Despite the increasing use of information technology in patient care, lack of effective communication remains a substantial barrier to patient safety and care transitions. The decentralized and fragmented nature of providing care without any source of integrated and centralized patient information is a major potential source of errors.

Communication difficulties in modern health care is not a new phenomenon. In 2000, the landmark Institute of Medicine report *To Err Is Human* reported that as many as 98,000 people died each year as the result of medical errors in the hospital setting (Kohn, Corrigan, & Donaldson, 2000). A 2004 report of 2455 sentinel events reported to the Joint Commission on Accreditation of Healthcare Organizations (now called The Joint Commission) noted that communications errors were the primary root cause in more than 70% of sentinel events in hospitals; 75% of the patients involved in these sentinel events died (Leonard, Graham, & Bonacum, 2004). Miscommunication is a key challenge leading to suboptimal care transitions.

▶ Models of Care Transitions in the Era of Value-Based Care

TABLE 33-1 describes characteristics and outcomes associated with six evidence-based care transitions interventions that have been implemented in various health systems in the United States.

TABLE 33-1	Summary of Evidence-Based Care Transitions Models and Outcomes			
Intervention	**Care Transitions Manager**	**Targeted Patient Setting and Population**	**Goal of Intervention**	**Transitions of Care-Related Outcomes for Intervention Group Versus Control Group**
Care Transitions Intervention (CTI) (Coleman, Parry, Chalmers, & Min, 2006)	Transition coach: advanced practice nurse (APN)	Older community-dwelling patients (≥ 65 years) admitted to the hospital with complex care needs	Reduce readmission rates	Lower 30-day readmission rate (8.3% versus 11.9%) and 90-day readmission rate (16.7% versus 22.5%) Lower 90-day and 180-day readmission rates for the same condition of index (5.3% versus 9.8% and 8.6% versus 13.9%, respectively) Lower mean hospital costs at 180 days
Transitional Care Model (TCM) (Naylor et al., 1994, 1999)	Transitional care nurse: APN	Older community-dwelling patients (≥ 70 years) admitted to the hospital with complex care needs	Improve patient and caregiver outcomes, reduce cost of care	Lower 2-week readmissions rate (4% versus 16%) and 6-week readmission rate (10% versus 23%) Lower readmission costs Lower charges for healthcare services after discharge
		Older community-dwelling patients (≥ 65 years) admitted to the hospital with complex care needs and at high risk for a poor discharge outcome	Reduce readmission rates	Lower readmission rate (20.3% versus 37.1%) Lower multiple readmission rate (6.2% versus 14.5%) Fewer hospital days per patient (1.53 versus 4.90 days) Increased time to first readmission 50% reduction in total Medicare costs at 24 weeks post discharge

(continues)

TABLE 33-1 Summary of Evidence-Based Care Transitions Models and Outcomes *(continued)*

Better Outcomes for Older Adults Through Safe Transitions (BOOST) (Hansen et al., 2013)	Individual physician mentor: MD	Hospitalized adults (≥ 18 years)	Reduce readmission rates of patients at high risk for readmission	Lower 30-day readmission rate (12.7% versus 14.7%)
Project Re-Engineered Discharge (Project RED) (Jack et al., 2009)	Nurse discharge advocate: RN	Hospitalized adults (≥ 18 years)	Minimize emergency department (ED) visits and readmission rates of diverse inpatient populations	Lower hospital utilization rate (0.314 versus 0.451 visit per person per month)
Guided Care Model (GCM) (Boult et al., 2013)	Guided care nurse: RN	Complex older ambulatory adults (≥ 65 years)	Improve quality of life and quality of care, reduce readmissions, lower costs of care	29% lower rates of home health care use No significant differences in hospital admissions or 30-day hospital readmissions
Geriatric Resources for Assessment and Care of Elders (GRACE) (Counsell et al., 2007; Counsell, Callahan, Tu, Stump, & Arling, 2009)	GRACE support team: APN (certified registered nurse practitioner [CRNP]) and licensed clinical social worker (LCSW)	Older community-dwelling patients (≥ 65 years) with annual income less than 200% of the federal poverty line who were receiving care in outpatient ambulatory-based health centers	Improve functional status, decrease ED visits not resulting in hospitalization, decrease costs of care	Lower cumulative 2-year ED visit rate per 1000 (1445 versus 1748) No significant differences in hospitalization rates For predefined high-risk group, lower rates of ED visits (848 versus 1314) and hospital readmissions (396 versus 705) per 1000
				No significant difference in mean 2-year costs For predefined high-risk group, lower cost during post-intervention (third) year ($5088 versus $6575) For predefined low-risk group, higher mean 2-year total costs ($13,307 versus $9654)

Who Manages Complex Care Transitions?

A common theme of the interventions reviewed in this chapter is the use of a "care transitions manager" to help the patient navigate the transition. This individual often serves as an advocate or coach for the patient during the transitions process, and may also be the person who assesses the patient in the context of the care transition.

In a majority of the interventions reviewed here, registered nurses served as transitions managers. These nurses received specialized training or had already met specific training requirements prior to being selected for the role. For example, the Project Re-Engineered Discharge (Project RED) nurse discharge advocates (DAs) were nurses trained using a manual containing detailed scripts, observations of relevant clinical interactions, and simulated practice sessions. In the Guided Care Model (GCM), a guided care nurse was required to have three years of practice experience plus an interest in gerontologic nursing, enthusiasm for patient counseling, and comfort with electronic information technology and interdisciplinary practice. These nurses also completed an education program and demonstrated competencies during a practicum with simulated patients.

Other interventions used advanced practice nurses (APNs) in the role. The Care Transitions Intervention (CTI) used APNs as "transition coaches." Each transition coach was expected to show competence in medication review and reconciliation, experience in helping patient communicate their needs to different healthcare professionals, and the ability to shift from doing things for the patient to encouraging the patient to do as much as possible independently. Within the Transitional Care Model (TCM), a transitional care nurse led the transition. The APNs in this model were required to have at least one year of practice as a nurse specialist.

The GRACE intervention used a support team consisting of an advanced practice nurse—specifically, a certified registered nurse practitioner (CRNP)—plus a social worker to lead the transition. The Better Outcomes for Older Adults Through Safe Transitions (BOOST) invention chose a physician with specific expertise in care transitions (plus quality improvement skills and experience in process and improvement science and change management) to guide each project as an individual physician mentor.

As each of these models has been disseminated into practice, adopters of these models have employed other types of personnel as care transitions managers (e.g., social workers, peer health educators, community volunteers).

Targeted Patient Care Settings and Populations

The CTI, TCM, BOOST, and Project RED targeted hospitalized patients. CTI and TCM further narrowed their focus to community-dwelling adults age 65 and older. BOOST and Project RED targeted hospitalized adults in specific settings (chosen acute-care units in BOOST hospitals, and all inpatient adults on specified general medical units for Project RED). GCM and GRACE, like CTI and TCM, focused specifically on older adults receiving care in primary care clinics.

Goal of Interventions and Outcomes

The interventions all sought to minimize complications related to care transitions. Successes were demonstrated in all of the reviewed interventions. Four of the interventions—CTI, TCM, BOOST, and Project RED—focused primarily on managing the transition from hospital to home. These interventions all demonstrated statistically significant reductions in readmissions. CTI and TCM also demonstrated cost benefits in their intervention groups. Two of the interventions—GCM and GRACE—were multicomponent care models targeted at vulnerable populations of older adults in the ambulatory primary care setting, and managing care transitions was one element of a complex care model. In the GCM intervention group, lower rates of home health care use were realized through the intervention, although there were no significant differences between groups in hospital admissions or readmission. Studies evaluating the GRACE intervention showed significant differences in emergency department (ED) visits, hospital admissions, and costs in a predefined high-risk group that received the intervention.

▶ Patient Assessment in the Context of Transitional Care Models

TABLE 33-2 details the model-specific approaches to patient assessment. Overall, patient assessment reflects the specific nature and goals of each of the interventions.

▶ Patient Assessments

EXHIBIT 33-1 describes the Elder Assessment Instrument (EAI), which can be used to screen older adults for abuse.

Each of the models included a high-level assessment of which specific patients were eligible to receive the intervention—a determination that was usually based on age and presence of specific medical conditions or reasons for hospitalization. In CTI, the study investigators chose 11 qualifying diagnoses that indicated a high likelihood that patients would require either a skilled nursing home stay or home health services based on previous research (Gage, 1999). In TCM, the authors narrowed the population addressed from their first randomized clinical trial (Naylor et al., 1994) to their second trial (Naylor et al., 1999) to better target the patients who could most benefit from the intervention. The primary care–based interventions (GCM and GRACE) also used individualized requirements an attempt to identify high-risk patients. GCM used the Hierarchical Condition

Category (HCC) predictive model to identify patients in the top 25% of risk for using health services heavily in the coming year (as based on insurance claims submitted during the previous year). GRACE used the approach of identifying vulnerable patients with an income level cutoff of less than 200% of the federal poverty level. The investigators defined this population as those people qualifying for their state (Indiana) Medicaid insurance coverage or enrolled in the county medical assistance plan.

Each of the models employed additional standardized assessment tools to achieve its outcomes. The assessments used across interventions varied widely and were usually performed by care transitions managers. CTI focused on appropriate medication reconciliation in the context of the "four pillars" of self-management: medication management, use of a patient-centered personal health record, timely follow-up, and knowledge of "red flags." The transitions coach used the Medication Discrepancy Tool to reconcile medications, and a plan was made to address any discrepancies.

The transitional care nurse in the TCM intervention conducted individualized assessments of both the patient and the caregiver during the hospitalization. The TCN then used these assessments to create a personalized discharge plan. The TCN summarized this plan for review in a progress note in the patient's chart within 24 to 48 hours after hospital admission, making it available to all necessary team members for the duration of the hospitalization.

BOOST leveraged two key assessment tools: the 8P Risk Assessment and General Assessment of Preparedness. The Project RED discharge advocate created an individualized "after-hospital care plan" based on a detailed assessment and used a pharmacist assessment and telephone follow-up to reduce preventable adverse drug events and medication-related admissions.

GCM and GRACE both outlined specific in-home assessments used by their respective care transitions managers. In GCM, the GCN conducted a comprehensive assessment of the patient's

TABLE 33-2 Assessments

Intervention	High-Level Initial Eligibility Assessment	Additional Assessments
Care Transitions Intervention (CTI)	Community-dwelling patients 65 years or older admitted to the study hospital with 1 of 11 selected hospital admission diagnoses: 1. Stroke 2. Congestive heart failure 3. Coronary artery disease 4. Cardiac arrhythmias 5. Chronic obstructive pulmonary disease 6. Diabetes mellitus 7. Spinal stenosis 8. Hip fracture 9. Peripheral vascular disease 10. Deep vein thrombosis 11. Pulmonary embolism	During the CTI transition, the transition coach (TC) was responsible for assessing the patient's ability to self-manage his or her own care. After this assessment, the TC needed to coach the patient (at varying individual levels) to self-manage issues related to the CTI-based four pillars of transitional care: medication self-management, use of a dynamic patient-centered personal health record, timely primary care provider (PCP) and specialty follow-up after discharge, and knowledge of 'red flags. The Medication Discrepancy Tool (Smith, Coleman, & Min, 2004) was used by the TC to reconcile all of the patient's medication regimens at this first home visit. This tool was created specifically to capture transition-related medication discrepancies to promote patient safety during care transitions. When a medication discrepancy was identified, a plan was enacted for how to solve the problem. The Medication Discrepancy Tool (and other tools relating to the four pillars of CTI) are all available at the CTI website (https://caretransitions.org /tools-and-resources/).

(continues)

TABLE 33-2 Assessments *(continued)*

Intervention	High-Level Initial Eligibility Assessment		Additional Assessments
Transitional Care Model (TCM)	Patients 70 years or older being discharged from the hospital for selected medical and surgical cardiac diagnostic-related groups (DRGs). Medical DRGs: 1. Congestive heart failure (CHF) 2. Angina/myocardial infarction Surgical DRGs: 1. Coronary artery bypass graft 2. Cardiac valve replacement	Patients also had to meet one of the following criteria: 1. Age 80 or older 2. Inadequate support system 3. Multiple, active, chronic health problems 4. History of depression 5. Moderate-to-severe functional impairment 6. Multiple hospitalizations during the prior 6 months	The discharge planning protocol completed by the transitional care nurse (TCN) included both patient assessment and caregiver assessment protocols. ■ *Patient assessment:* Using data gathered from the patient (including sociodemographics, general health status, use of health and social services before hospitalization, perceived needs after discharge, functional status, mental status, self-esteem, perception of health status, and emotional status), the TCN completes a thorough assessment of the patient's discharge needs within 24 to 48 hours after the patient's admission. ■ *Caregiver assessment:* Using data gathered from the patient's caregiver (including sociodemographics, perceived needs after the patient's discharge, health status, functional status, and mental status), the TCN completes a thorough assessment of the caregiver's needs after discharge within 24 to 48 hours after the patient's admission. Based on these assessments, the TCN develops a preliminary discharge plan in collaboration with the patient, caregiver, physician, primary nurse, and other healthcare team members. A summary of the initial plan is recorded by the TCN in the patient's chart.

1.	CHF	
2.	Angina	
3.	Myocardial infarction	
4.	Respiratory tract infection	
5.	Coronary artery bypass graft	
6.	Cardiac valve replacement	

Patients 65 years or older admitted with one of the following diagnoses:

	7. Major small and large bowel procedure 8. Orthopedic procedures of lower extremities	7. Hospitalization in the past 30 days 8. Fair or poor self-rating of health 9. History of nonadherence to the therapeutic regimen
Better Outcomes for Older Adults Through Safe Transitions (BOOST)	Admission on the BOOST adult inpatient unit	Although all BOOST interventions are individualized, the Society of Hospital Medicine does provide tools to assist with general assessments related to transitions. For example, there are handouts for "8P Risk Assessment" and "General Assessment of Preparedness" (GAP) available. The 8P screening tool is used to identify a patient's risk of adverse events after discharge. The GAP tool is a simple checklist to identify patient concerns regarding their own transition. Both of these tools (and others) can be found on the BOOST website (http://www.hospitalmedicine.org/Web/Quality_Innovation/SHM _Signature_Programs/Mentored_Implementation/Web/Quality__Innovation /Mentored_Implementation/Project_BOOST/Project_BOOST.aspx).
Project Re-Engineered Discharge (Project RED)	Hospitalized adults older than age 18 years on the general medical service being discharged to home and who have a telephone	Intervention included three core elements: 1. Nurse discharge advocate (DA) 2. After-hospital care plan (AHCP) 3. Follow-up telephone call with pharmacist The DA completes all components of the RED intervention to create an individualized AHCP. Each component has different associated "DA responsibilities," in which the DA must assess each patient's individualized needs. These are explained in more detail on the Project RED website (www.bu.edu /fammed/projectred/index.html). Pharmacist assessments and weekly follow-up phone call focused on reducing preventable adverse drug events and medication-related admissions (Schnipper et al., 2006).

(continues)

TABLE 33-2 Assessments

(continued)

Intervention	High-Level Initial Eligibility Assessment	Additional Assessments
Guided Care Model (GCM)	Recruited patients of participating primary care physicians. Initial screening: 1. 65 years old or older ambulatory primary care setting 2. Complex patient based on being in upper quartile of Hierarchical Condition Category (HCC) score	During the initial home visit, the guided care nurse (GCN) performs an initial assessment of the patient's medical, function, cognitive, affective, psychosocial, nutritional, and environmental status using standardized instruments (Boyd et al., 2007): 1. Inventories of impairment in instrumental activities of daily living (IADLs) and activities of daily living (ADLs) 2. Nutrition Screening Initiative checklist 3. Mini-Mental State Examination 4. Get Up and Go test 5. Geriatric Depression Scale 6. CAGE alcoholism scale 7. Screening questions for hearing impairment, falls, and urinary incontinence The GCN also collaborates with the patient's PCP in performing clinical processes throughout the intervention period, several of which require routine individualized patient assessment: 1. Assessing the patient and the primary caregiver at home 2. Promoting patient self-management 3. Coaching the patient to practice healthy behaviors 4. Educating and supporting the caregiver 5. Facilitating access to community resources

Geriatric Resources for Assessment and Care of Elders (GRACE)	Recruited patients of participating primary care physicians:	Initial in-home comprehensive geriatric assessment includes:	The GRACE protocol annually assessed for 12 common geriatric conditions:
	1. 65 years old or older ambulatory primary care setting 2. Income less than 200% of the federal poverty line	1. Medical and psychosocial history 2. Medication review 3. Functional assessment 4. Review of social supports and advance directives Physical assessment focuses specifically on: 1. Orthostatic vital signs 2. Vision 3. Hearing 4. Gait and balance 5. Affect 6. Mental status A home safety evaluation is also performed. (Counsell, Callahan, Buttar, Clark, & Frank, 2006)	1. Advance care planning 2. Health maintenance 3. Medication management 4. Difficulty walking/falls 5. Chronic pain 6. Urinary incontinence 7. Depression 8. Hearing loss 9. Visual impairment 10. Malnutrition or weight loss 11. Dementia 12. Caregiver burden

EXHIBIT 33-1 Elder Assessment Instrument (EAI)

Purpose: To be used as a comprehensive approach for screening suspected elder abuse victims in all clinical settings.

Instructions: There is no "score" for this instrument. A patient should be referred to social services in any of the following circumstances: (1) if there is any positive evidence without sufficient clinical explanation, (2) whenever there is a subjective complaint by the older adult of elder mistreatment, or (3) whenever the clinician deems there is evidence of abuse, neglect, exploitation, or abandonment.

1. General Assessment	Very Good	Good	Poor	Very Poor	Unable to Assess
a. Clothing					
b. Hygiene					
c. Nutrition					

Additional comments:

2. Possible Abuse Indicators	No Evidence	Possible Evidence	Probable Evidence	Definite Evidence	Unable to Assess
a. Bruising					
b. Lacerations					
c. Fractures					
d. Various stages of healing of any bruises or fractures					
e. Evidence of sexual abuse					
f. Statement by older adult related to abuse					

Additional comments:

3. Possible Neglect Indicators	No Evidence	Possible Evidence	Probable Evidence	Definite Evidence	Unable to Assess
a. Contractures					
b. Decubiti					
c. Dehydration					

	No Evidence	Possible Evidence	Probable Evidence	Definite Evidence	Unable to Assess
d. Diarrhea					
e. Depression					
f. Impaction					
g. Malnutrition					
h. Urine burns					
i. Poor hygiene					
j. Failure to respond to warning of obvious disease					
k. Inappropriate medications (over/under)					
l. Repetitive hospital admissions due to probable failure of healthcare surveillance					
m. Statement by older adult related to neglect					

Additional comments:

4. Possible Exploitation Indicators	No Evidence	Possible Evidence	Probable Evidence	Definite Evidence	Unable to Assess
a. Misuse of money					
b. Evidence					
c. Reports of demands for goods in exchange for services					
d. Inability to account for money/property					
e. Statement by older adult related to exploitation					

Additional comments:

(continues)

EXHIBIT 33-1   Elder Assessment Instrument (EAI)   *(continued)*

5. Possible Abandonment Indicators	No Evidence	Possible Evidence	Probable Evidence	Definite Evidence	Unable to Assess
a. Evidence that a caretaker has withdrawn care precipitously without making alternative arrangements					
b. Evidence that older adult is left alone in an unsafe environment for extended periods of time without adequate support					
c. Statement by older adult related to abandonment					
Additional comments:					

Summary	No Evidence	Possible Evidence	Probable Evidence	Definite Evidence	Unable To Assess
Evidence of abuse					
Evidence of neglect					
Evidence of exploitation					
Evidence of abandonment					
Additional comments:					

Fulmer, T. (2003). Elder abuse and neglect assessment. *Journal of Gerontological Nursing, 29*(6), 4–5.
Reprinted by permission of SLACK, Inc.

medical, functional, cognitive, affective, psychosocial, nutritional, and environmental status using commonly recognized standardized instruments such as the Mini-Mental State Examination and the Geriatric Depression Scale. The GCN also collaborated with the patient's primary care provider (PCP) to continue routine assessments to promote self-care throughout the intervention period. The initial in-home assessment by the GRACE team included a comprehensive geriatric assessment, a geriatric-specific physical assessment, and an in-home safety evaluation. The GRACE team protocol also assessed 12 specific geriatric "conditions" on an annual basis.

INTRODUCTORY CASE RESOLUTION

The patient described in this case was cared for at a facility that blended elements of the evidence-based transitions models, including a transitions nurse and social worker, written instructions, close PCP follow-up, and a follow-up phone call from the transitions team. Combining elements from several models is not uncommon. A dedicated transition nurse, in collaboration with a trained social worker, performed the necessary assessments to determine the older adult's eligibility for the hospital's transitional care program. Given his age, new coronary disease, cognitive impairment, and previously inadequate home support system, the transitions team deemed him appropriate for the program.

The patient was seen by the transitions nurse on the day of discharge for further assessment of his ability to self-manage his care. His family was also invited and included in the assessment and evaluated for their caregiver needs. After being educated about the challenges facing the patient after discharge, his daughter was able to arrange her schedule to stay with the patient at his home during the immediate post-discharge period. The patient went home after receiving individualized written discharge instructions and a two-week supply of his new medications.

At the first follow-up visit three days after discharge, the patient's primary care provider reconciled all his medications in the outpatient electronic health record with the written discharge instructions and discharge summary and addressed all medication discrepancies and questions regarding new symptoms and side effects. The primary care physician had already received the patient's completed discharge summary, which was faxed to the outpatient office by the hospital transitions team on the day of discharge. The patient and his daughter received a phone call from the hospital transitions nurse seven days after discharge, in which they reviewed all of the patient's medications once more and discussed red flags indicating a worsening of his condition and which actions to take in response to those warning signs. The transitions nurse also provided them with a telephone number to reach an available nurse for questions 24 hours a day.

▶ Summary

For an older adult, a care transition is a dangerous time when consequential oversights may occur (and occur often), leaving already vulnerable patients more prone to adverse medical errors and **hospital readmission**. This is especially true with the transition from inpatient hospitalization to home. Paramount to a successful transition is a thoughtful **geriatric assessment** of the conditions that leave a patient at risk for complications related to the transition and the necessary medical interventions to avoid these complications (i.e., limiting complex medication regimens and superfluous follow-up while keeping in mind an individual patient's goals of care and what needs to be done to achieve these goals). Assessment in the context of care transitions needs to align with the nature and goals of the clinical model of care transitions management being deployed by a hospital, health system, or other entity. This approach enables prioritization of both the medical and nonmedical ("social") dilemmas that families and patients face during these critical times.

Clear, deliberate, and precise communication is key to ensure an effective transition that promotes patient safety as well as patient and caregiver well-being. Many of the interventions to improve care transitions described in this chapter, despite initially requiring increased investment of mental and financial efforts, led to system-wide cost savings and increased satisfaction for the providers, patients, and caregivers involved. There is no one intervention that is used widely to aid in this transition. However, best practices—which include assigning a dedicated care transitions manager, developing protocols for key care transitions processes, and ensuring successful communication among all healthcare providers and caregivers involved—will be central to ultimately making transitions safer. Future investigations are needed to evaluate more nuanced and scalable innovations in transitions of care.

▶ Additional Resources for Healthcare Professionals

Geriatric assessment is but one component of what is needed to ensure successful care transitions. As noted earlier (especially in the BOOST model), much of the "assessment" during care transitions should also focus on assessing health system characteristics contributing to suboptimal transitions, rather than solely considering patient characteristics. In this manner, a more comprehensive set of solutions can be developed.

For further information, we recommend visiting the National Transitions of Care Coalition (NTOCC) website at http://www.ntocc.org/, specifically its guidebook on implementing and evaluating a plan to improve on transitions of care (http://www.ntocc.org/Portals/0/PDF/Resources/ImplementationPlan.pdf).

References

Boult, C., Leff, B., Boyd, C. M., Wolff, J. L., Marsteller, J. A., Frick, K. D., . . . Scharfstein, D. O. (2013). A matched-pair cluster-randomized trial of guided care for high-risk older patients. *Journal of General Internal Medicine, 28*(5), 612–621. https://doi.org/10.1007/s11606-012-2287-y

Boyd, C. M., Boult, C., Shadmi, E., Leff, B., Brager, R., Dunbar, L., . . . Wegener, S. (2007). Guided care for multimorbid older adults. *Gerontologist, 47*(5), 697–704. Retrieved from http://www.ncbi.nlm.nih.gov/pubmed/17989412

Coleman, E. A. (2003). Falling through the cracks: Challenges and opportunities for improving transitional care for persons with continuous complex care needs. *Journal of the American Geriatrics Society, 51*(4), 549–555. https://doi.org/10.1046/j.1532-5415.2003.51185.x

Coleman, E. A., Parry, C., Chalmers, S., & Min, S.-J. (2006). The care transitions intervention: Results of a randomized controlled trial. *Archives of Internal Medicine, 166*(17), 1822–1828. https://doi.org/10.1001/archinte.166.17.1822

Counsell, S. R., Callahan, C. M., Buttar, A. B., Clark, D. O., & Frank, K. I. (2006). Geriatric Resources for Assessment and Care of Elders (GRACE): A new model of primary care for low-income seniors. *Journal of the American Geriatrics Society, 54*(7), 1136–1141. https://doi.org/10.1111/j.1532-5415.2006.00791.x

Counsell, S. R., Callahan, C. M., Clark, D. O., Tu, W., Buttar, A. B., Stump, T. E., & Ricketts, G. D. (2007). Geriatric care management for low-income seniors: A randomized controlled trial. *Journal of the American Medical Association, 298*(22), 2623–2633. https://doi.org/10.1001/jama.298.22.2623

Counsell, S. R., Callahan, C. M., Tu, W., Stump, T. E., & Arling, G. W. (2009). Cost analysis of the Geriatric Resources for Assessment and Care of Elders care management intervention. *Journal of the American Geriatrics Society, 57*(8), 1420–1426. https://doi.org/10.1021/nl061786n.Core-Shell

Forster, A. J., Murff, H. J., Peterson, J. F., Gandhi, T. K., & Bates, D. W. (2003). The incidence and severity of adverse events affecting patients after discharge from the hospital. *Annals of Internal Medicine, 138*(3), 161–167. https://doi.org/10.7326/0003-4819-138-3-200302040-00007

Gage, B. (1999). Impact of the BBA on post-acute utilization. *Health Care Financing Review, 20*(4), 103–126. https://doi.org/hcfr-20-4-103 [pii]

Hansen, L. O., Greenwald, J. L., Budnitz, T., Howell, E., Halasyamani, L., Maynard, G., . . . Williams, M. V. (2013). Project BOOST: Effectiveness of a multihospital effort to reduce rehospitalization. *Journal of Hospital Medicine*, *8*(8), 421–427. https://doi.org/10.1002/jhm.2054

Jack, B. W., Chetty, V. K., Anthony, D., Greenwald, J. L., Sanchez, G. M., Johnson, A. E., . . . Culpepper, L. (2009). A reengineered hospital discharge program to decrease rehospitalization: A randomized trial. *Annals of Internal Medicine*, *150*(3), 178–187. Retrieved from http://www.ncbi.nlm.nih.gov/pubmed/19189907

Jencks, S. F., Williams, M. V., & Coleman, E. A. (2009). Rehospitalizations among patients in the Medicare fee-for-service program. *New England Journal of Medicine*, *360*(14), 1418–1428. https://doi.org/10.1056/NEJMsa0803563

Kohn, L. T., Corrigan, J., & Donaldson, M. S. (2000). *To err is human: Building a safer health system*. Washington, DC: National Academy Press. Retrieved from http://www.ncbi.nlm.nih.gov/pubmed/25077248

Kuo, Y.-F., Sharma, G., Freeman, J. L., & Goodwin, J. S. (2009). Growth in the care of older patients by hospitalists in the United States. *New England Journal of Medicine*, *360*(11), 1102–1112. https://doi.org/10.1056/NEJMsa0802381

Leonard, M., Graham, S., & Bonacum, D. (2004). The human factor: The critical importance of effective teamwork and communication in providing safe care. *Quality & Safety in Health Care*, *13*(suppl 1), i85–i90. https://doi.org/10.1136/qhc.13.suppl_1.i85

Naylor, M. D., Brooten, D., Campbell, R., Jacobsen, B. S., Mezey, M. D., Pauly, M. V., & Schwartz, J. S. (1999). Comprehensive discharge planning and home follow-up of hospitalized elders: A randomized clinical trial. *Journal of the American Medical Association*, *281*(7), 613–620. Retrieved from http://www.ncbi.nlm.nih.gov/pubmed/10029122

Naylor, M. D., Brooten, D., Jones, R., Lavizzo-Mourey, R., Mezey, M., & Pauly, M. (1994). Comprehensive discharge planning for the hospitalized elderly: A randomized clinical trial. *Annals of Internal Medicine*, *120*(12), 999–1006. Retrieved from http://www.ncbi.nlm.nih.gov/pubmed/8185149

Schnipper, J. L., Kirwin, J. L., Cotugno, M. C., Wahlstrom, S. A., Brown, B. A., Tarvin, E., . . . Bates, D. W. (2006). Role of pharmacist counseling in preventing adverse drug events after hospitalization. *Archives of Internal Medicine*, *166*(5), 565. https://doi.org/10.1001/archinte.166.5.565

Smith, J. D., Coleman, E. A., & Min, S.-J. (2004). A new tool for identifying discrepancies in postacute medications for community-dwelling older adults. *American Journal of Geriatric Pharmacotherapy*, *2*(2), 141–147. Retrieved from http://www.ncbi.nlm.nih.gov/pubmed/15555490

CHAPTER 34

Assessment of Older Adults in Their Home

Sandra Atkins, W. June Simmons, and Aaron Hagedorn

CHAPTER OBJECTIVES

1. Understand the advantages of an in-home geriatric assessment.
2. Understand which domains are the priority for in-home assessments (i.e., which information is uniquely available in the home).
3. Describe approaches for gaining acceptance for a home visit.
4. Identify mechanisms for dealing with family members and potential exposure to dangers related to in-home assessment.

KEY TERMS

Motivational interviewing　　　Person–environment fit　　　Warm handoff

▶ Introduction

This chapter deals primarily with nonmedical assessment of older adults, focusing on domains that can be assessed only in the home. Other chapters of this text discuss specific assessments, such as behavioral health, functioning, or social support, that can also be administered in the home, but this chapter looks at information uniquely available via in-home assessment.

Performing assessments in the home provides a rich opportunity to interact with older adults in their own environment. In this context, one can observe coping skills, potential strengths, and resilience (McQuaide & Ehrenreich, 1997). Meeting in the home allows the older adult to share his or her reality and enhances the engagement between the person doing the assessment and the patient and family. This type of encounter can provide more time and an open environment that promote a stronger personal connection and engagement, both of which are often core to social work assessment (Dybicz, 2012). By encouraging an older adult to tell his or her life story while being guided by an assessment tool, one can develop a rapport and a culturally sensitive perspective of that client (Millender, 2011).

In addition to the environmental and personal observational opportunities, standardized assessments can be structured to gather facts for understanding key needs, values, and goals to support development of an appropriate care and service plan. Comprehensive assessments involve multidimensional observations of and by the client and caregivers that extend to person–environment interaction (Youdin, 2014).

The home is the environment where older adults spend the most time. Items in the home may reflect the personality, resources, and interests of the person. Home layout and design may impact quality of life, in the practical sense of either supporting or impeding mobility and functioning—that is, **person–environment fit**, as M. Powell Lawton suggested (Lawton, 1983). The home is an important environment for many older adults and can be as important an assessment subject as the patients themselves. Does the home offer supports, comforts, and accommodations, or does it present any unique functional or safety challenges? Does the home contribute to social isolation? Does the person feel comfortable going outside of the home?

▶ Why Is In-Home Assessment Important?

There are many reasons for choosing to assess an older adult in the home environment. First, it may be a necessity for those patients who are unable or unwilling, for any of a variety of reasons,

to leave the house. Second, some safety issues may be related to the home environment, such that they require in-person observation. Often having "eyes and ears" in the home setting provides access to information not gathered in an interview only. A home visit may also be a program requirement; for example, most states' Medicaid Home and Community Based Services [Medicaid §1915(c)] waivers require an initial and then at least annual in-home assessment by nurse and/or social worker. Likewise, Meals on Wheels programs usually require an in-home assessment to certify eligibility.

Increasingly, health plans and other managed care entities have established case management programs, although they typically rely on telephone calls. These calls can be complemented by a well-targeted in-home assessment for older adults who have one or more complex chronic conditions. Telephonic case managers (usually registered nurses [RNs]) can select plan members or patients who appear to have complex needs or who have deteriorating physical, cognitive, and/or mental health conditions and, therefore, are at risk for hospitalization or nursing home placement or even inappropriate emergency department use. Risk factors among community-dwelling older adults that may trigger a home visit may potentially include the following:

- Recent hospitalization(s)
- Lack of a caregiver, inadequate caregiver support, or caregiver burden or poor health
- Cognitive impairment, which can lead to nonadherence and other risks
- Recent history of falls
- Mobility impairment
- Incontinence
- Complex medication regimens (e.g., multiple chronic conditions, multiple prescribers, multiple daily doses and schedules)
- Depression or anxiety
- Poor adherence to special diets, medications, exercise, or treatments
- Low health literacy, when the patient must carry out self-care or monitoring activities at home

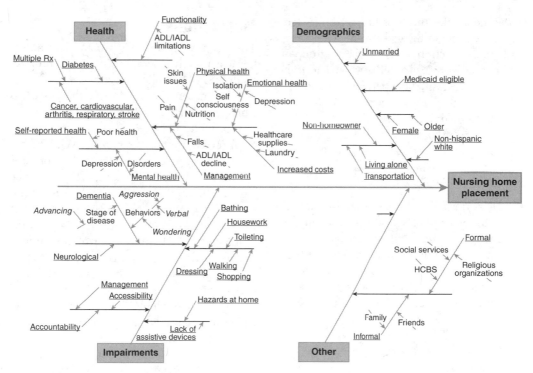

FIGURE 34-1 Patient characteristics correlated with nursing home placement.

- Lack of access to reliable or assisted transportation
- Financial needs related to ability to purchase nutritious food, pay for medications, and other issues

Many state Medicaid programs now require enrollment in a managed care health plan. Some have also initiated special programs for beneficiaries dually eligible for Medicare and Medicaid, where the health plan assumes the financial risk for long-term nursing home placement. These health plans need to assess members and address risk factors that may lead to patients' decline and nursing home placement. **FIGURE 34-1** summarizes the various patient factors that studies have identified as contributing to permanent nursing home placement, and that should therefore be reviewed in any assessment. For example, unmarried people who live alone in rented accommodations are at increased risk of nursing home placement. Caregiver factors, discussed in the *Caregiver Assessment* chapter, are also extremely important.

▶ Best Practices[1]

Anyone new to the practice of in-home assessments can benefit from the experience of seasoned experts in this area. Such an assessment is a very sensitive activity because the home is the client's personal space. It is important to remember that the home is where the older adult should be most in control, so the assessor should

---

1 Best practices and challenges were identified in a focus group that included four seasoned social workers in leadership positions within the Partners in Care Foundation.

let the client guide the assessor regarding where to sit and conduct the assessment. The points made in this section were raised by a group of senior social work leaders, all of whom had years of in-home assessment experience.

Photographs and other personal items in the setting or the condition of the home can be conversation starters that reveal a great deal about the person's interests, social support system, and values. General best practices for home visits include the following:

- *Don't rush.* Take time to establish rapport so the older adult will be more forthcoming about potentially uncomfortable subjects such as alcohol use, psychotropic medications, or abuse.
- *Ask permission.* This provides a sense of control to the older adult. Use phrases such as "Could you show me . . . ?" or "Is it okay if I look . . . ?"
- *The person has the right to be wrong.* The assessor should not use personal filters or standards to judge, but rather should elicit the older adult's perspective and preferences.
- *Confirm what the person says against observations.* An older adult may say he needs no help, but if the home is dirty and he has trouble getting out of a chair, he probably does need help.

▶ Assessment Domains: Priorities for the Home Visit

Time in the home is a precious resource, and one should go into the in-home assessment with clear priorities in mind. Many older adults may tire before a comprehensive assessment can be completed. Some of the work, such as structured interview questions, can be conducted by phone before and after the home visit, but other aspects must be done in the home. Unique opportunities impossible to seize anywhere except in the home are discussed next.

Medications

The top priority for a visit to an older adult's home is usually a comprehensive inventory of medications, including over-the-counter medications and supplements—even things such as Chinese herbal teas. Self-report and even brown-bag (bringing all medications to a central location) review are not as complete. While in the home, it is crucial to walk through to observe and inquire about medications, as they are often stored in multiple places such as the refrigerator, next to an easy chair, or in the bedroom. Before proceeding with this investigation, the home visit staff should ask permission to look in cupboards, drawers, and other places to find out-of-sight medications. It is advisable to check each medication container for the date filled and an approximate number of pills remaining to gauge adherence. Note that some older adults mix multiple medications into a single container, or put new medications into a favorite bottle that is easier to open or more right-sized.

For each medication, it is important to ask certain key questions:

- What do you take this medication for/why do you take it?
- How much do you take at one time?
- How often do you take it?
- How long have you been taking this medication?
- Does it seem to be working for you?
- Have you experienced any adverse effects?

During a general discussion about medications, additional questions are important:

- Have you left any prescriptions unfilled or failed to refill a prescription:
  - Because you could not afford to pay for it?
  - Because you decided the risks were not worth the benefit?
  - Because you did not understand why it was prescribed?
- Have you stopped taking any medications on your own (i.e., without a doctor telling you to stop)?

Tools

Dr. Eric Coleman has developed the Medication Discrepancy Tool for the Care Transitions Intervention (http://caretransitions.org/all -tools-and-resources/). This tool is an excellent checklist of reasons why a person may not be taking medications as directed and includes an action plan for any discrepancies discovered. A structured, evidence-based program for identifying medication safety risks in a home visit is HomeMeds, which pairs trained paraprofessionals with software and pharmacist review to identify and resolve potential medication-related problems such as falls, dizziness, confusion, and gastrointestinal bleeding.

Note that a medication inventory and inquiry does *not* require a clinical background. This investigation focuses on copying information from medication bottles, asking structured questions, and documenting any discrepancies between medications as directed and as taken. Thus, alternative workforce deployment may be used to complete this assessment.

Fall Risk (Including Home Safety and Sanitation)

The second priority for a geriatric assessment home visit tends to be a fall-risk assessment, which should include a general evaluation of safety and sanitation for the house itself. The U.S. Centers for Disease Control and Prevention (CDC) sponsors and makes available the standard tools used in this domain, including the STEADI (Stopping Elderly Accidents, Deaths, and Injuries) toolkit (https://www.cdc .gov/steadi/materials.html). The CDC recommends beginning with three screening questions and proceeding with a more comprehensive assessment if the answer is yes to any or all of the questions:

- Have you fallen in the past year?
- Do you feel unsteady when standing or walking?
- Do you worry about falling?

Although this assessment can be done in clinic or office, the home is also a good place to conduct the Timed Up and Go (TUG) test, another element in the CDC STEADI toolkit. The TUG test has been correlated with a history of falls (Beauchet et al., 2011). It involves timing the older adult as he or she rises from a seated position, walks 3 meters, turns around, returns, and sits back down.

Fall Risk Factors in the House

The CDC also publishes a checklist for consumers, "Check for Safety," in English and Spanish and makes copies available for free (https://www .cdc.gov/steadi/patient.html). The checklist guides the patient or family member to look for hazards on floors, stairs, and steps, and in the kitchen, bathroom, and bedrooms. Examples of items to check while in the home include the following:

- Furniture—for example, too low or too high to get into or out of safely, chairs with casters likely to move when sitting down or getting up
- Loose rugs
- Uneven or slippery walking surfaces inside and outside the home
- Cords in pathways
- Inadequate lighting, especially on stairways
- Need for handrails, grab bars, and assistive devices to enhance safety

While searching for fall risks in the home, it is advisable to look for other potential health-related issues:

- Nonfunctioning equipment (e.g., heater, air conditioner, kitchen appliances)
- Broken windows, screens, and so on
- Presence or absence of functioning smoke and carbon monoxide detectors
- Stairs that may be barriers for mobility-impaired older adults

Family and Social Network

Understanding the social support system for at-risk older adults is critically important. There are many ways to supplement structured social and family caregiver assessment questions (discussed in the *Caregiver Assessment* chapter) with observations and conversation. For example, most people have photographs of loved ones that can be used as conversation starters. A picture of a grandchild could stimulate questions like "How old is she now?", "Where does he live?", or "When is the last time you saw her?" Answers—or the lack of photos or other indicators of social support in the home—can provide a gauge of social isolation. Beyond directly asking the older adult about others in the home, presence of others in the home may be indicated by cars in the driveway, cigarettes in an ashtray, or clothes in the closet.

If others are present during the in-home assessment, the assessor can observe the dynamics of their interactions with the older adult—body language can express stress or comfort, for example. When others are present, it is important to try to keep the focus on the older adult by asking the older adult the questions and, if someone else answers, redirecting the question for confirmation by the person being assessed. If the assessor perceives potential caregiver burden or burnout, it would be important to schedule a separate interview of the caregiver to fully assess the situation and offer support.

Other Unique In-Home Assessment Domains

Visiting an older adult's home can provide other insights that are important for designing appropriate care and service plans.

Sniff Test

After getting permission to walk around the home and open cabinets, the home visitor can derive information from the odors present. For example, bathroom or trashcan odors may indicate a need for housekeeping support. Although the older adult may be hesitant to answer a question about cigarette smoking, alcohol use, or marijuana use, telltale odors may provide missing information.

Visual Evaluation of the House

While in the home, it is important to observe for cleanliness, especially issues with potential for direct harm, such as signs of vermin infestation or mold in the bathroom or kitchen. Other insights can be gained by observing contents of trashcans; for example, empty liquor bottles or beer cans may help explain a fall and suggest the need for an intervention. Clutter can be a safety issue that requires intervention. If there are many lists and reminders throughout the home, cognitive impairment may be an issue. Used ashtrays in the home of a person using oxygen can indicate both a safety hazard and a potential irritant for a person with lung disease.

Skill Demonstration

Another unique opportunity typically available only through a home visit is verification that the older adult has crucial skills or abilities. This can range from demonstrating ability to carry out activities of daily living (ADLs), such as getting out of bed or going to the bathroom, to demonstrating medication management or blood pressure monitoring. As the assessment progresses, the home visitor can begin to perceive how the patient's answers to questions may be at odds with observed reality. For example, when assessing if the person is independent in bathing, the assessor might ask the older adult to demonstrate how she gets in and out of the tub or shower. For patients with diabetes, asking for a demonstration of glucometer use would be important.

Observing for Cognitive, Self-Care, or Sensory Problems

While carrying out the assessment and engaging in conversation, the home visit staff can observe for signs of cognitive impairment (e.g., repeating questions, forgetting why you are there) and problems with hearing or vision. For example, in the process of doing a medication inventory, home visit staff can ask the older adult to read a label and explain what it means. If the home visitor speaks loudly, slowly, and using clear diction, hearing loss may be suspected if the older adult asks for questions to be repeated or shows signs of straining to hear. The home visit is a good opportunity to observe grooming and cleanliness—people often clean up well to see the doctor but in their more relaxed home environment it should be possible to see them as they usually are.

Neighborhood Conditions

Although changing neighborhoods may not be possible, some potential interventions can increase personal safety in a questionable neighborhood. Home visitors can be on the lookout for adequate locks, window bars, and other security features, as they may be affordable for the older adult and/or family or paid for by health plans or subsidized social service programs.

▶ Practice Challenges

Many unique challenges to home assessment arise that may be less of a concern in the typical assessment that takes place in a clinic.

Gaining Access to the Home

The first and foremost challenge in carrying out an in-home assessment is getting agreement for a home visit, as many older adults or their family members are suspicious or afraid of strangers seeking access to their home. It is important to establish rapport from the very start to avoid any perception that you are trying to sell the older adult something, rob the client, or represent an authority that could inhibit freedom for the older adult or a loved one. Beginning with the name of a trusted referral source is essential.

Best Practices for Gaining Access

To ensure the best success in securing permission to make a home visit, the initial introduction should include the following elements:

- The name of the organization or person (e.g., doctor) on whose behalf the assessment will be done
- The relationship of the referral source to the older adult (e.g., your doctor)
- The reason for the visit
- What will happen during the visit
- What will be done after the visit
- The name and credentials of the person who will be visiting

Experienced social workers recommend proceeding slowly to gauge the person's reactions and anticipating and providing information to combat typical objections. Using **motivational interviewing** techniques can help establish rapport and elicit internal reasons why the older adult would benefit from the home visit. Establishing rapport may be easier when the caller knows the audience, the community, and the healthcare context.

Barriers to Gaining Access to the Home

Social workers and others attempting to arrange for an in-home assessment have identified numerous potential barriers to be aware of and prepared for.

Unable to Contact the Patient. It is fairly common to be unable to reach the person recommended for an in-home assessment. A system-level approach to minimize this problem is to have an excellent program intake form that includes emergency contact information so that if the older adult cannot be reached, an alternative contact is available.

A typical barrier to contact is the fact that many people screen their calls and will not pick up the phone if they are not certain about the identity of the caller. The best approach to use if this happens is a **warm handoff**, meaning that someone the patient knows and trusts places the call, and a telephone conference is organized among the third party, the person arranging for the home visit, and the older adult or his or her representative. After making the introduction, explaining the purpose, and encouraging the older adult to participate, the third party may disconnect.

Another issue is that some people may move or change phone numbers frequently. In this case, a strategy that can work well is to visit the home unannounced and engage the older adult (or other person who answers the door) in conversation until a sufficient degree of rapport develops and the visitor is invited inside. The home visitor must have a photo badge, a business card, and an explanatory handout explaining clearly the relationship of the home visitor to a familiar and trusted person or organization.

Language and Immigration Status. It is important to match outreach and home visit personnel to the language and culture of the older adult to be assessed. In addition, immigration status for anyone in the household can be a major issue causing refusal of a home visit. Explaining the fact that the visit is not tied to governmental or law enforcement agencies may be helpful, but ultimately establishing rapport and understanding through conversation will be required. It may also be helpful to offer to meet at a neutral location outside the home until trust has been established.

Family Reticence. When family members become caregivers, they can be extremely protective and refuse access. Again, it is crucial to thoroughly explain the purpose of the home visit and the potential benefit, engaging in conversation until a degree of comfort and rapport have been established. Scheduling the appointment when the family member can be present may also help reduce resistance. Working with the entire support system is important for older adults with functional or cognitive deficits or complex chronic conditions. If the caregiver will be present during the in-home assessment, the home visitor should request a few minutes alone with the older adult, especially if the family dynamic seems indicative of potential abuse.

Safety for In-Home Assessment Personnel

Making home visits exposes workers to potentially dangerous situations. It is crucial to provide training, tools, and equipment to keep staff as safe as possible. Internet searching on the phrase "safety checklist for home visits" will bring up many appropriate tools. Experienced social work supervisors[2] also provide the following advice.

Before the Visit

The best approach is to assign staff who know the neighborhood well, speak the dominant language, and reflect the population. When scheduling the home visit, ask if anyone on the property has animals, especially dogs. Ask about parking: Request permission to use the driveway, or otherwise ask for advice on the best place to park. If the home is in a rough neighborhood, schedule the visit for a mid-week morning. It is also important to gauge the possibility of danger within the home, so asking about others who live on the property and knowing about the older adult's history of mental illness or substance abuse is advisable. The home visitor should take precautions, including carrying legal defensive items. Working in pairs, though not a low-cost option, can be a good approach under certain circumstances.

On the Day of the Visit

A best practice is to drive by the home to observe the neighborhood before getting out of the car. Trust your instincts and reschedule the visit if you sense any danger. Match attire to the neighborhood standard, but avoid brightly colored or revealing clothes. If there is an incident outside, move to the safest location within the home, call the police, and then wait until you see the police before leaving. Leave nothing visible in the car.

Potential Abuse or Neglect

In addition to asking direct questions, the home visitor should look for bruising or sores on the older adult and observe for possible tension when others are present in the home. It may be necessary to notify adult protective services if there is good reason to suspect abuse or self neglect. Usually the staff member performing the home visit should discuss any suspected abuse or neglect with a supervisor to determine whether additional services could resolve the issue and to gain the perspective of other, more experienced staff.

Presence of Family Members

In most cases, especially when the patient has cognitive impairment, it can be extremely helpful to have a family member present. When making the appointment for the home visit, the assessor should ask if there is anyone the patient wants to invite to be present. At some point, it is a good idea to request a private moment to do a cognitive status assessment and ask questions about potential abuse. In some cases, a family member may pose a danger to the staff member doing the assessment—for example, a drug-abusing child or grandchild. In such a case, it may be advisable to stop the assessment and leave to avoid problems, returning another time when the family member is not present.

▶ Sample Assessment Tool or Approach

This chapter has sought to complement the other chapters of this text dealing with structured assessment tools. The domains discussed here are most appropriately supported by a checklist approach. Throughout this chapter, tools have been suggested to guide activities, interviews, and observations during a home visit. These include the CDC's STEADI toolkit, HomeMeds, and Dr. Eric Coleman's Medication Discrepancy Tool (**BOX 34-1–BOX 34-3**).

BOX 34-1 Suggested Questions on Living Arrangements, Environmental and Home Safety, Self-Care, and Neglect

Is this your only/permanent residence? Yes/No; if no:
- Where else do you live/sleep?
  - Address and relationship

Do you own or rent? (Linked to financial worries, ability to do home modifications)
- Own, no mortgage
- Own, paying mortgage
- Rent/contribute to rent, including board and care or assisted living facility
- Do not pay rent/mortgage because someone else is paying

Do you live alone? Yes/No
   If yes and the patient has ADL/IADL problems or cognitive or emotional problems, trigger the problem statement: "Member/patient lives alone and has ADL and/or IADL needs and/or cognitive impairment and/or mental/emotional/behavioral health issues."

(continues)

BOX 34-1 Suggested Questions on Living Arrangements, Environmental and Home Safety, Self-Care, and Neglect *(continued)*

If no, ask about household composition: Who else lives here?

- Spouse/partner
- Adult children: number, names, and contact information
- Other relative(s): number and relationship
- Children/minor(s) younger than age 18: number, relationship, and ages
- Friend(s)
- Paid caregiver
- Renter/home sharing
- Congregate living: group home, board and care, retirement home, assisted living

Do you provide care for any other household members? Yes/No

If yes, who (relationship): Trigger caregiver burden assessment.

- If doing an assessment for an insurance plan or medical group, ask if the person cared for is in the same plan/group.
  - If yes, identify name, insurance identification number, member identification number.

How likely is it that you will lose your housing in the next 6 months? 4: extremely, 3: very, 2: somewhat, 1: unlikely

- If 3 or 4, why?
- Trigger problem statement: Member/patient fears loss of housing because:
  - Cannot afford mortgage/rent, upkeep, and/or utilities
  - Person(s) I live with may decide to "kick me out"
  - My physical condition makes access difficult
  - Notes:

Do you feel you would be better off living someplace else? Yes/No

- If yes:
  - Why?
    - Safety concerns
    - Accessibility concerns
    - Cost
    - Need care
  - Where?
  - With whom?
  - Why aren't you there now?

If there is any mobility-related ADL/IADL deficit: Do you need to climb stairs to enter or leave your house? Yes/No

If yes, tie to next question.

Is there a landlord (apartment/building manager, homeowners association) whom we may contact if needed? Yes/No

If yes, identify name, phone number, and email.

Are you able to keep the temperature in your home at a comfortable level? Yes/No

- If no, is the problem:
  - Heating?
  - Cooling?
  - Both?

Do any of the appliances or plumbing fixtures (e.g., sink, toilet) not function properly? Yes/No

If yes, explain.

Inspired by MDS for Homecare.

BOX 34-2 Patient Self-Assessment: Fall Risk

How many times have you fallen in the past month?
How many times have you fallen in the past 3 months?
STEADI Patient Brochure: Please circle "Yes" or "No" for each statement.

		Why It Matters
Yes (2) No (0)	I have fallen in the past year.	People who have fallen once are likely to fall again. If age < 70 and answer is no, skip STEADI.
Yes (2) No (0)	I use or have been advised to use a cane or walker to get around safely.	People who have been advised to use a cane or walker may already be more likely to fall.
Yes (1) No (0)	Sometimes I feel unsteady when I am walking.	Unsteadiness and needing support while walking are signs of poor balance.
Yes (1) No (0)	I steady myself by holding onto furniture when walking at home.	This is also a sign of poor balance.
Yes (1) No (0)	I am worried about falling.	People who are worried about falling are more likely to fall.
Yes (1) No (0)	I need to push with my hands to stand up from a chair.	This is a sign of weak leg muscles, a major reason for falling.
Yes (1) No (0)	I have some trouble stepping up onto a curb.	This is also a sign of weak leg muscles.
Yes (1) No (0)	I often have to rush to the toilet.	Rushing to the bathroom, especially at night, increases the chance of falling.
Yes (1) No (0)	I have lost some feeling in my feet.	Numbness in the feet can cause stumbles and lead to falls.
Yes (1) No (0)	I take medicine that sometimes makes me feel light-headed or more tired than usual.	Side effects from medicines can sometimes increase the chance of falling.
Yes (1) No (0)	I take medicine to help me sleep or improve my mood.	These medicines can sometimes increase the chance of falling.
Yes (1) No (0)	I often feel sad or depressed.	Symptoms of depression, such as not feeling well or feeling slowed down, are linked to falls.

Total_____
Add up the number of points for each "yes" answer. If you scored 4 points or more, you may be at risk for falling. Discuss this brochure with your doctor.

This checklist was developed by the Greater Los Angeles VA Geriatric Research Education Clinical Center and affiliates and is a validated fall risk self-assessment tool [Rubenstein, L. Z., Vivrette, R., Harker, J. O., Stevens, J. A., & Kramer, B. J. (2011). Validating an evidence-based, self-rated fall risk questionnaire (FRQ) for older adults. *Journal of Safety Research, 42*(6), 493–499]. Adapted with permission of the authors.

BOX 34-3 The CDC Fall Risk Checklist

If fall risk is high, do a thorough home review looking for the following hazards:

- Loose rugs
- Electrical cords
- Cluttered house
- Unsafe stairs
- Inadequate lighting
- Phone accessibility
- Safety concern outside the home (e.g., cracks in the sidewalk)

Floors: Look at the floor in each room.	*What to do*
When you walk through a room, do you have to walk around furniture?	Ask someone to move the furniture so your path is clear.
Do you have throw rugs on the floor?	Remove the rugs or use double-sided tape or a nonslip backing so the rugs will not slip.
Are there papers, books, towels, shoes, magazines, boxes, blankets, or other objects on the floor?	Pick up things that are on the floor. Always keep objects off the floor.
Do you have to walk over or around wires or cords (e.g., lamp, telephone, or extension cords)?	Coil or tape cords and wires next to the wall so you will not trip over them. If needed, have an electrician put in another outlet.
Stairs and Steps: Look at the stairs you use both inside and outside your home.	*Only include this if the patient has stairs.*
Are there papers, shoes, books, or other objects on the stairs?	Pick up things on the stairs. Always keep objects off stairs.
Are some steps broken or uneven?	Fix loose or uneven steps.
Is a light over the stairway missing?	Have an electrician put in an overhead light at the top and bottom of the stairs.
Is there only one light switch for the stairs (only at the top or at the bottom of the stairs)?	Have an electrician put in a light switch at the top and bottom of the stairs. You can get light switches that glow.
Has the stairway light bulb burned out?	Have a friend or family member change the light bulb.
Is the carpet on the steps loose or torn?	Make sure the carpet is firmly attached to every step, or remove the carpet and attach nonslip rubber treads to the stairs.

Are the handrails loose or broken? Is there a handrail on only one side of the stairs?	Fix loose handrails or put in new ones. Make sure handrails are on both sides of the stairs and are as long as the stairs.
Kitchen: Look at your kitchen and eating area.	
Are the things you use often on high shelves?	Move items in your cabinets. Keep things you use often on the lower shelves (about waist level).
Is your step stool unsteady?	If you must use a step stool, get one with a bar to hold on to. Never use a chair as a step stool.
Bathrooms: Look at all your bathrooms.	
Is the tub or shower floor slippery?	Put a nonslip rubber mat or self-stick strips on the floor of the tub or shower.
Do you need some support when you get in and out of the tub or up from the toilet?	Have grab bars put in next to and inside the tub and next to the toilet.
Bedrooms: Look at all your bedrooms.	
Is the light near the bed hard to reach?	Place a lamp close to the bed where it is easy to reach.
Is the path from your bed to the bathroom dark?	Put in a nightlight so you can see where you are walking. Some nightlights go on by themselves after dark.

Other Observations: Checklist	No	Yes	Problem Statement/ Recommendation
Unpleasant smells: kitchen, bathroom, trash			
Urine smell			
Unable to demonstrate proper use of health self-monitoring devices (e.g., glucometer, blood pressure cuff)			
Unable to read/understand medication label			

(continues)

BOX 34-3 The CDC Fall Risk Checklist   *(continued)*

Other Observations: Checklist	No	Yes	Problem Statement/ Recommendation
Evidence of self-neglect			
Evidence of vermin (droppings or live specimens): roaches, termites, rodents			
Evidence of hoarding			
Evidence of memory loss (e.g., reminders around the house)			
Evidence of cutting or self-harm/self-mutilation			
Evidence of potential abuse			
Other household members pose potential threat			

Modified from CDC. (2017). Check for safety: A home fall prevention checklist for older adults. Retrieved from https://www.cdc.gov/steadi/pdf /STEADI_CheckforSafety_brochure-a.pdf

▶ Assessing the Geriatric Population Living with Homelessness

The geriatric population living with homelessness is growing in the United States; it is predicted to more than double by 2050, from more than 44,000 people in 2010 to nearly 93,000 in 2050 (Sermons & Henry, 2010). Older adults living with homelessness face more physical, psychological, and cognitive health challenges than the general geriatric population or the general population living with homelessness. Specifically, people in the chronically homeless population tend to be "old" at a younger age. Functional impairments occur in 30% of homeless adults in their 50s and early 60s, or approximately the same rate as in people 20 years older among non-homeless adults (Cimino et al., 2015).

Addressing the needs of homeless individuals is important for containing healthcare costs. For example, although people living with homelessness constitute only approximately 0.1% of the general population, they account for nearly 10% of those using emergency department services (Feldman et al., 2017). A study in Hamilton, Ontario, found that of homeless adults using emergency department services, 66% were older than age 50; of these persons, only 20% were female. Of emergency department visits, 28% were related to psychiatric diagnoses, including substance use disorder.

Conducting psychosocial assessments of the geriatric population living with homelessness poses a unique set of challenges, not the least of which is finding and connecting with these individuals in temporary settings such as emergency shelters, transitional shelters, transitional housing, substance abuse rehabilitation centers, or places such as their car or a tent on a street corner. Once the person has been located, the next challenge is to establish trust. This usually means showing up multiple times to demonstrate that there is sincere concern about the person's health and well-being. The use of community health workers who have a relatively close match to the homeless person's language, background, and culture may be helpful in creating rapport, as may use of evidence-based motivational approaches.

Psychosocial assessments for older adults experiencing homelessness should include sections that cover the following components:

- Physical functioning
- Cognitive/psychological status
- Caregiver/social supports, including the degree to which the homeless community is an important source of support
- Formal services used—past and present
- Housing status, including length of time the person has been homeless
- Legal/financial resources

Most assessment questions need not be unique to those living with homelessness. The assessments found elsewhere in this text should work well.

"Vulnerability" is a valuable concept in the assessment of homeless people. Vulnerability indices or assessments have been developed to measure the likelihood of an individual experiencing homelessness to pass away, or to continue to experience homelessness. The Vulnerability Assessment Tool is a validated, reliable measure developed in 2003 by the community-based homeless services organization Downtown Emergency Services Center (DESC) in Seattle, Washington, as "a structured way of measuring individual's vulnerability to continued instability." It is often used to target scarce resources to those at highest risk of continued vulnerability (DESC, 2017). The instrument covers 10 domains:

- Survival skills
- Basic needs
- Mortality risk
- Medical risks
- Organization/orientation
- Mental health
- Substance use
- Communication
- Social behaviors
- Homelessness

Many organizations that serve homeless adults, including primary and specialty care settings, incorporate the psychosocial assessment into an office visit. Governmental organizations such as the Veterans Administration conduct such assessments as part of standard policy and procedure (National Social Work Program, VA Care Management and Social Work Services, 2010). This is important because although the 20 million U.S. veterans make up only 6% of the total population, they constitute approximately 11% of the homeless population (National Coalition for Homeless Veterans, n.d.; U.S. Department of Veterans Affairs, 2017).

Providers working with older adults can look at solutions that have been identified by research as key factors in helping adults avoid or reduce the health risks associated with age and homelessness. Some elements that should be included in a psychosocial assessment conducted with this population, as well as interventions to consider within a care plan, include the following:

- Assisting a client in having a permanent address or P.O. box to use to receive mail from Social Security, Medicare, Medicaid, their health plan, and/or county mental health or social services
- Assisting with benefits advocacy to secure and enroll in the best possible coverage options (National Council on Aging, 2017; Substance Abuse and Mental Health Services Administration, 2016)
- Ensuring access to preventive health care, such as regular visits with a primary care provider and specialists if needed
- Accessing subsidies such as Section 8 housing or Shelter Plus Care through the local housing authority, to assist the client in obtaining safe and stable housing

Other resources include the Substance Abuse and Mental Health Administration (2016) and its homelessness programs and resources.

▶ Summary

The home is a person-in-environment opportunity to understand the context of the older adult, and an opportunity to see the person's inner and outer experiences, resources, and capabilities. An in-home assessment visit represents a substantial investment, often lasting 2 hours in the home, with the addition of travel time, documentation and follow-up bringing the total time required to 6–8 hours. Given this investment, it is important to use time in the home to best advantage—focusing on domains that can be assessed only in the home environment and domains where additional insights can be gained through the home visit. The usual priority areas will be (1) a hands-on medication inventory and adherence evaluation; (2) fall risk and home safety assessment; (3) interview about or observation of family caregivers or others in the home; and (4) a multisensory walk-through and review of self-care capacity, including demonstration of ability to follow instructions on a medicine bottle or to use equipment such as a glucometer or blood pressure cuff.

Making a home visit is an extremely sensitive assignment, requiring specially trained personnel who are given tools both to guide interactions and to protect themselves in an unfamiliar environment. These visits are best carried out by staff who are linguistically and culturally matched to the older adult and to the neighborhood, who are dressed conservatively and do not draw attention to themselves, and who are prepared and know ahead of time where to go. With this preparation and training, in-home assessments can build close relationships and yield unique insights into the everyday abilities and challenges of older adults. In this era of "whole person" care, nothing else is likely to bring health care so close to the values and preferences, abilities and challenges, and social support system of the older adult. The result should be care tailored to the most important needs of the person, supporting that individual in remaining safely at home and in the community for as long as possible.

References

Beauchet, O., Fantino, B., Allali, G., Muir, S. W., Montero-Odasso, M., & Annweiler, C. (2011). Timed Up and Go test and risk of falls in older adults: A systematic review. *Journal of Nutrition, Health, and Aging, 15*(10), 933–938.

Cimino, T., Steinman, M. A., Mitchell, S. L., Miao, Y., Bharel, M., Barnhardt, C. E., & Brown, R. T. (2015). Disabled on the street: The course of functional impairment in older homeless adults. *JAMA Internal Medicine, 175*(7), 1237–1239. Retrieved from http://www.ncbi.nlm.nih.gov/pmc/articles/PMC4494897/

Downtown Emergency Services Center (DESC). (2017). Vulnerability Assessment Tool. Retrieved from https://www.desc.org/what-we-do/vulnerability-assessment-tool/

Dybicz, P. (2012). The ethic of care: Recapturing social work's first voice. *Social Work, 57*(3), 271–280.

Feldman, B. J., Cologero, C. G., Elsayed, K. S., Abbasi, O. Z., Enyart, J., Friel, T. J., . . . Greenberg, M. R. (2017). Prevalence of homelessness in the emergency department setting., *Western Journal of Emergency Medicine, 18*(3), 366–372. Retrieved from https://www.ncbi.nlm.nih.gov/pmc/articles/PMC5391885/

Lawton, M. P. (1983). Environment and other determinants of well-being in older people. *The Gerontologist, 23*(4), 349–357.

McQuaide, S., & Ehrenreich, J. (1997). Assessing client strengths. *Families in Society: The Journal of Contemporary Social Services, 78*(2), 201–212.

Millender, E. (2011). Using stories to bridge cultural disparities, one culture at a time. *The Journal of Continuing Education in Nursing, 42*(1), 37–42.

National Coalition for Homeless Veterans. (n.d.). Background & statistics: FAQ about homeless veterans. Retrieved from http://nchv.org/index.php/news/media/background_and_statistics/

National Council on Aging. (2017). BenefitsCheckUp. Retrieved from https://www.benefitscheckup.org

National Social Work Program, VA Care Management and Social Work Services. (2010, November; revised 2013, August). *Overview of VA programs where social workers serve*. Retrieved from http://vasocialworkers.org/Documents/Overview%20of%20VA%20Programs%20Where%20Social%20Workers%20Serve.pdf

Sermons, M. W., & Henry, M. (2010, April). The demographics of homelessness series: The rising elderly population. *Research Matters*. Homelessness Research Institute. Retrieved from https://endhomelessness.org/resource/the-rising-elderly-population/

Substance Abuse and Mental Health Services Administration. (2016, April 22). Homelessness programs and resources. Retrieved from https://www.samhsa.gov/homelessness-programs-resources

U.S. Department of Veterans Affairs, National Center for Veterans Analysis and Statistics. (2017, August 31). Veteran population. Retrieved from https://www.va.gov/vetdata/Veteran_Population.asp

Youdin, R. (2014). *Clinical gerontological social work practice*. Springer Publishing Company.

CHAPTER 35

Aging in Place: Transitional Housing and Supported Housing Models

Kari Lane, Colleen Galambos, Lorraine Phillips, Lori Popejoy, and Marilyn Rantz

CHAPTER OBJECTIVES

1. Understand the definition and components of aging in place (AIP).
2. Envision AIP possibilities in the community.
3. Describe key assessment features of an AIP model.
4. Recognize future research directions related to AIP.

KEY TERMS

Aging in place (AIP)   Health   Older adults
Functional decline   Housing

▶ Introduction

Aging in place (AIP) is the ability to live in one's home and community safely, independently, and comfortably, regardless of age, income, or ability level (Centers for Disease Control and Prevention [CDC], 2017). The preference of many **older adults** is to age in place either within their own homes or within a range of affordable age-appropriate **housing** options located in the community in which they reside. A survey conducted by AARP (Keenan, 2010) found that 88% of adults older than age 65 wished to age in place at home, and 92% wished to remain in their communities in appropriate housing options designed for seniors. For these respondents, AIP means remaining in their homes and communities in familiar surroundings while living independently and affordably.

Typically, as adults age and experience **health** and **functional decline**, they experience housing transitions, such as moving from their independent home to assisted living and then to nursing home settings. Moving from home to an assisted living facility is often necessary due to structural inadequacies of the home, lack of in-home care resources, and social isolation. The care provided in assisted living facilities and nursing homes is dictated by state and federal regulations that define and prescribe what, how, and who provides care. These regulations also mandate building and safety standards; payment for care may also be determined through these regulatory standards (e.g., Medicare and Medicaid). Although regulations differ from state to state, they typically define a specific level of ability that a resident must maintain to remain in independent, assisted living, or skilled nursing environments. Regulations require that residents move to a higher level of care as their health deteriorates and their self-care abilities decline (Rantz, Marek, & Zwygart-Stauffacher, 2000).

As an alternative, comprehensive AIP models use care coordination to integrate health, housing, and supportive services to maintain (where needed) and increase functional independence while respecting older adults' preferences about where they want to live (Rantz, et al., 2014). According to AARP (Ball, 2017), there are five key components to successful AIP models for older adults:

1. Choice: Provide affordable healthcare and housing options aimed at meeting the diverse and changing needs.
2. Flexibility: Provide a range of services tailored to meet the changing needs that can be applied to a variety of housing options.
3. Entrepreneurship: Recognize and make the most of organized communities.
4. Mixed generations: Capitalize on all abilities to contribute to the community and resolve personal challenges through linking the needs and skills of different age groups.
5. Smart growth: Apply good community design principles to promote accessibility and livability.

A sixth component—care coordination—is also necessary to ensure that choice and flexibility are maintained while providing comprehensive, interdisciplinary, quality care tailored to meet the needs of the person who is aging in place. That component relies on a care manager, usually a registered nurse (RN), who coordinates care between multiple interdisciplinary teams to promote health and optimal functioning (Rantz et al., 2014).

Successful AIP programs offer a range of flexible services that are designed to meet the needs of each older person. AIP models create both healthcare and housing options that provide support where it is needed as defined by an individual's desire and ability to live independently.

🔍 CASE VIGNETTE

Mr. Jones, an 89-year-old male who lives at home alone, falls and sustains a hip fracture. He is admitted to the hospital and undergoes surgery. His hospital stay is prolonged by a period of delirium, in which his surgical incision opens, and he undergoes general anesthesia again to repair the damage. He is discharged to a skilled nursing facility for daily physical therapy, during which time he experiences another episode of delirium and becomes incontinent of urine. The family is trying to determine if he can return to his home to live independently. He can walk 30 feet with a walker before becoming fatigued and remains incontinent of urine. He is currently taking antibiotics for a urinary tract infection.

▶ Aging in Place

While many apartment housing sites are not designed for an AIP environment, models of these settings provide important economic benefits and are essential, especially for low-income persons (Carder, Weinstein, & Kohon, 2012). Apartment living is attractive to older adults for many reasons. In AIP models, individuals can choose where they should age in place while making the best decisions based on their economic situation, family, and health status. AIP is flexible and adjustments can be made in the services received. These adjustments may be a direct result of the health care required (such as physical therapy) and may be a strong motivator for the older person's improvement and continued independence. Healthcare services can be applied in any setting, but are typically provided in the person's community setting. For example, suppose Mr. Jones receives physical therapy in his home; once he completes the physical therapy, this service stops, thereby reducing costs.

Additionally, individuals may be involved in numerous community activities in AIP environments. Many communities provide services for older adults in conjunction with entrepreneurs or community partnerships—for example, social, physical, psychological, housing, congregate meals, and transportation activities. Often these services are linked with intergenerational and smart growth activities (Baker, Webster, Lynn, Rogers, & Belcher, 2017; Ball, 2017). Engaging all generations in activities (e.g., local ballgames, events, daycare facilities housed within congregate apartment settings, older adults reading to youngsters at their schools) has been shown to have many benefits for all age groups. Smart growth activities can include encouraging older adults to serve on community boards to promote accessibility within the larger community.

Finally, many older adults appreciate the care coordination aspects of AIP. As older adults develop one or more chronic illnesses, many find they are in need of care coordination to assist with communicating concerns to physicians and to ensure that all physicians (not just their primary care provider) are aligned with the healthcare plan (Rantz et al., 2014).

TigerPlace: A Model

The University of Missouri's (MU) AIP is one such initiative. MU collaborated with Americare Systems, Inc., Sikeston, MO, to build an ideal housing community that encompasses the AIP model, called TigerPlace. TigerPlace was built following the passage of state legislation in 1999 and 2001 that allowed a facility with apartments to be built to nursing home standards and to be licensed as an intermediate care facility, but operated as independent housing with services. TigerPlace operates the nursing services under a series of waivers. It provides independent housing with health care, and support is added or removed as the individual requires it through the end of life. There is no need for the person to move or transition until the time of death (Rantz et al., 2011).

At TigerPlace, the wellness and healthcare component is provided by Sinclair Home Care, a home care agency operated by the MU Sinclair School of Nursing. Sinclair Home Care provides routine assessment, wellness activities, social work services, exercise classes, health promotion activities, and veterinary services (for residents with pets). Licensed nursing staff are on call 24 hours per day, 7 days a week, to assist with triaging any emergency situation. A wellness clinic is open during business hours Monday to Friday and for 4 hours on Saturday and Sunday. Residents can drop by to receive healthcare information and clinical care from an RN Care Coordinator during clinic hours. In AIP, comprehensive resident physical and psychosocial assessment is provided by an RN and social work team, who work with the resident's family and primary care provider to develop a comprehensive plan of care that is delivered by healthcare staff.

The focus of AIP at TigerPlace is to help residents maintain and regain independence and functional ability. The care coordination service has demonstrated that the residents at TigerPlace are able to age in place 1.8 years longer than a comparable nursing home admission (Rantz et al., 2015).

▸ Importance of Aging in Place

The aging of the baby boomer generation (born between 1946 and 1964) has been well described. The number of U.S. adults age 65 and older will nearly double to 89 million by 2050 (CDC, 2013). Those age 80 and older are expected to triple in number to 28 million (Joint Center for Housing Studies, 2014).

Additionally, U.S. seniors are expected to become more diverse. By 2050, the majority population of older non-Hispanic whites will account for 58% of the total U.S. population, representing a 20% decrease in this share since 2010 (CDC, 2013). Compared to Caucasians, the health and well-being of minority groups are more adversely impacted by health disparities including language barriers, poverty, and reduced access to healthcare services (CDC, 2013). Additionally, family traditions of persons of Hispanic and Asian descent are also different from those of Caucasians and African Americans, with Hispanic and Asian seniors being more likely to live in multigenerational housing (Joint Center for Housing Studies, 2014). As a result of increased poverty, minority groups are more likely to have lower rates of home ownership and fewer assets (Joint Center for Housing Studies, 2014).

The physical condition of seniors influences where and how well seniors live. Two out of every three older adults, regardless of race, have multiple chronic conditions and experience disorders related to substance abuse, mental illness, dementia, and developmental disabilities (CDC, 2017), all of which influence their ability to live independently and safely in their community-based homes. Poverty makes it difficult to find safe and affordable congregate or institutional housing options. Although programs such as Medicaid Home and Community-Based Services waivers can provide for home modifications and in-home services, service availability varies by region. For those older adults who are not eligible for Medicaid coverage, the costs of in-home care are substantial. While older adults face significant challenges in staying safely in their home with or without services and family support, adequate assessment of physical, psychosocial, and housing needs is essential to aging successfully in the home of choice (Kim, Gollamudi, & Steinhubl, 2017).

Approximately 835,000 individuals in the United States seek to age in place in residential care communities. These settings are a vital option in the continuum of long-term care that serves the needs of older adults and younger adults with disabilities who cannot live independently but do not require the skilled care provided in nursing homes (Rome & Harris-Kojetin, 2016). Residential care is largely a private pay service, although Medicaid may cover certain services for beneficiaries eligible for home and community-based services in these settings (National Center for Assisted Living, 2016).

Residential care communities are licensed and regulated at the state level and provide, at a minimum, housing, meals, personal assistance with activities of daily living (ADLs) and instrumental activities of daily living (IADLs), and supportive services. All states have at least one category of such licensing, but substantial state-to-state differences exist at these levels and in the terms used to refer to residential care (e.g., assisted living facility, residential care facility, rest homes, board and care homes, adult care homes, domiciliary care homes) (Carder, O'Keeffe, & O'Keeffe, 2015). The availability and complexity of healthcare services vary according to state regulation; they may be limited to basic services or they may extend to include social work, counseling, therapy, skilled nursing, dementia care, and pharmacy services. In the case of Mr. Jones, relocation from the skilled nursing facility to residential care with the full complement of services may best meet his current needs.

Older adults aging in residential care typically have multiple health and disabling conditions that require ongoing and expert geriatric evaluation and treatment. Across residential settings, 46% of residents have a diagnosis of cardiovascular disease, 40% Alzheimer's disease or other dementia, 23% depression, and 17% diabetes (Caffrey, Harris-Kojetin, & Sengupta, 2015). Complicating the quest to ensure quality of care in residential settings is the variation in registered nurse, licensed practical or vocational nurse, and aide hours per resident per day (Rome & Harris-Kojetin, 2016). Total registered nurse hours per resident per day varies from 0.04 hour in Louisiana to 1.03 hour in South Dakota, and the total hours across all staff levels varies from 1.69 hours in Nevada to 4.9 hours in Iowa. Additionally, states have differing dementia-specific training requirements, ranging from no requirements in many states to 8 or more hours annually in states such as California, Iowa, and Minnesota (National Center for Assisted Living, 2016). Because the extent to which residential communities may be equipped to manage residents' health problems depends largely on factors mandated by state regulations, geographical location influences the success of AIP in these settings.

While the federally regulated Minimum Data Set 3.0 resident assessment instrument is used in Medicare/Medicaid certified nursing homes, documentation in residential care communities is not standardized. That being said, the state of Maryland has developed the Assisted Living Resident Assessment Tool, which includes separate assessment forms for the healthcare practitioner and the assisted living manager, to systematically collect resident information for guiding care planning care and service delivery (Maryland Department of Health and Mental Hygiene, 2006). Assessment of older adults in residential settings should address these individuals' social, cognitive, physical, and emotional state, with the goal of optimizing health, function, independence, and quality of life (Maas & Buckwalter, 2006).

Returning to Mr. Jones, he remains at increased risk for falls due to his history of falling, mobility disability, and urinary incontinence. The CDC's Stopping Elderly Accidents, Deaths, and Injuries (STEADI) toolkit (CDC, National Center for Injury Prevention and Control, 2017) describes the components of a multifactorial fall risk assessment, including an examination of neurologic and cardiovascular function, postural dizziness/postural hypotension, visual acuity, incontinence, cognition, depression, and foot problems; a medication review to identify use of psychoactive medications and medications with anticholinergic side effects; and gait and balance testing using the Timed Up and Go test, 30-second chair stand, and a four-stage balance test to gauge fall risk. Although originally designed for community-based healthcare providers, the STEADI toolkit is easily administered in any clinical or residential setting, and provider resources are available at https://www.cdc.gov/steadi/.

Recently the Centers for Medicare and Medicaid Services (CMS) launched initiatives to develop, test, and evaluate measures geared toward meeting the Improving Medicare Post-Acute Care Transformation (IMPACT) Act's requirement for standardized patient assessment data across all post-acute care settings. This standardized assessment must address functional status, cognitive function and mental status, special services, treatments and interventions, medical conditions and comorbidities, impairments, and other categories identified by the Secretary of Health and Human Services (CMS, 2017). Collecting standardized and interoperable data that follow the person (e.g., from a skilled nursing facility to an assisted living facility) will support improved patient care practices, patient safety, care coordination, discharge planning, and comparison of quality across post-acute care settings. Although the standardized patient assessment data elements pertain to only a few specific quality domains in post-acute care settings, broadening the geriatric assessment to include these elements will help harmonize efforts of older adults' healthcare providers.

▶ Practice Challenges

AIP requires a continual focus on maintaining and regaining independence. Episodes of acute illness or exacerbation of chronic conditions are frequently accompanied by functional decline. Such a decline may be apparent in physical or cognitive function, or both, and require focused informal or formal rehabilitation. Informally, encouragement and reinforcement of the person's effort to increase mobility, regain stamina, and perform prior ADLs may be adequate to restore former functional capacity. In addition, more formal, outpatient services in the form of physical, occupational, speech, and cognitive therapies may be needed in some cases. Whatever the level of need, a continual focus on regaining independence is necessary for successful AIP.

This central focus on independence is often lost or even adversely reinforced by traditional long-term care settings. Traditional nursing home, assisted living, and supportive housing settings may, through their all-inclusive service packages, inadvertently reinforce dependence. For example, staff who are providing direct care may conclude that it is "easier" or faster to dress people or help with other ADLs, when, in fact, simple prompting or active teaching and encouragement to perform these daily activities would work as a first step, such that within a few days the person could be performing the activity with less help or alone. Residents in traditional settings may hold the view that "I pay for help, so I should use the help here!" In the AIP model of care at TigerPlace, regaining and maintaining independence results in incrementally lower healthcare service costs for each person. This approach, by design, reinforces that as much independence on the part of each person as possible is expected.

When new staff join AIP settings, the major focus on independence is sometimes challenging for them to embrace, especially if they have worked in traditional settings. Routine walking for exercise and pleasure is constantly encouraged through active teaching, reinforcement, and rehabilitation that helps to maintain and/or regain walking ability and stamina. Staff from other settings require much role modeling to demonstrate the teaching and gentle encouragement skills essential to this practice.

Families and residents also must readjust their expectations when moving into AIP settings. The commitment to providing care and services while needed, then withdrawing them as strength is regained, is a difficult concept to grasp, at least initially. It is common for residents to experience several increases, then decreases, in their healthcare service monthly bill while living at TigerPlace. Most people stay highly functional through the end of life, or until shortly before the end of life (Rantz et al., 2014) and overall length of stay is increased as compared to other settings (Rantz et al., 2015).

Because the AIP approach to long-term care differs so dramatically from the traditional nursing home, assisted living, and supportive housing settings, a clear marketing message about how AIP is different and why AIP can provide needed care and services through the end of life without transfer to traditional settings is essential. Leadership and other staff should clearly and continually explain the expectations of successful AIP, including providing tips on how to stay in place through the end of life and be functional and as independent as possible to the end. Primary care providers need education to understand the possibilities that AIP provides even when acute health events make it seem that a move is necessary. However, after experiencing the support and education provided by the RN care coordinator at TigerPlace, most primary care providers, as well as family and residents, fully embrace the possibilities and positive outcomes of AIP.

▶ Summary

AIP can be the best living environment for older adults when appropriate care coordination services are successfully wrapped around the individual. An RN care coordinator is key to successful management of the complex health-care needs of older adults. Other important considerations are individual choice, flexibility in programming and health care, involving the community via entrepreneurial smart growth opportunities, and mixed generational exposure. In this way, AIP promotes independence, active engagement, and functionality.

References

Baker, J. R., Webster, L., Lynn, N., Rogers, J., & Belcher, J. (2017). Intergenerational programs may be especially engaging for aged care residents with cognitive impairment: Findings from the Avondale intergenerational design challenge. *American Journal of Alzheimer's Disease and Other Dementias, 32*(4), 213–221. doi: 10.1177/1533317517703477

Ball, M. S. (2017). *Aging in place: A toolkit for local governments.* Retrieved from http://www.aarp.org/content/dam/aarp /livable-communities/plan/planning/aging-in-place-a -toolkit-for-local-governments-aarp.pdf

Caffrey, C., Harris-Kojetin, L., & Sengupta, M. (2015). Variation in residential care community resident characteristics, by size of community: United States, 2014. *NCHS Data Brief, 223*, 1–8.

Carder, P., O'Keeffe, J., & O'Keeffe, C. (2015). *Compendium of residential care and assisted living regulations and policy: 2015 edition.* Retrieved from https://aspe.hhs .gov/basic-report/compendium-residential-care-and -assisted-living-regulations-and-policy-2015-edition

Carder, P. C., Weinstein, J., & Kohon, J. (2012). *The health and housing specialist: An emerging job classification to support AIP in subsidized housing.* Report by the Institute on Aging at Portland State University, Portland, OR. Retrieved from https://www.pdx.edu/ioa/sites /www.pdx.edu.ioa/files/Health_and_Housing_Specialist _Final_Report_2012.pdf

Centers for Disease Control and Prevention (CDC). (2013). *Long-term care services in the United States: 2013 overview.* Retrieved from https://www.cdc.gov/nchs /data/nsltcp/long_term_care_services_2013.pdf

Centers for Disease Control and Prevention (CDC). (2014). *Operating characteristics of residential care communities, by community bed size: United States, 2012.* Retrieved from https://www.cdc.gov/nchs/products/databriefs /db170.htm

Centers for Disease Control and Prevention (CDC). (2017). Healthy places terminology. Retrieved from https:// www.cdc.gov/healthyplaces/terminology.htm

Centers for Disease Control and Prevention (CDC), National Center for Injury Prevention and Control. (2017). *STEADI initiative for health care providers.* Retrieved from https://www.cdc.gov/steadi/

Centers for Medicare and Medicaid Services (CMS). (2017). *Looking ahead: The IMPACT Act in 2017 call.* Retrieved from https://www.cms.gov/Outreach-and-Education /Outreach/NPC/National-Provider-Calls-and-Events -Items/2017-02-23-IMPACT.html

Joint Center for Housing Studies. (2014). *U.S. unprepared to meet the housing needs of its aging population.* Joint Center for Housing Studies of Harvard University. Retrieved from http://www.jchs.harvard.edu/us -unprepared-meet-housing-needs-its-aging-population

Keenan, T. A. (2010). Home and community preferences of the 45+ population. *AARP Public Policy Institute, 4*, 8.

Kim, K. I., Gollamudi, S. S., & Steinhubl, S. (2017). Digital technology to enable AIP. *Experimental Gerontologist, 88*, 25–31. doi: 10.1016/j.exger.2016.11.013

Maas, M. L., & Buckwalter, K. C. (2006). Providing quality care in assisted living facilities: Recommendations for enhanced staffing and staff training. *Journal of Gerontological Nursing, 32*(11), 14–22.

Maryland Department of Health and Mental Hygiene. (2006). *Maryland's Assisted Living Resident Assessment and Level of Care Scoring Tool.* Retrieved from http:// www.dhmh.maryland.gov/ohcq/AL/Docs/AL_Forms /al_tool_guide.pdf

National Center for Assisted Living. (2016). *Assisted living 2016 state regulatory review.* Retrieved from https:// www.ahcancal.org/ncal/advocacy/regs/Pages/Assisted LivingRegulations.aspx

Rantz, M. J., Lane, K. R., Phillips, L. J., Despins, L. A., Galambos, C., Alexander, G. L., . . . Miller, S. J. (2015). Enhanced RN care coordination with sensor technology: Impact on length of stay and cost in AIP housing. *Nursing Outlook, 63*, 650–655.

Rantz, M. J., Marek, K. D., & Zwygart-Stauffacher, M. (2000). The future of long-term care for the chronically ill. *Nursing Administration Quarterly, 25*, 51-58.

Rantz, M. J., Phillips, L., Aud, M., Marek, K. D., Hicks, L. L., Zaniletti, I., . . . Miller, S. J. (2011). Evaluation of aging in place model with home care services and registered nurse care coordination in senior housing. *Nursing Outlook, 59*(1), 37-46.

Rantz, M., Popejoy, L. L., Galambos, C., Phillips, L. J., Lane, K. R., Marek, K. D., . . . Ge, B. (2014). The continued success of registered nurse care coordination in a state evaluation of AIP in senior housing. *Nursing Outlook, 62*(4), 237–246.

Rome, V., & Harris-Kojetin, L. D. (2016). Variation in residential care community nurse and aide staffing levels: United States, 2014. *National Health Statistics Reports, 91*, 1–11.

CHAPTER 36

Thriving in Community

Sarah L. Szanton and Kali S. Thomas

CHAPTER OBJECTIVES

1. Describe the assessment of people in their homes.
2. Describe the assessment of the home environment to support aging in community.
3. Determine what matters to the older adult.

KEY TERMS

Aging in community   Aging in place

▶ Introduction

The vast majority of older adults want to age at home or in their neighborhood (Keenan, 2010). Aging in one's community provides access to community resources, social ties developed over decades, and an enhanced sense of control. These social ties and amenities are associated with decreased morbidity and mortality (Holt-Lunstad, Smith, & Layton, 2010; Ong, Uchino, & Wethington, 2016). Nevertheless, the home environment can be challenging for older adults, and navigating the environment can become more challenging due to changes with age such as physical shrinking, uneven gait,

and muscle weakness. Current geriatric assessment techniques in primary care do not routinely assess the ability to accomplish activities of daily living (ADLs), nor do they routinely assess how much doing these activities interacts with the home environment and with family support. In this chapter we describe what is important to assess and why, by highlighting exemplar programs with innovative assessments that can improve the ability of older adults to live meaningfully in their communities. We also present challenges in incorporating these programs or assessments into practice.

To support older adults and to prevent unnecessary relocation or healthcare utilization, it is important to assess both the person and his or her environment as well as the fit between person and environment (Lawton & Nahemow, 1973). Current geriatric assessment models are predominantly used within clinical settings. As more care and services are provided in the home and community, however, it will be important for geriatric assessment to occur within the contexts of these environments. Thus, best practices will include assessment in the context of home, person/environment fit, and family support.

▶ Models of Aging in Community

In medicine, there is currently a movement away from consideration to one disease or symptom at a time and toward consideration of patients' experiences as a whole within the context of their lives (Bayliss et al., 2014). This trend is particularly salient in geriatrics, where the majority of patients have more than one chronic condition and taking their goals and priorities for daily life into account is paramount (Grant, Adams, Bayliss, & Heisler, 2013).

The exemplars included in this chapter emphasize an approach consonant with the focus on what matters to older adults. These five different programs complete assessments aimed at advancing older adults' abilities to thrive in their communities: (1) the Veteran-Directed Home and Community Based Services Program, (2) Meals on Wheels, (3) Community **Aging in Place**, Advancing Better Living for Elders (CAPABLE), (4) Care of Persons with Dementia in Their Environments (COPE), and (5) New Ways for Better Days Tailored Activity Program for people with dementia. These programs are illustrative of innovative assessments and programs to allow older adults, at any point on the spectrum of function, to be able to age in the context of their communities and remain able to perform activities they define as mattering most to them. Research on these models has shown that improving the ability to accomplish these

activities saves healthcare resources (Ruiz et al., 2017; Veterans Affairs, 2017).

Veteran-Directed Home and Community Based Services Program

One way to assess not only patients but also their environment, the person–environment fit, and goals and activities that matter most to them, is through person-centered planning. The Veteran-Directed Home and Community Based Services Program (VD-HCBS), offered through the Veterans Health Administration in partnership with the Administration for Community Living, is an exemplar program designed to enable older adults to sustain community living through a person-centered, self-directed approach (Milliken, Mahoney, & Mahoney, 2016). In VD-HCBS, veterans are assigned a monthly budget based on the extent of their disability and need. The veteran, guided by a person-centered counselor at a local Aging and Disability Network Agency, identifies his or her own strengths, goals, preferences, needs, and desired outcomes. The person-centered counselor then works with the veteran to identify and access a unique mix of services to meet those needs and provides support during the planning, purchasing, and implementation of these goods and services (**FIGURE 36-1**).

The VD-HCBS's self-directed features differ from the traditional services model in which patients are assessed, asked questions, informed of resources, provided options, and must receive services during assigned hours. That is, the person-centered, self-directed approach is designed to promote the highest degree of autonomy, flexibility, and choice in allowing for consideration of personal preferences as well as veterans' health and safety needs, all while providing support to do the things most important to them. This practice of self-direction has spread across the United States and around the world because of its ability to improve quality of care and life satisfaction, improve access to care while controlling costs (Simon-Rusinowitz, Loughlin,

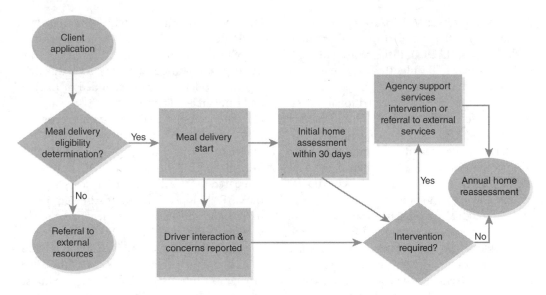

FIGURE 36-1 Innovative Assessment for Meals on Wheels Participants' Needs.

Ruben, Garcia, & Mahoney, 2010; Foster, Brown, Phillips, Schore, & Carlson, 2003), reduce unmet personal care needs, and increase participant satisfaction with care for both older adults and younger people with disabilities (Carlson, Foster, Dale, & Brown, 2007).

Meals on Wheels

Another example of a comprehensive in-home assessment is that provided by home delivered meals programs, generally referred to as "Meals on Wheels." These programs are found in many communities; are funded with a combination of federal, state, and local dollars; and vary in their assessment practices. Two exemplar programs utilize in-home comprehensive assessments that obtain an array of information to link clients with available resources: Meals on Wheels of Central Maryland and Meals on Wheels Inc. of Tarrant County.

For all clients who are eligible for services, Meals on Wheels of Central Maryland conducts an initial in-home assessment within 30 days of the client receiving home-delivered meals (Figure 36-1). This assessment covers the physical condition of the home as well as the client's

functional status (including unmet need for assistance), physical appearance, social support system, mental health, social–emotional well-being, food environment, ability to prepare meals, and financial status to determine whether other benefits or services may be needed. The findings from this assessment then inform the types of services and resources to which clients are linked and the additional referrals (e.g., targeted case management) that may be necessary. Clients are then reassessed as needed and annually, in their homes, and this process resumes.

In the Fort Worth, Texas, area, Meals on Wheels Inc. of Tarrant County provides case management and a registered dietician upon program entry. Similar to what happens in the Maryland program, a case manager screens the client for an expanded list of needs and preferences, including reviewing medications (dosing and frequency), observes for risks of falls and signs of dementia or depression, obtains hospital admissions and physician information, and gathers information about the client's caregiver and about the client's neighborhood. The client case manager also completes a comprehensive nutritional risk screening tool (Coulston, Craig, & Voss, 1996), a diabetes risk assessment (Lanza,

Albright, Zucker, & Martin, 2007), and a tool to measure ADLs and instrumental activities of daily living (IADLs). If the registered dietician (RD) on staff decides that the client needs an additional assessment, he RD visits the client and completes the Mini Nutritional Assessment to screen for malnutrition, a health literacy scale, and other scales measuring quality of life. Similar to the Maryland program, the RD also reviews the client's home food environment, including the neighborhood, pantry, cooking facilities, and ability to prepare food.

Although Meals on Wheels has a history of meal delivery and companionship, newer approaches to comprehensive assessment of the home and community resources underscore the vast opportunity to enhance person–environment fit through assessment and individualized planning.

Community Aging in Place, Advancing Better Living for Elders

The CAPABLE program seeks to improve one of the most costly, overlooked, and undertreated aspects of aging—namely, the inability to carry out everyday self-care activities. CAPABLE is an assessment-driven, individually tailored package of interventions delivered over 16 weeks by an occupational therapist (OT; 6 or fewer home visits), a registered nurse (RN; 4 or fewer home visits), and a handyman team (**TABLE 36-1**). Frail older participants learn and practice new strategies to manage functional difficulties in their homes; they use assistive devices and environmental improvements first with these health professionals, and then on their own. The OT focuses on self-care and function. The nurse focuses on the underlying medical/nursing issues that may be interfering with performance of ADLs and IADLs, such as pain, depression, strength/balance, and polypharmacy. The handyman team implements a work order constructed by the participant and the OT for the home to make it safer and more functional.

CAPABLE started as a research study in Baltimore, Maryland, and has been tested for efficacy in reducing disability (Szanton, Leff, Wolff, Roberts, & Gitlin, 2016) and depression as well as in decreasing healthcare utilization and expenses (Ruiz et al., 2017). As of this writing, the model has been expanded to 13 cities and rural areas in 8 states.

After completing the five-month program, 75% of participants had improved their performance of ADLs. On average, participants had difficulty with 3.9 out of 8.0 ADLs at baseline compared to 2.0 ADLs after the completion of the CAPABLE program. Approximately 53% of participants showed improvement in depressive symptoms (Szanton et al., 2016). The project also yielded approximately $20,000 in medical cost savings per person for the cost of the $3000 program—a more than six-fold return on investment in the two years after the patient received the program (Ruiz et al., 2017).

During the first visits of the OT and the RN, both of these clinicians elicit goals relating to function that the older adult prioritizes as important. These assessments start with what seem like conversations but are actually explorations of social support, memory, and other key indicators of ability to function at home. For the OT, this assessment starts with "Tell me about a typical day"; for the RN, it starts with "Tell me about your meals in the last day." This questioning elicits information on whether the client has enough food, whether anyone eats with the client, and whether the client has anything fresh. These questions are good rapport builders as well.

Whether one is implementing CAPABLE or simply attempting to do a high-quality home-based assessment, it is important to assess all ADLs and IADLs and to have the older adult prioritize their importance. ADLs include bathing, dressing, walking across a small room, dressing the upper body, dressing the lower body, getting on and off the toilet, eating, and grooming (Katz, Ford, Moskowitz, Jackson, & Jaffe, 1963). A thorough assessment will include how difficult each activity is; which devices the patient needs or uses, if any; and what priority it is for the patient to accomplish the ADL alone. Performing these assessments in the home setting

TABLE 36-1 Home Visits and Collaboration with CAPABLE Participants over a Four-Month Period

	OT Visit 1	OT Visit 2	After Visit 2	Visit 3	Visit 4	Visit 5	Visit 6
Occupational therapist (OT) and client together	Introduction; function-focused OT assessment. Fall risk and recovery education.	Determine client's functional goals, conduct home safety assessment, and identify necessary repairs or modifications.	Develop work order for home repairs/modifications and send it to the handyman.	Brainstorm and develop an action plan with the client for client-identified goal 1 (e.g., safely bathing, going upstairs, or preparing food).	Brainstorm and develop an action plan with the client for client-identified goal 2.	Brainstorm and develop an action plan with the client for identified goal 3; review the HM work and train the client on new assistive devices.	Wrap up, help the participant generalize solutions for future problems; review goals and client's achievement of them.
Handyman (HM)				HM visits the client's home, and reviews repairs/modifications and associated costs with the OT. Starts work and continues until it is complete.			

(continues)

TABLE 36-1 Home Visits and Collaboration with CAPABLE Participants over a Four-Month Period *(continued)*

	RN Visit 1	After RN Visit 1	RN Visit 2	RN Visit 3	RN Visit 4
Registered nurse (RN) and client together	Introduction; function-focused RN assessment including pain, mood, strength, balance, medication information, and primary care provider (PCP) advocacy/communication.	Make medication calendar for the client. Review the client's medications including side effects, interactions, and possible changes. Consult with the pharmacist if the client is on high-alert medications or more than 15 medications.	Determine goals in the RN domain together; start to brainstorm goals (e.g. pain on standing, fall prevention). Demonstrate CAPABLE exercises. Review medication calendar. Discuss patient/PCP communication. Develop correspondence to PCP.	Complete brainstorming/problem-solving process. Develop action plans for identified goals with the client. Assess PCP response to communication of client needs. Review/assess/troubleshoot exercise regimen.	Review progress and use of strategies for all target areas. Review RN section of flipbook that summarizes the program. Evaluate achievement of goals and readiness to change scale. Help the client generalize the brainstorming process for future health issues.

allows the provider to assess the interaction between person and environment, such as being able to witness the older adult needing to step over jagged linoleum in his or her kitchen to accomplish a task, or to reach up into a tall closet. Assessing the client's ability to perform IADLs in the home, such as doing laundry and managing medications, is useful because the home visitor can assess whether the washing machine is down treacherous steps or whether the older adult has pill boxes to manage medications.

Care of Persons with Dementia in Their Environments

The previous examples focused on older adults who can plan, prioritize, and act independently. One in 10 people older than age 65 has dementia, however, and this proportion increases to 30% after the age of 80 (Rocca et al., 2011). Fortunately, excellent assessments and evidence-based programs are available for people at all stages of cognitive abilities.

One example is Care of Persons with Dementia in Their Environments (COPE), which is designed to support people living with dementia at home and the care challenges faced by their family members. COPE is an individualized, caregiver-centric program that helps families identify and address their most significant care challenges, including the patient's functional decline, home safety concerns, and behavioral symptoms, and the caregiver's own feelings of being overwhelmed, distress, burden, or need for education and skills (Gitlin, Winter, Dennis, Hodgson, & Hauck, 2010). It involves up to 12 home sessions delivered by an occupational therapist and advanced practice nurse. The OT works with family caregivers to identify care challenges; assesses the person with dementia to identify functional abilities, interests, and preferences; and instruct families in ways to support daily function and engagement in activities. Families learn specific skills in communicating effectively, setting up daily routines and using activities, and modifying their home environment to make care easier and support

the function of the person with dementia. The nurse educates caregivers about dementia and common medical concerns and how to detect and monitor pain, dehydration, constipation, and other common issues; the nurse also obtains blood and urine samples to rule out underlying medical conditions such as undetected infection and refers the patient for further treatment if necessary.

New Ways for Better Days: Tailoring Activities for Persons with Dementia and Caregivers

New Ways for Better Days: Tailoring Activities for Persons with Dementia and Caregivers (TAP) is a program for people living with dementia who have behavioral symptoms such as agitation, apathy, irritability, aggression, repetitive vocalizations, and shadowing. This individualized, person-centric program provides people with dementia activities customized to their abilities and interests and instructs family members in their use as part of daily care routines. It involves up to eight home sessions delivered by an occupational therapist. The intervention unfolds in three phases:

- Phase I involves a novel assessment approach to identify preserved capabilities, physical functioning, and previous and current interests of the person with dementia.
- Phase II involves developing an "activity prescription" that specifies the person's capabilities, an activity, an activity goal and instructions for setting up the activity, and strategies for effectively involving the person living with dementia.
- Phase III involves instructing families in how to modify the prescribed activities for future cognitive and functional declines and how to generalize specific strategies (e.g., communication) to other care challenges.

TAP is being used in multiple countries (Scotland, Australia, Brazil, Chile, Italy, Hong Kong, and the United States) and in different settings (home, adult day, hospital, outpatient, nursing home). People with dementia and their families have been shown to experience a reduction in the number and frequency and severity of behaviors; improved engagement; improved quality of life and pleasure; reduced functional dependence; enhanced caregiver efficacy using activities; and reduction in caregiver time spent in daily care (Gitlin et al., 2008).

▶ Practice Challenges

Several practice challenges arise when assessing older adults in this comprehensive manner and at home. The first challenge is that of funding or reimbursement. In a practice world in which physicians and nurse practitioners are reimbursed a set amount for a short clinic visit, thorough person–environment home assessments pose a challenge to sustain financially. In 2017, the home assessor might be able to charge only $100 to $140 for this visit, depending on multiple factors. Second, when funding comes to the primary care providers only, it is difficult to have team members such as occupational therapists or registered dieticians provide the necessary assessments.

In addition, although these models are designed for older adults with some physical challenges, they are essentially preventive in nature. That is, they are designed to optimize function at any stage of functional decline as well as to maximize the home environment to support them. In doing so, they prevent hospitalization, rehospitalization, and nursing home admission (Ruiz et al., 2017; Thomas & Mor, 2013). As the organization of health care moves away from paying for visits and procedures and toward paying for keeping people well and out of high-cost utilization settings, programs that require team assessments, perhaps with screening first (e.g., Meals on Wheels, VD-HCBS, Independence at Home, CAPABLE, New Ways for Better Days, and COPE), will be seen as ways to address these dual needs of older adults and society and keep people as well as possible and thriving in their community.

A related challenge is the lack of a mechanism for consistently sharing these rich assessment data with healthcare providers, payers, or anyone else who might need it, such as family members. Much of this assessment is completed in silos, partly because use of information technology in healthcare and social services programs is much more limited than in other sectors (Gandhi, Khanna, & Ramaswamy, 2016). In addition, assessments primarily completed on paper are much more common when those assessments are performed outside the clinical setting. Further complicating the exchange of information is the general notion that social services programs are not yet recognized as valid contributors by the medical field; in turn, the value of integrating the rich information collected in many of these community-based programs is not seen.

Some of these assessments and services face the additional challenge of being considered a social service rather than a medical service. The United States lags behind all other industrialized nations in the balance of medical care to social services (Bradley, Elkins, Herrin, & Elbel, 2011). While some medical services are readily paid for, such as cardiac procedures, food provided through home-delivered meals has been considered a "social service" and has typically remained unfunded by medical programs, with the exception of some states' Medicaid 1915c waivers, demonstration projects, and a few innovative health plans. Similarly, home modifications, although inexpensive and relatively permanent, are not typically paid for with healthcare resources. This lack is also an opportunity, as just a small amount of spending in these areas may be able to leverage large healthcare returns. For example, the cost of CAPABLE is made back in the first quarter after the service is provided and continues for at least seven quarters after (Ruiz et al., 2017).

Recently, the bipartisan National Commission on Hunger recommended expanding Medicare managed care and Medicaid managed care plans to include coverage for meal delivery. Further, the move toward integration of social services and medical care is evidenced by the creation of programs such as Accountable Health Communities, which aim to better connect Medicare and Medicaid patients to community social services such as transportation and nutrition services, while reducing healthcare spending (Alley, Asomugha, Conway, & Sanghavi, 2016). As health systems begin to explore funding better patient connections to important nonmedical needs and integrating services provided by community-based organizations, it is possible that more money will flow toward innovative approaches to keeping older adults in their homes with enough mobility, food, and strength to use their home effectively.

▶ Summary

As the U.S. health system focuses more on patient goals and on delivering care that aligns with daily goals rather than just disease control goals, the programs highlighted in this chapter are poised to lead the way to **aging in community**. Home-based assessments have several inherent challenges in sharing information with health systems and in becoming integrated into payment streams. The move toward outcome-based payments aligns well with home-based assessment and care. In the end, house calls are not expensive, but they are priceless.

References

Alley, D. E., Asomugha, C. N., Conway, P. H., & Sanghavi, D. M. (2016). Accountable Health Communities--Addressing Social Needs through Medicare and Medicaid. *The New England Journal of Medicine*, *374*(1), 8–11. https://doi.org/10.1056/NEJMp1512532 [doi]

Bayliss, E. A., Bonds, D. E., Boyd, C. M., Davis, M. M., Finke, B., Fox, M. H., … Stange, K. C. (2014). Understanding the context of health for persons with multiple chronic conditions: Moving from what is the matter to what matters. *Annals of Family Medicine*, *12*(3), 260–269. https://doi.org/10.1370/afm.1643 [doi]

Bradley, E. H., Elkins, B. R., Herrin, J., & Elbel, B. (2011). Health and social services expenditures: associations with health outcomes. *BMJ Quality & Safety*, *20*(10), 826–831. https://doi.org/10.1136/bmjqs.2010.048363

Carlson, B. L., Foster, L., Dale, S. B., & Brown, R. (2007). Effects of cash and counseling on personal care and

well-being. *Health Services Research*, *42*(1 II), 467–487. https://doi.org/10.1111/j.1475-6773.2006.00673.x

Coulston, A. M., Craig, L., & Voss, A. C. (1996). Meals-on-wheels applicants are a population at risk for poor nutritional status. *Journal of the American Dietetic Association*, *96*(6), 570–573. https://doi.org/10.1016/S0002-8223(96)00157-5

Foster, L., Brown, R., Phillips, B., Schore, J., & Carlson, B. L. (2003). Improving the quality of Medicaid personal assistance through consumer direction. *Health Aff (Millwood) Suppl Web Exclusives*, 162–175.

Gandhi, P., Khanna, S., & Ramaswamy, S. (2016). A Chart That Shows Which Industries Are the Most Digital (and Why)? *Harvard Business Review*, 1–6.

Gitlin, L. N., Winter, L., Burke, J., Chernett, N., Dennis, M. P., & Hauck, W. W. (2008). Tailored activities to manage neuropsychiatric behaviors in persons with dementia and reduce caregiver burden: A randomized pilot study. *The American Journal of Geriatric Psychiatry*, *16*(3), 229–239. https://doi.org/10.1097/JGP.0b013e318160da72

Gitlin, L. N., Winter, L., Dennis, M. P., Hodgson, N., & Hauck, W. W. (2010). A biobehavioral home based intervention and the well-being of patients with dementia and their caregivers: The COPE randomized trial. *Journal of the American Medical Association*, *304*(9), 983–991. https://doi.org/10.1001/jama.2010.1253

Grant, R. W., Adams, A. S., Bayliss, E. A., & Heisler, M. (2013). Establishing visit priorities for complex patients: A summary of the literature and conceptual model to guide innovative interventions. *Healthcare (Amsterdam, Netherlands)*, *1*(3–4), 117–122. https://doi.org/10.1016/j.hjdsi.2013.07.008 [doi]

Holt-Lunstad, J., Smith, T. B., & Layton, J. B. (2010). Social Relationships and Mortality Risk: A Meta-analytic Review. *PLoS Med*, *7*(7), e1000316. https://doi.org/10.1371/journal.pmed.1000316

Katz, S., Ford, A. B., Moskowitz, R. W., Jackson, B. A., & Jaffe, M. W. (1963). Studies of Illness in the Aged. the Index of Adl: a Standardized Measure of Biological and Psychosocial Function. *JAMA: The Journal of the American Medical Association*, *185*, 914–919.

Keenan, T. A. (2010). *Home and Community Preferences of the 45+ Population*. Washington, D.C.: AARP. Retrieved from http://assets.aarp.org/rgcenter/general/home-community-services-10.pdf

Lanza, A., Albright, A., Zucker, H., & Martin, M. (2007). The diabetes detection initiative: a pilot program of selective screening. *American Journal of Health Behavior*, *31*(6), 632–642. https://doi.org/10.5555/ajhb.2007.31.6.632

Lawton, M. P., & Nahemow, L. (1973). Ecology and the Aging Process. In C. Eisdorfer & M. P. Lawton (Eds.), *The Psychology of Adult Development and Aging* (pp. 619–674). Washington, D.C.: American Psychological Association.

Milliken, A., Mahoney, E., & Mahoney, K. (2016). It Just Took the Pressure Off": Experiences of Caregivers in the

VD-HCBS Program. *Nursing Research*, 65(2), E25–E25. Retrieved from http://uml.idm.oclc.org/login?url=http://search.ebscohost.com/login.aspx?direct=true&db=c8h&AN=113905212&site=ehost-live

Ong, A. D., Uchino, B. N., & Wethington, E. (2016). Loneliness and health in older adults: A mini-review and synthesis. *Gerontology*, *62*(4), 443–449. https://doi.org/10.1159/000441651

Rocca, W. A., Petersen, R. C., Knopman, D. S., Hebert, L. E., Evans, D. A., Hall, K. S., … White, L. R. (2011). Trends in the incidence and prevalence of Alzheimer's disease, dementia, and cognitive impairment in the United States. *Alzheimer's & Dementia: The Journal of the Alzheimer's Association*, *7*(1), 80–93. https://doi.org/10.1016/j.jalz.2010.11.002

Ruiz, S., Snyder, L. P., Rotondo, C., Cross-Barnet, C., Colligan, E. M., & Giuriceo, K. (2017). Innovative Home Visit Models Associated With Reductions In Costs, Hospitalizations, And Emergency Department Use. *Health Affairs*, 36(3), 425–432. https://doi.org/10.1377/HLTHAFF.2016.1305

Simon-Rusinowitz, L., Loughlin, D. M., Ruben, K., Garcia, G. M., Mahoney, K. J. (2010). The benefits of consumer-directed services for elders and their caregivers in the cash and counseling demonstration and evaluation. *Public Policy & Aging Report, 20*, 27-31.

Szanton, S. L., Leff, B., Wolff, J. L., Roberts, L., & Gitlin, L. N. (2016). Home-Based Care Program Reduces Disability And Promotes Aging In Place. *Health Affairs*, *35*(9), 1558–1563. https://doi.org/10.1377/hlthaff.2016.0140

Thomas, K. S., & Mor, V. (2013). Providing more home-delivered meals is one way to keep older adults with low care needs out of nursing homes. *Health Affairs*, *32*(10), 1796–1802. https://doi.org/10.1377/hlthaff.2013.0390

Veterans Affairs, D. (2017). *A Comparison of a Veterans Directed Health Care Program vs. Community Nursing Home Placement*. Retrieved from https://nwd.acl.gov/docs/VDHCPaperFedPractRevision5_508.pdf

CHAPTER 37

Geriatric Assessment in Nursing Homes

Bernardo Reyes, Mandi Sehgal, Nancy A. Hodgson, and Joseph G. Ouslander

CHAPTER OBJECTIVES

1. Understand the key differences between assessments completed in nursing homes and those completed in other settings.
2. Describe the role of interprofessional teams in the assessment of nursing home patients.
3. Identify widely used assessment tools in nursing homes and discuss how to use relevant findings from such tools.

KEY TERMS

Assessment
Interprofessional

Long-term
Nursing facilities

Post-acute

▶ Introduction

Nursing facilities are complex, highly regulated, and dynamic settings of care. They are also commonly referred to as skilled nursing facilities (SNFs), as most nursing homes have all, or a portion, of their beds licensed for skilled care. The role of the nursing home has evolved over the last several decades from a facility that provided housing and supportive services to people who could not live in the community, to the nursing home of today that provides multiple types of care simultaneously, including skilled nursing, medical, and rehabilitative care to patients discharged from the hospital (**post-acute** care); **long-term** care for people with chronic medical, functional, and psychosocial conditions that preclude their living in a non-institutional setting; and end-of-life care, often in collaboration with an external hospice.

Patients (referring to those individuals in post-acute care) and residents (referring to those individuals in long-term care) in nursing homes generally have combinations of chronic health conditions and requirements for assistance with activities of daily living (ADLs) resulting in special medical, psychosocial, and functional needs. For these reasons, geriatric assessments in the nursing home setting extend beyond diagnosis and treatment of medical conditions, instead focusing on what residents can do, relative to what they are able to or wish to do. The ultimate goal of geriatric **assessment** in the nursing home is to obtain a comprehensive picture of the resident's social, psychological, medical, and functional capacities so as to create a comprehensive roadmap for treatment and long-term follow-up.

Most nursing homes are run as for-profit businesses, commonly organized into chains ranging from 5–10 facilities to more than 300 facilities. Nursing homes vary greatly in size and scope of services, with the average size being approximately 100 beds. The services range from post-acute care involving a short stay focused on post-hospitalization rehabilitation, to long-term residential care that supports quality of life through the end of life. The types of people who lived in nursing homes for long-term care in the past are now often living in assisted living facilities (ALFs); thus, many of the principles of assessment outlined in this chapter are relevant to that population as well. In addition to nursing homes, post-acute care is provided in a variety of settings including inpatient rehabilitation facilities and long-term acute care hospitals.

Nursing homes vary in the number of post-acute patients versus long-term care residents they serve at a given time. A typical 100- to 120-bed facility may have a post-acute census of 10–20 patients. Other nursing homes have a much higher post-acute census because of the favorable economics and contracts with Medicare managed care plans related to these patients' care; some of these facilities have waivers of the 3-day inpatient stay rule allowing patients to be admitted directly from home or an emergency department. Such facilities have a rapid turnover of patients with many admissions and discharges on a weekly basis, so they have a higher ratio of registered versus licensed practical nurses and nursing assistants. While the average length of stay of patients admitted for post-acute care is approximately 25 days, that stay is decreasing because of pressures exerted by value-based reimbursement, including Medicare managed care, bundled payments, and accountable care organizations. This shift has important implications for the timing and nature of assessments, which are discussed later in the chapter.

In contrast to post-acute care, long-term care refers to care provided over a sustained period to residents who have lost independence in one or more areas of functioning. This care can be socially based or provided as direct services to compensate for the functional losses; it can include rehabilitative efforts, though it is not intended to address the activities usually conducted as a part of primary medical care. Some post-acute patients who do not achieve their rehabilitative goals may become long-term care residents, whereas long-term care residents who have an acute illness requiring hospitalization can transiently become post-acute residents. In this situation, a new comprehensive assessment is required to adjust the goals for post-acute care. Long-term care residents generally live in a nursing home for an average of about two years, but some live in this setting for much longer.

▶ Goals of Assessment in the Nursing Home

The goals of assessment depend on the purpose of the nursing home stay and the context of the assessment. **FIGURE 37-1** illustrates the different types of patients and residents living in a nursing home. Some of the goals of care and assessment in one subgroup of these patients may be irrelevant and even inappropriate for other subgroups. For example, assessment of the ability

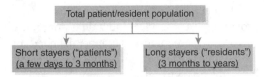

FIGURE 37-1 Different types of residents and patients in a nursing home.

to climb two stairs to get into a home or change levels in a home, or to shower safely without assistance, may be critical for a post-acute patient, but irrelevant to a long-stay resident. Similarly, repeated assessment and control of blood pressure or blood sugar may be important for an otherwise relatively healthy post-acute patient in the nursing home after a stroke or hip fracture, but inappropriate for a long-stay resident at the end of life.

While the domains of assessment in post-acute and long-term care are similar (**TABLE 37-1**), the focus of the assessment in post-acute care is on maximizing rehabilitation potential, whereas the focus of assessment for long-term care is on maximizing function and quality of life. The emphasis of each type of assessment varies, depending on whether it is an initial assessment, a reassessment, or an assessment of a change in condition.

▶ Roles of Interprofessional Team Members in Assessment

Care in a nursing home is highly **interprofessional**, for a number of reasons (**TABLE 37-2**). For example, nearly 80% of post-acute patients receive physical, occupational, and/or speech therapy. While most assessments are carried out by nurses, most hands-on nursing care is provided by certified nursing assistants. Geriatric assessments in the nursing home, therefore, are carried out by an interprofessional team with knowledge of age-related physiologic and psychologic changes,

TABLE 37-1 Assessment Domains: Post-Acute Care Versus Long-Term Care	
Post-Acute Care	**Long-Term Care**
Diagnoses	Diagnoses
Medical complexities	Health conditions
Other health conditions	Psychosocial well-being
Oral/nutritional status	Oral/dental status
Functional status	Physical function
Bowel/bladder continence	Bowel/bladder continence
Cognition	Cognition
Vision/communication	Communication/vision/hearing
Mood and behavior	Mood and behavior problems
Procedures/services	Special treatments and procedures
Rehabilitative prognosis	Activity pursuit patterns
Resources for discharge (including informal care)	Medication use
Home environment/safety	Goals of care
Transportation	Access to resources
Medication reconciliation	Health maintenance

TABLE 37-2 Rationale for an Interprofessional Team Approach in Geriatric Assessment
Growing heterogeneity of older population in nursing homes
Increasing prevalence of older adults with more complex needs related to chronic diseases
Complexity of skills and knowledge required to provide comprehensive care to residents
Specialization within health professions and fragmentation of disciplinary knowledge
Need for continuity of care and standard communication across treatment settings

and joint decisions about approaches to care, and providing direct services individually or jointly with other team members to meet the needs of the patient. The team members meet informally, formally, and virtually, and they use various structures and tools to meet, communicate, coordinate, and monitor care. The effectiveness of interprofessional teams depends on a number of factors, including the team members' knowledge of one another's roles; the scope of practice; mutual trust and respect among the team members; commitment in building relationships; and willingness to cooperate and collaborate.

Team membership usually includes a physician, a nurse, and a social worker. In addition, the interprofessional team in the nursing home should ideally include dieticians; speech, physical, and occupational therapists; social workers; pharmacists; dentists; certified nursing assistants; and medical subspecialists. Most importantly, the nursing home patient/resident and his or her significant others are central members of the team. Team members divide the work based on the team members' education and experience (**TABLE 37-3**).

and the ability to detect and remedy amenable problems at an early stage. At a practical level, interprofessional teams are involved in the assessment and planning of care, making independent

TABLE 37-3 Interprofessional Team Members and Their Role in Geriatric Assessments*	
Interprofessional Team Member	**Role in Assessment**
Nursing home patient/resident	Offers insights on daily routines, needs, abilities, interests, and preferences.
Patient/resident's family	Offers nuanced insights into the patient/resident's behavior and functional status. Helps the team define realistic goals, and shares effective strategies for interacting with the patient/resident.
Physician, nurse practitioner, or physician assistant	Assesses physical medicine and rehabilitative management needs.
Registered nurse (RN)	Assesses physical, emotional, spiritual, social, psychological, and cultural status.
Licensed practical nurse (LPN)	Assists the RN in the assessment of physical, social, and cultural status.

Interprofessional Team Member	Role in Assessment
Certified nursing assistant (CNA)	Assists the team assessing the daily physical and emotional needs of residents.
Dietician	Assesses ability for independent eating, and assesses preferences for foods that are ethnically and culturally appropriate, so as to prepare menus.
Social worker	Conducts a comprehensive, strengths-based assessment of the individual and the family support system.
Pharmacist	Assesses for the optimal pharmacotherapeutic regimen and monitors for adverse effects and interactions.
Speech therapist	Assesses speech and swallowing capacity.
Recreational therapist	Assesses the daily activity and recreational needs of the individual.
Occupational therapist	Assesses functional independence and safety in daily activities. Assesses the need for adaptive equipment for the individual so as to maximize functional independence.
Physical therapist	Assesses disability from acute or chronic disease or traumatic injuries, injury prevention, and physical fitness.
Administrator	Provides information regarding funding and available services. Works with the team to determine the best individualized care plan possible.
Clergy	Assesses spiritual, cultural, and emotional needs.

* Other members of the team that may contribute to comprehensive geriatric assessment include a dentist, respiratory therapist, optometrist, podiatrist, or orthoptist/prosthetist, depending on need.

▶ Standardized Assessments and Components

In most settings in which older adults receive care, geriatric syndromes such as frailty, functional impairment, falls, and dementia are frequently under-recognized and under-reported. In response to an Institute of Medicine report on the quality of care in U.S. nursing homes published in 1986, the federal government mandated a comprehensive assessment for all nursing home residents, known as the Minimum Data Set (MDS). There have been many additional efforts to standardize the approach to assessment of the older adult to improve the recognition of these syndromes such that an individualized plan of care can be implemented to ensure not only safety but also the highest level of function and quality of life. Many of these approaches are relevant to nursing home care.

Minimum Data Set

In the United States, geriatric assessment in the nursing home/long-term care setting consists initially of the Minimum Data Set. The MDS is a standardized assessment that is completed for all residents admitted to Medicare-certified nursing homes in the United States and for all residents admitted to Veteran Health Administration Community Living Centers (Saliba, 2012). The latest iteration of this assessment, MDS 3.0, is intended to facilitate better recognition of each resident's needs and inform care planning; it consists of multiple domains of resident health and function. The MDS is also used to generate publicly reported quality measures to determine reimbursement for post-acute Medicare fee-for-service beneficiaries.

The MDS 3.0 consists of direct resident interviews (when residents are able to make themselves understood at least some of the time) to assess several key domains of health, including cognition, mood, preferences for daily routines, preferences for activities, and pain. When residents are unable to make themselves understood, reliance on input from caregivers (family and those in the facility) is expected. An instruction manual accompanies the MDS 3.0, along with a publicly available training video, titled *Video on Interviewing Vulnerable Elders* (VIVE) (Picker Institute, 2012; Saliba et al., 2012).

MDS 3.0 does not include assessments of sexual function, spirituality, financial concerns, living situation, goals of care, and advanced care preferences, which are key components of a comprehensive geriatric assessment (**TABLE 37-4**). Additionally, MDS 3.0 incompletely addresses assessments of polypharmacy, goals of care, and social support, which are also considered key components of a comprehensive geriatric assessment (CGA).

Comprehensive Geriatric Assessment

The comprehensive geriatric assessment (CGA) serves as a more robust evaluation of an older adult, with the goal of developing a coordinated plan of care for the patient across multiple domains (Stuck, Siu, Wieland, Rubenstein, & Adams, 1993). This geriatric assessment has been shown to reduce disability, hospitalization, and institutionalization, and to improve quality of life (Rubenstein et al., 1984; Stuck et al., 1993). Many parts of the CGA are also included in MDS 3.0 (**TABLE 37-5**).

The CGA is often conducted in the outpatient setting (ambulatory or home), although it has some utility in the inpatient setting for those older adults who are admitted for specific reasons (e.g., hip fracture, pressure injuries, recurrent illness). The majority of CGAs are conducted using a patient-centered, interprofessional practice model consisting of a physician, nurse, social worker, and pharmacist, and including physical, speech, and occupational therapists, nutritionists, psychiatrists, psychologists, and dentists as indicated. The patient and his or her caregiver(s) are at the center of this team approach to care.

Limitations of the CGA are the time required for evaluation, coordination of the interprofessional team, and reimbursement. The CGA does not explicitly address concerns related to pain or preferences for activities or specific treatments, which are included as part of MDS 3.0.

Rapid Geriatric Assessment

The Rapid Geriatric Assessment (RGA; Morley, 2017) was developed to identify predisability in patients in hopes of intervening with a form of prevention prior to worsening illness. The RGA consists of four component assessments: the Simple "FRAIL" Questionnaire, a screening tool for fragility; the SARC-F Screen for Sarcopenia; the Simplified Nutritional Assessment Questionnaire (SNAQ); and the Rapid Cognitive Screen (RCS). Additionally, it includes a yes/no response question inquiring whether the patient has an advance directive (**FIGURE 37-2**). The scoring mechanisms for each of the individual assessments are included in the RGA (Morley, 2017).

TABLE 37-4 Components of the Comprehensive Geriatric Assessment and Corresponding Sections of the Minimum Data Set

Components of Comprehensive Geriatric Assessment	Links to MDS 3.0
Fall risk	Section G and GG: Balance during transfers and walking and mobility assessment Section J: Fall history
Cognitive impairment	Section C: Brief Interview for Mental Status (BIMS), confusion assessment method
Functional capacity	Section G and GG: ADL and self-care assessment
Mood	Section D: Patient Health Questionnaire (PHQ-9)
Polypharmacy*	Section N: Injections, insulin, psychoactive medications, antibiotics, anticoagulants, or diuretics
Nutrition	Section K: Swallowing/nutritional status
Incontinence (both urinary and fecal)	Section H: Bladder and bowel
Vision and hearing	Section B: Hearing, speech, and vision
Dentition	Section L: Oral/dental status
Social support*	Section F: Preferences for customary routine and activities

* MDS 3.0 does not include assessments of sexual function, spirituality, financial concerns, living situation, goals of care, and advanced care preferences, which are key components in the comprehensive geriatric assessment (CGA). MDS 3.0 incompletely addresses assessments of polypharmacy, goals of care, and social support, which are also considered key components of the CGA.
Note: The CGA does not explicitly address concerns around pain or preferences for activities or specific treatments, which are included as part of MDS 3.0.

Depending on the score on the assessment, the clinician may decide to pursue a plan of care to encourage prevention of further deterioration of illness. A training manual and video on how to administer the RGA are available from Saint Louis University's Gateway Geriatric Education Center (https://www.slu.edu/medicine /internal-medicine/geriatric-medicine/aging -sucessfully/).

Assessment of Acute Change in Condition

Changes in condition occur quite frequently in both post-acute patients and long-stay residents. The American Medical Directors Association's (n.d.) Society for Post-Acute and Long-Term Care Medicine have published guidelines for the management of acute changes in condition

TABLE 37-5 Comparison of Components of the Comprehensive Geriatric Assessment (CGA), Minimum Data Set 3.0 (MDS 3.0), and Rapid Geriatric Assessment (RGA)

Assessment Area	CGA	MDS 3.0	RGA
Functional capacity	√	√	
Fall risk	√	√	
Cognition (dementia/delirium)	√	√	√
Mood	√	√	
Behavior		√	
Polypharmacy	√		
Nutritional status	√	√	√
Incontinence (urinary/fecal)	√	√	
Sexual function	√		
Vision	√	√	
Hearing	√	√	
Speech		√	
Dentition	√	√	
Living situation	√		
Social support	√		
Financial concerns	√		
Goals of care	√		
Spirituality	√		
Advanced care preferences	√		√
Frailty			√
Sarcopenia			√

Assessment Area	CGA	MDS 3.0	RGA
Pain		√	
Preferences for customary routine and activities		√	
Pressure injuries	√	√	

Saint Louis University

Rapid Geriatric Assessment*

*there is no copyright on these screening tools and they may be incorporated into the electronic health record without permission and at no cost.

The simple "FRAIL" questionnaire screening tool
(3 or greater = frailty; 1 or 2 = prefrail)

Fatigue: Are you Fatigued?

Resistance: Cannot walk up one flight of stairs?

Aerobic: Cannot walk one block?

Illnesses: Do you have more than 5 illnesses?

Loss of weight: Have you lost more than 5% of your weight in the last 6 months?

Reproduced from Morley, J.E., Vellas, B., Abellan van Kan, G., Anker, S.D., Bauer, J.M., Bernabei, R., . . . Walston, J. (2013). Frailty consensus: A call to action. *The Journal of Post-Acute and Long-Term Care Medicine, 14*(6), 392–397, Copyright 2013, with permission from Elsevier.

Table I:SARC-F screen for Sarcopenia

Component	Question	Scoring
Strength	How much difficulty do you have in lifting and carrying 10 pounds?	None = 0 Some = 1 A lot or unable = 2
Assistance in walking	How much difficulty do you have walking across a room?	None = 0 Some = 1 A lot, use aids, or unable = 2
Rise from a chair	How much difficulty do you have transferring from a chair or bed?	None = 0 Some = 1 A lot or unable without help = 2
Climb stairs	How much difficulty do you have climbing a flight of ten stairs?	None = 0 Some = 1 A lot or unable = 2
Falls	How many times have you fallen in the last year?	None = 0 1-3 Falls = 1 4 or more falls = 2

Reproduced from Malmstrom, T.K., & Morley, J.E. (2013). Sarcopenia: The target population. *The Journal of Frailty & Aging, 2*(1), 55–56.

SNAQ (Simplified nutritional assessment questionnaire)

My appetite is
a. very poor
b. poor
c. average
d. good
e. very good

Food tastes
a. very bad
b. bad
c. average
d. good
e. very good

When I eat
a. I feel full after eating only a few mouthfuls
b. I feel full after eating about a third of a meal
c. I feel full after eating over half a meal
d. I feel full after eating most of the meal
e. I hardly ever feel full

Normally I eat
a. Less than one meal a day
b. one meal a day
c. two meals a day
d. three meals a day
e. more than three meals a day

Reproduced from Wilson, M.M.G., Thomas, D.R., Rubenstein, L.Z., Chibnall, J.T., Anderson, S., Baxi, A., . . . Morley, J.E. (2005). Appetite assessment: Simple appetite questionnaire predicts weight loss in community-dwelling adults and nursing home residents. Am J Clin Nutr 2005, 82, 1074–1081, American Society for Nutrition, American Society for Nutrition.

Rapid cognitive screen (RCS)

1. **Please remember these five objects. I will ask you what they are later.** [Read each object to patient using approx. 1 second intervals.]

Apple   Pen   Tie   House   Car

2. [Give patient pencil and the blank sheet with clock face.] **This is a clock face. Please put in the hour markers and the time at ten minutes to eleven o'clock.** [2 pts/hr markers ok; 2 pts/time correct]

3. **What were the five objects I asked you to remember?** [1 pt/ea]

4. **I'm going to tell you a story. Please listen carefully because afterwards, I'm going to ask you about it.**

Jill was a very successful stockbroker. She made a lot of money on the stock market. She then met Jack, a devastatingly handsome man. She married him and had three children. They lived in Chicago. She then stopped work and stayed at home to bring up her children. When they were teenagers, she went back to work. She and Jack lived happily ever after. What state did she live in? [1 pt]

Reproduced from Malmstrom, T.K., Voss, V.B., Cruz-Oliver, D.M., Cummings-Vaughn, L.A., Tumosa, N., Grossberg, G.T., & Morley, J.E. (2015). The Rapid Cognitive Screen (RCS): A point-of-care screening for dementia and mild cognitive impairment. *The Journal of Nutrition Health and Aging, 19*(7): 741–744.

Miscellaneous

Are you constipated? Y/N
Do you have worrisome incontinence? Y/N
Do you have an advanced directive? Y/N

FIGURE 37-2 Rapid Geriatric Assessment.

Stop and watch

Early warning tool

INTERACT
Version 4.0 tool

If you have identified a change while caring for or observing a resident, please **circle** the change and notify a nurse. Either give the nurse a copy of this tool or review it with her/him as soon as you can.

S	Seems different than usual
T	Talks or communicates less
O	Overall needs more help
P	Pain—new or worsening; Participated less in activities
a	Ate less
n	No bowel movement in 3 days; or diarrhea
d	Drank less
W	Weight change
A	Agitated or nervous more than usual
T	Tired, weak, confused, or drowsy
C	Change with skin color or condition
H	Help with walking, transferring, toileting more than usual

☐ Check here if no change noted
while monitoring high-risk patient

Patient/resident

Your name

Reported to   Date and time (am/pm)

Nurse response   Date and time (am/pm)

Nurse's name

FIGURE 37-3 The INTERACT "Stop and Watch" early warning tool.
Courtesy of INTERACT and Florida Atlantic University.

in the nursing home and made available tools for nurses to use before contacting a primary care provider (physician, nurse practitioner, or physician assistant) after an evaluation (https://paltc.org/product-store/know-it-all™-you-call -data-collection-system). Its Interventions to Reduce Acute Care Transfers (INTERACT) quality improvement program includes several tools for the identification, assessment, communication, and documentation of acute changes in a patient's or resident's condition, including the "Stop and Watch" early warning tool for direct care staff and families (**FIGURE 37-3**), the SBAR Communication Form and Progress Note for licensed nurses (**FIGURE 37-4**), and 10 care paths for assessment and management of common conditions associated with hospital transfers (see **FIGURE 37-5** for one example) (Ouslander, 2014). The INTERACT program is free for clinical use and can be found at http://www.pathway-interact.com/.

The assessments described in this section should be used as a guide in the development of a patient-centered plan of care. If, in the course of the patient/resident's illness, other issues arise,

SBAR Communication Form
and Progress Note for RNs/LPN/LVNs

INTERACT
Version 4.0 Tool

Before Calling the Physician / NP / PA / other Healthcare Professional:

☐ **Evaluate the Resident:** Complete relevant aspects of the SBAR form below
☐ **Check Vital Signs:** BP, pulse, and/or apical heart rate, temperature, respiratory rate, O_2 saturation and finger stick glucose for diabetics
☐ **Review Record:** Recent progress notes, labs, medications, other orders
☐ **Review an INTERACT Care Path** or **Acute Change in Condition File Card**, if indicated
☐ **Have Relevant Information Available when Reporting**
  (i.e. medical record, vital signs, advance directives such as DNR and other care limiting orders, allergies, medication list)

SITUATION

The change in condition, symptoms, or signs observed and evaluated is/are _____

This started on _____ / _____ / _____   Since this started it has gotten: ☐ Worse   ☐ Better   ☐ Stayed the same

Things that make the condition or symptom *worse* are _____

Things that make the condition or symptom *better* are _____

This condition, symptom, or sign has occurred before: ☐ Yes   ☐ No

Treatment for last episode *(if applicable)* _____

Other relevant information _____

BACKGROUND

Resident Description
This resident is in the facility for: ☐ Long-Term Care   ☐ Post Acute Care   ☐ Other: _____

Primary diagnoses _____

Other pertinent history *(e.g. medical diagnosis of CHF, DM, COPD)* _____

Medication Alerts
☐ Changes in the last week *(describe)* _____

☐ Resident is on *(Warfarin/Coumadin)* Result of last INR: _____   Date _____ / _____ / _____

☐ Resident is on other anticoagulant *(direct thrombin inhibitor or platelet inhibitor)*

Resident is on: ☐ Hypoglycemic medication(s) / Insulin   ☐ Digoxin

Allergies _____

Vital Signs

BP _____   Pulse _____ (or Apical HR _____) RR _____ Temp _____ Weight _____ lbs *(date _____ / _____ / _____)*

For CHF, edema, or weight loss: last weight before the current one was _____   on _____ / _____ / _____

Pulse Oximetry *(if indicated)* _____% on ☐ Room Air   ☐ O_2 (_____)

Blood Sugar *(Diabetics)* _____

Resident /Patient Name _____
(continued)

FIGURE 37-4 SBAR: situation, background, assessment, and recommendation (part of INTERACT).
Courtesy of INTERACT and Florida Atlantic University.

SBAR Communication Form
and Progress Note for RNs/LPN/LVNs (cont'd)

INTERACT®
Version 4.0 Tool

Resident Evaluation

Note: Except for Mental and Functional Status evaluations, if the item is not relevant to the change in condition check the box for "not clinically applicable to the change in condition being reported".

1. Mental Status Evaluation (compared to baseline; check all changes that you observe)

☐ Decreased level of consciousness (sleepy, lethargic)
☐ Increased confusion or disorientation
☐ Memory loss (new or worsening)

☐ New or worsened delusions or hallucinations
☐ Other symptoms or signs of delirium (e.g. inability to pay attention, disorganized thinking)
☐ Unresponsiveness

☐ Other (describe)
☐ No changes observed

Describe symptoms or signs _____

2. Functional Status Evaluation (compared to baseline; check all that you observe)

☐ Decreased mobility
☐ Needs more assistance with ADLs
☐ Falls (one or more)

☐ Swallowing difficulty
☐ Weakness (general)

☐ Other (describe)
☐ No changes observed

Describe symptoms or signs _____

3. Behavioral Evaluation

☐ Danger to self or others
☐ Depression (crying, hopelessness, not eating)
☐ Social withdrawal (isolation, apathy)

☐ Suicide potential
☐ Verbal aggression
☐ Physical aggression

☐ Personality change
☐ Other behavioral changes (describe)
☐ No changes observed

Describe symptoms or signs _____
☐ Not clinically applicable to the change in condition being reported

4. Respiratory Evaluation

☐ Abnormal lung sounds (rales, rhonchi, wheezing)
☐ Asthma (with wheezing)
☐ Cough (☐ Non-productive ☐ Productive)

☐ Inability to eat or sleep due to SOB
☐ Labored or rapid breathing
☐ Shortness of breath

☐ Symptoms of common cold
☐ Other respiratory changes (describe)
☐ No changes observed

Describe symptoms or signs _____
☐ Not clinically applicable to the change in condition being reported

5. Cardiovascular Evaluation

☐ Chest pain/tightness
☐ Edema
☐ Inability to stand without severe dizziness or lightheadedness

☐ Irregular pulse (new)
☐ Resting pulse >100 or <50

☐ Other (describe)
☐ No changes observed

Describe symptoms or signs _____
☐ Not clinically applicable to the change in condition being reported

6. Abdominal / GI Evaluation

☐ Abdominal pain
☐ Abdominal tenderness
☐ Constipation
   (date of last BM _____ / _____ / _____)
☐ Decreased/absent bowel sounds

☐ Distended abdomen
☐ Decreased appetite/fluid intake
☐ Diarrhea
☐ GI Bleeding (blood in stool or vomitus)
☐ Hyperactive bowel sounds

☐ Jaundice
☐ Nausea and/or vomiting
☐ Other (describe)
☐ No changes observed

Describe symptoms or signs _____
☐ Not clinically applicable to the change in condition being reported

Resident/Patient Name _____

(continued)

FIGURE 37-4 Continued
Courtesy of INTERACT and Florida Atlantic University.

SBAR Communication Form
and Progress Note for RNs/LPN/LVNs (cont'd)

INTERACT
Version 4.0 Tool

7. GU/Urine Evaluation
☐ Blood in urine
☐ Decreased urine output
☐ Lower abdominal pain or tenderness

☐ New or worsening incontinence
☐ Painful urination
☐ Urinating more frequently or urgency with or without other urinary symptoms

☐ Other *(describe)*
☐ No changes observed

Describe symptoms or signs _____
☐ Not clinically applicable to the change in condition being reported

8. Skin Evaluation
☐ Abrasion
☐ Blister
☐ Burn
☐ Contusion
☐ Discoloration

☐ Itching
☐ Laceration
☐ Pressure ulcer
☐ Puncture
☐ Rash

☐ Skin tear
☐ Splinter/sliver
☐ Wound *(describe)*
☐ Other *(describe)*
☐ No changes observed

Describe symptoms or signs _____
☐ Not clinically applicable to the change in condition being reported

9. Pain Evaluation

Does the resident have pain?
☐ No   ☐ Yes *(describe below)*

Is the pain?
☐ New   ☐ Worsening of chronic pain

Description/location of pain: _____

Intensity of Pain *(rate on scale of 1-10, with 10 being the worst)*: _____

Does the resident show non-verbal signs of pain (for residents with dementia)?

☐ No   ☐ Yes *(describe)* _____
                    (restless, pacing, grimacing, new change in behavior)

Other information about the pain _____
☐ Not clinically applicable to the change in condition being reported

10. Neurological Evaluation
☐ Abnormal Speech
☐ Decreased level of consciousness
☐ Dizziness or unsteadiness

☐ Seizure
☐ Weakness or hemiparesis

☐ Other neurological symptoms *(describe)*
☐ No changes observed

Describe symptoms or signs _____
☐ Not clinically applicable to the change in condition being reported

Advance Care Planning Information *(the resident has orders for the following advanced care planning)*
☐ Full Code   ☐ DNR   ☐ DNI *(Do Not Intubate)*   ☐ DNH *(Do Not Hospitalize)*   ☐ No Enteral Feeding   ☐ Other Order or Living Will *(specify)*

_____

Other resident or family preferences for care _____

_____

Resident/Patient Name _____
                                                                                    (continued)

FIGURE 37-4 Continued
Courtesy of INTERACT and Florida Atlantic University.

SBAR Communication Form
and Progress Note for RNs/LPN/LVNs (cont'd)

INTERACT
Version 4.0 Tool

APPEARANCE

Summarize your observations and evaluation: _____

_____

_____

REVIEW AND NOTIFY

Primary Care Clinician Notified:_____ Date ___/___/___ Time (am/pm)_____

Recommendations of Primary Clinicians *(if any)* _____

_____

_____

b. Check *all* that apply

Testing
- ☐ Blood tests
- ☐ EKG
- ☐ Urinalysis and/or culture

- ☐ Venous doppler
- ☐ X-ray
- ☐ Other *(describe)*
  _____

Interventions
- ☐ New or change in
  medication(s)
- ☐ IV or subcutaneous fluids

- ☐ Increase oral fluids
- ☐ Oxygen *(if available)*
- ☐ Other *(describe)*
  _____

☐ Transfer to the hospital (non-emergency) *(send a copy of this form)*   ☐ Call for 911   ☐ Emergency medical transport

Nursing Notes *(for additional information on the Change in Condition)*

_____

_____

_____

_____

_____

_____

Name of Family/Health Care Agent Notified:_____ Date ___/___/___ Time (am/pm)_____

Staff Name (RN/LPN/LVN) and Signature_____

Resident/Patient Name _____

FIGURE 37-4 Continued

Courtesy of INTERACT and Florida Atlantic University.

CARE PATH *Symptoms of shortness of breath (SOB)*

INTERACT
Version 4.0 tool

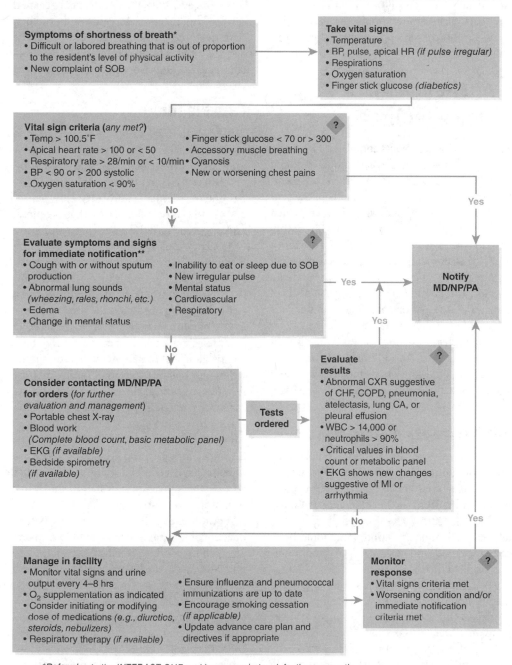

Symptoms of shortness of breath*
- Difficult or labored breathing that is out of proportion to the resident's level of physical activity
- New complaint of SOB

Take vital signs
- Temperature
- BP, pulse, apical HR *(if pulse irregular)*
- Respirations
- Oxygen saturation
- Finger stick glucose *(diabetics)*

Vital sign criteria (*any met?***)** ?
- Temp > 100.5°F
- Apical heart rate > 100 or < 50
- Respiratory rate > 28/min or < 10/min
- BP < 90 or > 200 systolic
- Oxygen saturation < 90%
- Finger stick glucose < 70 or > 300
- Accessory muscle breathing
- Cyanosis
- New or worsening chest pains

No

Yes

Evaluate symptoms and signs for immediate notification** ?
- Cough with or without sputum production
- Abnormal lung sounds *(wheezing, rales, rhonchi, etc.)*
- Edema
- Change in mental status
- Inability to eat or sleep due to SOB
- New irregular pulse
- Mental status
- Cardiovascular
- Respiratory

Yes

Notify MD/NP/PA

No

Yes

Evaluate results ?
- Abnormal CXR suggestive of CHF, COPD, pneumonia, atelectasis, lung CA, or pleural effusion
- WBC > 14,000 or neutrophils > 90%
- Critical values in blood count or metabolic panel
- EKG shows new changes suggestive of MI or arrhythmia

Consider contacting MD/NP/PA for orders *(for further evaluation and management)*
- Portable chest X-ray
- Blood work *(Complete blood count, basic metabolic panel)*
- EKG *(if available)*
- Bedside spirometry *(if available)*

Tests ordered

No

Yes

Manage in facility
- Monitor vital signs and urine output every 4–8 hrs
- O₂ supplementation as indicated
- Consider initiating or modifying dose of medications *(e.g., diuretics, steroids, nebulizers)*
- Respiratory therapy *(if available)*
- Ensure influenza and pneumococcal immunizations are up to date
- Encourage smoking cessation *(if applicable)*
- Update advance care plan and directives if appropriate

Monitor response ?
- Vital signs criteria met
- Worsening condition and/or immediate notification criteria met

*Refer also to the INTERACT CHF and lower respiratory infection care path
**Refer also to other INTERACT care paths as indicated by symptoms and signs

FIGURE 37-5 One of the INTERACT care paths for assessment and management of acute changes in condition.

Courtesy of INTERACT and Florida Atlantic University.

many distinct screening tools may be used to clarify the diagnosis. It is important to recognize that the needs and goals of care of patients with chronic, complex illness will likely change over time. These tools should serve as an adjunct to a coordinated team approach to care.

▶ Challenges and Opportunities

The results of assessments completed in nursing homes should be evaluated carefully. Depending on the setting or what triggered the assessment, the clinician should respond appropriately to such findings. During periodic assessments (such as those completed on a monthly or bimonthly basis, or a required quarterly MDS assessment), most of the actions triggered should be based on the longitudinal changes in the patient/resident's function and cognition and long-term goals of care. Sometimes laboratory abnormalities may be identified as well as changes in other markers of health such as nutritional status (either weight loss or weight gain). In addition, new drug–drug interactions and unnecessary medications could be identified at the time of these assessments.

Turning Assessment into Action

Continuous assessments, like those completed by CNAs and nurses, should trigger more immediate responses by clinicians than those from more holistic evaluations such as the CGA, because the findings from a CGA are often chronic in nature. Any change in condition should be at least monitored, and when necessary, communicated to the clinician.

A well-designed periodic assessment should include a predetermined action list in the event of a new condition or the worsening of a preexisting one. The actions should be proportional to the goals of care previously expressed by the patient and/or the patient's family, and should focus on providing quality of life and comfort when indicated. INTERACT, for example,

includes specific guidance on when to communicate changes to clinicians on an immediate versus a non-immediate basis.

Whatever the nature of the plan of care that results from these assessments, it should be patient centered and evidence based. **TABLE 37-6** lists examples of potential actions triggered by common findings from periodic assessments.

Care Planning

TABLE 37-7 shows the key assessments needed to construct a care plan for a post-acute patient or long-term care resident. There are two important aspects of care planning for nursing home patients/residents: (1) advance care planning and (2) the actual plan of care that is generated and updated from the assessments completed.

Advance care planning is a key component of geriatric care. In the post-acute patient or the long-term care resident, this type of planning is an ongoing process that should be adapted to the changing needs and the functional status of the patient. Effective person-centered care planning should take into consideration the personal values of the patient and should include, when necessary, the input of family members. As the members of the interprofessional team assess the resident/patient, the goals of care should drive care planning discussions as well. Many resources are available to assist with advance care planning, including those available in INTERACT, as well as other websites (e.g., http://eprognosis.ucsf.edu/ and https://prepareforyourcare.org/).

Another aspect of care planning is the list of actionable items that are aimed to recover the patient's premorbid functional level, especially after an acute event. The actionable items on this list correspond to specific deficits that are found during ongoing assessments and are aimed to promote functional independence and quality of life. The plan of care should be individualized and accompanied by clear goals and timetables. All elements that are included in the plan of care and the advance care planning should be based on the capabilities of the nursing home.

TABLE 37-6 Potential Actionable Items Found During Standard Assessments

Assessment	Findings	Action
MDS Frequency: At admission and periodic	Certified nursing assistant (CNA) reports coughing with meals or when swallowing medications.	Bedside swallow evaluation; speech therapy evaluation; modify diet consistency; evaluate which medications are essential.
	Medication: Resident received hypnotic as-needed (prn) medication five times in the last 7 days.	Discuss sleep hygiene issues. Assess for other reasons for insomnia, such as pain or nocturia.
	Resident reporting little interest or pleasure in doing things and feeling down, depressed, or hopeless.	Discuss possible causes of mood changes such as pain, hearing/visual impairment, or new psychosocial issues. Consider starting pharmacologic treatment.
	Resident received as-needed (prn) pain medication every day in the last 5 days.	Evaluate for acute illness or unreported injuries. Reassess pain needs—nonpharmacologic and pharmacologic.
	MDS: Change in the resident's usual performance using the 6-point scale.	Evaluate for acute illness, mood changes, and pain.
Rapid Geriatric Assessment	Patent reported not being able to ambulate for a city block and having more than five medical illness.	Reassess rehabilitation potential and goals. Potential for revision of discharge planning.
	Patient reported poor appetite, average taste for food, and having a meal per day.	Assess for acute illness including infection, dysphagia, or mood disorder. Evaluate medications.
CGA Frequency: At least once during a skilled nursing facility (SNF) stay	Capacity for medical decision making.	Review current status of healthcare proxy. Revise plan of care and discharge planning.
	Patient without family members or other means of social support.	Revise discharge planning. Identify healthcare proxy.
	Change in goals of care.	Revise medication list, plan of care, and disposition; consider hospice or palliative care.

Adapted from MDS 3.0 RAI Manual v1.15R October 1, 2017 Centers For Medicare & Medicaid Services. Retrieved from https://www.cms.gov/Medicare/Quality-Initiatives-Patient-Assessment-Instruments/NursinghomeQualityInits/MDS30RAIManual.html. Last Accessed March 12, 2018.

TABLE 37-7 Basic Elements to Consider When Building a Plan of Care

Comprehensive health assessment within 14 days of admission and at least one review within 90 days

Ongoing, regular assessments screening for change in condition (from the Minimum Data Set [MDS])

Services needed

Staff needs for providing services

Frequency of services

Equipment and supplies needs

Diet needs and food preferences

Role of Electronic Health Records in Assessments and Care Planning

Nursing homes are not eligible for Medicare's incentives for utilizing electronic health records (EHRs). Nonetheless, the payment reform initiatives undertaken by the Centers for Medicare and Medicaid Services (CMS) are encouraging nursing homes to move away from the inefficiencies and limited monitoring proficiencies of paper-based medical records. While nursing homes must report MDS data electronically to state and federal governments, most do not yet have well-functioning clinical electronic records. Nursing home EHRs are evolving from simple repositories of data to interacting assessment, care management, and decision support tools that provide live feedback to providers regarding potential changes in condition and even suggest adjustments of the plan of care if appropriate. Such capabilities might help to prevent adverse outcomes, including unnecessary acute hospital transfers, in the near future.

▶ Summary

Nursing homes are complex settings of care serving a variety of individuals, ranging from patients needing rehabilitation after an acute hospitalization to permanent residents of these facilities. Interprofessional-based assessments are the cornerstone of the care provided to these individuals. Several structured assessment tools can be used in these settings. Any changes in the plan of care should be person centered, meaning that they should consider patients' values and beliefs. Changes in condition as determined through assessment should trigger actions aimed at avoiding further complications in the early stages of acute illness and promoting quality of life and respect for the individual's dignity.

References

American Medical Directors Association. (2005). AMDA clinical practice guideline: Acute change of condition. [PDF document]. Retrieved from https://www.nhqualitycampaign.org/files/Acute_Change_in_Condition_Reference.pdf

Morley, J. L.-W. (2017). Rapid Geriatric Assessment: A tool for primary care physicians. *Journal of the American Medical Directors Association, 18*, 195–199.

Ouslander, J. B. (2014). The INTERACT quality improvement program: An overview for medical directors and primary care clinicians in long-term care. *Journal of the American Medical Directors Association, 15*, 162–170.

Picker Institute. (2012, March 12). *To reduce healthcare costs, try everything!* Retrieved from http://pickerinstitute.org/vive

Rubenstein, L. Z., Josephson, K. R., Wieland, G. D., English, P. A., Sayre, J. A., & Kane, R. L. (1984). Effectiveness of a geriatric evaluation unit: A randomized clinical trial. *New England Journal of Medicine, 31*, 1664–1670.

Saliba, D. B. (2012). Making the investment count: Revision of the Minimum Data Set for Nursing Homes, MDS 3.0. *Journal of the American Medical Directors Association, 13*, 602–610.

Saliba, D., Jones, M., Streim, J., Ouslander, J., Berlowitz, D., & Buchanan, J. (2012). Overview of significant changes in the Minimum Data Set for Nursing Homes Version 3.0. *Journal of the American Medical Directors Association, 13*, 595–601.

Stuck, A. E., Siu, A. L., Wieland, G. D., Rubenstein, L. Z., & Adams, J. (1993). Comprehensive geriatric assessment: A meta-analysis of controlled trials. *Lancet, 342*, 1032–1036.

CHAPTER 38

Emergency Department Assessment at the Time of Hospitalization

Teresita M. Hogan and Stacie Levine

CHAPTER OBJECTIVES

1. Discuss the emergency department (ED) as a critical access location for the management of older adult patients.
2. Describe the high-acuity, high-stress, and high-volume ED environment in terms of the need for rapid medical decision making.
3. Examine clinical assessment of older adults at the time of ED admission, including focused evaluation and documentation of geriatrics issues that impact the decision to hospitalize as well as ongoing hospital care.
4. Describe how medical decision making regarding admission should include consideration of high-risk conditions common in seniors.

KEY TERMS

Emergency department (ED)	Improvement	Older adult (OAs)
Hospital admission	Management	

▶ Introduction

The **emergency department (ED)** plays a critical role in the evaluation and treatment of **older adults (OAs)** in the United States. Today, the ED faces challenges associated with broad demographic changes in its patient population, increased severity of illness, diagnostic and treatment demands, and intense time pressures. As in all medical fields, providers in the ED are constantly asked to perform more frequent and complex tasks with fewer resources. Increasingly, EDs are used by primary and specialist physicians to provide expedited complex diagnostic testing and treatment, off-hours care, and as a coordination point in complex care transitions.

Within the U.S. healthcare system, OAs often require evaluation for a complex interplay of comorbidities, polypharmacy, social issues, and cognitive and functional impairment. These needs cab cause an age-based bias in the use of the ED as a portal for **hospital admission**. In fact, OAs are more likely to present to an ED with serious medical illness and more likely to need hospitalization (Baum & Rubenstein, 1987; Ettinger, Casani, Coon, Muller, & Piazza-Appel, 1987; Lowenstein, Crescenzi, Kern, & Steel, 1986). These facts confirm the idea that elder ED use is, in fact, appropriate and needed. A better system of coordinating care of OAs in the ED must be developed. Geriatricians, internists, and specialty physicians should better understand the functioning and demands of both the ED and emergency physicians (EPs) so as to best leverage the resources commanded by the ED for optimal care of OAs.

▶ Epidemiology

The ED currently manages more than one-fourth of all U.S. acute care outpatient visits (Schuur & Venkatesh, 2012; Smith et al., 2012), and 38% of all ED patient visits are made by OAs. The ED cared for more than 175 million OAs from 2001 to 2010 (Lo et al., 2017); this number increased by 25% through 2016, suggesting that ED use by OAs is outpacing the general demographic growth of this population. In addition, hospital admissions are now growing faster than outpatient visits. If these trends continue, they will place ever-increasing demands on hospitals in terms of both ED visits and hospitalizations (Pines, Mullins, Cooper, Feng, & Roth, 2013).

The ED is the major source of admissions to U.S. hospitals. More than 50% of U.S. nonobstetric hospitalizations are managed through the ED (Pitts, Niska, Xu, & Burt, 2008), with elder patients representing 32.5% to 57.3% of all general hospital admissions and 5.5% of all intensive care unit (ICU) admissions (Lo et al., 2017). There is a linear relationship between age and ED admission, with the odds of hospitalization increasing 2.9% for each year of age greater than 65 years (Greenwald et al., 2016). For every decade older than age 65 years, risk of ICU admission increases by 16% (Lo et al., 2017).

The determination of hospital admission versus discharge made in the ED establishes the course and cost of medical care for approximately 11 million elder patients annually (Schuur & Venkatesh, 2012). ED visits are associated with clinically meaningful functional decline within 6 months of the ED visit (Nagurney et al., 2017). Moreover, half of older adults utilize the ED in the last month of life, and 75% in the last 6 months of life (Smith, 2010). The critical role of EDs in care of this population highlights a need to improve systems of care and to better coordinate care between EDs and providers of both inpatient and outpatient care.

▶ Challenges to Geriatric Care in the ED

EDs were designed to care for one acute disease state, illness, or injury isolated in time with episodic use. This intent does not correspond to the complex, interwoven subacute issues evolving over longer periods and requiring care coordination that elder patients experience every day. OAs are at high risk of adverse health outcomes following an ED visit. At 3 months following such a visit, they experience a 5% mortality rate, a 20% hospitalization rate, and a 20% rate of repeat ED visits (Hastings, Schmader, & Sloane, 2007; McCusker, Cardin, & Bellavance, 2000; McCusker, Roberge, D., & Vadenboncoeur, 2009). These high death and utilization rates have been described as issues stemming from disease progression as well as from the coordination and navigation of the system of care, rather than being due to the specific care rendered in the ED (Schniter, Martin-Khan, & Gray, 2011). However, emergency care leaders are concerned that ED visits do not always fully address the pathology causing the visit, nor does the ED arrange outpatient intervention so as to prevent functional decline. In fact, many elders discharged from the ED experience clinically meaningful functional decline that is associated with increased mortality, institutionalization, and costs within 6 months after their ED visit (Nagurney et al., 2017). Although elder ED patients receive more medical testing, physician attention, and medical admissions, they suffer excess morbidity and mortality relative to younger adults (Aminzadeh & Dalziel, 2002; Wilber, Gerson, et al., 2006).

It is known that OAs with impaired functional status should be targeted for close medical surveillance and ready access to follow-up care when discharged from the ED. Yet most EDs do not routinely screen for, or readily identify, functional decline. One study demonstrated that 75% of the time functional status is ignored in the ED, leading to concerns about poor ED practice (Wilber, Blanda, & Gerson, 2006). In reality, functional decline among OAs is more likely to be a result of change in healthcare status or progression of existing disease, rather than a result of errant care in the ED (Schniter et al., 2011). Additional issues identified as adverse events resulting from deficient ED practice include the under-triage of OA illness severity, lack of recognition of geriatric syndromes and depression, adverse medication events, and poor communication among clinicians (Schniter et al., 2011).

ED Crowding and Boarding

Emergency department crowding describes the periodic mismatch between the supply of available healthcare staff and bed spaces in the ED and inpatient settings and the volume of patients needing these resources. Crowding results in long waits for evaluations and testing, and it places patients at considerable risk for adverse outcomes due to delay of evaluation and treatment. Lack of primary care is a major contributor to ED use and the overcrowded conditions found in 90% of U.S. EDs. Better coordination of ED use by primary care providers, either by direct admissions or through discussions with ED providers can help alleviate inappropriate use of ED resources. ED crowding and inadequate inpatient capacity have been identified by the Institute of Medicine as a public health crisis. Notably, mortality of admitted patients increases with increased ED boarding time (Singer, Thode, Viccellio, & Pines, 2011), with OAs being especially vulnerable to morbidity and mortality from prolonged waits for hospital beds.

Physicians diverting patients to the ED must understand the capacity of the ED at the time they are sending those patients for care. Care in clinics or by direct admission may at times be more appropriate for an individual, as well as safer for those patients already in the waiting room.

Boarding is the term used to describe the status of patients during the long wait for available inpatient beds after admission is requested. Boarding occurs largely due to limited hospital bed capacity. Boarders do not receive the same level of care from either the ED staff (who consider their work complete) or the inpatient staff (who have not yet accepted full responsibility for the patient) (Hollander & Pines, 2007).

The general internal medicine service serves as a safety valve by accepting ED admissions of more subspecialty patients when the specialty beds are full, thereby reducing ED boarding. However, delay of discharge of general medicine patients can be a major cause of boarding. Inpatient providers and EPs must work together to ease the burdens imposed by ED boarding and help improve quality throughout. This can is done by decreasing hospital length of stay and ensuring that patients are discharged home as soon as appropriate (Powell et al., 2012). Physicians who can affect the rate of discharge from the hospital can significantly improve ED boarding. Discussions among administration, those physicians accepting and discharging inpatients, and ED leadership may result in solutions to improve ED boarding and crowding. Review of specific hospital bed reservation policies, such as mandatory holding of beds for cardiac catheterization or other procedures, can smooth out the supply–demand relationship and thereby minimize delays in ED admissions (Levin et al., 2008). Better matching of total number of ED admissions to hospital discharges improves the next-day ED length of stay and reduces ED wait times; **improvements** in this admission–discharge ratio can enhance hospital system performance (Powell et al., 2012; Vermeulen et al., 2009).

Other strategies include development of inpatient full capacity protocols, inpatient discharge coordination, and surgical schedule smoothing (Handel et al., 2012). Surgical smoothing involves even distribution of cases throughout the week for better allocation of preoperative and postoperative beds, staff, and other resources to more effectively distribute resources required for care for these patients as well as resources needed for patients throughout the institution.

▶ Variability of the ED Admission Decision

The decision to admit patients to the hospital varies significantly from hospital to hospital, even when adjusting for patient demographic and presentation factors. This is likely due to variations in both hospital factors and physician behavior (Ismail & Pope, 2017). For instance, the ED may be used to admit patients for reasons other than true medical emergencies. Differences in ED admission rates have been identified with respect to patient gender, region of the United States, hospital size and type, patient race, and patient insurance (Greenwald et al., 2016). Hospital factors associated with increased admissions include smaller number of hospital beds, smaller physician staff size, and fewer total ED visits. Older patient populations and limited primary care access also result in higher rates of ED hospital admission (Studnicki, Platonova, & Fisher, 2012).

Admission decisions made by emergency physicians are influenced by both medical and nonmedical factors. Indeed, one survey of emergency physicians showed 51% of admissions were strongly or moderately influenced by nonmedical factors. Primary among them were lack of information on the patient's baseline condition, inadequate specialty care access, requirement for further diagnostics or procedures, and inadequate primary care access. These non-acuity-driven admissions are shorter and less costly than those admissions related to medical acuity, but lead to similar rates of ED readmissions and repeat hospitalization (Lewis Hunter, Spatz, Bernstein, & Rosenthal, 2016). Development of interdisciplinary protocols and pathways between geriatrician leaders and emergency providers can help decrease variability and improve both healthcare delivery and utilization in this population.

Assessment and Treatment of Common Geriatric Conditions at Admission

The most common complaints in OAs presenting to the ED are chest pain, shortness of breath, and abdominal pain, all of which clearly include life threats in their differential diagnoses. The complaints for which older patients are most often treated and discharged include essential hypertension, superficial injury, upper respiratory infections, sprains and strains, abdominal pain, back problems, lower respiratory disease, headache, diabetes without complication, open wounds, and subcutaneous tissue infections. The most common diagnoses leading to hospital admission include fluid and electrolyte disorders, coronary atherosclerosis and other heart disease, cardiac dysrhythmias, congestive heart failure, nonspecific chest pain, chronic obstructive pulmonary disease, hypertension, and abdominal pain (Owens et al., 2010).

There is a tension between the need for timely, expedited emergency throughput expected from EPs and a more complete assessment for common geriatric syndromes that impact morbidity and mortality in hospitalized elders. ED providers struggle with the necessity of more complete evaluations and view them as being more appropriately performed in the inpatient setting.

Even when limited to the subpopulation of high-risk elders, rather than all patients older than a given age, a comprehensive geriatric assessment (CGA) is time intensive and unlikely to be routinely performed by ED providers (Graf, Zekry, Giannelli, Michel, & Chevalley, 2011). In addition, a lack of rigorous evaluations with standard implementation tools have been documented in systematic reviews in the literature. This lack of effective tools has ruled out implementation of standard ED-based interventions targeted to reduce adverse outcomes in OAs (Karam, Radden, Berall, Cheng, & Gruneir, 2015). A potentially more feasible solution is to offer a multidisciplinary CGA in an ED observation unit, which may lead to targeted interventions (Southerland, Vargas, Nagaraj, Cure, & Caterino, 2017).

Brief geriatric assessments (BGA) have been attempted in the ED. One six-item BGA tool required only minutes to complete, yet had poor prognostic value for identification of elders at risk of prolonged hospital stay (Launay, de Decker, Kabeshova, Annweiler, & Beauchet, 2014). The Emergency Geriatric Screening (EGS) tool, which screens for cognition, falls, mobility, and activities of daily living, was feasible in one study and identified undetected geriatric syndromes while predicting some subsequent care needs (**FIGURE 38-1**) (Schoenenberger et al., 2014).

Cognition

In the discipline of emergency medicine, cognitive disorders are prioritized by beginning with extreme life threats of coma and stupor. These conditions occur in 5% to 9% of elders who visit the ED and require immediate evaluation and treatment (Han & Wilber, 2013). This care is followed by discovery and stabilization of immediate life threats characterized by the mnemonic WHHHIMPS: Wernicke's/Withdrawal, Hypoxia, Hypercarbia, Hypoglycemia, Hypertensive encephalopathy, Hyper/Hypothermia or Hypothyroidism, Intracerebral hemorrhage, Ischemic Stroke, Meningitis/encephalitis, Poisoning, and Status Epilepticus. After exhausting this list of dangerous issues, assessment and treatment can move to other less lethal problems.

Delirium is found in approximately 10% of elders who come to the ED (Elie et al., 2000; Hustey & Meldon, 2002), but is recognized only 35% of the time, with identification being more likely when the presentation is associated with a transient ischemic attack or stroke. Missed delirium may predispose providers to miss the patient's underlying medical issue and, therefore, is associated with higher morbidity and mortality rates (Chiovenda, Vincetelli, & Alegiani, 2002; Inouye, 2006). Currently, the appropriate **management** of symptoms of delirium in the ED remains unclear, with use of both nonpharmacologic and pharmacologic interventions being debated (Han & Wilber, 2013). A clinically useful acronym suggesting probable causes of delirium is DELIRUMS:

- Drugs
- Environment and Endocrine
- Low oxygen
- Infections
- Retention
- Ischemia (cardiac/vascular)
- Undernutrition
- Metabolic, Metastatic
- Subdural hematoma

Emergency geriatric screening (EGS) tool, consisting of short validated instruments for screening four domains (cognition, falls, mobility, and activities of daily living) [13, 19, 23].

Cognition

Instruction: Ask the patient the following questions. If the patient does not respond, the question is rated incorrect.

What day is today?	Incorrect*	Correct
What is the date today? (± 1 day is correct)	Incorrect*	Correct
What year is this?	Incorrect*	Correct
Spell "radio" backwards.	Incorrect	Correct
Evaluation consistent with impairment of cognition (if one single response was incorrect):	**Yes**	**No**

Falls

Instruction: Rate the following questions considering all availale sources (patient, proxy, observation, reports).

Did the patient present to the ED because of a fall?	Yes*	No
Did the patient have one or more falls during the last 12 months?	Yes	No
Evaluation consistent with patient history of falls (if one single response was yes):	**Yes**	**No**

Mobility

Instruction: Rate the following question considering all available sources (patient, proxy, observation, reports).

Did the patient require walking aids (cane, wheeled walker, or helping person) in- or outdoors before presenting to the ED?	Yes	No

Instruction: Rate the following questions according to the current situation in the ED.

Is the patient currently confined to bed?	Yes*	No
Does the patient currently need help (walking aids or helping person) to get out of bed?	Yes*	No
Does the patient need ≥20 seconds for the Timed Up and Go Test?	Yes	No
Evaluation consistent with impairment of mobility (if one single response was yes):	**Yes**	**No**

ADL

Instruction: Rate the following question considering all available sources (patient, proxy, observation, reports).

Did the patient require assistance for personal hygiene (sponge bath, tub bath, or shower) before presenting to the ED?	Yes*	No

Instruction: Rate the following questions according to the current situation in ED.

Is the patient currently confined to bed or does he need help (walking aid or helping person) to get out of bed?	Yes*	No
Does the patient require assistance (for direct help or instruction) for dressing (clothes or shoes)?	Yes*	No
Does the patient require assistance (for direct help or instruction) for toileting?	Yes*	No
Does the patient require assistance (for direct help or instruction) for feeding?	Yes	No
Evaluation consistent with impairment in ADL (if one single response was yes):	**Yes**	**No**

ADL = activities of daily living; ED = emergency department.
*If one of the responses marked with an asterisk applies, the rater may directly proceed to evaluating the domain (hierarchical structure).

FIGURE 38-1 Emergency Geriatric Screening (EGS) tool.

Reproduced from Schoenenberger AW, Bieri C, Ozgüler O, Moser A, Haberkern M, Zimmermann H, et al. A novel multidimensional geriatric screening tool in the ED: evaluation of feasibility and clinical relevance. *Am J Emerg Med*. 2014;32(6):623–8. Copyright 2014, with permission from Elsevier.

Other contributors to cognitive impairment, including dementia, occur in 15% to 40% of elders who visit the ED (Hustey, Meldon, Smith, & Lex, 2003), but are identified less than 50% of the time (Kakuma et al., 2003). In general, because dementia is considered to be a chronic condition, the diagnostic evaluation is not specifically viewed as an ED-relevant issue. Since 1996, several emergency medicine groups have called for routine formal evaluation of patients for cognitive impairment using specific tools like the Mini-Mental Status Exam (Sanders, 1996). To date, routine ED use of such tools has not been implemented.

The ideal tool to screen for cognitive impairment should be brief, usable by ED staff, and simple; require minimal equipment and training; and be highly sensitive and specific. Only a few tools have managed to meet this demanding list of criteria. The recommended screening tools to detect cognitive dysfunction in elder ED patients include the Brief Alzheimer's Screen, Short Blessed Test, Ottawa 3DY, and the caregiver-completed AD8 (Carpenter et al., 2003). The recommended delirium screening tools include the Confusion Assessment Method (CAM), the CAM-ICU, the 3D CAM, and the Delirium Triage Screen plus the Brief CAM (Inouye et al., 1990). In 2013, Han, Wilson, Vasilevskis, Shintani, and Schenelle, recommended use of the Delirium Triage Screen with the Brief CAM as valid and reliable and meeting most of the criteria for ED screening. Systematic reviews in the emergency medicine literature, however, have not found adequate validation of screening tools for cognitive impairment (LaMantia, Messina, Hobgood, & Miller, 2014). Further work is needed between geriatricians and emergency medicine professionals to determine the best method and timing of evaluation for cognitive disorders in this patient population.

Falls

Elder falls present the ominous combination of high prevalence, significant morbidity and mortality, increased healthcare utilization, and substantial excess cost. Recognition of and intervention to protect at-risk elders is considered to be a high-priority area for emergency medicine, yet prior efforts to address one or more of these issues have met with variable results. Fortunately, there are promising developments in this area that may improve the care of elders who are vulnerable to falls.

As many as 33% of elderly patients who suffer falls and are discharged home from the ED experience trauma-related functional decline within 3 months (Sirois et al., 2013). Even falls without injury result in loss of mobility and social participation (Lo, Brown, Sawyer, Kennedy, & Allman, 2014). Elder falls are the leading cause of injury deaths in persons older than age 65, and more than one-third of those individuals require ED revisits (Liu, Obermeyer, Chang, & Shankar, 2015). In one study, 35% of elderly patients who experienced a fall had one or more ED presentations, and 20.3% were found to have had one or more hospital admissions in the preceding 12 months. Fall-related ED presentation led directly to hospital admission in 42.7% of the cases, with the majority of these patients (78.0%) then receiving acute care only. The hospital length of stay was 14.4 days for men and 13.7 days for women; the remaining patients underwent further inpatient rehabilitation, with that length of stay being 35.6 days for men and 30.1 days for women (Close et al., 2012).Older patients presenting to the ED after a fall had high injury rates, high admission rates, and often prolonged hospitalization.

The additional healthcare costs among elders who experience falls range from $3500 to $11,000 for non-injurious falls to $27,000 to $39,507 for those patients with serious injury (Woolcott, Khan, Mitrovic, Anis, & Marra, 2012; Wu, Keeler, Rubenstein, Maglione, & Shekelle, 2010). Based on 2012 data, the cost of the typical ED elder evaluation in the wake of a fall is $1200, with this cost rising to $12,000 for each hospital admission. ED decisions to admit or discharge a patient who falls control the course and cost of care for approximately 11 million older adults in the United States annually (Schuur & Venkatesh, 2012).

The ED is a convenient location to screen, evaluate, and risk-stratify older adults at risk for many geriatric syndromes (Carpenter et al., 2014). Approximately one-third are revealed to have fallen previously, so detection in the ED can prompt referral to falls prevention programs (Bell, Talbot-Stern, & Hennessy, 2000).

The Geriatric Emergency Department (GED) guidelines for optimal care of older adults who fall have been enthusiastically endorsed by multiple prominent emergency medicine and geriatric physician and nursing organizations (**BOX 38-1**). Even so, much ED care is discordant with these recommendations (Tirrell et al., 2015). Most older patients who visit the ED do not receive any guideline-directed falls management (Salter et al., 2006). Even when ED fall-risk evaluation occurs, fewer than 15% of patients discharged from the ED receive follow-up instructions to address these issues (Carpenter & Lo, 2015). When elderly patients who visit the ED for falls do not receive guideline care, their morbidity, mortality, utilization, and cost profiles are significantly worse compared to their peers who do receive such care (Platts-Mills et al., 2016). The magnitude of the economic and social costs of falls in older adults underscores the need for active research and interventions in the field of elder ED falls.

Pain

Pain is the symptom most frequently reported by ED patients (Cordell et al., 2002). Unfortunately, pain in the OA population is often inadequately managed (Todd et al., 2007). One reason for this inadequacy is the significant variability in the assessment, reassessment, and treatment of OAs' pain in the ED (Hwang, Richardson, Harris, & Morrison, 2010; Platts-Mills et al., 2012; Platts-Mills et al., 2016).

The Society for Academic Emergency Medicine and the American College of Emergency Physicians have developed quality improvement (QI) indicators for pain management of ED elders (Terrell et al., 2009) (**BOX 38-2**). These guidelines list goals that ED providers should attain in care of elders with pain. All too often, however, pain protocol improvements are not sustained without routine monitoring, thereby implying that education should be linked with quality metrics and staff feedback for lasting effect. Hogan, Howell, Cursio, Wong, & Dale (2016) linked staff education and pain protocols to quality monitoring with reporting back to staff members, and demonstrated significant reductions in final pain score and intensity as well as increased both pain reassessment and analgesic administration to implementation of such protocols.

BOX 38-1 Geriatric Emergency Department (GED) Guidelines for Optimal Care of Older Adults Who Fall

1. Increase the detection of life-threatening events precipitating the fall.
2. Identify the cause of the fall as an acute condition, a progression of preexisting disease, or an accelerated general decline. Initiate treatment and ensure appropriate disposition.
3. Evaluate and treat post-fall traumatic injuries.
4. Provide urgent medication review and reconciliation.
5. Provide timely physical therapy evaluation and referral to outpatient therapy as needed.
6. Develop and operationalize an ED elder fall risk assessment protocol appropriate for the resources found at each institution.
7. Develop and operationalize linkage to elder services to decrease fall risk and enhance patient safety.
8. Optimize transitions of care through interdisciplinary communications and standardized referral protocol development.

BOX 38-2 Pain Management of Older Adults in the ED

1. A formal pain assessment should be documented within 1 hour of the patient's arrival.
2. If the patient remains in the ED longer than 6 hours, a second pain assessment should be documented.
3. If the patient receives pain treatment in the ED, a pain reassessment should be documented prior to discharge home.
4. For patients with moderate to severe pain, pain treatment should be initiated or a reason why treatment was not initiated should be documented.
5. Meperidine (Demerol) should be avoided.
6. If a patient is prescribed opioid analgesic upon discharge, a bowel regimen should always be provided.

Data from Terrell, K. M., Hustey, F. M., Hwang, U., Gerson, L. W., Wenger, N. S., & Miller, D. K. (2009). Quality indicators for geriatric emergency care. *Academic Emergency Medicine, 16*(5), 441–449.

Medication Management

The average OA is prescribed from three to six medications daily, and older patients experience adverse drug events at a rate double that found among younger patients (Budnitz et al., 2006). EPs do not routinely screen for adverse drug reactions or drug–drug interactions; moreover, although 10% to 16% of OA present with adverse drug events, only half of these problems are correctly diagnosed in the ED (Hohl, Lord, Colacone, & Pépin, 2005). In addition, 31% of OAs who visit the ED are on a Beers-identified potentially inappropriate mediation (Beers, 1997; Hohl, Dankoff, Colacone, & Afilalo, 2001), yet a startling 13% of elder patents receive at least one Beers-listed prescription in the ED and 20% receive more than one such potentially inappropriate prescription drug at discharge (Caterino, Emond, & Camargo, 2004).

Published minimal geriatric competencies for emergency medicine residents recommend training in selection and dosing of medications, identification of potential drug interactions, and proper explanation of newly prescribed medications when discharging seniors (Hogan et al., 2010).

Elder Mistreatment

Elder abuse or neglect is defined as any action against an OA that results in harm or risk of harm and is carried out by a person in an expected trusting relationship or when the OA is targeted based on age or disability. This mistreatment may include physical, verbal, sexual, neglect, and financial exploitation (Dong, 2015). Estimates of elder mistreatment prevalence in community-dwelling OAs range from 5% to 10% (Lachs & Pillemer, 2015).

Elder abuse may result in physical injuries or illnesses that prompt an emergency evaluation; thus, EDs are an important setting for identifying this problem. Unfortunately, failure to identify and document elder mistreatment is commonplace; the proportion of documented cases presenting through EDs today is significantly lower than previous estimates (0.013%) (Evans, Hunold, Rosen, & Platts-Mills, 2017).

A number of explanations have been offered for the delays and failure to detect elder abuse. Physician factors include lack of formal training in assessment of elder mistreatment, lack of knowledge of the steps required to report it, and lack of documentation of the diagnosis in the medical record (Jones, Veenstra, Seamon, & Krohmer, 1997). Patients may be unable to self-report abuse or neglect due to cognitive issues, or because they fear retribution by the perpetrators. In addition, the presentation of conditions that may result from abuse, such as falls and fractures, commonly occur from accidental injuries or trauma, making it difficult to make the diagnosis (Gibbs, 2014).

Assessing patients for abuse takes time and requires caution: The provider must consider the risk of false accusation when abuse is not present. To overcome these challenges, a team-based approach that engages emergency medical services, triage providers, nurses, radiologists and technicians, social workers, and care managers has been proposed. The *Recognizing Mistreatment in Older Adults* chapter provides more details.

Elder mistreatment and neglect have been associated with higher rates of hospitalization. One population-based prospective study demonstrated that elder abuse is associated with increased rates of hospitalization in instances of both suspected and confirmed abuse (Dong & Simon, 2013b). Psychological abuse, financial exploitation, and caregiver neglect are each independently associated with higher rates of hospitalization. The risk of hospitalization increases when patients are subjected to two or more forms of abusive acts—a relationship that holds across different levels of sociodemographic, socioeconomic, and health-related or psychosocial factors, as well as across various levels of comorbidity and cognitive or physical impairment.

Elder mistreatment is also associated with higher rates of admission to skilled nursing facilities (SNFs), and with stays in these institutions often lasting more than 30 days (Dong & Simon, 2013a). Psychological abuse, physical abuse, financial exploitation, and caregiver neglect have each been associated with an increased rate of SNF admission, though neglect conferred the highest risk for SNF admission. This information could be useful in decreasing length of stay and planning for hospital discharge in victims of such abuse.

Geriatric Trauma

The overall discussion of the emergency evaluation and management of geriatric trauma is beyond the scope of this chapter. Instead, the focus here is on determinants of immediate and in-hospitalization morbidity and mortality, and the role of geriatrics providers in the care of geriatric trauma patients. Trauma is the seventh leading cause of elder mortality, with standing height falls being a leading mechanism of elder trauma. Age itself has been identified as a risk factor for poor

outcomes in trauma patients, although it is unclear whether the differences in older individuals' outcomes reflect decreased physiologic reserve, associated preexisting conditions, or other factors.

Aggressive trauma care, including early injury management and rehabilitation, can result in good outcomes for elder trauma victims. The American College of Surgeons' Trauma Quality Improvement Program (TQIP) has developed Geriatric Trauma Management Guidelines that recommend geriatric consultation for injured OAs. Early consultation increases adherence to the TQIP guidelines, as evidenced by quality indicators such as higher rates of delirium diagnosis, documentation of patients' living situation, code status, documentation in the form of a medications list, and recommendation of physical therapy (Southerland, Gure, et al., 2017). Furthermore, the addition of multidisciplinary geriatric medicine in the care of OA trauma victims reduces hospital-acquired complications such as functional decline, falls, delirium, and death (Fallon et al., 2006).

The EAST Geriatric Trauma Guidelines, published in 2003, provide evidence-based recommendations that could be used to guide medical decision making in care of geriatric trauma patients (Jacobs et al., 2003). According to these guidelines:

- As many as 85% of elder trauma patients will return to independent function.
- Advanced patient age should lower the threshold for emergency medicine service providers to divert patients to Level 1 trauma centers.
- Elders should be preferentially diverted to Level 1 trauma centers, should they exist, to increase survival.
- Age itself is not predictive of poor outcomes and, therefore, should not be used as the sole criterion for determining or limiting advanced care.
- A Glasgow Coma Scale (GCS) score of 8 or less, especially if persistent for more than 72 hours, is associated with a dismal prognosis.
- Presence of an arterial base deficit of 6 or less within 1 hour of admission is associated with

66% mortality and of itself may suggest occult shock, the need for intensive care, greater extent of shock, and inadequacy of resuscitation.

- Post-injury complications are more severe in OAs than those in younger patients, so targeted preventive therapies should be instituted.
- Class III evidence shows that both an initial respiratory rate of less than 10 breaths per minute and a trauma score of less than 7 are each associated with a 100% mortality rate. Consideration of early palliation exists for these patients; however, this evidence is only level III, which limits its applicability to individual patients.
- There is no literature to support any specific age older than which in-hospital mortality can be predicted with any confidence.
- A profound perfusion deficit may be present in "stable"-appearing elder trauma patients secondary to low cardiac output, suggesting early invasive hemodynamic monitoring may improve survival (Gubler et al., 1997).

Data from Jacobs, D. G., Plaisier, B. R., Barie, P. S., Hammond, J. S., Holevar, M. R., Sinclair, K. E., . . . EAST Practice Management Guidelines Work Group. (2003). Practice Management Guidelines for Geriatric Trauma: The EAST Practice Management Guidelines Work Group. *The Journal of Trauma: Injury, Infection, and Critical Care, 54*(2), 391–416.

Consideration of preexisting conditions (PECs) has some ability to predict the likelihood of adverse outcomes in elder trauma patients. Interestingly, the effect of PECs becomes progressively less pronounced with advancing age. PECs are found in 30% of trauma patients older than 65 years (McMahon, Schwab, & Kauder, 1996), and 69% of those older than 75 years (Kauder & Schwab, 1990). In a study of almost 8000 trauma patients, Milzman et al. (1992) found a threefold mortality increase in patients with PECs. Gubler et al. (1997) examined 9424 elder trauma patients and discovered a 5-year mortality increase of 2 to 8.4 times in this population depending on the number and severity of PECs. It is uncertain which specific PECs have predictive value in this context.

The Injury Severity Score (ISS) is the most widely studied measure of anatomic or physiologic severity of illness; it is a predictor of poor outcomes in elder trauma studies. However, the ISS has limited early prognostic capability due to the delays in data points required to calculate the score.

Cardiac, infectious, and pulmonary complications are all predictive of poor geriatric trauma outcomes. Preventable complications contribute to 32% to 62% of elder trauma deaths (Pellicane, Byrne, & DeMaria, 1992). Prevention of such complications is, therefore, imperative.

Taken together, optimal care of the geriatric trauma patient requires the support of a multidisciplinary team that engages geriatrics experts alongside the trauma team.

Risk Assessment for Adverse Outcomes

Attempts to risk-stratify OAs at risk for poor outcomes on either discharge from the ED or admission to the hospital from the ED are not new. Many studies have looked at predictors from both usual care parameters and use of various screening tools. To date, most show that further study is warranted before reliable predictors can be recommended (Aminzadeh & Dalziel, 2002). Risk stratification instruments to date have been impractical, inaccurate, and unreliable; they do not accurately distinguish high- or low-risk subsets (Carpenter et al., 2015).

The Identification of Seniors at Risk (ISAR) is one of the most commonly cited risk screening tools in the ED (**FIGURE 38-2**). A prospective study utilizing ISAR screening identified high-risk patients who were older, using more medications, and requiring urgent ED care, and who had longer ED lengths of stay. The ISAR predicted ED returns but was not predictive of hospital admission or readmission rates in 30 or 180 days (Tavares, Sa-Couto, Bolz, & Capezuti, 2017).

Other tools include the Modified Early Warning Score (MEWS) and the VitalPac Early Warning Score (VIEWS), which incorporates physiologic parameters such as vital signs, level of consciousness, and urine output into a prediction

ISAR	Yes	No
1) Before the illness or injury that brought you to the emergency department, did you need someone to help you on a regular basis?	1	0
2) Since the illness or injury that brought you to the emergency department, have you needed more help than usual to take care of yourself?	1	0
3) Have you been hospitalized for one or more night during the past six months (excluding a stay in the emergency department)?	1	0
4) In general, is your sight good?	0	1
5) In general, do you have serious problems with your memory?	1	0
6) Do you take more than three different medications every day?	1	0

FIGURE 38-2 Identification of Seniors at Risk (ISAR).

Reproduced from McCusker, J., Bellavance, F., Cardin, S., Trepanier, S., Verdon, J., & Ardman, O. (1999). Detection of older people at increased risk of adverse health outcomes after an emergency visit: The ISAR screening tool. *Journal of the American Geriatrics Society, 47*(10), 1229–1337.

model. Both the MEWS and VIEWS scoring systems can predict requirement of hospitalization and in-hospital mortality of older ED patients (Dundar et al., 2016). The high-sensitivity C-reactive protein-to-albumin ratio is higher in elders experiencing all-cause hospital mortality and may serve as a surrogate marker of disease severity (Oh et al., 2017). The Palliative Performance Scale (PPS) may predict survival in older patients admitted to the hospital from the ED, but has yet to be prospectively studied (Babcock, Gould Kuntz, Kowalsky, Calitri, & Kenny, 2016).

▶ The Future of Geriatric ED Care: Geriatric Emergency Department Guidelines

To address both the severity of illness and the poor outcomes experienced by elderly patients, ED leaders and staff alike have recognized OAs as a distinct ED population requiring specific policies, protocols, procedures, personnel, and equipment for optimal care. EDs have strategically implemented such specific changes for optimal elder care. Some EDs have implemented so many specific elder changes that they consider themselves "centers of excellence" in elder emergency care and designate themselves as "senior friendly" or "geriatric emergency departments" (GEDs) (Hogan, Olade, & Carpenter, 2014). Recommended GED features are detailed in the Geriatric Emergency Department Guidelines (Cordell et al., 2002). These features are considered so important to the future of elder emergency care that the external validation of hospitals implementing elder care initiatives will soon occur. Accreditation of GEDs by the American College of Emergency Physicians will begin in 2018 (Carpenter et al., 2017). While this is an important step, major improvements in care of OAs who present to the ED requires a multipronged approach that incorporates education and system-wide changes.

▶ Summary

Over one-quarter of all acute care visits in the U.S. are managed in the high stress, time limited ED environment, which is not conducive to the evaluation of the complex interwoven subacute conditions so often present in older adults. Implementation of the Geriatric Emergency Department Guidelines can help improve an EDs focus on the most high yield older adult issues. This guideline implementation may decrease ED variability in assessment and treatment, and improve both interdisciplinary cooperation and transitions of care.

Cognitive disorders, falls, medication management, pain control, elder mistreatment, and risk assessment for adverse outcomes are high impact targets where enhanced communication and collaboration between geriatricians and emergency physicians can enhance ED care for our vulnerable older adult population.

References

Aminzadeh, F., & Dalziel, W. B. (2002). Older adults in the emergency department: A systematic review of patterns of use, adverse outcomes, and effectiveness of interventions. *Annals of Emergency Medicine, 39*(3), 238–247.

Babcock, M., Gould Kuntz, J., Kowalsky, D., Calitri, N., & Kenny, A. M. (2016). The Palliative Performance Scale predicts three- and six-month survival in older adult patients admitted to the hospital through the emergency department. *Journal of Palliative Medicine, 19*(10), 1087–1091.

Baum, S. A., & Rubenstein, L. Z. (1987). Old people in the emergency department: Age-related differences in emergency department use and care. *Journal of the American Geriatrics Society, 35*, 398–404.

Beers, M. H. (1997). Explicit criteria for determining potentially inappropriate medication use by the elderly: An update. *Archives of Internal Medicine, 157*, 1531–1536.

Bell, A. J., Talbot-Stern, J. K., & Hennessy, A. (2000). Characteristics and outcomes of older patients presenting to the emergency department after a fall: A retrospective analysis. *Medical Journal of Australia, 21*(4), 179–182.

Budnitz, D. S., Pollock, D. A., Weidenbach, K. N., Mendelsohn, A. B., Schroeder, T. J., & Annest, J. L. (2006). National surveillance of emergency department visits for outpatient adverse drug events. *Journal of the American Medical Association, 296*, 1858–1866.

Carpenter, C. R., Bassett, E. R., Fischer, G. M., Shirshekan, J., Galvin, J. E., & Morris, J. C. (2003). Four sensitive screening tools to detect cognitive dysfunction in geriatric emergency department patients: Brief Alzheimer's Screen, Short Blessed Test, Ottawa 3DY, and the caregiver-completed AD8. *Academic Emergency Medicine, 18*(4), 374–384.

Carpenter, C. R., Hwang, U., Biese, K., Carter, D., Hogan, T. M., Karounos, M., . . . Stern, M. (2017). ACEP accredits geriatric emergency care for emergency departments. *ACEP Now, 36*(4).

Carpenter, C. R., & Lo, A. X. (2015). Falling behind? Understanding implementation science in future emergency department management strategies for geriatric fall prevention. *Academic Emergency Medicine, 22*(4), 478–480.

Carpenter, C. R., Shelton, E., Fowler, S., Suffoletto, B., Platts-Mills, T. F., Rothman, R. E., & Hogan, T. M. (2015). Risk factors and screening instruments to predict adverse outcomes for undifferentiated older emergency department patients: A systematic review and meta-analysis. *Academic Emergency Medicine, 22*(1), 1–21.

Carpenter, C. R., Rosenberg, M., Christensen, M., & Blanda, M. (2014). Geriatric emergency medicine guidelines for staffing, training, protocols, infrastructure, and quality improvement. *Emergency Medicine Reports, 35*, 1–12.

Caterino, J. M., Emond, J. A., & Camargo, C. A. (2004). Inappropriate medication administration to the acutely ill elderly: A nationwide emergency department study, 1992–2000. *Journal of the American Geriatrics Society, 52*, 1847–1855.

Chiovenda, P., Vincetelli, G. M., & Alegiani, F. (2002). Cognitive impairment in elderly ED patients: Need for multidimensional assessment for better management after discharge. *American Journal of Emergency Medicine, 20*, 332–335.

Close, J. C., Lord, S. R., Antonova, E. J., Martin, M., Lensberg, B., Taylor, M., . . . Kelly, A. (2012). Older people presenting to the emergency department after a fall: A population with substantial recurrent healthcare use. *Emergency Medicine Journal, 29*(9), 742–747.

Cordell, W. H., Keene, K. K., Giles, B. K., Jones, J. B., Jones, J. H., & Brizendine, E. J. (2002). The high prevalence of pain in emergency medical care. *American Journal of Emergency Medicine, 20*(3), 165–169.

Dong, X. Q. (2015). Elder abuse: Systematic review and implications for practice. *Journal of the American Geriatrics Society, 63*, 1214–1238.

Dong, X., & Simon, M. A. (2013a). Association between reported elder abuse and rates of admission to skilled nursing facilities: Findings from a longitudinal population based cohort study. *Gerontology, 59*(5), 464–472. doi: 10.1159/000351338

Dong, X. Q., & Simon, M. A. (2013b). Elder abuse as a risk factor for hospitalization in older persons. *JAMA Internal Medicine, 173*(10), 911–917. doi: 10.1001/jamainternmed.2013.238

Dundar, Z. D., Ergin, M., Karamercan, M. A., Ayranci, K., Colak, T., Tuncar, A., . . . Gul, M. (2016). Modified Early

Warning Score and VitalPac Early Warning Score in geriatric patients admitted to emergency department. *European Journal of Emergency Medicine, 23*(6), 406–412.

Elie, M., Rousseau, F., Cole, M., McCusker, J., Primeau, F., & Bellavance, F. (2000). Prevalence and detection of delirium in elderly emergency department patients. *Canadian Medical Association Journal, 163*, 977–981.

Ettinger, W. H., Casani, J. A., Coon, P. J., Muller, D. C., & Piazza-Appel, K. (1987). Patterns of use of the emergency department by elderly patients. *Journal of Gerontology, 42*, 638–642.

Evans, C. S., Hunold, K. M., Rosen, T., & Platts-Mills, T. F. (2017). Diagnosis of elder abuse in U.S. emergency departments. *Journal of the American Geriatrics Society, 65*(1), 91–97.

Fallon, W., Rader, R., Zyzanski, S., Mancuso, C., Martin, B., Breedlove, L., . . . Campbell, J. (2006). Geriatric outcomes are imporved by a geriatric trauma consultation service. *Journal of Trauma and Acute Care Surgery, 61*(5), 1040–1046.

Gibbs, L. M. (2014). Understanding the medical markers of elder abuse and neglect: Physical examination findings. *Clinics in Geriatric Medicine, 30*, 687–712.

Graf, C. E., Zekry, D., Giannelli, S., Michel, J. P., & Chevalley, T. (2011). Efficiency and applicability of comprehensive geriatric assessment in the emergency department: A systematic review. *Aging Clinical and Experimental Research, 23*(4), 244–254. doi: 10.3275/7284

Greenwald, P. W., Estevez, R. M., Clark, S., Stern, M. E., Rosen, T., & Flomenbaum, N. (2016). The ED as the primary source of hospital admission for older (but not younger) adults. *American Journal of Emergency Medicine, 34*(216), 943–947.

Gubler, K. D., Davis, R., Koepsell, T., Soderberg, R., Maier, R. V., & Rivara, F. P. (1997). Long-term survival of elderly trauma patients. *Archives of Surgery, 132*, 1010–1014.

Han, J. H., Wilson, A., Vasilevskis, E. E., Shintani, A., & Schnelle, J. F. (2013). Diagnosing delirium in older emergency department patients: Validity and reliability of the delirium triage screen and the brief confusion assessment method. *Academic Emergency Medicine, 62*(5), 457–465.

Han, J. H., & Wilber, S. T. (2013). Altered mental status in older patients in the emergency department. *Clinics in geriatric medicine, 29*(1), 101–136.

Handel, D. A., Ginde, A., Raja, A., Rogers, J., Sullivan, A. F., Espinola, J. A., & Camargo, C. A. Jr. (2012). Implementation of crowding solutions from the American College of Emergency Physicians Task Force report on boarding. *International Journal of Emergency Medicine, 21*(4), 279–286.

Hastings, S. N., Schmader, K. E., & Sloane, R. J. (2007). Adverse health outcomes after discharge from the emergency department: Incidence and risk factors in a veteran population. *Journal of General Internal Medicine, 22*, 1527.

Hogan, T. M., Howell, M. D., Cursio, J. F., Wong, A., & Dale, W. (2016). Improving Pain Relief in Elder Patients (I-PREP): An emergency department education and quality intervention. *Journal of the American Geriatrics Society, 64*(12), 2566–2571.

Hogan, T. M., Losman, E. D., Carpenter, C. R., Sauvigne, K., Irmiter, C., Emanuel, L., & Leipzig, R. M. (2010). Development of geriatric competencies for emergency medicine residents using an expert consensus process. *Academic Emergency Medicine, 17*(3), 316–324.

Hogan, T. M., Olade, T. O., & Carpenter, C. R. (2014). A profile of acute care in an aging America: Snowball sample identification and characterization of united states geriatric emergency departments in 2013. *Academic Emergency Medicine, 21*(3), 337–346.

Hohl, C. M., Dankoff, J., Colacone, A., & Afilalo, M. (2001). Polypharmacy, adverse drug-related events, potential adverse drug interactions in elderly patients presenting to an emergency department. *Annals of Emergency Medicine, 38*, 666–671.

Hohl, C. M., Lord, V., Colacone, A., & Pépin, J. (2005). Emergency physician recognition of adverse drug-related events in elder patients presenting to an emergency department. *Academic Emergency Medicine, 12*, 197–205.

Hollander, J. E., & Pines, J. M. (2007). The emergency department crowding paradox: The longer you stay, the less care you get. *Annals of Emergency Medicine, 50*(5), 497–499.

Hustey, F. M., & Meldon, S. W. (2002). The prevalence and documentation of impaired mental status in elderly emergency department patients. *Annals of Emergency Medicine, 39*, 248–253.

Hustey, F. M., Meldon, S. W., Smith, M. D., & Lex, C. K. (2003). The effect of mental status screening on the care of elderly emergency department patients. *Annals of Emergency Medicine, 41*(5), 678–686.

Hwang, U., Richardson, L. D., Harris, B., & Morrison, R. S. (2010). The quality of emergency department pain care for older adult patients. *Journal of the American Geriatrics Society, 58*(11), 2122–2128.

Inouye, S. K. (2006). Delirium in older persons. *New England Journal of Medicine, 354*, 1157–1165.

Inouye, S. K., van Dyck, C. H., Alessi, C. A., Balkin, S., Seigal, A. P., & Horwitz, R. I. (1990). Clarifying confusion: The confusion assessment method: A new method for detection of delirium. *Annals of Internal Medicine, 113*(12), 941–948.

Ismail, S. A., & Pope, I. (2017). Risk factors for admission at three urban emergency departments in England: A cross-sectional analysis of attendances over 1 month. *BMJ Open, 22*(6), e011547.

Jacobs, D. G., Plaisier, B. R., Barie, P. S., Hammond, J. S., Holevar, M. R., Sinclair, K. E., . . . & EAST Practice Management Guidelines Work Group. (2003). Practice management guidelines for geriatric trauma: The EAST Practice Management Guidelines Work Group. *Journal of Trauma and Acute Care Surgery, 54*(2), 391–416.

Jones, J. S., Veenstra, T. R., Seamon, J. P., & Krohmer, J. (1997). Elder mistreatment: National survey of emergency physicians. *Annals of Emergency Medicine, 30*(4), 473–479.

Kakuma, R., Fort, D., Galbaud, G., Arsenault, L., Perrault, A., Platt, R. W., . . . & Wolfson, C. (2003). Delirium in older emergency department patients discharged home: effect on survival. *Journal of the American Geriatrics Society, 51*(4), 443–450.

Karam, G., Radden, Z., Berall, L. E., Cheng, C., & Gruneir, A. (2015, July 14). Efficacy of emergency department-based interventions designed to reduce repeat visits and other adverse outcomes for older patients after discharge: A systematic review. *Geriatrics and Gerontology International, 15*(9), 1107–1117. [Epub ahead of print]. doi: 10.1111/ggi.12538

Kauder, D. R., & Schwab, C. W. (1990). Comorbidity in geriatric patients. *Advances in Trauma, 5.*

Lachs, M. S., & Pillemer, K. A. (2015). Elder abuse. *New England Journal of Medicine, 373*, 1947–1956.

LaMantia, M. A., Messina, F. C., Hobgood, C. D., & Miller, D. K. (2014). Screening for delirium in the emergency department: A systematic review. *Annals of Emergency Medicine, 53*(5), 551–560.

Launay, C. P., de Decker, L., Kabeshova, A., Annweiler, C., & Beauchet, O. (2014). Screening for older emergency department inpatients at risk of prolonged hospital stay: The brief geriatric assessment tool. *PLoS One, 9*(10), e110135. doi: 10.1371/journal.pone.0110135

Levin, S. R., Dittus, R., Aronsky, D., Weinger, M. B., Han, J., Boord, J., & France, D. (2008, August 29). Optimizing cardiology capacity to reduce emergency department boarding: A systems engineering approach. *American Heart Journal, 156*(6), 1202–1209. [Epub ahead of print]. doi: 10.1016/j.ahj.2008.07.007

Lewis Hunter, A. E., Spatz, E. S., Bernstein, S. L., & Rosenthal, M. S. (2016). Factors influencing hospital admission of non-critically ill patients presenting to the emergency department: A cross-sectional study. *Journal of General Internal Medicine, 31*(1), 37–44. doi: 10.1007/s11606-015-3438-8

Liu, S. W., Obermeyer, Z., Chang, Y., & Shankar, K. N. (2015). Frequency of ED revisits and death among older adults after a fall. *American Journal of Emergency Medicine, 33*(8), 1012–1018.

Lo, A. X., Brown, C. J., Sawyer, P., Kennedy, R. E., & Allman, R. M. (2014). Life-space mobility declines associated with incident falls and fractures. *Journal of the American Geriatrics Society, 62*, 919–923.

Lo, A. X., Flood, K. L., Biese, K., Platts-Mills, T. F., Donnelly, J. P., & Carpenter, C. R. (2017). Factors associated with hospital admission for older adults receiving care in U.S. emergency departments. *Journals of Gerontology, 72*(8), 1105–1109.

Lowenstein, S. R., Crescenzi, C. A., Kern, D. C., & Steel, K. (1986). Care of the elderly in the emergency department. *Annals of Emergency Medicine, 15*, 528–535.

McCusker, J., Cardin, S., & Bellavance, F. (2000). Return to the emergency department among elders: Patterns and predictors. *Academic Emergency Medicine, 7*, 249–259.

McCusker, J., Roberge, D., & Vadenboncoeur, A. (2009). Safety of discharge of seniors from the emergency department to the community. *Healthcare Quarterly, 12*, 24–32.

McMahon, D. J., Schwab, C. W., & Kauder, D. (1996). Comorbidity and the elderly trauma patient. *World Journal of Surgery, 20*, 1113–1120.

Milzman, D. P., Boulanger, B. R., Rodriguez, A., Soderstrom, C. A., Mitchell, K. A., & Magnant, C. M. (1992). Pre-existing disease in trauma patients: A predictor of fate independent of age and injury severity score. *Journal of Trauma, 32*, 236–243.

Nagurney, J. M., Fleischman, W., Han, L., Leo-Summers, L., Allore, H. G., & Gill, T. M. (2017, January 6). Emergency department visits without hospitalization are associated with functional decline in older persons. *Annals of Emergency Medicine, 69*(4), 426–433. [Epub ahead of print]. doi: 10.1016/j.annemergmed.2016.09.018

Oh, J., Kim, S. H., Park, K. N., Oh, S. H., Kim, Y. M., Kim, H. J., & Youn, C. S. (2017). High-sensitivity C-reactive protein/albumin ratio as a predictor of in-hospital mortality in older adults admitted to the emergency department. *Clinical and experimental emergency medicine, 4*(1), 19.

Owens, P. L., Barrett, M. S., Gibson, T. B., Andrews, R. M., Weinick, R. M., & Mutter, R. L. (2010). Emergency department care in the United States: A profile of national data sources. *Annals of Emergency Medicine, 56*(2), 150–165.

Pellicane, J. V., Byrne, K., & DeMaria, E. J. (1992). Preventable complications and death from multiple organ failure among geriatric trauma victims. *Journal of Trauma, 33*, 440–444.

Pines, J. M., Mullins, P., Cooper, J. K., Feng, L. B., & Roth, K. E. (2013). National trends in emergency department use, care patterns, and quality of care of older adults in the United States. *Journal of the American Geriatrics Society, 61*(1), 12–17.

Pitts, S. R., Niska, R., Xu, J., & Burt, C. W. (2008, August 6). *National Hospital Ambulatory Medical Care Survey: 2006 emergency department summary. National Health Statistics Reports, 7.* Hyattsville, MD: Department of Health and Human Services, National Center for Health Statistics.

Platts-Mills, T. F., Esserman, D. A., Brown, D. L., Bortsov, A. V., Sloane, P. D., & McLean, S. A. (2012). Older US emergency department patients are less likely to receive pain medication than younger patients: Results from a national survey. *Annals of Emergency Medicine, 60*(2), 199–206.

Platts-Mills, T. F., Flannigan, S. A., Bortsov, A. V., Smith, S., Domeier, R. M., Swor, R. A., . . . Lee, D. C. (2016). Persistent pain among older adults discharged home from the emergency department after motor vehicle crash: a prospective cohort study. *Annals of Emergency Medicine, 67*(2), 166–176.

Powell, E. S., Khare, R. K., Venkatesh, A. K., Van Roo, B. D., Adams, J. G., & Reinhardt, G. (2012). The relationship between inpatient discharge timing and emergency department boarding. *Journal of Emergency Medicine, 42*(2), 186–196.

Salter, A. E., Khan, K. M., Donaldson, M. G., Davis, J. C., Buchanan, J., Abu-Laban, R. B., . . . McKay, H. A. (2006). Community-dwelling seniors who present to the emergency department with a fall do not receive Guideline care and their fall risk profile worsens significantly: A 6-month prospective study. *Osteoporosis International, 17*(5), 672–683.

Sanders, A. B. (1996). Emergency care of the elder person. *American Journal of Emergency Care, 15*(2), 205–206.

Schniter, L., Martin-Khan, M., & Gray, L. (2011). Negative health outcomes and adverse events in older people attending emergency departments: A systematic review. *Australasian Emergency Nursing Journal, 14*(3), 141–162.

Schoenenberger, A. W., Bieri, C., Özgüler, O., Moser, A., Haberkern, M., Zimmermann, H., . . . Exadaktylos, A. (2014). A novel multidimensional geriatric screening tool in the ED: Evaluation of feasibility and clinical relevance. *The American Journal of Emergency Medicine, 32*(6), 623–628.

Schuur, J. D., & Venkatesh, A. K. (2012). The growing role of emergency departments in hospital admissions. *New England Journal of Medicine, 367*(5), 391–393.

Singer, A. J., Thode, H. C., Viccellio, P., & Pines, J. M. (2011). The association between length of emergency department boarding and mortality. *Academic Emergency Medicine, 18*(12), 1324–1329.

Sirois, M. J., Émond, M., Ouellet, M. C., Perry, J., Daoust, R., Morin, J., . . . & Allain-Boulé, N. (2013). Cumulative incidence of functional decline after minor injuries in previously independent older Canadian individuals in the emergency department. *Journal of the American Geriatrics Society, 61*(10), 1661–1668.

Smith, A. K., Schonberg, M. A., Fisher, J., Pallin, D. J., Block, S. D., Forrow, L., & McCarthy, E. P. (2010). Emergency department experiences of acutely symptomatic patients with terminal illness and their family caregivers. *Journal of Pain and Symptom Management, 39*(6), 972–981.

Smith, A. K., McCarthy, E., Weber, E., Cenzer, I. S., Boscardin, J., Fisher, J., & Covinsky, K. (2012). Half of older Americans seen in emergency department in last month of life; most admitted to hospital, and many die there. *Health Affairs, 31*(6), 1277–1285.

Southerland, L. T., Gure, T. R., Ruter, D. I., Li, M. M., & Evans, D. C. (2017). Early geriatric consultation increases adherence to TQIP Geriatric Trauma Management Guidelines. *Journal of Surgical Research, 216*, 56–64.

Southerland, L. T., Vargas, A. J., Nagaraj, L., Cure, T. R., & Caterino, J. M. (2017). An emergency department observation unit is a feasible setting for multidisciplinary geriatric assessments in compliance with the geriatric emergency department guidelines. *Journal of Emergency Medicine.* [Epub ahead of print]. http://dx.doi.org/10.1111/acem.13328

Studnicki, J., Platonova, E. A., & Fisher, J. W. (2012). Hospital-level variation in the percentage of admissions originating in the emergency department. *American Journal of Emergency Medicine, 30*(8), 1441–1446.

Tavares, J. P., Sa-Couto, P., Bolz, M., & Capezuti, E. (2017). Identification of Seniors at Risk (ISAR) in the emergency room: A prospective study. *International Emergency Nursing, 35*, 19–24.

Terrell, K. M., Hustey, F. M., Hwang, U., Gerson, L. W., Wenger, N. S., & Miller, D. K. (2009). Quality indicators for geriatric emergency care. *Academic Emergency Medicine, 16*(5), 441–449.

Tirrell, G., Sri-on, J., Lipsitz, L. A., Camargo, C. A. Jr., Kabrhel, C., & Liu, S. W. (2015). Evaluation of older adult patients with falls in the emergency department: Discordance with national guidelines. *Academic Emergency Medicine, 22*(4), 461–467.

Todd, K. H., Ducharme, J., Choiniere, M., Crandall, C. S., Fosnocht, D. E., Homel, P., & Tanabe, P. (2007). Pain in the emergency department: Results of the pain and emergency medicine initiative (PEMI) multicenter study. *The Journal of Pain, 8*(6), 460–466.

Vermeulen, M. J., Ray, J. G., Bell, C., Cayen, B., Stukel, T. A., & Schull, M. J. (2009). Disequilibrium between admitted and discharged hospitalized patients affects emergency department length of stay. *Annals of Emergency Medicine, 54*(6), 794–804.

Wilber, S. T., Blanda, M., & Gerson, L. W. (2006). Does functional decline prompt emergency department visits and admission in older patients? *Academic Emergency Medicine, 13*, 680–682.

Wilber, S. T., Gerson, L. W., Terrell, K. M., Carpenter, C. R., Shah, M. N., Heard, K., & Hwang, U. (2006). Geriatric emergency medicine and the 2006 Institute of Medicine reports from the Committee on the Future of Emergency Care in the US health system. *Academic Emergency Medicine, 13*(12), 1345–1351.

Woolcott, J. C., Khan, K. M., Mitrovic, S., Anis, A. H., & Marra, C. A. (2012). The cost of fall related presentations to the ED: A prospective, in-person, patient-tracking analysis of health resource utilization. *Osteoporosis International, 23*(5), 1513–1519.

Wu, S., Keeler, E. B., Rubenstein, L. Z., Maglione, M. A., & Shekelle, P. G. (2010). A cost effectiveness analysis of a proposed national falls prevention program. *Clinics in Geriatric Medicine, 26*(4), 751–766.

CHAPTER 39

The Older Adult Driver

George W. Rebok, Vanya C. Jones, Annie C. Harmon, and David B. Carr

CHAPTER OBJECTIVES

1. Describe the common medical conditions and medications associated with impaired driving performance in older adults.
2. Explain the impact of cognitive impairment and dementia on older adult drivers.
3. Describe the medical fitness-to-drive approach to evaluating older drivers.
4. Discuss the consequences of driving cessation and mobility resources in older adult drivers.

KEY TERMS

Cognitive impairment   Medical fitness-to-drive   Older adult driver

▶ Introduction

The automobile is the most important source of transportation for older adults. The ability to drive or be driven is crucial for older persons to maintain an important link with society. Functional assessment, which can include driving ability, is an important domain for clinicians who are involved in providing geriatric care. Clinicians should determine whether their patients are currently driving, provide information on healthy driving behaviors, assess medical conditions or visual/cognitive domains that

may place their patients at increased risk for a motor vehicle injury or driving cessation, and intervene and treat medical illnesses, when possible, that can impair driving skills.

Some clinicians may be reluctant to address driving habits. However, one could argue that impaired driving skills should not be viewed any differently from the prevention, detection, and improvement of impaired mobility such as walking, which can also result in a fall and subsequent injury. Epidemiologic studies have identified risk factors for driving cessation and motor vehicle crash or injury in older adults (Marottoli et al., 1998). There is still a need to validate current risk factors and to determine whether modification of these risk factors provides a benefit to the patient or society. While awaiting further investigation in this area, the clinician should not delay in assessing or assisting older adults in an attempt to maintain or improve driving skills. When driving retirement occurs, clinicians who care for older adults should be ready to assist with suggestions for acceptable alternative modes of transportation.

▶ Older Drivers

An 84-year-old male is brought in by the family for further evaluation of cognitive decline. The daughter relates a 2-year history of short-term memory loss, characterized by repetition, difficulty in naming, impaired ability to recall recent events, and being lost on two occasions while driving to unfamiliar destinations. The daughter is concerned about her father's safety behind the wheel given a recent at-fault crash. The patient has no insight into his deficits. He has a history of osteoarthritis with restricted range of motion, longstanding diabetes, hypertension, and generalized anxiety disorder. His medications include metformin, nifedipine, atenolol, and alprazolam as needed. During the review of systems, the patient complains of neck and lower back pain, daytime somnolence, and dizziness. His examination is nonfocal, but he does have severely limited range of motion for his neck. His rapid pace walk reveals that he covers 20 feet in 12 seconds. His psychometric test profile reveals an abnormal clock-drawing task and a Trail Making Test part B that takes him 210 seconds to complete.

This older adult probably has Alzheimer's disease, which along with his daytime somnolence,

comorbidities, and use of alprazolam, places him at a very high risk for medically impaired driving. The recommendation to stop driving was resisted. The family and the patient agreed to an on-the-road test by a driving rehabilitation specialist after the alprazolam was discontinued and sleep apnea was ruled out. It became obvious in traffic that the patient could not drive safely, as he was not attentive to other vehicles and had significant difficulties with lane maintenance. The occupational therapist recommended no further driving.

In the office follow-up visit with the physician, the recommendation to stop driving was given verbally and in writing to the patient and daughter. Alternative means of transportation were discussed, along with referral to a gerontologic care manager. The daughter was available for assisting with the majority of the patient's trips. The car was removed from the premises. The patient eventually moved into an assisted living environment, where he had meal and medication oversight provided.

▶ Behaviors and Characteristics of Older Drivers

Mobility—specifically driving—is associated with freedom, safety, and access to the world (Satariano et al., 2012). Driving is the most common, reliable, and preferred source of transportation for older adults (Chihuri et al., 2016). In the United States, the number of drivers older than age 65 and the number of miles driven by older adults are increasing annually (Centers for Disease Control and Prevention [CDC], 2015; U.S. Department of Transportation, 2016). In 2015, 18% of all licensed drivers in the United States were older than 65, up from 14% in 1999 (U.S. Department of Transportation, 2016). Along with increases in the number of older drivers on the roadways, older adults are maintaining their driving status longer and driving farther (U.S. Department of Transportation, 2016). For example, since the mid-1990s, the number of licensed drivers older than age 70 has increased by approximately 6% and their mileage per year has increased approximately 40% (Insurance Institute for Highway Safety & Highway Loss Data Institute, 2014). If this trend continues, the number of older drivers will double by the year 2030 (Goodwin et al., 2015).

Changes in driving status often have negative consequences for older adults (Curl, Stowe, Cooney, & Proulx, 2014; Edwards, Lunsman, Perkins, Rebok, & Roth, 2009). Research on mobility for older adults (older than 65 years of age) has found that changes in driving are associated with reduced quality of life, isolation, and poor health outcomes (CDC, 2015; Edwards, Lunsman, et al., 2009; Mezuk & Rebok, 2008; Sims, Ahmed, Sawyer, & Allman, 2007). Transportation is also a potential source of healthcare disparities for older adults. For example, access to a private car is a significant factor in access to health care (Sammer, 2012). Individuals with a license and a private car have up to two times as many healthcare visits as individuals without a license (Pesata, Pallija, & Webb, 1999; Sammer, 2012). Millions of Americans, of all ages, do not obtain health care in a given year because of the lack of access to transportation (Wallace, Hughes-Cromwick, & Mull, 2006). For older adults, access to a car and health often go beyond healthcare access (Marottoli et al., 2000). That is, driving maintains access to life outside of a home, health care, and quality of life (Edwards, Myers, et al., 2009; Marottoli et al., 2000; Oxley & Whelan, 2008; White et al., 2016).

Crashes and Older Adults

In the United States, drivers older than age 85 have the highest rate of fatal crashes per miles driven when compared to all other age groups, including teenagers, and crash risks increase past age 60 (Insurance Institute for Highway Safety & Highway Loss Data Institute, 2014). Furthermore, the age 70 or older driver is more likely to die in a crash when compared to members of younger age groups (Cheung & McCartt, 2011).

The risk for motor vehicle crashes (MVC) and the flood of older drivers onto U.S. roads make it urgent to understand the complex issue of aging and driving. Older-driver crashes are related to slowed perception and response, lack of recognition of changes in these abilities, or lack of awareness that these abilities can be influenced by medication use, poor vision, and frailty (Li, Braver, & Chen, 2003; Sims et al., 2007). Although there are challenges for longevity for drivers beyond age 70 years, the crash rate of older drivers in 2015 was 26% lower than the crash rate in 1997 (Insurance Institute for Highway Safety & Highway Loss Data Institute, 2017). It has been suggested that these reductions in crash risk are attributable to factors such as older adults living healthier lives for longer periods and the availability of more services to train/adapt older adults in safe driving (Cicchino & McCartt, 2014).

Older-Driving Safety Behaviors

Older adults typically adhere to the main crash prevention countermeasures that driving safety experts promote for crash and injury reduction in all driving groups, including not drinking and driving, not speeding, and wearing seat belts (CDC, 2015; Stutts, Martell, & Staplin, 2009; U.S. Department of Transportation, 2016). Older adults also modify their behavior to drive during the most optimal conditions (e.g., good weather, not in rush hour, and on local roads instead of highways) (Molnar et al., 2015).

▶ Older Drivers at Risk for a Motor Vehicle Crash

Common diseases in older drivers that have been noted to affect driving ability include, but are not limited to, visual impairment, diabetes mellitus, seizure disorders, Alzheimer's disease, cerebrovascular accidents, depression, cardiovascular disease, sleep disorders, arthritis and related musculoskeletal disorders, and alcohol and drug use (Charlton et al., 2010; Hetland &

Carr, 2014; National Office for Traffic Medicine, 2017). More studies are needed to examine the effect of multiple illnesses on the driving task, although interestingly one study of comorbidity indices that measured increasing burden actually showed more relevance for younger or middle-aged drivers than for older adults (Papa et al., 2014).

Diseases should be graded as to their severity and ability to affect driving errors or the human factors related to MVC. For instance, diabetes has a potential to affect the three important domains of driving: (1) perception (e.g., from retinopathy or cataract), (2) cognition (e.g., from hypoglycemia), and (3) motor response (e.g., from neuropathy). Thus, a clinician may have to make a determination as to the severity of the disease and the impact on the intrinsic factors and weigh these findings within the context of a patient who may have comorbidities. Doing so becomes more difficult in older drivers, who may be dealing with multiple mild to moderate diseases (e.g., visual impairment, mild **cognitive impairment**, and arthritis).

Diseases or syndromes that can impair consciousness, such as angina, arrhythmias, diabetes, seizures, syncope, transient ischemic attacks, cerebrovascular accidents, and arthritis, should be assessed for severity to determine whether the disease has the potential to impact driving. Polypharmacy is not uncommon in older adults. Many common medication classes have been studied and noted to either increase the crash risk or impair driving skills when assessed by simulators or road tests. These classes include, but are not limited to, narcotics and benzodiazepines (Drummer et al., 2004), antihistamines, antidepressants, antipsychotics, hypnotics, alcohol, and muscle relaxants. One study that focused on older drivers noted that long-acting benzodiazepines are associated with increased crash rates (Hemmelgarn, Suissa, Huang, Boivin, & Pinard, 1997). Another report suggests that a significant number of older adults may be driving while intoxicated or under the influence of other medications (Higgins, Wright, & Wrenn, 1996; Johansson, Bryding, Dahl, Holmgren, & Viitanen, 1997).

Many studies published in the literature have validated screening tools to assist clinicians with fitness-to-drive decisions for older adults or those with specific diseases. In addition, many screens of functional abilities can easily be adopted by clinicians in the office setting. However, brief screens should not be used as the only measure to evaluate driving privileges. Static visual acuity has not been consistently linked to motor vehicle safety outcomes, but visual fields and contrast sensitivity have been shown to be important constructs (Owsley, 2011; Owsley & McGwin, 2010). The majority of states have minimum visual acuity and field requirements to license drivers, and there are certainly potential health and crash benefits from screening for and treating cataracts in older adults (Owsley et al., 2002).

The American Geriatrics Society/National Highway Traffic Safety Administration updated guideline recommends that physicians also consider evaluating joint range of motion, manual motor strength, and adopt the rapid pace walk for risk prediction (Pomidor, 2016). Visual and cognitive screens include tools that assess visuospatial and executive function skills, particularly those pertaining to planning and foresight, such as the clock drawing test and mazes (Carr, Barco, Wallendorf, Snellgrove, & Ott, 2011), and those that tap into visual search and processing speed/attention such as Trail Making Test parts A and B (Roy & Molnar, 2013). The Mini-Mental State Examination (MMSE) has not been shown to be an accurate predictor of driving risk (Joseph et al., 2014), although an evidence-based review suggested that scores less than 24 might serve as a red flag in persons with dementia (Iverson et al., 2010). The Driving Health Inventory with UFOV (useful field of view) is a computerized battery that has been validated prospectively with MVC risk in older adults in a license renewal setting (Staplin, Gish, & Wagner, 2003). More studies and larger samples of medically impaired drivers with specific medical conditions (e.g., dementia, stroke) in clinical settings are needed to determine the utility of these tests, their feasibility of administration, the appropriate cutoff values, and their association with impaired driving outcomes.

Although physicians may have some reluctance in addressing driving issues in the office because of perceived liability risk and concern over patient acceptance of this topic, many recognize the importance of assessing driving skills (Bogner, Straton, Gallo, Rebok, & Keyl, 2004). Clinicians should also incorporate an injury control approach into their health maintenance practice for older adults. Important driving issues that the clinician should discuss with the older driver include using a seat belt, limiting alcohol consumption, refraining from using a cellular phone while driving, obeying the speed limit, and enrolling in refresher courses, such as the Driving Safety Programs offered by AARP or the American Automobile Association (AAA).

▶ Normal Aging, Preclinical Alzheimer's Disease, Mild Cognitive Impairment, and Dementia

There is growing interest in studying the driving abilities of older adults with dementia, particularly those in the earliest stages of the disease when they are most likely to be driving actively (Yamin, Stinchcombe, & Gagnon, 2016). Brain autopsy studies of older drivers who died in motor vehicle crashes have found that many have pathology consistent with Alzheimer's disease (AD), although the individuals may not have been diagnosed with the disease prior to the crash (Gorrie, Rodriguez, Sachdev, Duflou, & Waite, 2007; Johansson, Bogdanovic, Kalimo, Winblad, & Viitanen, 1997; Viitanen et al., 1998). A driving questionnaire administered to older adults with varying degrees of cognitive impairment (cognitively normal, mild cognitive impairment, early AD) identified a relationship

between amyloid burden as measured by positron emission topography and driving risk; this relationship was evident in the preclinical stage of AD (Ott et al., 2017). Recent cross-sectional and longitudinal studies have found associations with preclinical AD and driving errors as measured on a performance-based road test (Roe, Babulal, et al., 2017; Roe, Barco, et al., 2017). Thus, preclinical AD may explain some of the increased crash risk associated with older adults, although other explanations may be plausible, such as cerebral small-vessel disease or physical frailty (Bond et al., 2017; Carr et al., 2016).

Dementia is one of the major medical illnesses that contributes to the increased crash rate in older adults (Odenheimer, 1993). This relationship may not be surprising given the prevalence of dementia of the Alzheimer's type, which doubles every 5 years over the age of 65 years (Cummings, 2004; van der Flier & Scheltens, 2005). One study that administered cognitive tests to older adults during driver license renewal revealed that a significant number of drivers older than age 80 demonstrated some degree of cognitive impairment (Stutts, Stewart, & Martell, 1998). Studies in tertiary referral centers have revealed an increased crash rate in drivers with dementia of the Alzheimer's type in comparison with controls, although there have been exceptions. Larger population-based studies that are able to identify cognitively impaired drivers by brief cognitive screens have found modest increases in crash rates among **older adult drivers** (Foley, Wallace, & Eberhard, 1995). Nevertheless, it is often difficult to find associations between cognitive and visual impairment and crashes because of the infrequent occurrence of these events, along with the reduction in the number of trips made over time with aging.

More studies are needed on the benefits and risks of screening of cognitively impaired older drivers (Carr & Ott, 2010). There is also a need for more research on how advanced in-vehicle technologies can assist with the maintenance of safe driving and independent functioning in those individuals with mild cognitive impairment and dementia (Eby et al., 2016). Finally, the efficacy of different intervention approaches, including combinations of interventions (e.g., pharmacotherapy and cognitive training), needs to be explored (Anstey, Eramudugolla, Ross, Lautenschlager, & Wood, 2016). Promising preliminary data have shown the beneficial effects of cholinesterase inhibitors on cognitive domains critical to safe driving on a simulated driving task in individuals with dementia (Daiello et al., 2010) as well as the benefits of cognitive training (Ball, Edwards, Ross, & McGwin, 2010; Edwards, Lunsman, et al., 2009; Ross, Freed, Edwards, Phillips, & Ball, 2016) and exercise interventions targeting driving-related abilities in older adults (Marmeleira, Godinho, & Fernandes, 2009; Marottoli et al., 2007).

▶ Assessing Driving Skills

Many health professionals and organizations may assist in the education, training, or assessment of the older driver. These include, but are not limited to, subspecialists in the field of medicine (e.g., neurology and cardiology), neuropsychologists, occupational therapists, physical therapists, courses such as the AARP Smart Driver online course, the medical advisory board of the state or driver improvement office, and insurance companies. A driving simulator may also play a role in assessing driving abilities (Rebok & Keyl, 2004). Although some studies have indicated their results are correlated with crash risk (Lee, Lee, Cameron, & Li-Tsang, 2003), there is insufficient evidence for recommending clinical application of simulators to replace on-road driving assessments, and simulators may not be available in many centers (Eramudugolla, Price, Chopra, Li, & Anstey, 2016). In recent years, however, simulator technology has advanced and become more affordable, to the point that it is considered a safer alternative to on-road assessment and training (Casutt, Theill, Martin, Keller, & Jancke, 2014; Classen & Brooks, 2014; Freund, Gravenstein, Ferris, & Shaheen, 2002).

Road performance tests have traditionally been considered the standard by which to evaluate driving skills (Freund et al., 2002). For example, the Washington University Road Test (WURT) has been used as a major outcome measure of driving fitness in several studies of older drivers (Carr et al., 2011; Hunt et al., 1997). Road tests have some limitations because they are often scored subjectively, the road conditions may vary, and the tests may be performed in a car on a driving course that is unfamiliar to the subject. Even so, road tests have been advocated by several authors as the preferred method to assess driving competency (Stutts & Wilkins, 2003), and impairment in these tests has been correlated with an increase in future crash risk (Keall & Frith, 2004).

Occupational therapists, often based at rehabilitation centers, may have specific training and experience in evaluating drivers with medical impairments. The therapist may be able to assist in modifications to the vehicle that could enable its safe and timely operation by the older driver.

The physical therapist can be an indispensable member of the driving rehabilitation team. Large studies on older adult drivers in the community indicate that back pain and arthritis (Foley et al., 1995; Hu, Trumble, Foley, Eberhard, & Wallace, 1998), along with the use of pain medications (Tuokko, Beattie, Tallman, & Cooper, 1995), are associated with increased crash rates. Thus, limitations in muscle strength caused by pain or disuse or restrictions in range of motion of joints such as the hands, feet, and neck may play an important role in driving impairment. Interventions to improve muscle strength and joint function have the potential to improve driving skills such as braking speed (Sayers & Gibson, 2012).

Even if medically impaired patients pass a road test, a question of how closely to monitor the patient over time will always exist. Repeat road tests can be expensive, but when drivers with Alzheimer's disease who pass road tests are followed longitudinally, skills can be expected to decline in the presence of chronic disease (Molnar et al., 2015).

▶ Driving Retirement

Many older drivers have been driving longer than their physicians have been practicing medicine. Hence, it is important for health professionals to discuss the issues related to reducing or stopping driving in a sensitive manner, offering individualized counseling based on a patient's functional abilities and resources to help the individual remain engaged as a non-driver. The physician can play an important role in driving cessation by giving realistic and clear feedback about the patient's current functional skills and abilities that affect driving safety.

Ideally, patients and providers will begin conversations about driving before cessation is compulsory, allowing patients to gather resources and prepare emotionally for a non-driving future. Research shows that the process of driving reduction and cessation occurs over years, giving clinicians multiple opportunities to integrate fitness-to-drive into otherwise routine visits (Dobbs, Carr, & Morris, 2002). Having an ongoing dialogue about driving safety and encouraging planning for alternatives to maintain community mobility after driving cessation engages the patient in the process, facilitating not only solutions, but also better acceptance of the situation. These discussions should be documented in the patient's chart.

When counseling older adults on driving cessation, the physician should be ready to suggest alternative transportation resources, both public and private. However, it is not enough to simply list nearby non-driving transportation options. While options must be available where patients live and wish to travel, availability is only one of the five A's of senior mobility described by the Beverly Foundation and the American Public Transportation Association. Other critical factors include how acceptable, affordable, accessible, and adaptable alternative modes of transportation are for each individual. Such a holistic approach reveals consistent environmental, physical, and social barriers to driving cessation, especially in rural areas.

Even in parts of the United States where public and specialized transportation options are available, older adults strongly prefer rides with family members or friends to any other mode of transportation for convenience and comfort (Collia, Sharp, & Giesbrecht, 2003). In addition, use of personal vehicles allows older adults to avoid numerous barriers to using public alternatives. For example, the physical and cognitive decrements that limit driving also impair the ability to navigate public transportation, especially for older adults who have never or infrequently used public options. Patients with greater impairment require a higher level of service (e.g., wheelchair lifts, door-through-door assistance), which are often offered only with specialized public or private transportation. Local communities, societies, retirement centers, or local church groups may use funds or volunteers to provide transportation services to physicians' offices, grocery stores, and meetings.

A small subset of older adults who are advised to stop driving because of health reasons may continue to drive despite this advice. This possibility can be minimized through early and ongoing conversations about driving safety and transportation alternatives, especially when discussions are framed by the five A's (availability, acceptability, affordability, accessibility, and adaptability). Understanding the internal and external pressures motivating older adults to continue driving against medical or legal recommendations, such as fear of dependence (especially in rural areas), being responsible for others' transportation (Byles & Gallienne, 2012; Choi, Mezuk, Lohman, Edwards, & Rebok, 2013), and not having friends or family to provide rides (Johnson, 2008), yields insights into developing pragmatic and effective solutions for former drivers.

▸ Ethical, Legal, and Policy Issues

As mentioned earlier, some patients may refuse to stop driving despite advice from a family member or a clinician. The patient may request a referral for another opinion. This option should be reserved for only questionable cases because some evaluations (private or state) may be cursory or superficial.

The clinician may consider writing a letter to the state Department of Motor Vehicles (DMV) requesting both written and road tests to evaluate driving safety for the patient if the risk is unclear and if a driving evaluation by a driving rehabilitation specialist (DRS) is not possible. In Missouri, only 3% of older adults referred for a **medical fitness-to-drive** evaluation were able to retain their license (Eby, Molnar, Shope, Vivoda, & Fordyce, 2003). If the clinician believes that the patient is not safe to drive, then a letter can be written that should state this recommendation without the need for additional testing. Most states will honor the physician recommendation, although the driver can appeal. The American Academy of Neurology recommends that state laws should allow for voluntary reporting from the physician, and should provide for both physician anonymity and civil immunity (Bacon, Fisher, Morris, Rizzo, & Spanaki, 2007). Clinicians need to know the specific statutes in their state; updated information can be obtained from the state licensing authority. The Insurance Institute for Highway Safety and Highway Loss Data Institute (2017) also has a website that is updated on specific laws related to older drivers.

Some older adult drivers do not have insight into their own illness, such as patients suffering from Alzheimer's disease. Unfortunately, primary care physicians may not recognize that their older adult patients who drive have significant cognitive impairment. The spouse, family, physician, occupational therapist, and DMV may need to work together to keep those individuals judged to be unsafe from driving. In situations in which the patient does not have insight into his or her driving limitations, these efforts may include involving the police or DMV to confiscate the driver's license or involving family members to remove access to car keys, move the automobile off the premises, change door locks, file down the ignition keys, or disable the battery cable.

An elegant and useful guide from the Hartford Insurance Company should be available in physicians' offices to address this important issue and may be helpful to the driver with cognitive impairment and his or her spouse. Copies can be sent free of charge, and the order form is available on the company's website.

▸ Future Trends in Older Adult Mobility

Current research and studies on older drivers have focused on methods to identify the medically impaired driver who is at risk for a motor vehicle crash or at risk for driving cessation. A comprehensive, step-by-step approach appears to be the most appropriate method to assess older adult drivers when safety issues or functional impairment have been raised or identified. Physicians should take an active role in assessing their patients' risk for injury while driving. Referral to other professionals or organizations may be helpful in the evaluation and treatment process as well as in the maintenance of the driving skills of older adults.

A myriad of websites are available to assist with older driver mobility. New safety features should be considered when purchasing new cars (https://mycardoeswhat.org), and older adults have endorsed having some of these options in their vehicles (*Business Wire*, 2012). These in-vehicle technologies may allow medically impaired older adults to drive more safely and for a longer span (Miller, 2013). A recent review of different types of technologies (e.g., crash avoidance systems, in-vehicle information systems) revealed that older adults recognize the benefits of such systems and appreciate that these systems help them avoid crashes, improve the ease and comfort of driving, and expand travel to places that older adults might typically avoid (Eby et al., 2016).

In addition to resources for older driver mobility, AAA has many tools for senior drivers that can assist with decisions in regard to driving safety, such as Roadwise Rx (http://www.roadwiserx.com) for medication review and vehicle ergonomics (AAA Senior Driving, 2017). A list of additional older driver resources can be found in **Appendix 39A**.

▶ Summary

Public policy efforts focused on the routine assessment of senior drivers during license renewal have already been initiated in some states. In fact, questionnaires have indicated that older adults are willing to undergo some tests to promote safer driving for the public but do not reach consensus on which measures should be instituted (Dobbs et al., 2002). The efficacy of routine screening measures during license renewal, such as vision tests and road tests, is in question because in-person license renewal appears to be the only measure in the United States associated with a decreased crash risk in older adults (Grabowski, Campbell, & Morrisey, 2004). By comparison, road tests administered in other countries may be more efficacious and should be studied (Keall & Frith, 2004). More work is needed on the utility of educational programs that have the potential to improve driving skills (Eby et al., 2003; Owsley, McGwin, Phillips, McNeal, & Stalvey, 2004). Research on the type of screening and the utility and feasibility of the screening measures during license renewal to decrease the crash rate is still needed.

Lastly, the age of driverless cars is upon us; it is being powered by the on-demand mobility industry, with many tech giants offering various options (Fox News, 2013; Matus & Heck, 2015). This may eventually be an option for extending the driving life spans for older adults.

References

AAA Senior Driving. (2017). Find the right vehicle for you. Retrieved from http://seniordriving.aaa.com/maintain-mobility-independence/car-buying-maintenance-assistive-accessories/smartfeatures/

Anstey, K. J., Eramudugolla, R., Ross, L. A., Lautenschlager, N. T., & Wood, J. (2016). Road safety in an aging population: Risk factors, assessment, interventions, and future directions. *International Psychogeriatrics, 28*(3), 349–356. doi: 10.1017/S1041610216000053

Bacon, D., Fisher, R. S., Morris, J. C., Rizzo, M., & Spanaki, M. V. (2007). American Academy of Neurology position statement on physician reporting of medical conditions that may affect driving competence. *Neurology, 68*(15), 1174–1177. doi: 10.1212/01.wnl.0000259514.85579.e0

Ball, K., Edwards, J. D., Ross, L. A., & McGwin, G., Jr. (2010). Cognitive training decreases motor vehicle collision involvement of older drivers. *Journal of the American Geriatrics Society, 58*(11), 2107–2113. doi: 10.1111/j.1532-5415.2010.03138.x

Bogner, H. R., Straton, J. B., Gallo, J. J., Rebok, G. W., & Keyl, P. M. (2004). The role of physicians in assessing older drivers: Barriers, opportunities, and strategies. *Journal of the American Board of Family Practice, 17*(1), 38–43.

Bond, E. G., Durbin, L. L., Cisewski, J. A., Qian, M., Guralnik, J. M., Kaspere, J. D., & Mielenz, T. J. (2017). Association between baseline frailty and driving status over time: A secondary analysis of the National Health and Aging Trends Study. *Injury Epidemiology, 4*(1), 9. doi: 10.1186/s40621-017-0106-y

Business Wire. (2012). New research by the Hartford and MIT AgeLab reveals top ten car technologies for mature drivers. Retrieved from http://www.businesswire.com/news/home/20120918005454/en/Research-Hartford-MIT-AgeLab-Reveals-Top-Ten

Byles, J., & Gallienne, L. (2012). Driving in older age: A longitudinal study of women in urban, regional, and remote areas and the impact of caregiving. *Journal of Women and Aging, 24*(2), 113–125. doi: 10.1080/08952841.2012.639661

Carr, D. B., Barco, P. P., Babulal, G. M., Stout, S. H., Johnson, A. M., ... Roe, C. M. (2016). Association of functional impairments and co-morbid conditions with driving performance among cognitively normal older adults. *PLoS One, 11*(12), e0167751. doi: 10.1371/journal.pone.0167751

Carr, D. B., Barco, P. P., Wallendorf, M. J., Snellgrove, C. A., & Ott, B. R. (2011). Predicting road test performance in drivers with dementia. *Journal of the American Geriatrics Society, 59*(11), 2112–2117. doi: 10.1111/j.1532-5415.2011.03657.x

Carr, D. B., & Ott, B. R. (2010). The older adult driver with cognitive impairment: "It's a very frustrating life." *Journal of the American Medical Association, 303*(16), 1632–1641. doi: 10.1001/jama.2010.481

Casutt, G., Theill, N., Martin, M., Keller, M., & Jancke, L. (2014). The Drive-Wise Project: Driving simulator training increases real driving performance in healthy older drivers. *Frontiers in Aging Neuroscience, 6,* 85. doi: 10.3389/fnagi.2014.00085

Centers for Disease Control and Prevention (CDC). (2015). *Motor vehicle safety: Older adult drivers.* Retrieved from http://www.cdc.gov/motorvehiclesafety/older _adult_drivers/index.html

Charlton, J., Koppel, S., Odell, M., . . . Devlin, A., Langford, J., O'Hare, M., . . . Scully, M. (2010). *Influence of chronic illness on crash involvement of motor vehicle drivers* (2nd ed.). Retrieved from http://www.monash.edu.au/miri/research /reports/muarc300.pdf

Cheung, I., & McCartt, A. T. (2011). Declines in fatal crashes of older drivers: Changes in crash risk and survivability. *Accident Analysis & Prevention, 43*(3), 666–674. doi: 10.1016/j.aap.2010.10.010

Chihuri, S., Mielenz, T. J., DiMaggio, C. J., Betz, M. E., DiGuiseppi, C., Jones, V. C., & Li, G. (2016). Driving cessation and health outcomes in older adults. *Journal of the American Geriatrics Society, 64*(2), 332–341. doi: 10.1111/jgs.13931

Choi, M., Mezuk, B., Lohman, M. C., Edwards, J. D., & Rebok, G. W. (2013). Gender and racial disparities in driving cessation among older adults. *Journal of Aging and Health, 25*(8 suppl), 147S–162S. doi: 10.1177/0898264313519886

Cicchino, J. B., & McCartt, A. T. (2014). Trends in older driver crash involvement rates and survivability in the United States: An update. *Accident Analysis & Prevention, 72,* 44–54. doi: 10.1016/j.aap.2014.06.011

Classen, S., & Brooks, J. (2014). Driving simulators for occupational therapy screening, assessment, and intervention. *Occupational Therapy in Health Care, 28*(2), 154–162. doi: 10.3109/07380577.2014.901590

Collia, D. V., Sharp, J., & Giesbrecht, L. (2003). The 2001 National Household Travel Survey: A look into the travel patterns of older Americans. *Journal of Safety Research, 34*(4), 461–470.

Cummings, J. L. (2004). Alzheimer's disease. *New England Journal of Medicine, 351*(1), 56–67. doi: 10.1056 /NEJMra040223

Curl, A. L., Stowe, J. D., Cooney, T. M., & Proulx, C. M. (2014). Giving up the keys: How driving cessation affects engagement in later life. *Gerontologist, 54*(3), 423–433. doi: 10.1093/geront/gnt037

Daiello, L. A., Ott, B. R., Festa, E. K., Friedman, M., Miller, L. A., & Heindel, W. C. (2010). Effects of cholinesterase inhibitors on visual attention in drivers with Alzheimer disease. *Journal of Clinical Psychopharmacology, 30*(3), 245–251. doi: 10.1097/JCP.0b013e3181da5406

Dobbs, B. M., Carr, D. B., & Morris, J. C. (2002). Evaluation and management of the driver with dementia. *Neurologist, 8*(2), 61–70.

Drummer, O. H., Gerostamoulos, J., Batziris, H., Chu, M., Caplehorn, J., Robertson, M.D., & Swann, P. (2004). The involvement of drugs in drivers of motor vehicles killed in Australian road traffic crashes. *Accident Analysis & Prevention, 36*(2), 239–248.

Eby, D. W., Molnar, L. J., Shope, J. T., Vivoda, J. M., & Fordyce, T. A. (2003). Improving older driver knowledge and self-awareness through self-assessment: The driving decisions workbook. *Journal of Safety Research, 34*(4), 371–381. doi: 10.1016/j.jsr.2003.09.006

Eby, D. W., Molnar, L. J., Zhang, L., St. Louis, R. M., Zanier, N., Kostyniuk, L. P., & Stanciu, S. (2016). Use, perceptions, and benefits of automotive technologies among aging drivers. *Injury Epidemiology, 3*(1), 28. doi: 10.1186/s40621 -016-0093-4

Edwards, J. D., Lunsman, M., Perkins, M., Rebok, G. W., & Roth, D. L. (2009). Driving cessation and health trajectories in older adults. *Journals of Gerontology, Series A: Biological Sciences and Medical Sciences, 64*(12), 1290–1295. doi: 10.1093/gerona/glp114

Edwards, J. D., Myers, C., Ross, L. A., Roenker, D. L., Cissell, G. M., McLaughlin, A. M., & Ball, K. K. (2009). The longitudinal impact of cognitive speed of processing training on driving mobility. *Gerontologist, 49*(4), 485–494. doi: 10.1093/geront/gnp042

Eramudugolla, R., Price, J., Chopra, S., Li, X., & Anstey, K. J. (2016). Comparison of a virtual older driver assessment with an on-road driving test. *Journal of the American Geriatrics Society, 64*(12), e253–e258. doi: 10.1111 /jgs.14548

Foley, D. J., Wallace, R. B., & Eberhard, J. (1995). Risk factors for motor vehicle crashes among older drivers in a rural community. *Journal of the American Geriatrics Society, 43*(7), 776–781.

Fox News. (2013). *Five future transportation technologies that will actually happen.* Retrieved from http://www. foxnews.com/tech/2013/11/27/five-future-transportation- technologies-that-will-actually-happen.html

Freund, B., Gravenstein, S., Ferris, R., & Shaheen, E. (2002). Evaluating driving performance of cognitively impaired and healthy older adults: A pilot study comparing on-road testing and driving simulation. *Journal of the American Geriatrics Society, 50*(7), 1309–1310.

Goodwin, A., Thomas, L., Kirley, B., Hall, W., O'Brien, N., & Hill, K. (2015). *Countermeasures that work: A highway safety countermeasure guide for state highway safety offices* (8th ed.). DOT HS 812 202. Washington, DC: National Highway Traffic Safety Administration. Retrieved from https:// www.ghsa.org/sites/default/files/2016-12/812202 -CountermeasuresThatWork8th_0.pdf

Gorrie, C. A., Rodriguez, M., Sachdev, P., Duflou, J., & Waite, P. M. (2007). Mild neuritic changes are increased in the brains of fatally injured older motor vehicle drivers. *Accident Analysis & Prevention, 39*(6), 1114–1120. doi: 10.1016/j.aap.2007.02.008

Grabowski, D. C., Campbell, C. M., & Morrisey, M. A. (2004). Elderly licensure laws and motor vehicle fatalities.

Journal of the American Medical Association, 291(23), 2840–2846. doi: 10.1001/jama.291.23.2840

Hemmelgarn, B., Suissa, S., Huang, A., Boivin, J. F., & Pinard, G. (1997). Benzodiazepine use and the risk of motor vehicle crash in the elderly. *Journal of the American Medical Association, 278*(1), 27–31.

Hetland, A., & Carr, D. B. (2014). Medications and impaired driving. *Annals of Pharmacotherapy, 48*(4), 494–506. doi: 10.1177/1060028014520882

Higgins, J. P., Wright, S. W., & Wrenn, K. D. (1996). Alcohol, the elderly, and motor vehicle crashes. *American Journal of Emergency Medicine, 14*(3), 265–267. doi: 10.1016/s0735-6757(96)90172-2

Hu, P. S., Trumble, D. A., Foley, D. J., Eberhard, J. W., & Wallace, R. B. (1998). Crash risks of older drivers: A panel data analysis. *Accident Analysis & Prevention, 30*(5), 569–581.

Hunt, L. A., Murphy, C. F., Carr, D., Duchek, J. M., Buckles, V., & Morris, J. C. (1997). Reliability of the Washington University Road Test: A performance-based assessment for drivers with dementia of the Alzheimer type. *Archives of Neurology, 54*(6), 707–712.

Insurance Institute for Highway Safety & Highway Loss Data Institute. (2014, February 20). *Fit for the road: Older drivers' crash rates continue to drop.* Retrieved from http://www.iihs.org/externaldata/srdata/docs/sr4901.pdf

Insurance Institute for Highway Safety & Highway Loss Data Institute. (2017). *Older drivers.* Retrieved from http://www.iihs.org/iihs/topics/laws/olderdrivers

Iverson, D. J., Gronseth, G. S., Reger, M. A., Classen, S., Dubinsky, R. M., & Rizzo, M. (2010). Practice parameter update: Evaluation and management of driving risk in dementia: Report of the Quality Standards Subcommittee of the American Academy of Neurology. *Neurology, 74*(16), 1316–1324. doi: 10.1212/WNL.0b013e3181da3b0f

Johansson, K., Bogdanovic, N., Kalimo, H., Winblad, B., & Viitanen, M. (1997). Alzheimer's disease and apolipoprotein E epsilon 4 allele in older drivers who died in automobile accidents. *Lancet, 349*(9059), 1143–1144. doi: 10.1016/S0140-6736(97)24016-X

Johansson, K., Bryding, G., Dahl, M. L., Holmgren, P., & Viitanen, M. (1997). Traffic dangerous drugs are often found in fatally injured older male drivers. *Journal of the American Geriatrics Society, 45*(8), 1029–1031.

Johnson, J. E. (2008). Informal social support networks and the maintenance of voluntary driving cessation by older rural women. *Journal of Community Health Nursing, 25*(2), 65–72. doi: 10.1080/07370010802017034

Joseph, P. G., O'Donnell, M. J., Teo, K. K., Gao, P., Anderson, C., Probstfield, J. L., . . . Yusuf, S. (2014). The Mini-Mental State Examination, clinical factors, and motor vehicle crash risk. *Journal of the American Geriatrics Society, 62*(8), 1419–1426. doi: 10.1111/jgs.12936

Keall, M. D., & Frith, W. J. (2004). Association between older driver characteristics, on-road driving test performance, and crash liability. *Traffic Injury Prevention, 5*(2), 112–116. doi: 10.1080/15389580490435006

Lee, H. C., Lee, A. H., Cameron, D., & Li-Tsang, C. (2003). Using a driving simulator to identify older drivers at inflated risk of motor vehicle crashes. *Journal of Safety Research, 34*(4), 453–459.

Li, G., Braver, E. R., & Chen, L. H. (2003). Fragility versus excessive crash involvement as determinants of high death rates per vehicle-mile of travel among older drivers. *Accident Analysis & Prevention, 35*(2), 227–235. doi: 10.1016/S0001-4575(01)00107-5

Marmeleira, J. F., Godinho, M. B., & Fernandes, O. M. (2009). The effects of an exercise program on several abilities associated with driving performance in older adults. *Accident Analysis & Prevention, 41*(1), 90–97. doi: 10.1016/j.aap.2008.09.008

Marottoli, R. A., Allore, H., Araujo, K. L., Iannine, L. P., Acampora, D., Gottschalk, M., . . . Peduzzi, P. (2007). A randomized trial of a physical conditioning program to enhance the driving performance of older persons. *Journal of General Internal Medicine, 22*(5), 590–597. doi: 10.1007/s11606-007-0134-3

Marottoli, R. A., de Leon, C. F. M., Glass, T. A., Williams, C. S., Cooney, L. M., Jr., & Berkman, L. F. (2000). Consequences of driving cessation: Decreased out-of-home activity levels. *Journal of Gerontology: Social Sciences, 55B*(6), S334–S340. doi: 10.1093/geronb/55.6.S334

Marottoli, R. A., Richardson, E. D., Stowe, M. H., Miller, E. G., Brass, L. M., Cooney, L. M. Jr., Tinetti, M. E. (1998). Development of a test battery to identify older drivers at risk for self-reported adverse driving events. *Journal of the American Geriatrics Society, 46*(5), 562–568. doi: 10.1111/j.1532-5415.1998.tb01071.x

Matus, J., & Heck, S. (2015). *Understanding the future of mobility.* Retrieved from https://techcrunch.com/2015/08/08/understanding-the-future-of-mobility/

Mezuk, B., & Rebok, G. W. (2008). Social integration and social support among older adults following driving cessation. *Journals of Gerontology, Series B: Psychological Sciences and Social Sciences, 63*(5), S298–S303.

Miller, M. (2013). New technology helps older drivers keep the keys longer. Retrieved from https://www.reuters.com/article/us-column-miller-cars-idUSBRE98G05I20130917

Molnar, L. J., Eby, D. W., Zhang, L., Zanier, N., Louis, R. M. S., & Kostyniuk, L. P. (2015). Self-regulation of driving by older adults: A synthesis of the literature and framework. *Aging, 20*, 227–235.

National Office for Traffic Medicine. (2017). *Sláinte agus Tiomáint medical fitness to drive guidelines (group 1 and 2 drivers).* Retrieved from https://www.rcpi.ie/traffic-medicine/medical-fitness-to-drive-guidelines/

National Safety Council. (2017). *Home page.* Retrieved from https://mycardoeswhat.org/

Odenheimer, G. L. (1993). Dementia and the older driver. *Clinics in Geriatric Medicine, 9*(2), 349–364.

Ott, B. R., Jones, R. N., Noto, R. B., Yoo, D. C., Snyder, P. J., Bernier, J. N., . . . Roe, C. M. (2017). Brain amyloid in preclinical Alzheimer's disease is associated with increased driving risk. *Alzheimer's & Dementia (Amsterdam), 6,* 136–142. doi: 10.1016/j.dadm.2016.10.008

Owsley, C. (2011). Aging and vision. *Vision Research, 51*(13), 1610–1622. doi: 10.1016/j.visres.2010.10.020

Owsley, C., & McGwin, G., Jr. (2010). Vision and driving. *Vision Research, 50*(23), 2348–2361. doi: 10.1016/j.visres.2010.05.021

Owsley, C., McGwin, G., Jr., Phillips, J. M., McNeal, S. F., & Stalvey, B. T. (2004). Impact of an educational program on the safety of high-risk, visually impaired, older drivers. *American Journal of Preventive Medicine, 26*(3), 222–229. doi: 10.1016/j.amepre.2003.12.005

Owsley, C., McGwin, G., Jr., Sloane, M., Wells, J., Stalvey, B. T., & Gauthreaux, S. (2002). Impact of cataract surgery on motor vehicle crash involvement by older adults. *Journal of the American Medical Association, 288*(7), 841–849.

Oxley, J., & Whelan, M. (2008). It cannot be all about safety: The benefits of prolonged mobility. *Traffic Injury Prevention, 9*(4), 367–378. doi: 10.1080/15389580801895285

Papa, M., Boccardi, V., Prestano, R., Angellotti, E., Desiderio, M., Marano, L., . . . Paolisso, G. (2014). Comorbidities and crash involvement among younger and older drivers. *PLoS One, 9*(4), e94564. doi: 10.1371/journal.pone.0094564

Pesata, V., Pallija, G., & Webb, A. A. (1999). A descriptive study of missed appointments: Families' perceptions of barriers to care. *Journal of Pediatric Health Care, 13*(4), 178–182. doi: 10.1016/S0891-5245(99)90037-8

Pomidor, A. (Ed.). (2016). *Clinician's guide to assessing and counseling older drivers* (3rd ed.). Washington, DC: National Highway Traffic Safety Administration. Retrieved from https://geriatricscaronline.org/ProductAbstract/clinicians-guide-to-assessing-and-counseling-older-drivers-3rd-edition/B022

Rebok, G. W., & Keyl, P. M. (2004). Driving simulation. *Gerotechnology: Research and Practice in Technology and Aging,* 191.

Roadwise Rx. (2016). Home page. Retrieved from http://www.roadwiserx.com/

Roe, C. M., Babulal, G. M., Head, D. M., Stout, S. H., Vernon, E. K., Ghoshal, N., . . . Fierberg, R. (2017). Preclinical Alzheimer's disease and longitudinal driving decline. *Alzheimer's & Dementia: Translational Research & Clinical Interventions, 3*(1), 74–82.

Roe, C. M., Barco, P. P., Head, D. M., Goshal, N., Selsor, N., Babulal, G. M., . . . Morris, J. C. (2017). Amyloid imaging, cerebrospinal fluid biomarkers predict driving performance among cognitively normal individuals. *Alzheimer Disease and Associated Disorders, 31*(1), 69–72. doi: 10.1097/WAD.0000000000000154

Ross, L. A., Freed, S. A., Edwards, J. D., Phillips, C. B., & Ball, K. (2017). The impact of three cognitive training programs on driving cessation across 10 years: A randomized controlled trial. *The Gerontologist, 57*(5), 838–846. doi: 10.1093/geront/gnw143

Roy, M., & Molnar, F. (2013). Systematic review of the evidence for Trails B cut-off scores in assessing fitness-to-drive. *Canadian Geriatrics Journal, 16*(3), 120–142. doi: 10.5770/cgj.16.76

Sammer, G. (2012). Wirkungen und Risiken einer City-Maut als zentrale Säule eines städtischen Mobilitätskonzepts. *Zukünftige Entwicklungen in der Mobilität,* 479–491.

Satariano, W. A., Guralnik, J. M., Jackson, R. J., Marottoli, R. A., Phelan, E. A., & Prohaska, T. R. (2012). Mobility and aging: New directions for public health action. *American Journal of Public Health, 102*(8), 1508–1515. doi: 10.2105/AJPH.2011.300631

Sayers, S. P., & Gibson, K. (2012). Effects of high-speed power training on muscle performance and braking speed in older adults. *Journal of Aging Research, 2012,* 426278. doi: 10.1155/2012/426278

Sims, R. V., Ahmed, A., Sawyer, P., & Allman, R. M. (2007). Self-reported health and driving cessation in community-dwelling older drivers. *Journals of Gerontology, Series A: Biological Sciences and Medical Sciences, 62*(7), 789–793. doi: 10.1093/gerona/62.7.789

Staplin, L., Gish, K. W., & Wagner, E. K. (2003). MaryPODS revisited: Updated crash analysis and implications for screening program implementation. *Journal of Safety Research, 34*(4), 389–397.

Stutts, J., Martell, C., & Staplin, L. (2009). Identifying behaviors and situations associated with increased crash risk for older drivers, No. HS-811 093. Retrieved from https://rosap.ntl.bts.gov/view/dot/1880

Stutts, J. C., Stewart, J. R., & Martell, C. (1998). Cognitive test performance and crash risk in an older driver population. *Accident Analysis & Prevention, 30*(3), 337–346.

Stutts, J. C., & Wilkins, J. W. (2003). On-road driving evaluations: A potential tool for helping older adults drive safely longer. *Journal of Safety Research, 34*(4), 431–439.

Tuokko, H., Beattie, B. L., Tallman, K., & Cooper, P. (1995). Predictors of motor vehicle crashes in a dementia clinic population: The role of gender and arthritis. *Journal of the American Geriatrics Society, 43*(12), 1444–1445.

U.S. Department of Transportation, Federal Highway Administration, Office of Highway Policy Information. (2016). Highway Statistics 2015. Retrieved from https://www.fhwa.dot.gov/policyinformation/statistics/2015/dl20.cfm

van der Flier, W. M., & Scheltens, P. (2005). Epidemiology and risk factors of dementia. *Journal of Neurology, Neurosurgery, and Psychiatry, 76*(suppl 5), v2–v7. doi: 10.1136/jnnp.2005.082867

Viitanen, M., Johansson, K., Bogdanovic, N., Berkowicz, A., Druidc, H., Erikssond, A., . . . Kalimoai, H. (1998). Alzheimer changes are common in aged drivers killed in single car crashes and at intersections. *Forensic Science International, 96*(2–3), 115–127.

Wallace, R., Hughes-Cromwick, P., & Mull, H. (2006). Cost-effectiveness of access to nonemergency medical transportation: Comparison of transportation and health care costs and benefits. *Transportation Research Record: Journal of the Transportation Research Board, 1956,* 86–93. doi: 10.3141/1956-11

White, M. N., King, A. C., Sallis, J. F., Frank, L. D., Saelens, B. E., Conway, T. L., . . . Kerr, J. (2016). Caregiving, transport-related, and demographic correlates of sedentary behavior in older adults: The Senior Neighborhood Quality of Life Study. *Journal of Aging and Health, 28*(5), 812–833. doi: 10.1177/0898264315611668

Yamin, S., Stinchcombe, A., & Gagnon, S. (2016). Comparing cognitive profiles of licensed drivers with mild Alzheimer's disease and mild dementia with Lewy bodies. *International Journal of Alzheimer's Disease, 2016,* 6542962. doi: 10.1155/2016/6542962

Appendix 39A

Physician and Caregiver Resources for Older Drivers

Administration on Aging (AOA): https://www.acl.gov/node/408

American Medical Association (AMA), Physician's Guide to Assessing and Counseling Older Drivers: https://one.nhtsa.gov/people/injury/olddrive/OlderDriversBook/pages/Contents.html

American Occupational Therapy Association (AOTA): www.aota.org/olderdriver

Association for Driver Rehabilitation Specialists (ADED): www.aded.net

At the Crossroads: A Guide to Alzheimer's Disease, Dementia, and Driving: https://s0.hfdstatic.com/sites/the_hartford/files/cmme-crossroads.pdf

Automobile Association of America (AAA): https://seniordriving.aaa.com

DriveABLE: www.driveable.com

Family and Friends Concerned About an Older Driver: https://one.nhtsa.gov/people/injury/olddrive/FamilynFriends/faf_index.htm

Family Conversations with Older Drivers: https://www.thehartford.com/resources/mature-market-excellence/family-conversations-with-older-drivers

Insurance Institute for Highway Safety (IIHS): http://www.iihs.org/iihs/topics/t/older-drivers/topicoverview

Mayo Clinic Health Information: https://www.mayoclinic.org/

National Highway Traffic Safety Administration (NHTSA): www.nhtsa.dot.gov

Educational Material and Courses for Older Drivers

AARP Driver Safety Program: www.aarp.org/families/driver_safety

Alternative Transportation Options

AAA Foundation for Traffic Safety: https://aaafoundation.org

American Public Transportation Association: www.apta.com

AOA Eldercare: www.eldercare.gov

Community Transportation Association: www.ctaa.org

Local Agency on Aging: https://www.payingforseniorcare.com/longtermcare/find_aging_agencies_adrc_aaa.html

CHAPTER 40

Advance Care Planning Through the Incorporation of Values History Discussions

David Doukas and Stephen Hanson

CHAPTER OBJECTIVES

1. Be able to use advance directives, including the living will, durable powers of attorney for health care, physician orders for life-sustaining treatment, the family covenant, and the Values History, to help patients guide their medical treatment.
2. Determine which types of advance directives are appropriate for a patient based on the patient's prognosis and familial/social conditions.
3. Understand the moral reasons that support the use of advance directives.

KEY TERMS

Advance directives	Decision making	End-of-life
Autonomy		

▶ Introduction

Geriatric assessment requires an examination of the present and preparation for the future. Patients need to consider their long-term care options, as well as health directives for a broad array of interventions. The prerequisite for such conversation and **decision making** is an adequate disclosure of the information necessary to the patient regarding advance care planning. Physicians, along with the other members of the care team, are responsible for addressing future health concerns as part of their fiduciary responsibility for managing their patients' medical conditions, and for taking ownership of the task of initiating discussions on **advance directives**. The latter task considers both the respect due to each patient and the possibility of eliminating therapeutic interventions that would not be beneficial to the patient given his or her unique circumstances. While physicians may be reluctant to discuss advance directives because of their own discomfort, they can also influence the comfort level of the patients and families by leading such a discussion (Doukas, Gorenflo, & Coughlin, 1991). Unfortunately, even when discussions of end-of-life treatments are integrated into the medical care of hospitalized patients, stated preferences are not routinely translated into physician's orders (SUPPORT Investigators, 1995).

Both living wills and durable powers of attorney for health care (DPA-HC) address preferences for future health care. Since their advent, physician orders for life-sustaining treatment (POLST) forms have been developed that identify those treatments allowable or refused by the patient in a future of incapacity or terminal illness. The Patient Self-Determination Act of 1990 was intended to enhance use of advance directives and DPA-HCs by requiring healthcare institutions that receive Medicare and Medicaid funds to ask patients if an advance directive has been signed. Although studies revealed that signing rates increased in the wake of this law, the universal execution of the advance directive did not (Teno et al., 1997).

Advance directives have a sound ethical foundation, but they often fail to assess or acknowledge people's values in their formulation, execution, and implementation. People view their lives and health care as part of their remembrances of loved ones lost and perceive how their own mortality can be influenced through the use of advance directives. The Centers for Medicare and Medicaid Services (CMS) has been helpful in encouraging development of advance directives since the passage of the Affordable Care Act: It has enacted regulations that allow physicians and other advanced practice clinicians to engage patients in 30-minute incremental blocks for advance care planning purpose (U.S. Department of Health and Human Services, 2016). This type of planning can be done within the reimbursement mechanisms regulating both inpatient and outpatient medicine, so that now any clinicians who might have been reluctant to have these conversations due to time constraints can be paid for their effort.

In the late 1980s, Doukas and McCullough proposed to make this process more systematic by using an instrument that both assesses and acknowledges the values of patients in end-of-life healthcare planning, the Values History (Doukas, Lipson, & McCullough, 1989; Doukas & McCullough, 1988, 1991; Doukas & Reichel, 1993). The Values History is an **autonomy**-enhancing instrument that seeks to engage the patient in an in-depth, longitudinal discussion of the patient's values and healthcare preferences that are to be carried out when decision making by the patient is no longer possible. It asks the patient to identify values and preferences before the patient can no longer speak for himself or herself. As such, the Values History is intended to serve as extension of the living will and DPA-HC, while also fulfilling the mandate of the Patient Self-Determination Act to inform patients about their right to refuse future medical therapy (including documenting their choices regarding the use of advance directives) (Omnibus Budget Reconciliation Act, 1990). The Values History eases this process by addressing relevant values that underlie the informed consent process for these directives.

These values and preferences are to be discussed first in the outpatient setting, with additional Values History discussions occurring with changes of health status. This approach decreases the probability of encountering uncertainty about the person's preferences for **end-of-life** care, and enables the healthcare team to apply the patient's values and preferences regarding respect, communication, and benefit. Addressing values and preferences when discussing advance directives is an essential aspect of geriatric care. Patients need to understand that their own values and preferences are what drive their future care and, importantly, recognize how they themselves can frame future decisions through the use of their advance directives. By extension, the physician is the steward of this process of informed consent, whereby the patient needs to first be informed about opportunities for future care, along the right to accept or refuse such care based on the patient's own values. This process can then be safeguarded within the electronic medical record and the hospital record, and can be implemented by the family, physician, and inpatient hospital team.

▶ The Living Will

The living will is a written statement (or witnessed oral declaration, as allowed in applicable law) that documents a person's competent decision to withhold or withdraw artificial means of health care in present or future circumstances of terminal illness (and, in many states, irreversible comatose and vegetative states) when the person can no longer make decisions. The living will allows the person to decide in advance which life-prolonging therapies in the treatment of a terminal disease process and its complications should not be administered. The individual is free to change or revoke any aspect of the living will, and in many states can even revoke the

living will entirely at any time, including when he or she is later incapacitated. Physicians and family members cannot revoke a validly executed living will.

Sometimes the language of the living will is unclear about which particular medical procedures are to be refused, since this document is often created prior to any specific knowledge of the circumstances that led to the patient's incapacity. This lack of precision can lead to misinterpretation of what the person has refused (Eisendrath & Jonsen, 1983). Physician interpretation or misinterpretation of the person's intent as well as his or her assessment of the probability of recovery can shade the likelihood of advance directive implementation (Eisendrath & Jonsen, 1983).

As a legal statutory instrument (in all states but Michigan), living wills allow competent persons to exercise autonomous control over their future medical care in anticipation of future incapacity. As noted earlier, ethics and the law of informed consent doctrine require that patients be informed about medically reasonable therapies and the alternative of no intervention at all. The informed consent doctrine states that patients have the right to accept or refuse any therapy, and this right to accept or decline potentially life-sustaining medical therapies can be indicated in a living will. End-of-life treatment options should be discussed by doctors with their patients, especially with older adults who may be faced with end-of-life decisions. Living wills should be based on the patient's values regarding future medical treatment and care. Nevertheless, in some cases, the patient may have received the living will form from an attorney, a doctor's office, or an Internet download, and filled it out, signed it, and had it witnessed without the opportunity to address their own fundamental values regarding explicit end-of-life preferences. To understand the patient's reasoning and motivation in executing a living will, more information is required than the instrument itself typically includes. This information can be obtained via the Values History.

▶ The Durable Power of Attorney for Health Care

The durable power of attorney for health care is a legal document that transfers the power of medical decision making from the patient to an agent (who can be a relative or other trusted individual) either contemporaneously with or prior to the onset of incapacity, or whose effect comes into force when the patient lacks decision-making capacity. Its durability derives from the fact that the agent's decision-making power continues throughout the patient's incapacity. The agent should not be the physician, as there is the obvious potential of conflict of interest in the decision-making process. All jurisdictions provide for the DPA-HC as a valid form of decision making.

The scope of the DPA-HC transcends the narrow end-of-life confines of the living will, as it allows a proxy decision maker the flexibility to make a wide range of medical decisions for a loved one who is now incapacitated, or to make decisions of a person who wishes to waive autonomously his or her own right to make decisions. Those decisions are expected to be based on conversations previously held between the patient and the proxy regarding future health care. The duty of the DPA-HC agent upon the patient's incapacity is to consider the medically reasonable options and then select the options that most closely adhere to the previously discussed or written preferences of the individual—a process called the substituted judgment standard. If the patient's preferences are not known, decisions should be based on the patient's best interests—a process referred to as the best interest standard.

The surrogate decision maker authorized by the DPA-HC is able to be more flexible in addressing medical decisions than the limited details that may be discussed in the generic, often state-created, form of the living will. Although the living will avoids the potential stress of placing the decision-making burden on another's shoulders, the DPA-HC (or a combination of a living will and DPA-HC) may be a better approach because it can accommodate a wider spectrum of future medical conditions and possible medical responses. Physicians can also attempt to free the proxy from any moral burden by highlighting the fact that the agent's job is to convey the patient's values and preferences, rather than make the decisions alone. Patients may feel more confident using a DPA-HC to voice and enforce their interests, rather than using a more concrete living will to indicate a preference for specific medical treatments or refusals without such flexibility.

The main objection to the DPA-HC is uncertainty about whether the agent has a sufficient understanding of all of the patient's many healthcare preferences—and whether the agent and patient have *ever* had a discussion of end-of-life treatment at all (Wanzer et al., 1984). Often patients are reluctant to discuss their values, much less their specific preferences about terminal care, with their agent.

▶ The Family Covenant

The use of the family covenant in eldercare has been advocated by one of the authors and John Hardwig (Doukas & Hardwig, 2003) in end-of-life treatment advance planning. The family covenant is a healthcare agreement in which the patient selects family members and other loved ones to be included in the information-sharing and decision-making processes involved in treatment selection both before and after incapacity. The patient makes the determination of who is to be included in this process, with the basis of selection founded upon love and trust between the patient and those persons of family and/or acquaintance who can reflect reliably the values and treatment preferences of the patient. The family covenant transcends the narrow scope of DPA-HC documents with an appreciation that families often are very relevant in these decisions, that families often make deliberative decisions as a cohesive whole, and that the patient may regard this cohesive whole as more important in selecting a designated agent (Doukas & Hardwig, 2003). This model is more accepting of alternative models of family based decision making that are held as valued in many parts of the world (Doukas & Hardwig, 2003).

The family covenant model begins with an agreement that endures over time concerning to whom information should flow and how decisions can be made. The passage of time allows for the accumulation of trust, thereby strengthening the relationship and allowing for ongoing discussion, deliberation, and decision making. The family covenant can then be used as a method to discuss advance directives and other relevant advance care planning options, such as those described previously.

▶ The Values History

The Values History (**Appendix 40A**) was first published in the literature (in the first *Handbook of Geriatric Assessment* in 1988) as a means to identify better end-of-life healthcare values and treatment preferences based on those values (Doukas & McCullough, 1988). This instrument is intended to complement the living will and DPA-HC, rather than replace them. The Values History asks the individual to identify and discuss his or her values and beliefs regarding terminal care; this step is followed by considering end-of-life treatment decisions in advance, given these values. It also asks the individual to consider under which parameters these decisions apply, and in which circumstances his or her values would support changing the treatment decisions for the individual. Through this articulation of end-of-life values, the patient's perspective becomes better understood by the patient, his or her family, and his or her physician, and this understanding can be documented by appending the Values History to the individual's living will and DPA-HC. The intended effect is to enhance communication

as well as the implementation of the treatment preferences when appropriate.

Preamble

The preamble articulates the premise of the Values History: to supplement the person's other advance directive(s). These values and preferences guide physicians when an individual without decision-making capacity is terminally ill, irreversibly comatose, in a persistent vegetative state, or otherwise when a qualified patient under applicable advance directive law, and the withholding or withdrawing of life-sustaining measures is being contemplated. As with other advance directive instruments, the Values History is changeable and revocable, per the individual's own jurisdiction, as long as the person is able to voice his or her preferences.

Values Section

The person first identifies life values relevant to the treatment decisions that must be made. The foundation of this section is a thought-provoking query as to whether the length of life or the quality of life is more important to the patient. Identifying those values *most* important to him or her from a list of 13 end-of-life values (based on commonly held precepts of communication, respect for patient decision making, benefit, and avoidance of harm) then follows this first choice, as it may have great bearing when considering these values. Other values can be added to this list, as it is not intended to be comprehensive, but rather just serves as a starting point for facilitating communication. These identified values can then help the individual formulate his or her treatment preferences in regard to end-of-life medical care.

Preferences Section

The Preferences section contains a list of medical interventions, with acute care decisions appearing first, followed by chronic care treatment options. This listing allows for decisions regarding intervention when advanced cardiac life support (ACLS protocols) versus longitudinal care may be invoked in the hospital, nursing, rehabilitation, and home settings. Many preference statements introduce the concept of a "trial of intervention," limited by either time or benefit (N.B.: this was a new concept in 1988) (Doukas & McCullough, 1988). This nuanced approach allows for a therapy to be used for a designated period of time or to ascertain whether medical benefit is present and continued after a therapy is initiated, and helps to break down barriers of artificial constraints that are forced as a "yes" or "no" decision point into touch points that more realistically capture the relevance aspects of either time or benefit.

Discussing cardiopulmonary resuscitation (CPR) is fundamental in considering end-of-life care, as withholding or stopping resuscitation in dire circumstances will usually result in death. Many physicians, hospitals, and, importantly, patients presume that this medical therapy will be provided. Code status is of particular importance in chronic and critical illness where such decisions are increasingly relevant. Such orders can also be used in out-of-hospital do not resuscitate (DNR) orders, which are allowed in many states for patients in home and hospice care. Respirator and endotracheal intubation discussions help to clarify the unifying concept of ACLS resuscitation: If ACLS protocols are to be used, they must be used in compliance with established standards. "Partial codes" are not condoned in an individual's treatment preferences, as they may set up false hopes for treatment benefit where there is none.

Each subsequent chronic care directive is based in the context of future long-term recuperative or vegetative care. The chronic care treatment options include total parenteral nutrition, intravenous hydration/medication, all medications for the treatment of illnesses by other routes (e.g., oral or by intramuscular injection), enteral feeding tubes, and dialysis. The physician should make it clear that pain medications will always be prescribed as needed.

Preferences then follow addressing autopsy, proxy negation, and organ donation. The investigation of the causes of death may be very important for some persons, such as when autopsy might help clarify genetic familial disease risks. The person is given an opportunity to add any other medical preferences not otherwise addressed.

The unique and singularly helpful proxy negation directive, grounded within the Values History, allows the individual to name those persons who are to be excluded from the individual's healthcare decision making in the future. This proactive omission preference is useful when family members have a different philosophy or religious belief regarding medical care or have a conflict of interest.

The last directive encourages the person to consider a gift of life by filling out a uniform donor card (specific to the individual's state), allowing for the postmortem use of organs in transplantation, medical therapy, and medical research or education. Families are encouraged to respect this personal decision, as well as that of autopsy.

Clinical Use of the Values History

All competent adult patients should be offered the living will, the DPA-HC, and the Values History, and all three instruments should be part of geriatric assessment. POLSTs should be offered only if a patient has a specific need to guide treatment outside the medical setting, so they are not a necessary part of all geriatric assessments.

In the primary care office, preliminary questioning on end-of-life care should be initiated by the physician. This discussion usually begins with the DPA-HC designation, as it is often an easier task to identify a proxy decision maker. This take-off point is where the family covenant can then be introduced to identify boundaries set by the patient on who should be included in discussions on medical care and treatment decision. Often, this would be the appropriate moment to identify any relevant identifiable proxy negation.

The next step would be to discuss the living will in the context of future terminal illness or irreversible incapacity. When the patient signs (i.e., executes) his or her living will and/

or DPA-HC, this event should be documented within the medical record, with copies also placed in the medical record, along with an appropriate note discussing the conversations that led to these decisions as well as patient-expressed delineations of how the family can or should have a place in the patient's future health care. Such discussions should be made in a flexible, non-time-constrained fashion such that the patient's deeply held values regarding future end-of-life care can be carefully examined, and clarified, between the physician and the patient, and if allowed by the patient, by relevant family members or other loved ones. This process is also now reimbursed by CMS in both the outpatient and inpatient settings.

The physician's next step would be to introduce the Values section of the Values History. Subsequently, the physician should discuss the preferences listed in the Values History. These discussions should be rooted in the context of the person's own medical problems. For example, the physician should explain the lack of benefit of CPR to someone with conditions that generally reduce the chances of successful CPR. The acute care treatment options (e.g., CPR, intubation, and ventilation) should also be discussed early, with the patient's signature being obtained on the Values History to demonstrate the patient's consent to use of this document.

The remainder of the Values History can be discussed during follow-up visits as part of other health maintenance examinations, with documentation of subsequent decisions as they are articulated. Each treatment preference should be individually signed and dated as agreed to over time. The physician should document these treatment preferences in the medical record for that date. Treatment preferences should be rooted in the patient's values from the Values section, as well as other relevant concerns that are likely to arise in discussion. The preparation of a POLST may be appropriate in the context of this discussion if indicated by a patient's specific medical condition and preferences.

Values-based discussion allows for a more meaningful understanding of the individual's reasoning while also probing for dissonant value–preference statements or any other inconsistencies in the patient's value structure regarding healthcare treatment. Also, any impediments to the person's ability to formulate an informed consent may be gleaned through this process. The physician could thereby help the person therapeutically to restore his or her decision-making capacity. Throughout this evolving advance directive informed consent process, the law and ethics of informed consent require the physician to presume that persons are able to consent to these decisions unless unable to do so.

The Values History preserves respect for the patient by allowing the DPA-HC agent as well as other identified family covenant members to use the patient's values and preferences as a basis for healthcare decision making in the event of future incapacity. The patient should understand that this respect is best secured in advance to help his or her significant others help him or her in the future. If the individual has no advance directive or proxy, the physician should inform him or her that signing these documents would best ensure that his or her wishes would be carried out. Five states (California, Delaware, Michigan, Missouri, and New York) have had case law arise in which "clear and convincing" standards of evidence (i.e., explicit written or oral declarations) were required before withholding or withdrawing life-prolonging care. Every patient must understand that making no decision *is a decision*—in that treatment against his or her own values may be imposed if no advance directive is executed.

▶ POLST/MOLST Forms

A newer form of advance directive is the physician (or medical) order for life sustaining treatment (POLST or MOLST, although other similar acronyms—COLST, MOST, POST, or TPOPP [transportable physician orders for patient preferences] — are used in different states for similar documents). The POLST guides emergency medical personnel in a crisis and is generally meant for persons who have serious health conditions, who wish to avoid some or all life-sustaining treatments, and who reside in long-term care facilities or otherwise outside of a hospital. The POLST is created by *a patient and a clinician* knowledgeable about the patient's condition, and signed by a physician or other clinician as a standing medical order (Hanson & Doukas, 2016). Such portable medical orders are often meant to prevent the instigation of undesired burdensome medical treatments. They may also be completed to ensure medical treatment is in concert with a patient's religious views. A POLST may also be completed to ensure aggressive life-saving care is provided—though since that is the norm in an emergency situation, it may not be necessary in all cases.

Since whether a given treatment is perceived as overly burdensome, or a religious preference, is a highly personal decision, not all persons need a POLST. Generally, only patients with serious illnesses, for whom their healthcare providers "would not be surprised if they died within a year" are appropriate candidates for a POLST (National POLST Paradigm, n.d.). As these forms are medical orders, they are to be followed by medical professionals in circumstances where emergency decisions about life-sustaining care might have to be made, even outside of the hospital setting.

POLST forms are printed in a bright color—the recommended national standard is a bright pink—and require a clinician's signature to be valid. Thus, unlike the other forms of advance directives, a patient cannot complete a valid POLST himself or herself. It is therefore imperative upon clinicians to engage in discussions about these orders with patients who might benefit from a POLST well ahead of the actual need for the orders.

At time of this text's publication, all states (except South Dakota, although the state does have an out-of-hospital DNR directive that can direct EMS personnel not to engage in CPR; South Dakota Department of Health, 2017) either had a POLST program or were developing one (National POLST Paradigm, n.d.). The stage of development of the program varies from state to state, but even in states with clear law creating a POLST, the acceptance of them as valid orders in various healthcare institutions varies widely. Further, some states have forms that differ from the general norm (National POLST Paradigm, n.d.). Due to these potentially shifting factors, providers should familiarize themselves with their local state and institutional policies, and should keep up-to-date with those laws and policies in case of changes. They should also consider ensuring that persons who might encounter a patient's POLST—such as home care providers, nursing home staff, and other out-of-hospital providers—understand what the POLST means and will abide by the patient's stated preferences. A guide to state programs and the status of those programs can be found at POLST.org (National POLST Paradigm, n.d.).

Each state's POLST form is different, but the standard elements of a POLST include three major sections plus a signature space. The first section identifies the decision to request or refuse CPR if the patient has no pulse or is not breathing. The second section contains directives for medical interventions if the patient has a pulse and is breathing. The choices here normally include an option for comfort care only, including a preference to avoid transfer to the hospital, an option for basic treatment that may include hospitalization but avoidance of intensive care unit (ICU) treatment, and an option requesting any medically appropriate treatment, including transfer to an ICU. Some state's forms include explicit instructions for particular types of treatment, such as antibiotic use or dialysis, or specific directions about transfer to hospital. The third section (which may be combined with the second section) contains directives about preferences for artificial nutrition, usually including the option to request it, refuse it, or allow it for a time-limited trial period.

Since the POLST is a medical order, it must also include a section for the signature of the clinician creating the order. Which clinicians are capable of legally signing a POLST will differ

CASE EXEMPLAR

Mr. Bob Harris comes into Dr. Zelda Smith's office for an extended appointment for assessment of his abilities. Mr. Harris, who is 78 years old, is widowed and living alone. Dr. Smith asks Mr. Harris whether he has an advance directive. He replies, "Yes, after my wife's death I signed a living will and one of those health care proxies (a DPA-HC). My son John is the proxy." Dr. Smith asks what John understands about Mr. Harris's end-of-life values and preferences. He replies, "John will know what to do," but indicates that he has never engaged in any specific conversations on end-of-life treatment, as both he and his son have been a bit reluctant to talk about it. Mr. Harris also states that he has an estranged daughter, Betty, with whom he has had no contact for 9 years; they have sharply different views on health, life, and religion.

Dr. Smith uses this opportunity to initiate a conversation about advance directive values, with an emphasis on asking why Mr. Harris had executed his advance directives. His responses, which reflect the trauma of seeing his wife die, then stimulate a discussion on his own quality of life and other associated values. Dr. Smith discusses the Values History with Mr. Harris. Mr. Harris completes the Values section and addresses several acute care preferences by initialing each and signing the form.

Over the next two physician appointments, John joins Dr. Smith and Mr. Harris in discussing the remainder of the Preferences section of the Values History. Mr. Harris also lists Betty in the proxy negation so that she will not attempt to usurp John's role at some later date. Also, they agree on the POLST form preferences (for their state) that reflect his Values History values and preferences. All three parties recognize how this discussion will help in the future, and the completed copies of the forms are placed in his medical chart, with Mr. Harris keeping the originals and his son having a copy. This duplication allows for ready use in case of hospitalization and to assist the proxy to help with decision making, which in turn will help Dr. Smith with the writing of orders in the hospital.

from state to state. POLST.org (http://polst.org/elements-polst-form/) discusses the suggested structure of POLST forms, but practitioners should seek out their own state's specific POLST form.

▶ Barriers to Using Advance Directives

Potential barriers may arise in using any advance directive. First, as noted previously, the physician may delay initiating advance directive discussions with the person until the "right time" (Doukas et al., 1991). This delay of informed consent may hinder good surrogate decisions about future health care. Both the physician and the patient can lose a valuable opportunity to discuss values regarding end-of-life care if the patient becomes ill and decisions need to be made in the absence of helpful discourse on values and preferences.

Patient ambivalence or wariness in discussing advance directives can be a barrier as well. Physicians should attempt continued sensitive discussion, particularly regarding what may happen if no advance directive is ever signed.

Family members may sometimes impede the execution of an advance directive if no attempt is made to engage them during its development. A family member may disagree with a patient's refusal of medical therapies and attempt to circumvent the refusal. In such circumstances, it is helpful to acknowledge the family member's concerns and values and to inform him or her that advance directives are intended to safeguard the patient's autonomy and dignity. Of note, the family covenant helps to identify proactively the family members whom the patient considers relevant in medical decision making, as well as which persons should not be part of these discussions or subsequent decisions. Such information, when documented in the medical records, can help the patient and physician identify who has "standing" to speak for the patient when incapacity occurs.

▶ Legal Considerations

All states now have an advance directive statute (either living will, DPA-HC, or both), and many have either POLST or MOLST forms. Almost all of these statutes allow for directives to be appended to them (Society for the Right to Die, 1985). If a state does not have a statute with this stipulation, it is still prudent to append the Values History to an advance directive, as competently held values and preferences will enhance any future questions regarding the legal and moral weight of the values and preferences articulated. Organ donation statutes vary according to jurisdiction, and seeking the applicable organ donor card from the Department of Motor Vehicles and attaching it to the Values History is strongly recommended.

▶ Summary

Advance directives are a pivotal aspect of documenting advance care planning. The Values History is an important complement to formal advance directives that helps to understand the patient's living will and the DPA-HC better, and can help articulate the patient's values and preferences through the POLST. The Values History supplements, rather than replaces, these advance directives. Through its completion, all parties can gain a deeper level of meaning of what the patient wants in the future.

The greatest utility of the Values History is to facilitate discussion prior to the patient's incapacity regarding basic healthcare values and value-based preferences. A longitudinal conversation best approximates the ethical preference that informed consent be a *process* rather than an event (Doukas, 1999). So, too, should the Values History be considered merely a template to spur and facilitate an ongoing discussion of values and preferences that can then safeguard the patient's future healthcare wishes. The Values History, when coupled with contemporaneous statutory advance directives, preserves the patient's future autonomy and dignity by communicating core health values and translating these values into preferences that the physician can implement when appropriate.

References

Doukas, D. J. (1999). Ask them and they will tell you: Advance directives in patient care. *American Family Physician, 59*, 530–533.

Doukas, D., Gorenflo, D., & Coughlin, S. (1991). The living will: A national survey. *Family Medicine, 123*, 354–356.

Doukas, D. J., & Hardwig, J. (2003). Using the family covenant in planning end-of-life care: Obligations and promises of patients, families, and physicians. *Journal of the American Geriatrics Society, 51*, 1–4.

Doukas, D., Lipson, S., & McCullough, L. (1989). Value History. In W. Reichel (Ed.), *Clinical aspects of aging* (3rd ed., pp. 615–616). Baltimore, MD: Williams & Wilkins.

Doukas, D., & McCullough, L. (1988). Assessing the Values History of the aged patient regarding critical and chronic care. In J. Gallo and W. Reichel (Eds.), *The handbook of geriatric assessment* (1st ed., pp. 111–124). Rockville, MD: Aspen.

Doukas, D., & McCullough, L. (1991). The Values History: The evaluation of the patient's values and advance directives. *Journal of Family Practice, 3*, 145–153.

Doukas, D., & Reichel, W. (1993). *Planning for uncertainty: A guide to living wills and other advance directives for health care.* Baltimore, MD: Johns Hopkins University Press.

Eisendrath, S., & Jonsen, A. (1983). The living will: Help or hindrance? *Journal of the American Medical Association,* 2054–2058.

Hanson, S. S., & Doukas, D. J. (2016). Advance care planning. In C. Arenson, J. Busby-Whitehead, S. Durso, M. F. Singh, L. Mosqueda, D. Swagerty, & W. Reichel (Eds.), *Reichel's care of the elderly* (7th ed., pp. 781–796). Cambridge, UK: Cambridge University Press.

National POLST Paradigm. (n.d.). State programs. Retrieved from http://polst.org/programs-in-your-state/

Omnibus Budget Reconciliation Act, Public Law No. 101–508 §§4206, 4751 (1990).

Society for the Right to Die. (1985). *The physician and the hopelessly ill patient: Legal, medical, and ethical guidelines.* New York, NY: Author.

South Dakota Department of Health. (2017). Comfort One (DNR). Retrieved from http://doh.sd.gov/providers/ruralhealth/ems/advanced-directives.aspx

SUPPORT Investigators. (1995). A controlled trial to improve outcomes for seriously ill hospitalized patients: The study to understand prognoses and preferences for outcomes and risks of treatment. *Journal of the American Medical Association, 274,* 1591–1598.

Teno, J. M., Lynn, J., Wenger, N., Phillips, R. S., Murphy, D. P., Connors, A. F. Jr., . . . Knaus, W.A. (1997). Advance directives for seriously ill hospitalized patients: Effectiveness with the Patient Self-Determination Act and the SUPPORT intervention. *Journal of the American Geriatric Society, 45,* 500–507.

U.S. Department of Health and Human Services, Centers for Medicare and Medicaid Services. (2016). 42 CFR Parts 405, 410, 411, 414, 425, 495, [CMS-1631-P], RIN 0938-AS40; Medicare Program; Revisions to Payment Policies under the Physician Fee Schedule and Other Revisions to Part B for CY 2016.

Wanzer, S., Adelstein, J., Cranford, R., Federman D. D., Hook, E. D., Moertel C. G., . . . van Eys, J. (1984). The physician's responsibility toward hopelessly ill patients. *New England Journal of Medicine, 310,* 955–959.

Appendix 40A

The Values History

Patient name: _____

This Values History serves as a set of my specific value-based directives for various medical interventions. It is to be used in healthcare circumstances when I may be unable to voice my preferences. These directives shall be made a part of the medical record and used as supplementary to my living will and/or durable power of attorney for health care.

I. Values Section

Values are things that are important to us in our lives and our relationships with others—especially loved ones. There are several values important in decisions about terminal treatment and care. This section of the Values History invites you to identify your most important values.

A. Basic Life Values

Perhaps the most basic values in this context concern length of life versus quality of life. Which of the following two statements is the most important to you?

_____ 1. I want to live as long as possible, regardless of the quality of life that I experience.

_____ 2. I want to preserve a good quality of life, even if this means that I may not live as long.

B. Quality-of-Life Values

There are many values that help us to define for ourselves the quality of life that we want to live. Review this list (and feel free to either elaborate on it or add to it), and circle those values that are most important to your definition of quality of life.

1. I want to maintain my capacity to think clearly.
2. I want to feel safe and secure.
3. I want to avoid unnecessary pain and suffering.
4. I want to be treated with respect.
5. I want to be treated with dignity when I can no longer speak for myself.
6. I do not want to be an unnecessary burden on my family.
7. I want to be able to make my own decisions.
8. I want to experience a comfortable dying process.
9. I want to be with my loved ones before I die.
10. I want to leave good memories of me to my loved ones.
11. I want to be treated in accord with my religious beliefs and traditions.

12. I want respect shown for my body after I die.
13. I want to help others by making a contribution to medical education and research.
14. Other values or clarification of values above: _____

II. Preferences Section

Some directives involve simple yes or no decisions. Others provide for the choice of a trial of intervention. Use the values identified above to explain why you made the choice you did. The information will be very useful to your family, healthcare surrogate (or proxy), and healthcare providers.

Initials/Date

___ ___ 1. I want to undergo cardiopulmonary resuscitation.

_____ Yes

_____ No

Why? _____

___ ___ 2. I want to be placed on a ventilator. (Please note: If you answer NO to CPR #1, then the default is NO on this item as well, as this option is part of the treatment of cardiopulmonary resuscitation.)

_____ Yes

_____ Trial for the time period of

_____ Trial to determine effectiveness using reasonable medical judgment

_____ No

Why? _____

___ ___ 3. I want to have an endotracheal tube used to perform items 1 and 2. (Please note: If you answer NO to CPR #1, then the default is NO on this item as well, as this option is part of the treatment of cardiopulmonary resuscitation.)

_____ Yes

_____ Trial for the time period of

_____ Trial to determine effectiveness using reasonable medical judgment

_____ No

Why? _____

___ ___ 4. I want to have total parenteral nutrition administered for my nutrition.

_____ Yes

_____ Trial for the time period of

_____ Trial to determine effectiveness using reasonable medical judgment

_____ No

Why? _____

___ ___ 5. I want to have intravenous medication and hydration administered; regardless of my decision, I understand that intravenous hydration to alleviate discomfort or pain medication will not be withheld from me if I so request them.

_____ Yes

_____ Trial for the time period of

_____ Trial to determine effectiveness using reasonable medical judgment

_____ No

Why? _____

___ ___ 6. I want to have all medications used for the treatment of my illness continued; regardless of my decision, I understand that pain medication will continue to be administered, including narcotic medications.

_____ Yes

_____ Trial for the time period of

_____ Trial to determine effectiveness using reasonable medical judgment

_____ No

Why? _____

___ ___ 7. I want to have nasogastric, gastrostomy, or other enteral feeding tubes introduced and administered for my nutrition.

_____ Yes

_____ Trial for the time period of

_____ Trial to determine effectiveness using reasonable medical judgment

_____ No

Why? _____

___ ___ 8. I want to be placed on a dialysis machine.

_____ Yes

_____ Trial for the time period of

_____ Trial to determine effectiveness using reasonable medical judgment

_____ No

Why? _____

___ ___ 9. I want to have an autopsy done to determine the cause(s) of my death.

_____ Yes

_____ No

Why?_____

___ ___ 10. I want to be admitted to the intensive care unit if necessary. (Please note: If you answer NO to CPR #1, then the default in some hospitals is NO on this item as well, as refusing cardiopulmonary resuscitation means you also refuse intensive care unit treatment.)

_____ Yes

_____ No

Why? _____

___ ___ 11. If I become a patient in a long-term care facility or if I receive care at home and experience a life-threatening change in health status, I want 911 called in case of a medical emergency. (Add your state-required "At Home DNR order" here, if applicable.)

_____ Yes

_____ No

Why? _____

__ __ ___ 12. Other directives: _____

I consent to these directives after receiving honest disclosure of their implications, risks, and benefits by my physician, free from constraints and being of sound mind.

_____	_____
Signature	Date
_____	
Witness	
_____	
Witness	

___ ___ 13. Proxy negation:

I request that the following persons NOT be allowed to make decisions on my behalf in the event of my disability or incapacity: _____

_____	_____
Signature	Date
_____	
Witness	
_____	
Witness	

___ ___ 14. Organ donation:

Specific state version inserted/attached here

Modified from Doukas, D., & McCullough, L. (1991). The values history: The evaluation of the patient's values and advance directives. *The Journal of Family Practice, 32*(2), 145-153. Reprinted with permission from *The Journal of Family Practice*. © 2018, Frontline Medical Communications Inc.

CHAPTER 41

Clinical Assessment of Older Persons with Developmental Disabilities

Christine McDonough and Kara Peterik

▶ Introduction

People with **developmental disabilities (DD)** present with a wide range of conditions. *Developmental disability* is a term that was introduced

in the 1960s, and it encompasses various conditions that share onset early in life and, therefore, long duration of impact with developmental implications (Crocker, 2006). The Rehabilitation Act Amendments of 1978 provided a definition of developmental disability that has been widely used (PL 95-602):

> A severe, chronic disability of a person which (A) is attributable to a mental or physical impairment or combination of mental or physical impairments; (B) is manifested before the person attains the age of twenty-two; (C) is likely to continue indefinitely; (D) results in substantial functional limitations in three or more of the following areas of major life activity: (i) self-care, (ii) receptive and expressive language, (iii) learning, (iv) mobility, (v) self-direction, (vi) capacity for independent living, and (vii) economic sufficiency; and (E) reflects the person's need for a combination and sequence of special interdisciplinary, or generic care, treatment, or other services which are life-long or extended duration and are individually planned and coordinated.

Although this definition has endured, several elements have been added to the Patient's Bill of Rights since 1979, and amendments and acts have been passed to increase protections and to integrate important societal goals such as inclusion in the community, independence, and financial productivity (Crocker, 2006).

Developmental disability includes genetic and acquired conditions causing chromosomal changes as well as conditions caused by environmental exposures and pregnancy-related conditions. Down syndrome, congenital heart disease, cerebral palsy, seizure disorders, and neurologic disorders such as neural tube defects are some examples. The term **intellectual disabilities (ID)** has largely replaced *mental retardation* and includes autism spectrum disorders as well as Down syndrome and other congenital disorders, representing a large proportion of the people with developmental disabilities.

Ultimately, DD/ID refers to the people growing, working, playing, and having relationships who have a wide range of physical, cognitive, behavioral, mental health, social, and environmental challenges. These individuals are increasingly reaching older age, and experiencing substantial barriers to access to community integration, education, financial productivity, independence, and healthcare services. On the one hand, **older adults** with DD require tailored, patient-centered care that reflects the specific challenges and opportunities they face, and evidence shows that **assessment** tailored to specific health characteristics improves care (Lennox et al., 2007). On the other hand, similar to the general population, for a large proportion of people with DD, the non-specialty-based community medical system is capable of providing appropriate medical care (Crocker, 2006).

▶ Developmental Disabilities Are Important to Geriatric Clinical Assessment

The topic of DD when performing **geriatric** assessment is of critical importance for several reasons. First, there is an ethical imperative to provide high-quality care to older adults with DD. Second, the number of adults with ID/DD is increasing. Estimates based on the 2010 U.S. Census suggest that there were more than 850,000 community-dwelling adults age 60 and older with developmental disabilities when these data were collected (Factor, Heller, & Janicki, 2012). This number is expected to increase to 1.4 million by 2030.

Third, there are known disparities in health and health care for people with DD. For example, people with DD experience worse health, more impairments and functional limitations, and shorter life expectancy (Balogh et al., 2016; Ouellette-Kuntz et al., 2005). Among the other risk factors associated with reduced life expectancy in individuals with DD are severe motor and functional impairment for people with cerebral palsy, refractory seizures associated with seizure disorders/epilepsy, chronic upper respiratory infection, heart conditions, choking, reduced mobility, and eating and toileting difficulties (Service, Tyler, & Janicki, 2006).

▶ Disparities in Care and Health Are Substantial

In 2002, the U.S. Surgeon General published a report titled "Closing the Gap: A National Blueprint to Improve the Health of Persons with Mental Retardation." This report, which included input from the DD community, reported that people with mental retardation experience "more difficulty finding, getting to and paying for appropriate health care" (U.S. Department of Health and Human Services, 2002). Disparities are worse for people with mental retardation from minority communities, and estimates indicate that the proportion of the total U.S. population accounted for by non-Hispanic Caucasians will decrease to 54% by 2050 (Factor et al., 2012); thus, minority subpopulations are expected to grow in the near term. Needs of people with DD who are from minority populations often go undetected due to the different cultural norms about care and because of language barriers (Factor et al., 2012). Pursuing cultural competency for the populations served and providing care in the patient's native language or via translation are two strategies with the potential to improve care for this particularly vulnerable segment of the population with DD.

Eliminating health disparities for people with disabilities is an ongoing goal of the national *Healthy People* initiative. Indeed, one of the 2020 goals is to "maximize health, prevent chronic disease, improve social and environmental living conditions, and promote full community participation, choice, health equity, and quality of life among individuals with disabilities of all ages" (U.S. Department of Health and Human Services, 2017).

Whereas older adults with DD experience the same overall physical process of aging as do adults without DD, biological, physical, and social factors may combine to produce earlier development of chronic health conditions in these individuals than in other adults (Factor et al., 2012). However, compared to other patient populations, people with DD are subject to different levels of health risks, exhibit different clinical presentations, and may not match the usual expectation of the clinical course of a health condition.

▶ Geriatric Care for People with DD Should Be Tailored Based on Their Conditions

Life expectancies vary depending on the specific conditions underlying DD. Risk factors for decreased life expectancy include severe seizure disorders, heart conditions, severe physical and intellectual impairments and associated health conditions, and chronic respiratory infections (Service et al., 2006). In addition, people with DD are at elevated risk for earlier development of some geriatric syndromes and other chronic conditions:

- At age 60, the prevalence of Alzheimer's-type dementia among adults with Down syndrome is estimated to be as high as 50%, compared to the population prevalence of 6% (Janicki & Dalton, 2000; Service et al., 2006; Zigman & Lott, 2007).

- Osteoporosis has been found to occur earlier in life for people with DD, potentially due to use of antiseizure medications and the presence of vitamin D insufficiency (Service et al., 2006; Tyler, Snyder, & Zyzanski, 2000).

- Some individuals with DD are vulnerable to seizure disorders and their sequelae, including increased risk of unexpected death, social impacts, and seizure-related injuries (Service et al., 2006).

- Obesity rates of people with intellectual development disabilities (IDD) in the United States range from 21% to 33.6% (Stancliffe et al., 2011); other research has found obesity rates high as 70% in adults with Down syndrome (Rimmer & Wang, 2005). Individuals with IDD tend to be sedentary, not achieving levels of appropriate physical activity (Mann, Zhou, McDermott, & Poston, 2006; Peterson, Janz, & Lowe, 2008; Seekins, Traci, Bainbridge, & Humphries, 2005).
- In many countries, the chief cause of death for people with ID is cardiovascular disease (Haveman et al., 2009).
- People with ID have a higher risk of falls.
- People with ID are at higher risk of being abused.
- Dental conditions are among the most common problems for people with ID (Haveman et al., 2009).
- Women with DD experience menopause earlier than those without DD (Coppus et al., 2010).
- People with neuromuscular disorders (e.g., cerebral palsy) are more likely to experience sarcopenia, osteoporosis, arthritis, and pain (Strax, Luciano, Dunn, & Quevedo, 2010).

Additionally, Haveman et al. (2009) include declines in mobility, increases in pain, increases in visual and hearing impairment, and changes to bowel and bladder function as signs of aging in those persons with ID.

The concept of aging should be carefully considered in the context of the lived experience of people with DD. Aging within the biological context refers to the processes of growth, maturation, and deterioration of body structures and functions (Haveman et al., 2009). The two key mechanisms for aging are believed to be genetic programming to complete maturation and initiate aging, and social, behavioral, psychological, and environmental impacts on the body (Haveman et al., 2009). Environmental factors that relate to specific events in time

also influence individuals with DD. Historical societal treatment of people with DD has had profound impacts on aging within this subpopulation, and local history may reveal relevant issues. For example, more recent interventions can have more durable impacts over time on younger people with DD compared to their predecessors. Prior policies, such as institutionalization, in the United States will have affected the health and functioning of large numbers of older adults today, as will prior trends in service provision and policies.

Haveman and Stöppler have advanced the concept of *functional aging* related to their work in the area of ID (Haveman, 2004; Haveman & Stöppler, 2004). They and others have found that for people with ID, aging is meaningful within the context of changes in functional ability—in particular, "being able to do things and participate in activities; nutrition; and hygiene and self-care" (Haveman et al., 2009). This relationship, combined with increases in risk of disorders for people with DD, makes the concept of functional aging particularly valuable in the context of clinical assessment. Chronological age may not be as useful as a trigger for assessment of specific issues in individuals with DD as it is in the general population. Therefore, a key component of clinical assessment of older adults with DD should be developing an understanding of their physical, cognitive, social, and behavioral function so that changes can be detected and addressed in a timely manner. Functional decline should be recognized as an important indicator of potential health conditions and aging. Understanding of function is a relatively new aspect of clinical care, and the theory and methods for its assessment continue to evolve. There are many available measures, which are discussed in other chapters of this text. Clinicians may need to use a "rolling" approach to assessment, whereby selected domains of functioning are addressed at each visit, to feasibly build a strong understanding of the specific patient's baseline status (Service et al., 2006).

A key role for clinicians in the care of people with DD is to support their autonomy.

Geriatric caregivers will be familiar with age-related biases that can undermine older adults' opportunities to make choices and determine their own paths. The assumptions and biases that limit self-determination for older adults are in play throughout life for people with DD. Therefore, it is critical that clinicians understand their patients' capabilities and respect their rights. Janicki and Ansello (2000) introduced the term *assisted autonomy* to describe supported self-determination through negotiation and decision making with the assistance of others. The need for assisted autonomy in many cases underlines the importance of developing a collaborative relationship with the patient and key caregiver(s) (Service et al., 2006).

▶ Challenges to Providing High-Quality Care for Older Adults with DD

One important modifiable source of health disparities in older adults with DD is the rate at which health conditions—for example, arthritis, hypertension, heart disease, chronic obstructive pulmonary disease (COPD), diabetes, cerebrovascular disease, atherosclerosis, and cancer—go unrecognized. More frequent clinical assessment may be appropriate to effectively evaluate the likelihood of new health conditions or changes in functional status that require intervention. Unfortunately, people with DD often report having difficulty finding clinicians who will provide care (e.g., dentistry, gynecology, ophthalmology, mental health), experiencing long wait times, and finding the physical environment in which care is delivered difficult or impossible to access (Ward, Nichols, & Freedman, 2010). People with ID are more likely to report unmet needs for health/mental care, prescription medications, and dental care than the general population (Anderson, Larson, Lakin, & Kwak, 2003; Krahn, Hammond, & Turner, 2006; Parish, Moss, & Richman, 2008).

Although some of these access issues require financial and policy changes, some may be within the purview of clinicians and their institutions. Physicians report limited experience and comfort interacting with people with DD, insufficient training in issues specific to DD, inadequate reimbursement for necessary care, and restraints on time (Reichard & Turnbull, 2004). Whereas clinical practice guidelines often provide critical knowledge to support consistent quality care, the lack of inclusion of content related to the health needs of people with DD further intensifies the challenges facing healthcare providers (Haveman et al., 2009). Other important reasons for limited quality of care include a primary clinical focus on DD, at the expense of strategic planning for prevention and management of secondary conditions so critical to function and participation; lack of appropriate professional training; and social barriers such as poverty.

▶ Clinical Assessment

In general, clinicians should use the same principles and approaches described throughout this text when assessing older adults with DD. This section highlights those aspects of assessment that may require adjustment for people with DD. In particular, assessment of pain, cognitive ability, mental health, physical function, and social support are domains of key importance for people with DD.

Medical, Developmental, and Functional History

Existing physical, cognitive, mental health, and behavioral impairments may complicate the diagnostic process for older adults with DD. Therefore, a thorough understanding of patients' medical and functional history and current status is critical to establishing their clinical needs and identifying clinically significant changes at their earliest presentation. Keep in mind that in addition to the history provided by the patient, information from a caregiver, a guardian, and/or family members plays an important role in many cases (Deb, Matthews, Holt, & Bouras, 2001). The following medical, social, and functional history should be taken:

- History of DD: Cause of DD, history in family, developmental milestones
- Psychosocial history: Personality and behavior; principal relationships (support/ caregivers and social); current and previous levels of interpersonal interactions with others in the family, at school, or at work; daily and weekly routines; living situation (in own home, with family, in an assisted living residence)
- Education, school, and job history: Important life events and academic level reached
- Medical history:

  - Past, present, and recurrent illnesses
  - Drug history: Past, recent changes, and current medications; adverse event history; known allergies and past reactions; substance and alcohol use
  - Physical: Spasticity; functional ability level and limitations
  - Cognitive: Ability level and limitations
  - Communication: Ability level and how the person communicates pain or discomfort
  - Psychiatric and behavioral: Diagnoses, contact with psychiatric services, assessment of risk to self and/or others
  - Vision and hearing
  - Forensic: Problems with the law (patient, family, friends)
  - History of present complaint

Knowing the older adult's history allows the clinician to detect new health conditions and changes in function.

Pain Assessment

Self-report is the current gold standard for assessing the patient's experience of pain (Baldridge & Andrasik, 2010). People with DD may have difficulty describing, locating, and rating the severity of their pain, and clinicians may face challenges in understanding these patients due to lack of familiarity with the specific patient with DD and his or her cognitive and communication functioning (Baldridge & Andrasik, 2010). Even so, clinicians should attempt to obtain self-reports of pain, if possible, and also consider observed or reported behavior changes such as self-injurious behavior, aggression, nonverbal vocal expressions, agitation, and facial expressions (Herr & Garand, 2001). The American Society for Pain Management Nursing recommends using a hierarchical approach for nonverbal patients: (1) obtain a self-report (elicit yes/no responses, vocalizations, hand grasp or eye blink), (2) look for potential causes of pain (e.g., pathological sources, procedures that knowingly cause iatrogenic pain), (3) observe patient behaviors (de Knegt et al., 2013; Herr, Coyne, McCaffery, Manworren, & Merkel, 2011), (4) obtain a caregiver/ family proxy report of behavior or activity changes, and (5) attempt an analgesic trial.

Chan, Hadjistavropoulos, Williams, and Lint-Martindale (2014) developed the observation-based Pain Assessment Checklist for Seniors with Limited Ability to Communicate (PACSLAC-II), a 31-item checklist for older adults with communication difficulties. The checklist is broken into six sections: facial expressions, verbalizations and vocalizations, body movements, changes in interpersonal interactions, changes in activity patterns or routines, and mental status changes. De Knegt et al. (2013) note that visual analog or numeric rating scales assessing pain correlate with observational scales, and suggest that using both types of scales can provide a more complete assessment of pain.

Cognitive Assessment

Screening and assessment tools for the detection of dementia in the general population are usually not appropriate for people with ID because of floor effects in the measures (Deb, Hare, Prior, & Bhaumik, 2007). Alternative approaches fall into two categories: caregiver reports and those that involve the direct assessment of the individual (Strydom et al., 2009).

Caregiver/Informant Assessments

The Dementia Screening Questionnaire for Individuals Intellectual Disabilities (DSQIID) is an observer-rated dementia screening tool developed for adults with ID. This 53-item checklist has acceptable internal consistency, and good test–retest and interrater reliability. DSQIID takes approximately 10–15 minutes to complete and can be done at home or in a clinic (Deb et al., 2007).

The Adaptive Behaviour Dementia Questionnaire (ABDQ) is a 15-item tool that assesses for changes in adaptive behavior to screen for Alzheimer's dementia in adults with Down syndrome. It has acceptable reliability and validity. Its reported positive predictive value is 89% and the negative predictive value is 94%, with an accuracy rate of 92% (Prasher, Farooq, & Holder, 2004).

The Cambridge Examination for Mental Disorders of Older People with Down Syndrome and others with Intellectual Disability (CAMDEX-DS) (Ball, Holland, Huppert, Treppner, & Dodd, 2006) is a semi-structured interview of caregiver/informants modified from the CAMDEX, which was developed for early diagnosis and measurement of dementia in general older adult populations. The CAMDEX-DS asks for a history of cognitive and activities of daily living (ADLs) and mood and functional decline over time.

Direct Assessment of Persons with ID

The Cambridge Cognitive Examination—Down Syndrome version (CAMCOG-DS version; Ball, Holland, Hon, et al., 2006) is the neuropsychological component of the CAMDEX-DS and is adapted from CAMCOG, a brief neuropsychological battery used to assess cognitive function. It is usually administered by a mental health professional as a direct assessment with persons with ID.

Mental Health Assessment

Little is known about "usual" psychological development across the lifespan in persons with ID. Many individuals with ID have restricted social roles and networks (Service et al., 2006). The Vanderbilt Kennedy Center for Excellence in Developmental Disabilities (n.d.) developed a comprehensive toolkit for primary care providers that provides guidance on assessing behavioral and mental issues in adults with IDD. This toolkit included several checklists and assessment tools to guide the care of behavioral and mental health problems for adults with IDD in a primary care setting.

The psychiatric assessment schedule for adults with developmental disabilities (PAS-ADD) (Moss, Ibbotson, Prosser, Patel, & Simpson, 1997) provides both a 25-item screening checklist, which untrained persons can use to identify mental health issues in adults with ID, and a structured clinical interview, which requires training to administer. The PAS-ADD clinical interview uses information from both the patient and a key informant. Either interview can produce research diagnoses, so the PAS-ADD can be used with nonverbal patients.

Functional Assessment

The most common challenges in assessment of physical function are associated with severe physical limitations (e.g., requiring wheelchair or assistive devices to get around) and cognitive/communication limitations. When feasible, clinicians should use measures recommended in the *Physical Assessment* and *Mobility Assessment* chapters (e.g., Timed Up and Go, 6-minute walk tests), documenting necessary adjustments (e.g., assistive device use, rest periods) for future comparison. The PULSES profile tool is a comprehensive assessment that is used to evaluate ADLs in older and chronically ill persons. Specifically, it evaluates physical condition, upper limb function, lower limb function, sensory components, excretory function, and mental and emotional status (Granger, Sherwood, & Greer, 1977; Moskowitz, 1985). It can be used to assist in program and rehabilitation planning.

Self-report measures that account for use of a wheelchair or other assistive device, such as the Activity Measure for Post-Acute Care (AM-PAC) (Haley et al., 2004) and the Patient-Reported Outcome Measurement Information System (PROMIS) (Rose, Bjorner, Becker, Fries, & Ware, 2008) physical function scales, may be helpful for patients who are able to provide self-reports of their functional ability. In combination with history and observation, administration of a self-report measure by a proxy (e.g., the caregiver) can provide useful information. Evidence indicates that proxy-reported function is moderately correlated with self-report (median correlations: 0.60–0.70), and that caregiver proxies tend to report more limited function (Andresen, Vahle, & Lollar, 2001; Hilari, Owen, & Farrelly, 2007; Horowitz, Goodman, & Reinhardt, 2004; Sneeuw, Sprangers, & Aaronson, 2002).

Social/Social Support Assessment

Older adults with DD and their social support networks face special challenges in regard to aging in place and engaging in society. Most persons with DD live with their families (25% in their own home, 60% with family, and 12% in a formal residence facility) (Factor et al., 2012). During the assessment of persons with DD, clinicians should consider the potential impact of financial issues, guardianship, decision-making support, residential planning, vocational support, and needs for community involvement.

Because there is wide variation by state in the resources provided for people with disabilities, clinicians should conduct a social support scan of their area, including the DD and aging services systems. The Administration for Community Living (2017) supports a range of programs, including Aging and Disability Networks. Examples of DD services networks include state Councils of DD, Disability Advocacy Agencies, and University Centers for Excellence in DD. Some of the aging services networks include the National Respite Network, National Council on Aging Senior Centers, Centers for Independent Living, Eldercare Locator, Community Service and Employment Program, Long-Term Care Ombudsman, and Elder Abuse programs. In many cases, it will be helpful to provide a referral to a social worker for full assessment and development of a plan for support services.

▶ Preventive Health

In addition to the guidance provided throughout this text, detailed recommendations for preventive health for older adults with DD have been published by Service et al. in 2006 and Sullivan et al. in 2011 (**TABLE 41-1**). These guidelines address timing and frequency of preventive health assessments. Although many recommendations are similar to those for older adults without DD, these guidelines address conditions for which adults with DD are at increased risk. Specific conditions that adults with DD are at a higher risk of developing include: cardiac disease, obesity, dental disease, gastrointestinal and feeding disorders (e.g., GERD and *H. Pylori* infection), osteoporosis, and endocrine disorders (e.g., thyroid disease and diabetes in adults with Down syndrome). Screening for these secondary conditions is imperative in adults with DD.

TABLE 41-1 Healthcare Guidelines for Older Adults with Developmental Disabilities*

Condition	Clinical Assessment
Sensory Impairment Visual impairment Hearing impairment	Vision and hearing impairments can be overlooked in adults with DD. Visual acuity test, glaucoma screen, and ophthalmoscopy every 1–2 years. Perform otoscopy and audiometry every 1–2 years.
Cardiovascular Hypertension Atrial fibrillation Physical activity Hyperlipidemia	Cardiac disorders are common in adults with DD. They are at risk for developing coronary artery disease due to lack of physical activity, smoking, and possibly from the use of certain psychotropic medicines. Check blood pressure annually. Assess heart rhythm. Review physical activity habits and provide exercise counseling if needed. Order a fasting lipid profile every 5 years, and more frequently if the patient is taking atypical antipsychotic medications or has diabetes.
Diabetes	Screen annually after age 45. Adults with Down syndrome are at a higher risk of developing diabetes.
Thyroid Disease	Perform a thyroid-stimulating hormone (TSH) test annually. Consider a TSH test if there is an unexplained change in behavior or level of functioning. Adults with DD have a higher risk of developing thyroid disease than the general population.
Cancer Screening Colon cancer Breast cancer Cervical cancer Skin cancer Prostate cancer Ovarian cancer Lung cancer	At age 50, screen with one of the following strategies: Conduct fecal occult blood testing yearly along with flexible sigmoidoscopy every 3 years; colonoscopy every 10 years; or flexible sigmoidoscopy every 5 years or fecal occult blood testing yearly. Perform mammography every 1–2 years and clinical breast exam yearly. No screening is necessary if the woman has no history of sexual intercourse. No screening is necessary for a woman with hysterectomy for noncancer indications. May cease Pap smears after age 65 if the woman has no history of human papillomavirus (HPV) or abnormal Pap smears and has three documented normal Pap smears. Perform an annual Pap smear if the woman tests positive for HPV. Perform clinical skin examination. Screening by prostate-specific antigen (PSA) is controversial. Discuss the risks, benefits, and limitations. No adequate screening methodologies are available, including bimanual pelvic examinations and CA-125 monitoring. No adequate screening methodologies are available. Provide smoking cessation counseling for current smokers.

(continues)

TABLE 41-1 Healthcare Guidelines for Older Adults with Developmental Disabilities* *(continued)*

Condition	Clinical Assessment
Dental Disease	Perform an annual oral exam. Refer patient to a dentist for regular dental care, including cleaning every 6 months or as recommended by a dentist. Dental disease is a common health issue in adults with DD because they can have difficulty maintaining an oral hygiene routine.
Nutritional Issues Obesity Malnutrition Osteoporosis	Measure height, weight, and body mass index (BMI) annually. Perform nutrition screening. Osteoporosis tends to occur earlier in adults with DD than the general population. There are several risk factors that impact adults with DD including limited mobility, higher risk of falls, specific genetic syndromes (e.g., Down and Prader-Willi), and long-term use of certain drugs (e.g., glucocorticoids, anticonvulsants). Assure that the individual has daily intake of 1500 mg calcium and 800 IU vitamin D. Consider bone mineral density (BMD) screening earlier and at regular intervals for high-risk patients. Check serum vitamin D (OH) levels at regular interviews.
Mental Health Depression Sleep Social isolation Abuse/neglect Substance abuse	Screen annually or sooner for behaviors or emotions that may indicate depression. Assess for sleep interval changes. Assess for changes in social network. Screen annually. Behavioral changes that may indicate signs of abuse include unexplained change in weight, aggression, withdrawal, depression, avoidance, poor self-esteem, inappropriate attachment or sexualized behavior, sleep or eating disorders, and substance abuse. Screen for alcohol, drug, and tobacco use.
Functional Changes Cognitive impairments Mobility impairments Falls Incontinence	Screen for changes in cognitive function. Screen for changes in mobility. Evaluate fall risk annually. Screen for changes in continence.
Immunizations Tetanus/diphtheria Pneumococcal Influenza Hepatitis B	Primary series and booster every 10 years. Give at age 65 and review indications for booster. Annually. Primary series and review indications for booster.

Condition	Clinical Assessment
Advance Planning Advance directives	Review and updated advance directives and specify a person to assist with decision making.
Medication Review	Review medications at regular intervals with patients and caregivers to assure adherence and evaluate for side effects or interactions.

* Modified slightly from Service et al. (2006) and Sullivan (2011).

Modified from Service, K. P., Tyler, C. V. J., & Janicki, M. P. (2006). Geriatrics. In I. L. Rubin & A. C. Crocker (Eds.), *Medical Care for Children & Adults with Developmental Disabilities* (pp. 575–590). Baltimore, MD: Paul H. Brookes Publishing Co.

▶ Summary

Getting to know your older patients with DD and their support network is the key to tailoring the assessment and management plan to meet their unique needs. The usual geriatric care principles and preventive care, combined with supported autonomy, serve as the foundation from which adjustments are made based on the specific cause of DD, patient abilities, and related conditions.

References

Administration for Community Living. (2017, October 10). Programs: Overview. Retrieved from https://www.acl.gov/programs

Anderson, L. L., Humphries, K., McDermott, S., Marks, B., Sisirak, J., & Larson, S. (2013). The state of the science of health and wellness for adults with intellectual and developmental disabilities. *Intellectual and Developmental Disabilities, 51*(5), 385–398.

Anderson, L. L., Larson, S. A., Lakin, K. C., & Kwak, N. (2003). *Health insurance coverage and health care experiences of persons with disabilities in the NHIS-D. DD Data Brief* (Vol. 5). Minneapolis, MN: University of Minnesota, Research and Training Center on Community Living.

Andresen, E. M., Vahle, V. J., & Lollar, D. (2001). Proxy reliability: Health-related quality of life (HRQoL) measures for people with disability. *Quality of Life Research, 10*(7), 609–619.

Baldridge, K. H., & Andrasik, F. (2010). Pain assessment in people with intellectual or developmental disabilities. *American Journal of Nursing, 110*(12), 28–35.

Ball, S. L., Holland, A. J., Hon, J., Huppert, F. A., Treppner, P., & Watson, P. C. (2006). Personality and behaviour changes mark the early stages of Alzheimer's disease in adults with Down's syndrome: Findings from a prospective population-based study. *International Journal of Geriatric Psychiatry, 21*(7), 661–673.

Ball, S., Holland, T., Huppert, F., Treppner, P., & Dodd, K. (2006). *The Cambridge examination for mental disorders of older people with Down's syndrome and others with intellectual disabilities.* Cambridge, UK: Cambridge University Press.

Balogh, R., McMorris, C. A., Lunsky, Y., Ouellette-Kuntz, H., Bourne, L., Colantonio, A., & Gonçalves-Bradley, D. C. (2016). Organising healthcare services for persons with an intellectual disability. *Cochrane Database of Systematic Reviews, 4*, CD007492.

Chan, S., Hadjistavropoulos, T., Williams, J., & Lints-Martindale, A. (2014). Evidence-based development and initial validation of the pain assessment checklist for seniors with limited ability to communicate-II (PACSLAC II). *Clinical Journal of Pain, 30*(9), 816–824.

Coppus, A. M. W., Evenhuis, H. M., Verberne, G.-J., Visser, F. E., Eikenlenboom, P., van Gool, W. A., & van Duijn, C. M. (2010). Early age at menopause is associated with increased risk of dementia and mortality in women with Down syndrome. *Journal of Alzheimer's Disease, 19*, 545–550.

Crocker, A. C. (2006). The developmental disabilities. In I. L. Rubin & A. C. Crocker (Eds.), *Medical care for children and adults with developmental disabilities* (2nd ed., pp. 15–23). Baltimore, MD: Paul H. Brookes Publishing.

Deb, S., Hare, M., Prior, L., & Bhaumik, S. (2007). Dementia screening questionnaire for individuals with intellectual disabilities. *British Journal of Psychiatry, 190*(5), 440–444.

Deb, S., Matthews, T., Holt, G., & Bouras, N. (2001). *Practice guidelines for the assessment and diagnosis of mental health problems in adults with intellectual disability.* Cheapside, UK: Pavilion/The Ironworks.

de Knegt, N. C., Pieper, M. J., Lobbezoo, F., Schuengel, C., Evenhuis, H. M., Passchier, J., & Scherder, E. J. (2013). Behavioral pain indicators in people with intellectual disabilities: A systematic review. *Journal of Pain, 14*(9), 885–896.

Factor, A., Heller, T., & Janicki, M. (2012). *Bridging the aging and developmental disabilities service networks: Challenges and best practices.* Chicago, IL: Institute on Disability and Human Development, University of Illinois at Chicago.

Granger, C. V., Sherwood, C. C., & Greer, D. S. (1977). Functional status measures in a comprehensive stroke care program. *Archives of Physical Medicine and Rehabilitation, 58,* 555–561.

Haley, S. M., Coster, W. J., Andres, P. L., Ludlow, L. H., Ni, P., Bond, T. L., . . . Jette, A. M. (2004). Activity outcome measurement for postacute care. *Medical Care, 42* (1 Suppl.), I49–I61.

Haveman, M. J. (2004). Disease epidemiology and aging people with intellectual disabilities. *Journal of Policy and Practice in Intellectual Disabilities, 1,* 16–23.

Haveman, M. J., Heller, T., Lee, L. A, Maaskant, M. A, Shooshtari, S., & Strydom, A. (2009). *Report on the state of science on health risks and ageing in people with intellectual disabilities.* Dortmund, Germany: IASSID Special Interest Research Group on Ageing and Intellectual Disabilities/Faculty Rehabilitation Sciences, University of Dortmund.

Haveman, M. J., & Stöppler, R. (2004). *Altern mit geistiger Behinderung.* Stuttgart, Germany: Kohlhammer Verlag.

Herr, K., Coyne, P., McCaffery, M., Manworren, R., & Merkel, S. (2011). Pain assessment in the patient unable to self-report: Position statement with clinical practice recommendations. *Pain Management Nursing, 12*(4), 230–250.

Herr, K., & Garand, L. (2001). Assessment and measurement of pain in older adults. *Clinics in Geriatric Medicine, 17*(3), 457–478.

Hilari, K., Owen, S., & Farrelly, S. J. (2007). Proxy and self-report agreement on the Stroke and Aphasia Quality of Life Scale-39. *Journal of Neurology, Neurosurgery, and Psychiatry, 78*(10), 1072.

Horowitz, A., Goodman, C. R., & Reinhardt, J. P. (2004). Congruence between disabled elders and their primary caregivers. *Gerontologist, 44*(4), 532–542.

Janicki, M. P., & Ansello, E. F. (Eds.). (2000). *Community supports for aging adults with lifelong disabilities.* Baltimore, MD: Brookes Publishing.

Janicki, M. P., & Dalton, A. J. (2000). Prevalence of dementia and impact on intellectual disability services. *Mental Retardation, 38,* 276–288.

Krahn, G. L., Hammond, L., & Turner, A. (2006). A cascade of disparities: Health and health care access for people with intellectual disabilities. *Mental Retardation and*

Developmental Disabilities Research Reviews, 12, 70–82. PubMed: 16435327

Lennox, N., Bain, C., Rey-Conde, T., Purdie, D., Bush, R., & Pandeya, N. (2007). Effects of a comprehensive health assessment programme for Australian adults with intellectual disability: A cluster randomized trial. *International Journal of Epidemiology, 36*(1), 139–146.

Mann, J., Zhou, H., McDermott, S., & Poston, M. B. (2006). Healthy behavior change of adults with mental retardation: Attendance in a health promotion program. *American Journal of Mental Retardation, 111*(1), 62–73.

Moskowitz, E. (1985). PULSES profile in retrospect. *Archives of Physical Medicine and Rehabilitation, 66,* 647–648.

Moss, S., Ibbotson, B., Prosser, D., Patel, P., & Simpson, N. (1997). Validity of the PAS-ADD for detecting psychiatric symptoms in adults with learning disability (mental retardation). *Social Psychiatry and Psychiatric Epidemiology, 32,* 344.

Ouellette-Kuntz, H., Garcin, N., Lewis, M. E., Minnes, P., Martin, C., & Holden, J. J. (2005). Addressing health disparities through promoting equity for individuals with intellectual disability. *Canadian Journal of Public Health, 96*(Suppl. 2), S8–S22.

Parish, S. L., Moss, K., & Richman, E. L. (2008). Perspectives on health care of adults with developmental disabilities. *Intellectual and Developmental Disabilities, 46*(6), 411–426.

Peterson, J. J., Janz, K. F., & Lowe, J. B. (2008). Physical activity among adults with intellectual disabilities living in community settings. *Preventive Medicine, 47*(1), 101–110.

Prasher, V., Farooq, A., & Holder, R. (2004). The Adaptive Behaviour Dementia Questionnaire (ABDQ): Screening questionnaire for dementia in Alzheimer's disease in adults with Down syndrome. *Research in Developmental Disabilities, 25*(4), 385–439.

Reichard, A., & Turnbull, H. R. III. (2004). Perspectives of physicians, families, and case managers concerning access to health care by individuals with developmental disabilities. *Mental Retardation, 42*(3), 181–194.

Rimmer, J. H., & Wang, E. (2005). Obesity prevalence among a group of Chicago residents with disabilities. *Archives of Physical Medicine and Rehabilitation, 86*(7), 1461–1464.

Rose, M., Bjorner, J. B., Becker, J., Fries, J. F., & Ware, J. E. (2008). Evaluation of a preliminary physical function item bank supported the expected advantages of the Patient-Reported Outcomes Measurement Information System (PROMIS). *Journal of Clinical Epidemiology, 61*(1), 17–33.

Seekins, T., Traci, M. A., Bainbridge, D., & Humphries, K. (2005). Secondary conditions risk appraisal for adults. In W. M. Nehring (Ed.), *Health promotion for persons with intellectual and developmental disabilities* (pp. 325–342). Washington, DC: American Association on Mental Retardation.

Service, K. P., Tyler, C. V. J., & Janicki, M. P. (2006). Geriatrics. In I. L. Rubin & A. C. Crocker (Eds.), *Medical care for children and adults with developmental disabilities* (pp. 575–590). Baltimore, MD: Paul H. Brookes Publishing.

Sneeuw, K. C. A., Sprangers, M. A. G., & Aaronson, N. K. (2002). The role of health care providers and significant others in evaluating the quality of life of patients with chronic disease. *Journal of Clinical Epidemiology, 55*(11), 1130–1143.

Stancliffe, R. J., Lakin, K. C., Larson, S., Engler, J., Bershadsky, J., Taub, S., . . . Ticha, R. (2011). Overweight and obesity among adults with intellectual disabilities who use intellectual disability/developmental disability services in 20 U.S. States. *American Journal of Intellectual & Developmental Disability, 116*(6), 401–418.

Strax, T. E., Luciano, L., Dunn, A. M., & Quevedo, J. P. (2010). Aging and developmental disabilities. *Physical Medicine and Rehabilitation Clinics of North America, 21*, 419–427.

Strydom, A., Lee, L. A, Jokinen, N., Shooshtari, S., Raykar, V., Torr, J., . . . Maaskant, M. A. (2009). *Report on the state of science on dementia in people with intellectual disabilities*. Dortmund, Germany: IASSID Special Interest Research Group on Ageing and Intellectual Disabilities.

Sullivan, W. F., Berg, J. M., Bradley, E., Cheetham, T., Denton, R., Heng, J., . . . McMillan, S. (2011, May). Primary care of adults with developmental disabilities: Canadian consensus guidelines. *Canadian Family Physician, 57*, 541–553.

Tyler, C. V., Snyder, C. W., & Zyzanski, S. (2000). Screening for osteoporosis in community dwelling adults with mental retardation. *Mental Retardation, 38*(4), 316–321.

U.S. Department of Health and Human Services. (2002). *Closing the gap: A national blueprint to improve the health of persons with mental retardation. Report of the Surgeon General's Conference on Health Disparities and Mental Retardation*. Rockville, MD: U.S. Department of Health and Human Services, Public Health Service, Office of the Surgeon General.

U.S. Department of Health and Human Services. (2017). Disability and health. *Healthy People 2020*. Retrieved from https://www.healthypeople.gov/2020/topics-objectives /topic/disability-and-health

Vanderbilt Kennedy Center for Excellence in Developmental Disabilities. (n.d.). Health care for adults with intellectual and developmental disabilities: Toolkit for primary care providers: Behavioral and mental issues. Retrieved from http://vkc.mc.vanderbilt.edu/etoolkit/mental -and-behavioral-health/

Ward, R. L., Nichols, A. D., & Freedman, R. I. (2010). Uncovering health care inequalities among adults with intellectual and developmental disabilities. *Health & Social Work, 35*(4), 280–290.

Zigman, W. B., & Lott, I. T. (2007). Alzheimer's disease in Down syndrome: Neurobiology and risk. *Mental Retardation and Developmental Disabilities Research Reviews, 13*(3), 237–246.

CHAPTER 42

Assessing Disaster Preparedness and Response

Carmel Bitondo Dyer, Amber M. Zulfiqar, Garima Arora, and Renee Flores

CHAPTER OBJECTIVES

1. Explain why older people who are community-dwelling and nursing home residents are more vulnerable to the effects of disasters.
2. Describe the types of disaster and the best practices for each.
3. Identify the psychiatric, ethical, and social needs of elderly victims of disasters.

KEY TERMS

Post-traumatic stress   Preparedness   Vulnerability

▶ Introduction

On September 1, 2005, three days after Hurricane Katrina pummeled Louisiana and the Gulf Coast, the city of Houston prepared to receive displaced victims. The old Astrodome stadium and associated buildings were readied to meet both the healthcare and custodial needs of tens of thousands of people. A large MASH unit was erected, and Texas Medical Center hospital personnel, trauma experts, and City of Houston health officials stood ready to serve. But this disaster did not yield mass injuries; instead, these victims suffered from a lack of food and water, medications, shelter, and exposure to the elements—and the majority were older than age 65.

Many of the elderly victims were nursing home residents or frail older adults without local family—and many were impoverished. For a variety of reasons, these individuals were unable to leave in advance of the hurricane; they were the most vulnerable members of the community.

Prior to this event, little attention had been focused on the needs of older patients in disasters. Hurricane Katrina opened the eyes of the public health and governmental officials, and alerted many disciplines of the healthcare community to the threat posed to this subpopulation. This chapter outlines why older adults are more vulnerable in disasters, describes the best medical and surgical practices in such cases, and addresses the psychiatric, social, and ethical needs of this segment of the population.

▶ Why Community-Dwelling Older People and Nursing Home Residents Are More Vulnerable to the Effects of Disasters

In 2009, approximately 40 million people living in the United States, or one in eight Americans, were 65 years or older. As a consequence of declining fertility and increased longevity, the number of older adults is anticipated to become an even greater proportion of U.S. population in the future, with this group accounting for one in every five Americans by 2030. Older adults are among the most heterogeneous U.S. population subgroups, ranging from bedridden demented patients to marathon runners, and from community-dwelling elders to nursing home residents. Some are highly functional, whereas others need caregivers to help them with their activities of daily living (ADLs), such as bathing, dressing, eating, medication administration, and transportation. The elderly population as a whole has proved to be the most vulnerable subgroup during disasters due to decreased mobility, multiple comorbidities, frailty, social isolation, and a high level of dependency (De Lepeleire, Iliffe, Mann, & Degryse, 2009;

Iliffe et al., 2007; Melis et al., 2008; Rockwood, 2005). Lack of food and water, fluctuating temperature extremes, and high levels of stress during disasters can play a role in exacerbating illnesses and increasing infection rates (Eisenman, Cordasco, Asch, Golden, & Glik, 2007).

Some elderly individuals require frequent access to routine health; interruptions can result in increased morbidity and mortality following disasters. Similarly, depending on medicine and medical equipment such as oxygen, dialysis machines, or even a simple assistive device like a walker or cane may pose problems during evacuations (Uscher-Pines, Vernick, Curriero, Lieberman, & Burke, 2009). In general, frail elders are more vulnerable than their healthier counterparts during a disaster. They are less likely to have household disaster **preparedness** supplies or an emergency evacuation plan, and have less ability to take care of themselves during and after disasters (Eisenman et al., 2007).

Pets play an important role for older adults during disasters. Separation distress can threaten seniors' well-being as well as increase the likelihood of risky behaviors to save pets. The strength of this attachment varies, but seniors with limited social support and economic distresses are especially vulnerable in this regard (Thompson et al., 2014). In one study of older adults, the mental plan of these elders was geared toward protecting their animals from harm and ensuring pet survival. This same study showed that among households with physically frail and disabled individuals, 75% considered pets' survival a major planning concern (Thompson, Trigg, & Smith, 2017). Concern for pets has been known to influence behaviors during disasters, including refusal to evacuate.

For all vulnerable populations, the Arnold formula (i.e., risk = hazard × **vulnerability**/manageability) becomes particularly pertinent. Fragility—a widely recognized state of reduced physiologic reserve or "homeostenosis"—increases vulnerability to stressors in the older population, particularly those stressors that result from disasters. In the face of such stressors, frail elders are more likely to have delayed recovery from illness and higher risk of hospitalization with potentially worse outcomes. Two key precipitants of poor outcomes are immobility and depression. Risk factors for harm during disasters include sensory deficits, cognitive impairment, and age-related changes in thermoregulation. The place and type of residence, language barriers, and circumstances that limit effective communication place older populations at increased risk (Aldrich & Benson, 2008; Fernandez, Byard, Lin, Benson, & Barbera, 2002).

Frailty, due to older adults' lack of physiological reserves, makes survival during disasters more precarious. There is often a fine line between "frail" and "not frail," such that under extreme stress even a robust elder can become frail. Thus, the potentially vulnerable elderly make up an even larger percentage of the U.S. population. **TABLE 42-1** details the physiologic changes and geriatric syndromes that make disaster preparedness, evacuation, and care after a disaster event much more difficult for the elderly.

TABLE 42-1 Challenges in a Disaster Setting, by Condition or Syndrome

Cognitive Disorders

- May not remember to pack necessary effects, including medications
- May become disoriented in an unfamiliar setting such as a shelter
- New behavioral problems may arise or otherwise controlled behaviors may be exacerbated
- Missed doses of dementia medications can cause a rapid deterioration in function

Depression

- May manifest as a cognitive disorder
- May not be able to effectively extricate themselves or easily negotiate new situations
- May be more prone to post-traumatic stress disorder

Delirium

- Health professionals often miss delirium or mistake it for a dementing illness
- Potential risk factor for death due to underlying acute medical illness

Functional Impairment

- Lack of mobility hampers evacuation
- Lack of assistive devices is common in disaster situations
- Must be assessed early on in a disaster (e.g., with the SWiFT Screening Tool) to be sure that basic activities of daily living can be achieved
- May not be able to drive or access public transportation

(continues)

TABLE 42-1 Challenges in a Disaster Setting, by Condition or Syndrome	*(continued)*
Vision and Hearing Impairment	
■ Relief workers often rely on signs to communicate with large numbers of people ■ May misplace hearing aids or batteries may run low, so that the person is unable to hear instructions in noisy situations	
Susceptibility to Exploitation and Abuse	
■ May be prone to exploitation by proprietary owners of nursing homes, apartment landlords, and individuals ■ A subset of volunteers, who supposedly come to assist the elderly, may try to take advantage of older adults	

Data from Federal Emergency Management Agency (FEMA). (2017). *Preparing for disaster for people with disabilities and other special needs.* Retrieved from https://www.fema.gov/media-library/assets/documents/897

Mortality in Disasters

Older adults are highly susceptible to death during a natural disaster (Fernandez et al., 2002). Of the 38 people who died during evacuation from New Orleans to Houston during Hurricane Katrina in 2005, the Harris County Medical Examiner's Office noted that 64% (23 of 36 cases) were older than 60 years. All but 4 were classified as natural deaths. Other deaths were classified as suicide (2), accidental (1), and homicide (1). It was later determined that more than 1000 adults died in New Orleans; of those who perished, more than 75% were older adults. The deaths associated with Hurricane Rita from September 18 to 26, 2005, included more accidents. The Medical Examiner's Office identified 45 cases related to the events surrounding that hurricane evacuation. Of the Rita-related deaths, in 64% of cases (29 of 45), the decedents were older than 60 years. Seven of the fatalities were found to be caused by hyperthermia (classified as accidental), and 4 of those individuals were older than 60 years. Most of the deaths were classified as natural and caused by chronic medical problems that were probably exacerbated by the evacuation process. Clearly, older adults experience higher mortality rates than younger, more

able-bodied evacuees (Knowles & Garrison, 2006; Spiegel, 2006; Stephens et al., 2007).

▶ Types of Disasters

Inhabitants of every region in the world are subject to natural disasters. For the millions of people who have disabilities, either physical or cognitive, including older adults, disasters such as hurricanes and tornados and acts of terrorism present indisputable challenges. Healthcare professionals can and should help elders plan ahead to cope with these events (U.S. Census 2010, 2017).

Hurricanes

Hurricanes often become life-threatening as well as property-threatening disasters due to the flooding and high winds associated with these storms. When a hurricane looms, it is important to have both a disaster action plan and disaster supplies in place. For those who shelter in place, physical labor is required to prepare for an incoming hurricane, and older adults should plan for the time and help needed for boarding up windows and doors. They may also need help storing loose lawn furniture, supplies, bicycles, and other items prior to the storm. For those who will need to evacuate, understanding designated routes and having a full tank of gas are essential. Manual wheelchairs, medication supply kits, and disaster kits should also be prepared ahead of time. Older adults should be given community information on shelters identified as "special needs" sites and should understand their community's plan to support medical equipment that requires power sources (American Red Cross, 2017a).

Earthquakes and Tornados

The mantra "Drop, cover, and hold on" is important for older adults to remember during an earthquake. Frail elders may be less steady on their feet, and many injuries during an earthquake occur due to falling or moving around, resulting in head injuries and fractures. Bedbound elders should remain in the bed, with a covering over their head to protect them from flying objects and glass. All older adults should stay indoors until the tremors stop and then leave by way of stairs, rather than an elevator. If a gas leak is noted, they should leave the house or building and move as far away as possible.

If outdoors during an earthquake, the person should identify a spot to drop to the ground and remain on the ground until the tremors stop. It is important to stay clear of trees, power lines, streetlights, and buildings. Drivers in vehicles should stop, pull to the side of the road, and avoid bridges and overpasses. If near mountains or hills, elders should be watchful for falling rocks and landslides (American Red Cross, 2017b).

Like earthquakes, tornados can demolish homes and entire buildings. Tornados can hurl debris in the air that can become a lethal weapon. Any disaster plan should include a safe place in the home to shelter, such as a basement, storm cellar, or another interior space with no windows. If in a multifloor building, the elder should go to an area without window exposure (lower floors are preferred). In any disaster,

elevators should be avoided. Mobile home residents should make their way to the nearest shelter in advance, as unstable homes can be hurled into the air during tornados (American Red Cross, 2017d).

Acts of Terrorism

The unbridled attacks on the World Trade Center and Pentagon on September 11, 2001, underscore the need for the elder population to be ready to withstand unpredicted crises. Such unexpected acts of terror have raised awareness of these potential threats within and outside of the United States. In 2003, the Department of Homeland Security was established and recognized the need for disaster preparedness for the United States as a whole, as well as for especially vulnerable populations (Torgusen & Kosberg, 2006). Older adults with mobility issues cannot be expected to respond quickly to these sudden events. As in the case of natural disaster, underlying illness can be exacerbated by the direct effects of a terrorist attack as well as by the mental stress associated with this type of disaster (International Society for Traumatic Stress Studies, 2016).

▶ Best Practices in Disaster Management

Best practices for disaster management include using a rapid assessment tool, assembling an emergency supply kit, maintaining an medical information sheet, ensuring pet care, and registering with the Disaster Response Registry.

Rapid Assessment Tool

Geriatric assessment is the cornerstone of geriatric care—something that is true during disasters as well as under normal circumstances. A tool that can be rapidly employed is needed to appropriately triage and provide services and care for older adults during disasters. Following

Hurricane Katrina, a tool was developed to quickly triage those seniors most in need of services through a brief, targeted geriatric assessment. The domains covered included cognition, social and medical needs, and ability to perform activities of daily living. The SWiFT (Seniors Without Families Triage) Screening Tool is intended to assist older adults without family members who need assistance.

Prior to their arrival in Houston in the wake of Hurricane Katrina, some older adults were actively separated from their families for ease of evacuation. The SWiFT Screening Tool was used to identify the most vulnerable elders without family members who could advocate for them. This tool is divided into three levels of ability, and assigns a time frame for interventions with suggested interventions by level (Dyer, Regev, Burnett, Festa, & Cloyd, 2008).

Emergency Supply Kit

An emergency supply kit should always be at the ready, easily accessible by the older adult, and updated on a regular basis. **TABLE 42-2** lists the recommended contents of this supply kit.

Medical Information Checklist and Other Documents

It is crucial to have copies of medical information to assist emergency workers. Medical information checklists should include personal information such as emergency contacts (including copies of any medical power of attorney, advance directives, or living will), copies of insurance records, Social Security cards, and identification cards. Names and contact information of primary care physicians and specialists should be included, along with medication lists detailing medication names, dosages, and instructions for administration (Sollitto, 2017).

Other important documents to have on hand include the home ownership title. This will enable access to Federal Emergency Management Agency (FEMA) or other community resources

---

TABLE 42-2 Emergency Supply Kit
■ Seven-day supply of water (1 gallon per person per day), nonperishable food, and essential kitchen accessories such as a manual can opener and cooking utensils
■ Flashlight, portable battery-powered radio/transistor radio and extra batteries
■ Fully charged cell phone and extra battery
■ First aid kit that includes hygiene supplies such as hand sanitizer and toilet paper
■ Matches in a waterproof container
■ Whistle
■ Extra clothing and blankets
■ Photocopies of identification and cash (as ATMs will not work in a power outage)
■ Medication supply kit: prescription medications (in original bottles if possible), hearing aids, eye glasses, oxygen
■ Six gallons of gasoline and ½ tank of gas in vehicle

Reproduced from Langan, J., & Palmer, J. (2012). Listening to and learning from older adult Hurricane Katrina survivors. *Public Health Nursing, 29*(2), 126–135.

(e.g., long-term recovery groups) during recovery. Low-income and elderly persons who have fixed incomes, limited economic funds, and no insurance may have to rely on FEMA for assistance in the aftermath of a disaster (personal communication, Tracy Odvody-Figueroa, attorney and disaster assistance team manager, 2017).

Pet Care

The American Red Cross does not permit animals in disaster shelters unless they are designated service animals. When they have pets, older adults should keep a list of pet medical records, pet-friendly hotels, boarding facilities, and veterinarians and local animal shelters that provide refuge to animals in the event of an emergency. Animals also need emergency kits of essential supplies, including medications, safety equipment such as leashes, food and water, toys if easily transportable, and current photos in the event that the pet becomes lost (American Red Cross, 2017c). In addition, it is important for older adults to have the proper identification for the pet, along with veterinary and immunization records (Federal Emergency Management Agency, 2011).

Disaster Response Registry

An important step to prepare for the event of a disaster is to sign on to the Disaster Response Registry. This registry provides the opportunity for frail elders to identify themselves as vulnerable and potentially in need of assistance during a disaster. The Disaster Response Registry assists with distributing emergency relief supplies and other services to distressed individuals (US Legal, 2017).

▶ Psychiatric, Ethical, and Social Needs of Elderly Victims of Disasters

The geriatric population has a unique vulnerability during disasters due to the interplay among the biological, psychological, and social changes associated with aging (Claver, Dobalian, Fickel, Ricci, & Mallers, 2013). A disproportionate burden is placed on the elderly not only during an actual disaster, but also during the recovery phase. It is the ethical responsibility of healthcare professionals to promote emotional well-being and recovery of the older adults during disasters.

Evacuation

Psychosocial concerns for older adults in a disaster requiring evacuation include poor social support systems, living alone, death of spouse or significant other, financial constraints, loss of sense of autonomy and independence, concerns about personal safety during the evacuation process, trepidation about "no personal control" over the occurrence/outcome of the disaster, fear of the unknown, distress about the loss of valued and cherished possessions, worries about abandoning pets, and anxieties about the process of recovery in the aftermath (Duggan, Deeny, Spelman, & Vitale, 2010; Sakauye, Streim, Kennedy, & Kirwin, 2009; Somes & Donatelli, 2012a, 2012b, 2014).

As disasters in the recent history all over the world have shown, the triage system during calamities is most commonly based on ambulation and ability to understand commands under stress. Due to multiple medical comorbidities, sensory decline (e.g., hearing loss, vision loss), cognitive decline, and impaired mobility, the elderly fall short on many measures of these established triage systems. This calls for a separate triage system for older adults, such as the SWiFT Screening Tool (see **FIGURE 42-1** for the SWiFT Screening Tool and **FIGURE 42-2** for the SWiFT Level Tool in Disaster Preparedness). Elderly persons may be classified as either 1) living independently with minimal medical issues and no need for assistance with ADLs or 2) living independently, in assisted living, with family caregivers, with home health, with major medical issues and needing assistance with ADLs or 3) the frailest, living in healthcare facilities (Banks, 2013). The last group are completely dependent on the caregiving facility during the evacuation process and, therefore, are the most vulnerable and at the greatest risk for adverse outcomes (Brown, Rothman, & Norris, 2007; Claver et al., 2013).

Recovery Phase

The concerns about the elderly population continue during the recovery phase. Medical issues can be exacerbated during a disaster, requiring higher levels of care, sometimes from an already strapped system (Aldrich & Benson, 2008). Preexisting psychiatric issues such as depression, anxiety, and cognitive disorders also make recovery challenging for the elderly due to worsening of prior symptoms and the possible onset

Current date:		Worker's name:	
Name:		DOB:	

Do you have family or friends with you here?	☐Y ☐N	Confirmed? ☐Y ☐N

<table>
<tr>
<td>Level 1:
<u>Health/mental health priority</u>

<u>Goes to social work booth in medical clinic</u></td>
<td colspan="2">A. Do you have any of the following medical problems:

☐Y ☐N Diabetes
☐Y ☐N Heart disease
☐Y ☐N High blood pressure
☐Y ☐N Memory
☐Other
Note:

B. Do you take medicine?
☐Y ☐N
Do you have your medicine?
☐Y or ☐N
If "no," treat as level 1</td>
<td>C. Do you need someone to help you with:
☐Y ☐N Walking
☐Y ☐N Eating
☐Y ☐N Bathing
☐Y ☐N Dressing
☐Y ☐N Toileting
☐Y ☐N Medication administration
Any checks, treat as level 1
Do you use something to help you get around:
☐Cane
☐Walker
☐Wheel chair
☐Bath bench</td>
</tr>
<tr>
<td>D. Where are you right now?

If senior cannot or does not answer correctly treat as level 1</td>
<td>E. Name 3 ordinary items and have them repeat them; for example, "apple, table, penny."</td>
<td>F. What year is it?

If senior cannot/does not answer correctly treat as level 1</td>
<td>G. Ask them to repeat the three items you previously mentioned.

If more than one item is missed, treat as level 1.</td>
</tr>
<tr>
<td>Level 2:
<u>case management needs</u>

<u>Is referred to a case manager</u></td>
<td>A. Ask them what their major need is right now.</td>
<td>B. Do you have a plan for where you will go when you leave here?
☐Yes ☐No</td>
<td>C. Income/entitlements

Are you on:
☐Y ☐N Medicare
☐Y ☐N Medicaid
☐Y ☐N SSI
☐Y ☐N Social security
☐Y ☐N Food stamps
☐Y ☐N V A benefits
☐Y ☐N Section 8 housing funds
Do you have your documents?
☐Yes ☐No</td>
</tr>
<tr>
<td>Level 3: Only
<u>needs to be linked to family or friends</u>

<u>Directed to Red Cross volunteer</u></td>
<td>A. Family

Do you need help to find your family/friends?
☐ Yes ☐No</td>
<td>B. Names:

Relationship:

Location:</td>
<td>Where is the senior located?</td>
</tr>
</table>

FIGURE 42-1 SWiFT Screening Tool. ©

Reproduced from Dyer, C. B., Regev, M., Burnett, J., Festa, N., & Cloyd, B. (2008). SWiFT: A rapid triage tool for vulnerable older adults in disaster situations. *Disaster Medicine and Public Health Preparedness*, 2(Suppl. 1), S45–S50, reproduced with permission.

Swift level tool in disaster preparedness		
Swift level	Explanation	Preparatory steps
1	Cannot perform at least one basic ADL (activities of daily living: eating, bathing, dressing, toileting, walking, continence) without assistance	Evacuate early rather than late depending on the circumstance. If possible, keep with family member, companion, or caregiver. Receives assistance in gathering all assistive devices, including eye glasses, walkers, hearing aids, list of medicines, names of doctor(s), family contact telephone number, and important papers, so they are accessible.
2	Trouble with instrumental activities of daily living (i.e., finances, benefits management, assessing resources)	Gather, with assistance if necessary, all assistive devices, including eye glasses, walkers, hearing aids, list of medicines, names of doctor(s), family contact telephone numbers, and important papers, so they are accessible.
3	Minimal assistance with ADL and instrumental activities of daily living	Advise individuals to have all assistive devices, including walkers, eye glasses, hearing aids, list of medicines, names of doctor(s), family contact telephone numbers, and important papers together and accessible.

FIGURE 42-2 SWiFT Level Tool in Disaster Preparedness.

Reproduced from Dyer, C. B., Regev, M., Burnett, J., Festa, N., & Cloyd, B. (2008). SWiFT: A rapid triage tool for vulnerable older adults in disaster situations. *Disaster Medicine and Public Health Preparedness, 2* (Suppl 1), S45–S50, reproduced with permission.

of these symptoms from exposure to a stressful situation (Parker et al., 2016). The lifetime experiences of the elderly might have included traumatic events (particularly war veterans or Holocaust survivors) and exposure to this trauma can worsen their **post-traumatic stress** disorder (PTSD), trigger suppressed symptoms, or cause a secondary stress response. Antecedent drug and/or alcohol use may worsen or relapse subsequent to trauma (Oe et al., 2016). Due to baseline reduced social connectedness, some elderly individuals require significant social support to mitigate stress and help with recovery.

The addition of post-impact social isolation and financial issues due to loss of family or the loss of homes and possessions increase the need for encompassing care even after returning to the community. It is also necessary for healthcare professionals to ensure that seniors are not abused or exploited during the recovery phase, especially if there is a lack of decision-making capacity or the existence of a power of attorney or guardianship. Significantly, unmet social and psychological needs can have deleterious effects on physical health (Torgusen & Kosberg, 2006).

Evacuation protocols should incorporate training for first responders about frailty and dementia, as well as training on de-escalation of anxiety and agitated behaviors. Formal and informal caregivers are encouraged to plan for and practice disaster preparedness drills. Disaster preparedness policies, protocols, and programs are especially important in nursing home and assisted living settings, and basic requirements for preparedness training can be set by these facilities. Ensuring access to safe and adequate transportation must be a major consideration. Implementing geriatric-specific triage protocols, having systems and procedures in place to help keep track of the elderly, and establishing pre-assigned and separate shelters for them (which allow for family members and/or pets to stay with them) are also of significant importance.

Planning and preparedness should also address the personal responsibilities of caregivers (whether at a facility, as home health aides, or even for family members). Ethical concerns about caregivers who are worried about themselves and their family's safety versus caring for or abandoning patients are real. Psychological impacts of "vicarious traumatization" (Cunningham, 2004), compassion fatigue (Adams, Figley, & Boscarino, 2008), secondary stress, and burnout plague first responders, caregivers, and post-disaster relief personnel (Labrague et al., 2017; Morgan, 2016). To guard against these possibilities turning into reality, healthcare providers should employ strategies that include detachment, empathic communication, the provision of support, and remaining aware of the patients' physical and mental reactions (Oe et al., 2016).

The aftermath of disaster requires significant social and psychological support. Involvement of specially trained geriatric social workers and community case managers can help. Training should aim at ensuring access to and receipt of available aid (e.g., FEMA, American Red Cross); restarting Supplemental Security Income (SSI); preventing exploitation; providing psychological support in the case of any family deaths, financial loss, loss of home or possessions, and worsening of medical issues; and managing cultural issues, among other concerns. The fields of disaster psychiatry, disaster debriefing/therapy, crisis management, and project management should be tapped during the training. Provision of psychological first aid to health professionals and support staff is essential to the entire planning process (Brown et al., 2009).

▶ Summary

A coordinated effort is paramount to achieve optimal disaster preparedness for elderly patients. Involvement of gerontologic experts (e.g., medical providers, nurses, social workers) is an obvious choice when undertaking such preparation. However, preplanning involving the community (i.e., for homebound individuals and first responders), healthcare facilities, and hospitals at local, regional, national, and international levels should also be explored. Adult protective services agency personnel and older adults themselves can help with these community-based plans (Banks, 2013). Personal protection plans should include age-appropriate recommendations and account for disability, mobility, and cognitive issues. **BOX 42-1** details suggested components of best practices for older disaster victims.

BOX 42-1 Best Practices for Response to Disaster

1. Develop a simple, inexpensive, cohesive, integrated, and efficient federal tracking system for elders and other vulnerable adults that can be employed at the state and local levels during disasters.
2. Designate separate shelter areas for elders and other vulnerable adults.
3. Involve gerontologists (e.g., geriatricians, geriatric nurse practitioners, gerontologic social workers, or other aging experts) in all aspects of emergency preparedness and care delivery.
4. Involve region-specific social services, medical and public health resources, volunteers, and facilities in pre-event planning for elders and vulnerable adults.
5. Involve gerontologists (e.g., geriatricians, geriatric nurse practitioners, gerontologic social workers, or other aging experts) in the training and education of front-line workers and other first responders about frail adults' unique needs.

6. Utilize a public health triage system like the SWiFT Screening Tool for elders and other vulnerable populations in pre- and post-disaster situations.
7. The personnel charged with overseeing elders and vulnerable adults should maintain a clear line of communication with the shelter's central command. Communication within the shelter should involve technology such as cell phones and walkie-talkies.
8. Provide protection from abuse and fraud for elders and other vulnerable adults.
9. Develop coordinated regional plans for evacuations of residents of long-term care facilities and for homebound persons with special needs (e.g., ventilator-dependent adults).
10. Conduct drills and research on disaster preparedness plans and the use of a triage tool, such as SWiFT, to ensure their effectiveness and universality.

References

Adams, R. E., Figley, C. R., & Boscarino, J. A. (2008). The Compassion Fatigue Scale: Its use with social workers following urban disaster. *Research on Social Work Practice, 18*(3), 238–250.

Aldrich, N., & Benson, W. F. (2008). Disaster preparedness and the chronic disease needs of vulnerable older adults. *Preventing Chronic Disease, 5*(1), A27.

American Red Cross. (2017a). Be Red Cross ready: Hurricane safety checklist. Retrieved from https://www.redcross .org/images/MEDIA_CustomProductCatalog/m4340160 _Hurricane.pdf

American Red Cross. (2017b). Earthquake safety. Retrieved from http://www.redcross.org/get-help/prepare-for-emergencies /types-of-emergencies/earthquake#Before

American Red Cross. (2017c). Pet fire safety. Retrieved from http://www.redcross.org/get-help/how-to-prepare-for -emergencies/types-of-emergencies/fire/pet-fire-safety

American Red Cross. (2017d). Tornado safety. Retrieved from http://www.redcross.org/get-help/prepare-for-emergencies /types-of-emergencies/tornado

Banks, L. (2013). Caring for elderly adults during disasters: Improving health outcomes and recovery. *Southern Medical Journal, 106*(1), 94–98.

Brault, M. W. (2012). Americans With Disabilities: 2010 *Current Population Reports, Household Economic Studies* (Vol. P70-131). Washington, DC: US Census Bureau.

Brown, L. M., Bruce, M. L., Hyer, K., Mills, W. L., Vogxaiburana, E., & Polivka-West, L. A. (2009). A pilot study evaluating the feasibility of psychological first aid for nursing home residents. *Clinical Gerontologist, 32*(3), 293–308.

Brown, L. M., Rothman, M., & Norris, F. (2007). Issues in mental health care for older adults during disasters. *Generations, 31*(4), 25–30.

Claver, M., Dobalian, A., Fickel, J. J., Ricci, K. A., & Mallers, M. H. (2013). Comprehensive care for vulnerable elderly veterans during disasters. *Archives of Gerontology and Geriatrics, 56*, 205–213.

Cunningham, M. (2004). Teaching social workers about trauma: Reducing the risk of vicarious traumatization in the classroom. *Journal of Social Work Education, 40*(2), 305–317.

De Lepeleire, J., Iliffe, S., Mann, E., & Degryse, J. (2009). Frailty: An emerging concept for general practice. *British Journal of General Practice, 59*(562), 177–182.

Duggan, S., Deeny, P., Spelman, R., & Vitale, C. T. (2010). Perceptions of older people on disaster response and preparedness. *International Journal of Older People Nursing, 5*, 71–76.

Dyer, C. B., Regev, M., Burnett, J., Festa, N., & Cloyd, B. (2008). SWiFT: A rapid triage tool for vulnerable older adults in disaster situations. *Disaster Medicine and Public Health Preparedness, 2*(Suppl. 1), S45–S50.

Eisenman, D. P., Cordasco, K. M., Asch, S., Golden, J. F., Glik, D. (2007). Disaster planning and risk communication with vulnerable communities: Lessons from Hurricane Katrina. *American Journal of Public Health, 97*, S109–S115.

Federal Emergency Management Agency (FEMA). (2011). Pet/service animal preparedness. Retrieved from https:// emilms.fema.gov/IS909/assets/12_Pets&ServiceAnimals.pdf

Federal Emergency Management Agency (FEMA). (2017). *Preparing for disaster for people with disabilities and other special needs.* Retrieved from https://www.fema .gov/media-library/assets/documents/897

Fernandez, L. S., Byard, D., Lin, C. C., Benson, S., & Barbera, J. A. (2002). Frail elderly as disaster victims: Emergency management strategies. *Prehospital Disaster Medicine, 17*(2), 67–74.

Iliffe, S., Kharicha, K., Harari, D., Swift, C., Gillmann, G., & Stuck, A. E. (2007). Health risk appraisal in older people 2: The implications for clinicians and commissioners of social isolation risk in older people. *British Journal of General Practice, 57*(537), 277–282.

International Society for Traumatic Stress Studies. (2016). *Mass disasters, trauma, and loss.* Retrieved from https:// www.istss.org/ISTSS_Main/media/Documents/ISTSS _MassDisasterTraumaandLoss_English_FNL.pdf

Knowles, R., & Garrison, B. (2006). Planning for the elderly in natural disasters. *Disaster Recovery Journal, 19*(4). Retrieved from https://www.drj.com/journal/fall-2006 -volume-19-issue-4/planning-for-elderly-in-natural -disasters.html

Labrague, L. J., Hammad, K., Gloe, D. S., McEnroe-Petitte, D. M., Fronda, D. C., Obeidat, A. A., . . . Mirafuentes, E. C. (2017). Disaster preparedness among nurses: A systematic review of literature. *International Nursing Review*.

Langan, J., & Palmer, J. (2012). Listening to and learning from older adult Hurricane Katrina survivors. *Public Health Nursing, 29*(2), 126–135.

Melis, R., van Eijken, M., Teerenstra, S., van Achterberg, T., Parker, S. G., Borm, G. F., . . . Rikkert, M. G. M. O. (2008). Multidimensional geriatric assessment: Back to the future: A randomized study of a multidisciplinary program to intervene on geriatric syndromes in vulnerable older people who live at home (Dutch EASYcare Study). *Journals of Gerontology, Series A: Biological Sciences and Medical Sciences, 63*(3), 283–290.

Morgan, P. M. (2016). The psychological impact of mass casualty incidents on first responders: A systematic review. *Journal of Emergency Management, 14*(3), 213–226.

Oe, M., Fuiji, S., Maeda, M., Nagai, M., Harigane, M., Miura, I., . . . Abe, M. (2016). Three-year trend survey of psychological distress, post-traumatic stress, and problem drinking among residents in the evacuation zone after the Fukushima Daiichi Nuclear Power Plant accident: The Fukushima Health Management Survey. *Psychiatry and Clinical Neurosciences, 70*(6), 245–252.

Parker, G., Lie, D., Siskind, D. J., Martin-Khan, M., Raphael, B., Crompton, D., . . . Kisely, S. (2016). Mental health implications for older adults after natural disasters: A systematic review and meta-analysis. *International Psychogeriatrics, 28*(1), 11–20.

Rockwood, K. (2005). A global clinical measure of fitness and frailty in elderly people. *Canadian Medical Association Journal, 173*(5), 489–495.

Sakauye, K. M., Streim, J. E., Kennedy, G. J., & Kirwin, P. D. (2009). AAGP position statement: Disaster preparedness for older Americans: Critical issues for the preservation of mental health. *American Journal of Geriatric Psychiatry, 17*(11), 916–924.

Sollitto, M. (2017). Managing personal medical information. Retrieved from https://www.agingcare.com/articles/health -information-checklist-to-keep-caregivers-organized-136218 .htm

Somes, J., & Donatelli, N. S. (2012a). Disaster planning considerations involving the geriatric patient: Part I. *Journal of Emergency Nursing, 38*(5), 479–481.

Somes, J., & Donatelli, N. S. (2012b). Disaster planning considerations involving the geriatric patient: Part II. *Journal of Emergency Nursing, 38*(6), 563–567.

Somes, J., & Donatelli, N. S. (2014). Ethics and disasters involving geriatric patients. *Journal of Emergency Nursing, 40*(5), 493–496.

Spiegel, A. (2006). Katrina's impact on elderly still resonates. Retrieved from http://www.npr.org/templates/story /story.php?storyId=5239019

Stephens, K., Grew, D., Chin, K., Kadetz, P., Greenough, P. G., Burkle, S. L., . . . Franklin, E. R. (2007). excess mortality in the Aftermath of Hurricane Katrina: A preliminary report. *Disaster Medicine and Public Health Preparedness, 1*(1), 15–20.

Thompson, K., Every, D., Rainbird, S., Cornell, V., Smith, B., & Trigg, J. (2014). No pet or their person left behind: Increasing the disaster resilience of vulnerable groups through animal attachment, activities and networks. *Animals, 4*(2), 214–240. doi: 10.3390/ani4020214

Thompson, K., Trigg, J., & Smith, B. (2017). Animal ownership among vulnerable populations in regional south Australia. *Journal of Public Health Management and Practice, 23*(1), 59–63. doi: 10.1097/phh.0000000000000416

Torgusen, B. L., & Kosberg, J. I. (2006). Assisting older victims of disasters: Roles and responsibilities for social workers. *Journal of Gerontological Social Work, 47*(1–2), 27–44.

US Legal. (2017). Disaster response registry law and legal definition. Retrieved from https://definitions.uslegal .com/d/disaster-response-registry

Uscher-Pines, L., Vernick, J. S., Curriero, F., Lieberman, R., Burke, T. A. (2009). Disaster-related injuries in the period of recovery: The effect of prolonged displacement on risk of injury in older adults. *Journal of Trauma, 67,* 834–840.

Index

Note: Page numbers followed by *f* or *t* indicate material in figures or tables, respectively.

A

AARP Public Policy Institute, 326
AARP Smart Driver, 422
abandonment, 215
abdomen assessment, 257–258
ABDQ. *See* Adaptive Behaviour Dementia Questionnaire (ABDQ)
ability, writing and construction, 191–192
ACA. *See* Affordable Care Act (ACA)
accountable care organization (ACO), 43, 84, 153
Accountable Health Community (AHC), 96
ACE. *See* acute care for elders (ACE)
ACLS protocols. *See* advanced cardiac life support (ACLS) protocols
ACO. *See* accountable care organization (ACO)
ACOVE. *See* Assessing Care of Vulnerable Elders (ACOVE)
ACP. *See* advance care planning (ACP)
acting, importance of, 3–4
Active Aging Framework, 25
active listening, 75
activities of daily living (ADLs), 370, 384
  ability to accomplish, 373
  ability to carry, 354
  assessment of, 267
  difficulties on, 107
  family caregivers, 82–83
  history of cognitive and, 267
  inability to perform, 266
  Katz Index of Independence in, 234

Lawton instrumental, 235
  need for assistance in, 232
  personal assistance with, 368
  problems in performing, 234
Activity Measure for Post-Acute Care (AMPAC), 316t, 455
acts of terrorism, 465
acute alcohol, 293
acute care for elders (ACE), 135, 166, 168
acute pain, 271t
AD. *See* Alzheimer's disease (AD)
Adaptive Behaviour Dementia Questionnaire (ABDQ), 454
addict, 294
adherence packaging, 310–311
ADLs. *See* activities of daily living (ADLs)
Administration of Community Living (ACL), 278, 455
admission decisions, 404
Adult Protective Services (APS), 221
advance care planning (ACP), 142, 146, 180, 181, 432–433
  barriers to using advance directives, 439–440
  durable power of attorney for health care, 434
  family covenant, 434–435
  goals of care, 182
  legal considerations, 440
  living will, 433
  POLST/MOLST forms, 437–439
  potential value of, 181
  Values History. *See* Values History
advance directives, 180, 432
  barriers to using, 439–440
  forms, 184
  use of, 432
Advanced Activities of Daily Living (AADL) tool, 233

advanced cardiac life support (ACLS) protocols, 436
advanced care planning, 15
  advance directives, 180
  best practices in, 182–183
  conversation, 182
  documentation, 182–183
  importance of, 180–181
  Medicare coverage of, 17
  overview, 179–180
  practice challenges, 183–184
  tools for, 183
advanced practice nurses (APNs), 335
adverse outcomes, risk assessment for, 411–412
Affordable Care Act (ACA), 85, 145, 432
age/aging, 373. *See also* older adults (OAs)
  of baby boomer generation, 368
  concept of, 450
  health and life expectancy, 22–23
  natural consequence of, 197–198
Age-Friendly Cities and Communities, 20
age-friendly health systems, 31–32
  aim, purpose, and expected benefits, 33–34
  challenges of, 33
  characteristics of, 32
  concept design, 32
  definition of, 32
  initiatives, 36
  prototype model, 34–36
  scale-up design and social movement, 36–38
  spread of, 37
  steps, 38–39
age-friendly initiatives
  design and development of, 37
  evaluation of, 26

age-friendly locality, 26
age-friendly prototype, 34
    interventions and actions, 35*t*
Aging and Disability Evidence-
        Based Programs and
        Practices (ADEPP)
        program, 278
aging in place (AIP), 365–367
    approach to long-term care, 370
    care coordination aspects of, 367
    environment, 367
    importance of, 368–369
    models, 366, 370
    practice challenges of, 370
    programs, 366
    settings, 370
    TigerPlace, 367–368
AGS Beers Criteria, 236
AIP. *See* aging in place (AIP)
alcohol, 293
    consumption guidelines for, 292
    consumption, patterns of, 292
    immediate effects of, 292
    screening instruments, 295
    use, 291, 298
        disorder, 292
        potential chronic effects of, 293
Alcohol, Smoking and Substance
        Involvement Screening Test
        (ASSIST), 295
Alcohol Use Disorders Identification
        Test (AUDIT), 295–297
alcoholic, 294
alprazolam, 418
alternative payment models, 153
Alzheimer's and Dementia Care
        (ADC), 172–173
Alzheimer's dementia, 236, 237
Alzheimer's disease (AD), 418, 419,
        421, 422
    prevalence of, 104
American Automobile Association
        (AAA), 421, 425
American Geriatrics Society (AGS),
        7, 68, 236, 420
American Medical Association, 222
American Public Transportation
        Association, 423
American Recovery and
        Reinvestment Act, 137
American Red Cross, 466
American Society for Pain
        Management Nursing, 452
AMPAC. *See* Activity Measure for
        Post-Acute Care (AMPAC)
anemia, 327

annual wellness visit (AWV), 142,
        145–146
anorexia of aging, 324
anticipation of needs, 4
anxiety, 249, 282
anxiety disorders, 293
APNs. *See* advanced practice
        nurses (APNs)
appetite, 324–325
APS. *See* Adult Protective
        Services (APS)
Ariadne Labs Serious Illness Care
        programs, 184
Arnold formula, 462
arthritis, 419
Assessing Care of Vulnerable Elders
        (ACOVE)
    quality indicators, 158–159
    researchers, 158
assessment, 337–341*t*, 448. *See also*
        specific types
    into action, 398, 399*t*
    and care plans, 66
        contextual frame of older
            adults, 66–68
        person-centered care, 68–69
        planning, 70–72
        timing and nuance of
            ascertaining goals in,
            69–70
    clinical, 286
    general guidelines for, 104–105
    geriatric, 384
    instruments for, 106
    of mobility, 313
    of older adults, 106, 369
    tools, 284, 319
    types and purposes of, 120*t*
assessment data, 55–56
    adherence to treatment, 58
    communication problems, 59
    coordination between physicians
        using EHRs, 57
    coordination with caregivers and
        family members, 57
    future possibilities, 58–59
    geriatric access to electronic
        patient portals, 56–57
    hiding/suppressing notes, 61
    patient satisfaction measures,
        57–58
    patient-friendly terminology, 58
    physician resistance, 59
    practical application, 61
    presbycusis, 57
    privacy and security concerns, 61

    psychiatry/behavioral health
        issues, 61
    technical savvy, 59
    test results, obtaining, 58
    understanding terminology, 60
assisted autonomy, 451
assisted living facilities (ALFs), 384
Assisted Living Resident Assessment
        Tool, 369
asthma, environmental triggers
        for, 89
atrial fibrillation, 249
atrioventricular (A-V) block, 249
at-risk alcohol use, risk factors for,
        293
at-risk drinking, 292, 293
attitudes, 107
autonomy, 432
average life expectancy, 67
avoidable harms in older adult
        patients, 33

B

baby boomer, 3
    aging of, 206
BADLs. *See* basic activities of daily
        living (BADLs)
balance assessment, 260–261
barbiturates, 293
basic activities of daily living
        (BADLs), 126–127
Beers Criteria for Potentially
        Inappropriate Medication
        Use in Older Adults,
        306–308
behavioral economics, 42
behavioral health services, 299
Behavioral Risk Factor Surveillance
        System (BRFSS), 20
beliefs, 107
    and attitudes, 103
Benjamin Rose Institute Care
        Consultation model, 160
benzodiazepines, 293
best practice treatment, 59
Better Outcomes for Older Adults
        Through Safe Transitions
        (BOOST)
    invention, 335
    model of care, 170
BGA. *See* brief geriatric
        assessments (BGA)
Bipartisan Policy Center, 153–154

blood pressure (BP), 248
    assessment and control of, 385
    for hypertension monitoring, 58
    measurement, 247
    monitoring, 354
    orthostatic, 158
    postural, 247
boarding, 403–404
body mass index (BMI), 249
BOOST. *See* Better Outcomes for
    Older Adults Through Safe
    Transitions (BOOST)
bothersome pain, 266
BP. *See* blood pressure (BP)
brain failure, 210
breasts assessment, 258
BRFSS. *See* Behavioral Risk Factor
    Surveillance System (BRFSS)
BRI Care Consultation
    intervention, 278
brief geriatric assessments
    (BGA), 405
broader policy changes, 96
bundled payment, 43
    models, 84

C

CAM. *See* Confusion Assessment
    Method (CAM)
Cambridge Cognitive Examination-
    Down Syndrome version
    (CAMCOG-DS version), 454
cannabis, 291, 293, 294
cardiopulmonary resuscitation
    (CPR), 436
care, dimension of, 283
Care of Persons with Dementia
    in Their Environments
    (COPE), 374, 379
care planning, 2, 70
    assessment and. *See* assessment
        and care plans
    implementation of, 53
    process, 66
care transitions, 331
    complex, 335
    evidence-based models of, 332
    manager, 335
    model, 168, 169t, 170
Care Transitions Intervention
    (CTI), 335
Caregiver Advise, Record, and
    Enable (CARE) Act, 85–86

caregivers, 82, 232, 275
    abuse, 244
    assessment, 275, 277
        demographics and
            prevalence, 276
        practice challenges, 278
        practices, 276–277
        where to start, 277–278
    formal, 238
    informal, 238
    negative outcomes for, 276
    role of, 232
CARET. *See* Comorbidity Alcohol
    Risk Evaluation Tool
    (CARET)
CCM. *See* chronic care management
    (CCM)
CDT. *See* Clock Drawing
    Test (CDT)
Center to Advance Palliative
    Care, 184
Centers for Medicare and Medicaid
    Services (CMS), 43, 68,
    126, 432
central pain, 272t
cerebral palsy, 448
certified registered nurse
    practitioner (CRNP), 335
CGA. *See* comprehensive geriatric
    assessment (CGA)
charitable giving, 22
cholinesterase inhibitors, 421
chronic alcohol, 293
chronic care management (CCM),
    142, 146
    models, 161
chronic care model, 150
Chronic Disease Self-Management
    Program, 75
chronic illnesses, 325
chronic medical illness, 209–210
chronic obstructive pulmonary
    disease (COPD), 66, 74,
    276, 311, 317, 325
chronological age, 450
civic engagement, 22
CLCs. *See* community living centers
    (CLCs)
clinical assessment, developmental
    disability (DD), 286,
    447–448, 448–449
    challenges to providing
        high-quality care, 451
    cognitive assessment, 454
    disparities in care and health are
        substantial, 449

functional assessment, 454–455
geriatric care for people,
    449–451
medical, developmental,
    and functional history,
    451–452
mental health assessment, 454
pain assessment, 452
preventive health, 455
social/social support
    assessment, 455
clinical barriers, 71
clinical care, 16
clinicians, key resources for, 287
clock drawing, 192
Clock Drawing Test (CDT), 109
cognition, 405–407
cognitive ability, individual's level
    of, 267
cognitive assessment, 454
    dementia and cognitive impair-
        ment, 186
    differential diagnosis, 186–187,
        187t
    mental status examination. *See*
        mental status examination
    overview, 185–186
    practical considerations, 193–194
    pre-assessment process, 187–188
    test selection, 188
cognitive capacity, decline of, 186
Cognitive Capacity Screen, 190
cognitive function assessment,
    108–109
cognitive impairment, 110, 192, 236,
    269, 420, 424
    degrees of, 421
    routine screening for, 188
    screen for, 407
    setting of, 311
cognitive problems, 354–355
cognitive screening, 158
collaborative care, 126
collaborative team care, 158
co-management, 159, 160–161
communication skills, 242
Community Aging in Place,
    Advancing Better Living
    for Elders (CAPABLE)
    model, 174, 374, 376–379,
    377–378t
community assessment, domains
    of, 152t
community care workers, 153
community living centers
    (CLCs), 53

community team-based geriatric care
  domains of community assessment, 151–152, 152*t*
  overview, 149–151
  targeting and assessment, 151–152
  team-based care for older adults, 153
community team-based models, 153
community-based homes, 368
community-based teams, effective assessment for, 152
community-dwelling elders, 350, 462
comorbidity, 126–127
  among chronic conditions, 127*f*
Comorbidity Alcohol Risk Evaluation Tool (CARET), 295
competencies, 15
complex care management, 151
complex care transitions, 335
comprehensive assessments, 350
Comprehensive Care for Joint Replacement (CJR) Model, 43
comprehensive geriatric assessment (CGA), 150, 388, 390*t*, 405
  limitations of, 388
compromised functional ability, 127
Confusion Assessment Method (CAM), 407
congenital heart disease, 448
consciousness, attention and level of, 190–191
construction ability, 192
COPD. *See* chronic obstructive pulmonary disease (COPD)
COPE. *See* Care of Persons with Dementia in Their Environments (COPE)
coping skills, 349
Cornell Scale for Depression in Dementia, 204
coronary artery disease, 206*t*
coronary atherosclerosis, 405
CPR. *See* cardiopulmonary resuscitation (CPR)
crashes, and older adults, 419
CRNP. *See* certified registered nurse practitioner (CRNP)
crowding, 403–404
CTI. *See* Care Transitions Intervention (CTI)
cultural beliefs, 107
cultural competence, 103, 104

D

daily life
  course of, 25
  goals and priorities for, 374
daily living needs, 68
DC. *See* dementia care (DC)
DD. *See* developmental disability (DD)
death-denying culture, 180
deaths, rates of, 180
decision making, 432
  evidence-based, 3
  healthcare, 436
  medical, 2, 3
  process of, 194
  shared, 3, 3*f*, 10, 134
decisional balance, 298–299
dehydration, 324
delirium, 185–186, 186, 327, 405
  deficit indicative of, 191
  management of symptoms of, 405
Delirium Triage Screen, 407
delirum, 405
dementia, 129, 185, 186, 243, 266, 325, 421
  care and coding, 146
  diagnosis of, 193–194
  epidemic, 185
  individuals with, 421
  patients with, 210
  risk for, 186
dementia care (DC), 142
Dementia Screening Questionnaire for Individuals Intellectual Disabilities (DSQIID), 454
demographic trends, 19–20
  age-friendly cities and communities, 25–26
  charitable giving, 22
  civic engagement, 22
  current and projected aging population growth, 20–21
  disparities in health and life expectancy, 22–24
  gender and sexual orientation, 23
  healthy aging, 20
  income and education, 24
  race and ethnicity, 23–24
  social and economic capital, 21–22
  social network, 24
  spending and working, 21–22
  volunteerism, 22
Department of Motor Vehicles (DMV), 424

deprescribing, medication, 309
  stepwise approach to, 309*t*
depression, 206, 207, 282, 293, 325, 327
  assessment, 197–198
    Beck depression inventory, 203
    challenges and best practices in, 205–206
    differential diagnosis of, 209–210
    Geriatric Depression Scale, 203–204
    of late-life disorders, 198–205
    patient health questionnaire, 200, 201–202*f*
    purpose of, 200
    recommendations for practice, 210–211
  clinical levels of, 205
  consequences of, 207
  diagnosis of, 187
  prevalence and incidence rates of, 109
  recognition of, 110
  screening of, 210
  symptoms of, 204, 205, 209
  unipolar, 209
depressive disorder, 197, 209
  burden of, 198
  diagnosis of, 159
  medical conditions and medications associated with, 206*t*
  occurrence of, 197
developmental disability (DD), 447, 448–449
  algorithm for clinical assessment of people with, 453*f*
  assessing older adults with, 451
  clinical assessment. *See* clinical assessment, developmental disability (DD)
  definition of, 448
  disparities in health and health care for, 448, 451
  guidelines for older adults with, 456–458*t*
  historical societal treatment of people with, 450
  history of, 452
  primary clinical focus, 451
DHQ. *See* Diet History Questionnaire (DHQ)
diabetes mellitus, 419
Diagnostic and Statistical Manual of Mental Disorders (DSM-V) criteria, 186, 198, 292
  for major depressive disorder, 199*t*

diagnostic interview, 205
Diet History Questionnaire
    (DHQ), 328
DIF. *See* differential items
    functioning (DIF)
differential items functioning
    (DIF), 108
dimension of care, 283
direct care providers, 153
disability, 129–130, 266
disaster, 461–462
    acts of terrorism, 465
    earthquakes, 465
    elderly victims, 461–462
    emergency supply kit, 466, 466*t*
    evacuation, 467
    hurricanes, 464–465
    medical information checklist
        and documents, 466
    mortality in, 464
    pet care, 466–467
    practices for response, 470–471
    preparedness policies, 469
    psychiatric, ethical, and social
        needs of elderly victims of,
        467–470
    rapid assessment tool, 465–466
    recovery phase, 467–470
    response registry, 467
    risk factors for harm during, 463
    setting, challenges in, 463–464*t*
    tornados, 465
    types of, 464–465
    vulnerable to effects of,
        462–464
discipline-specific individuals, 16
discrimination, 93
disease management, 1
distress, 282
dizziness, 248
DMV. *See* Department of Motor
    Vehicles (DMV)
do not resuscitate (DNR)
    orders, 436
documentation, 182–183
Down syndrome, 448
driving competency, 422
Driving Health Inventory, 420
driving impairment, role in, 422
driving rehabilitation specialist
    (DRS), 424
Driving Safety Programs, 421
driving skills, 417
drowsiness, 187
DRS. *See* driving rehabilitation
    specialist (DRS)
drug–drug interactions, 307

drugs
    addicts, 294
    interactions with diseases, 236
    screening instruments, 295–296
    use disorder, 292
dually eligible individuals, 117
    functional limitations among, 117*f*
    healthcare spending for, 119
durable powers of attorney for
        health care (DPA-HC),
        432, 434
dying process, 179
Dynamic Gait Index (DGI), 316*t*
dysarthria, 191
dyslipidemia, 160
dysthymia, 198

E

EAI. *See* Elder Assessment
    Instrument (EAI)
ears assessment, 252–253
earthquakes, 465
EAST Geriatric Trauma
    Guidelines, 410
economic insecurity, 116
economic security, 116
ED. *See* emergency department (ED)
ED assessment. *See* emergency
    department (ED)
    assessment
elder abuse, 409
    signs of, 250
Elder Assessment Instrument (EAI),
    222–225, 342–344
elder mistreatment (EM), 215–216,
    409–410
    approach for readers, 227
    assessment for, 217–221
    causes of, 217
    clinical assessment for, 227
    clinical interview, 219
    clinical screening for, 226
    definition of, 215–216
    documentation, 221
    instrument, 222–225
    laboratory and imaging studies,
        219–220
    medical and social consequences
        of, 217
    patient–caregiver interaction,
        218–219
    physical examination of, 219
    practice challenges of, 226
    questions to assess for, 220*f*

    reporting to authorities, 221–222
    risk and vulnerability, 217, 218*f*
    scope and consequences of,
        216–217
    tools for formal screening,
        222–226
elderly individuals, 248
electrolyte disorders, 405
electronic health records (EHRs),
    59, 137, 144, 158, 159,
    160, 400
    adoption of, 128
    system, 56
elevated prevalence, 94
EM. *See* elder mistreatment (EM)
emergency department (ED)
        assessment, 402
    admission decision, 404–412
    challenges to geriatric care in,
        402–403
    cognition, 405–407
    crowding and boarding, 403–404
    elder mistreatment, 409–410
    epidemiology of, 402
    falls, 407–408
    geriatric emergency department
        guidelines, 412
    geriatric trauma, 410–411
    medication management, 409
    pain, 408
    readmissions, 404
    risk assessment for adverse out-
        comes, 411–412
    treatment of common geriatric
        conditions at admission,
        404–405
emergency evacuation plan, 462
Emergency Geriatric Screening
    (EGS) tool, 405, 406*f*
emergency medical services
    (EMS), 183
emergency physicians (EPs), 402
emergency supply kit, 466, 466*t*
emotional burden, 276
EMS. *See* emergency medical
    services (EMS)
encephalopathy, 186
end-of-life
    care, 433
    decisions, 180
    preferences, 180, 182–183
    treatment options, 433
Epidemiologic Catchment Area
    Program, 193
ethnic grouping, 106
ethnic minorities, 104
ethnic prejudice, 93

evacuation, 467
 during hurricane, 464
 problems during, 462
 protocols, 469
evidence-based care transitions
  interventions, 332,
  333–334t
evidence-based decision making, 3
evidence-based education, 151
evidence-based geriatric care,
  fundamentals of, 33
evidence-based hierarchical
  approach, 265
evidence-based models, 32
 geriatrics models of care. See
  geriatrics models of care
 overview, 165–166
eye contact, 243
eyes assessment, 251–252

F

FACIT-Sp-12 tool, 286
fall risk, 293, 359
 assessment, 353
 checklist, 360–362
falls, 327, 407–408
false-positive detection, 210
familismo, 110
Family Caregiver Alliance (2012)
  website, 277
family caregivers (FCs), 81, 166, 236
 demand for, 82
 effective support for, 276
 and healthcare professionals, 86–87
 hospital readmissions and, 85
 implications for, 84–85
 of older adults, 82–83
 perform complex, medical/
  nursing tasks, 83
 presence of, 276
 view of, 276
family context, 81
 CARE Act, 85–86
 family caregivers. See family
  caregivers
family covenant model in eldercare,
  434–435
family members, presence of, 357
family reticence, 356
family-centered care, 81
fatigue, 327
FCs. See family caregivers (FCs)
Federal Emergency Management
  Agency (FEMA), 466

Federal Interagency Forum on
  Aging-Related Statistics, 21
fee for service (FFS), 42, 44
FEMA. See Federal Emergency
  Management Agency
  (FEMA)
fever, defined, 249
FFQ. See food frequency
  questionnaire (FFQ)
FICA tool, 284, 286
financial exploitation, 215, 220f
fluency, 191
Folstein Mini-Mental State
  Examination, 192
food, 324–325
 insecurity, 326
 intake, 324
 lack of, 462
food frequency questionnaire
  (FFQ), 328
formal caregivers, 238
formal coaching, 161
formal religious affiliation, 282
fragmented care, 117
frailty, 165–166, 266, 325, 327
Framingham Heart Study, 248
function, 231
functional ability, 450
functional aging, 450
Functional Assessment of
  Chronic Illness Therapy-
  Spiritual Well-being
  (FACIT-Sp-12), 285
functional assessment of older
  adults, 107–108, 231–232,
  232, 238, 241
 and best practices, 232–233
 case exemplar, 237–238
 elements of, 232
 tools, 233–237
Functional Assessment Staging Test
  (FAST scale), 236–237
functional decline, 366
functional decline and
impairment, 327
functional impairment, 110, 275, 276
functional limitations, 14
functional skills, 423
functional well-being, 232

G

gaining access, home
 barriers to, 355–356
 best practices for, 355

gait assessment, 260–261
gait speed, 315t
GAO. See General Accountability
  Office (GAO)
GCM. See Guided Care Model
  (GCM)
GCN. See guided care nurse
  (GCN)
GDS. See Geriatric Depression
  Scale (GDS)
GEDs. See Geriatric Emergency
  Departments (GEDs)
GEM. See Geriatric and Evaluation
  Management (GEM)
General Accountability Office
  (GAO), 51
genetic differences, 104
genitourinary system and rectal
  examination, 258–259
Geriatric and Evaluation
  Management (GEM), 51,
  170, 172
 model of care, 172
geriatric assessment, 7, 15, 133, 345,
  383–384, 465–466
 of acute change in condition,
  389–398
 care planning, 398, 400
 challenges and opportunities,
  398–400
 comprehensive geriatric assessment (CGA), 388
 goals of, 384–385
 INTERACT care paths, 397f
 interprofessional team approach
  in, 386–387t
 Minimum Data Set, 387–388,
  389t, 390t
 models of, 374
 multiculturalism and. See multiculturalism and geriatric
  assessment
 plan of care, elements, 400t
 Rapid Geriatric Assessment
  (RGA), 388–389, 390–391t
 role of electronic health
 records, 400
 roles of interprofessional team
  members, 385–386
 SBAR, 393–397f
 standard assessments, 399t
 standardized assessments and
  components, 387
 turning assessment into
  action, 398
 types of residents and
  patients, 385f

geriatric care, 283, 324, 417
  challenges to, 402–403
  future directions of, 15–17
  historical perspectives of, 14–15
  models of, 34
  overview of, 9–10
  for people, 449–451
  principles with examples, 10–14
geriatric caregivers, 450–451
Geriatric Depression Scale (GDS),
    203–204, 237
  in geriatric depression assess-
    ment, 204
  limitation of, 204
  Short Form score, 237
Geriatric Emergency Departments
    (GEDs), 408, 412
geriatric evaluation unit (GEU), 51
geriatric evaluations, 52
geriatric health conditions, 14
geriatric hospitals, 50
Geriatric Interdisciplinary Team
    Training (GITT)
  advance care planning, 146
  annual wellness visit (AWV),
    145–146
  chronic care management, 146
  dementia care and coding, 146
  description of, 142–143
  financial challenges, 143
  implementation of, 145
  Medicare codes, 144
  overview, 142
  program for, 142
  teams, 144–145
  workforce challenges, 143–144
Geriatric Interprofessional
    Team Transformation in
    Primary Care (GITT-PC),
    141–142
  components of, 142
geriatric patient, 241
  physical assessment of, 241
geriatric primary care (GPC), 52
Geriatric Research, Education,
    and Clinical Centers
    (GRECCs), 50
Geriatric Resources for Assessment
    and Care of Elders
    (GRACE), 15
  intervention, 335
  model, 172
  team protocol, 345
geriatric syndromes, 244, 449, 463
  assessment and management
    of, 15
geriatric trauma, 410–411

geriatrics
  basic tenet of, 149
  foundational element of, 149
  principles of, 15
  review of systems, 245–246t
geriatrics models of care, 166
  care transitions models, 168–170
  community-based models, 170–173
  components of, 166
  home care models of care, 174
  hospital-based models, 166–168
  long-term care-based models,
    174–175
  strategies to implement, sustain,
    and disseminate, 175–176
GeriPACT, 52
  benefits of, 52
  management, 53
gerontologic nursing, 335
GEU. See geriatric evaluation unit
    (GEU)
GITT. See Geriatric Interdisciplinary
    Team Training (GITT)
GITT-PC model, 144, 146
Glasgow Coma Scale (GCS) score,
    410–411
Global Age-Friendly Cities and
    Communities project, 25
global budget, 43
GRACE. See Geriatric Resources
    for Assessment and Care of
    Elders (GRACE)
GRECCs. See Geriatric Research,
    Education, and Clinical
    Centers (GRECCs)
guided care model, 172
Guided Care Model (GCM), 335
guided care nurse (GCN), 172
guideline-based care, benefits and
    harms of, 10

H

HADS. See Hospital Anxiety and
    Depression Scale (HADS)
hair assessment, 250–251
harm reduction approach, 299
Hartford Insurance Company, 424
HBPC. See home-based primary
    care (HBPC)
head assessment, 251
"heads in beds" mindset, 42
healing relationships, 3
health, 366
  documentation of, 2

Health Insurance Portability
    and Accountability Act
    (HIPAA), 137
health maintenance organizations
    (HMOs), 180
health systems, 32
healthcare. See also patients
  decision making, 436
  delivery models, 15
  evidence-based models of, 32
  heterogeneity of, 9–10
  on per capita basis, 15
  person-centered decision-making
    in, 3f
  policy, development of, 15
  power of attorney, 180
  provider, 151–152
  system, 3, 16, 94–96
  utilization, 185
HealthLeads program's healthcare
    system, 95, 95f
healthy aging, 20, 96, 97f
Healthy People 2020, 90, 232,
    266, 449
hearing function, 233
heart assessment, 255–256
heavy drinking, 292
HELP. See Hospital Elder Life
    Program (HELP)
heroin, 294
heterosexual older adults, 93
Hierarchical Condition Category
    (HCC) predictive
    model, 336
hip surgeries, 44
HIPAA. See Health Insurance
    Portability and
    Accountability Act
    (HIPAA)
HMOs. See health maintenance
    organizations (HMOs)
home care models of care, hospital
    at home, 174
home-based primary care (HBPC),
    51, 53
  demonstration program, 53
  model, 174
homelessness, geriatric population
    living with, 362–363
homeostenosis, 462
homosexuality, 247
HOPE tool, 284
hopelessness, 207
hospital
  admission, 402
  readmission, 345
  setting, medical errors in, 332

Hospital Anxiety and Depression
    Scale (HADS), 205
Hospital Elder Life Program
    (HELP), 15, 168
hospital-based models,
    166–168, 167*t*
hospitalization rate, 403
"hot spotting" approach, 151
household disaster preparedness, 462
housing, 365
hurricane, 464–465
    Katrina, 461–462, 464,
        465–466, 466
    Rita, 464
hypertension, 160
hypomania, 209

I

IADLs. *See* instrumental activities of
    daily living (IADLs)
ICU. *See* intensive care unit (ICU)
ID. *See* intellectual disabilities (ID)
IDD. *See* intellectual development
    disabilities (IDD)
Identification of Seniors at Risk
    (ISAR), 411, 412*f*
IHI. *See* Institute for Healthcare
    Improvement (IHI)
illness, diagnosis and treatment
    of, 90
imagine planning, death, 180
immigration, 356
improvements
    in admission, 404
    model for, 37, 38*f*
    process of, 142
Improving Medicare Post-Acute
    Care Transformation
    (IMPACT) Act, 369
Improving Mood-Promoting Access
    to Collaborative Treatment
    (IMPACT), 159–160
informal caregivers, 238
informed consent doctrine, 433
in-home assessment, 349–350
    best practices of, 351–352
    domains of, 352–355
    fall risk, 353
    family and social network,
        353–354
    geriatric population living with
        homelessness, 362–363
    importance of, 350–351

medications, 352
patient characteristics, 351*f*
practice challenges, 355–357
sample assessment tool or
    approach, 357–362
tools, 353
in-home care resources, 366
Injury Severity Score (ISS), 411
Institute for Healthcare
    Improvement (IHI), 16, 34
instrumental activities of daily living
    (IADLs), 82–83, 107,
    126–127, 233, 237, 244, 368
intellectual development disabilities
    (IDD), 117, 450
intellectual disabilities (ID), 448
intellectual functions, 188, 189
intensive care unit (ICU), 181, 402
    treatments, 438
INTERACT program. *See*
    Interventions to Reduce
    Acute Care Transfers
    (INTERACT) program
interdisciplinary protocols,
    development of, 404
Interdisciplinary Team Training
    in Geriatrics (ITTG)
    programs, 51
interdisciplinary teams, 150
interpersonal assessment
    approach, 267
interprofessional, 142
interprofessional care (IPC), 126
interprofessional collaboration
    (IPC), 135
interprofessional education
    (IPE), 137
interprofessional team,
    high-functioning
    creating and maintaining,
        135–136
    evidence for effectiveness of
        teams, 134–137
    frequency, timing, location,
        structure, and etiquette of
        meetings, 136
    individual to responsible for
        meetings, 136
    interprofessional education, 137
    meetings to, 136–137
    membership, 136
    overview, 133–134
    purpose of, 136
    team effectiveness, measuring, 139
    team-building programs,
        138*t*, 139

technology's role in changing
    teamwork, 137
    training, 137–139
Interventions to Reduce Acute Care
    Transfers (INTERACT)
    program, 174–175, 175*t*
intracranial hemorrhage, 189
IPC. *See* interprofessional care
    (IPC); interprofessional
    collaboration (IPC)
ISAR. *See* Identification of Seniors
    at Risk (ISAR)
ISH. *See* isolated systolic
    hypertension (ISH)
isolated systolic hypertension
    (ISH), 248
ISS. *See* Injury Severity Score (ISS)

J

Joann Briggs Institute, 250
John A. Hartford Foundation, 34,
    67, 161, 181
Joint Commission on Accreditation
    of Healthcare
    Organizations, 332

K

Katrina hurricane, 461–462, 464,
    465–466, 466
Katz Index, 233, 234
"know–do" gap, 36
Kokmen Short Test of Mental Status,
    190
Korotkoff sounds, 248

L

language, 191, 356
large-scale social change, 38, 39*f*
late-life depression (LLD), 197
    assessment of, 198, 199, 210
    overview of, 198
    pharmacologic treatment of, 211
    treatment of, 211
late-life disorders, 198–205
Late-Life Function and Disability
    Instrument (LLFDI),
    316*t*, 317

Lawton Instrumental Activities of Daily Living Scale, 233, 235
leadership, 370
length of stay (LOS), 135
lethargy, 187
licensed drivers, 418
life expectancy, 2f, 14
    disparities in, 91
    risk factors, 449
lifespace questionnaire, 316t
living will, 180, 433
LLD. See late-life depression (LLD)
longevity dividend, 20
longevity for drivers, 419
longitudinal care, 53
long-term care
    assessment for, 385
    post-acute care vs., 385t
    residents, 384
long-term memory, 190
long-term services and supports (LTSS), 82, 117, 118
    dominant source of payment for, 119
    expenditures, 119f
    programs, 115–116, 120
long-term supports and services, 127
LOS. See length of stay (LOS)
Lown Institute, 4
LTSS. See long-term services and supports (LTSS)
lungs assessment, 255–256

M

MAI. See Medication Appropriateness Index (MAI)
major depressive disorder (MDD), 198
    diagnosing, 203–204
    lower rates of, 207
malnutrition, 324
    consequences of, 327
    risk for, 328
manic depression, 209
Maslow's hierarchy of needs, 323–325
mass customization of care, 46, 47f
MCC. See multiple chronic conditions (MCC)
MDD. See major depressive disorder (MDD)

MDS. See Minimum Data Set (MDS)
Meals on Wheels program, 350, 374, 375–376, 375f
Medicaid, 118t
    administrative processes, 119
    assessment data, 121
    funds, 432
    misalignments in, 119
    programs, 116, 310, 351
Medicaid Home and Community Based Services, 350, 368
medical assessment, 75
medical care, advances in, 117
medical comorbidity, 206
medical decision making, 2, 3
medical fitness-to-drive evaluation, 424
medical management, 1
medical needs, 2
medical/nursing tasks, 82–83
Medicare, 91, 118t, 175
    administrative processes, 119
    annual wellness visit, 128
    assessment data, 121
    beneficiaries, 181, 310
    codes, 143–144
    coverage of advanced care planning, 17
    fee-for-service approach, 126
    fee-for-service beneficiaries, 127
    funds, 432
    health maintenance organizations (HMOs), 150
    inpatient readmissions, 85
    insured population, 21
    misalignments in, 119
    payment codes, 181
    programs, 15, 116
    and value-based purchasing, 84–85
Medicare Coordinated Care Demonstration, 151
Medication Appropriateness Index (MAI), 307–308
    elements of, 308, 308t
medication assessment in older adults, 236, 305–306
    adherence, 310
    challenges, 310–311
    deprescribing, 309
    goal of, 305
    importance of polypharmacy, 306
    management, 336, 409
    reconciliation process, 307t
    stepwise approach to deprescribing, 309t
    tools, 306–310

Medication Discrepancy Tool, 336
medication reconciliation, 306, 310
    process for, 306, 307t
medication-related adverse effects, 306
memory
    assessment of, 190
    second component of, 190
    self-reports of, 190
mental health assessment, 454
mental status examination, 188–189, 190
    attention and level of consciousness, 190–191
    components of, 191
    higher cognitive functions, 189–190
    language, 191
    memory, 190
    standardized brief assessments, 192–193
    writing and construction ability, 191–192
mental status screening instruments, 193
mental status testing, fundamental beginning to, 191
metabolic disturbances, 206t
MEWS. See Modified Early Warning Score (MEWS)
Mill Act, 51
Mini Cog test, 109, 192
Mini-Mental State Examination (MMSE), 108–109, 407, 420
    screening, 192
Minimum Data Set (MDS), 369, 387–388, 389t, 390t
Mini-Nutritional Assessment-Short Form (MNA-SF), 327–328
mixed and undetermined pain, 272t
MMSE. See Mini-Mental State Examination (MMSE)
MNA-SF. See Mini-Nutritional Assessment-Short Form (MNA-SF)
mobility, 241, 276, 313, 418. See also mobility assessment
    characteristics of, 317
    disability, 317
    higher-level, 314
    impairments and suggested measures, 317, 318t
    problems, 314
    selection of, 317

mobility assessment, 313
  challenges, 319–320
  clinical characteristics of, 317
  definition and epidemiology, 314
  measures of, 314–317,
    317, 318*t*
  "one size fits all" approach
    to, 314
  performance and self-report-
    based tools, 315–316*t*
MoCA. *See* Montreal Cognitive
  Assessment (MoCA)
models of care, 166
Modified Early Warning Score
  (MEWS), 411
Montreal Cognitive Assessment
  (MoCA), 109, 192, 236
mood assessment scale, 204–205
mood symptoms, 199
morbidity, 186
mortality, 135, 186
  in disasters, 464
motivational interviewing
  techniques, 355
motor vehicle crashes (MVC),
  419, 420
MU Sinclair School of Nursing, 367
multiculturalism and geriatric
  assessment, 103–104
  communication with ethnically
    diverse older adults, 106
  depression assessment, 109–110
  eliciting beliefs and attitudes
    about illness, 107
  heterogeneity within older ethnic
    minority groups, 104–105
  reliability, validity, and use of
    instruments for ethnic
    minorities, 105–106
  selected domains of, 107–109
  social and economic issues in,
    110–111
multimorbidity, 157, 306
multiple chronic conditions
  (MCC), 74
musculoskeletal system, 256–257
MVC. *See* motor vehicle crashes
  (MVC)

N

nails assessment, 250–251
National Health and Aging Trends
  Study, 244

National Health and Nutrition
  Examination Survey
  (NHANES), 248, 325
National Institute on Alcohol Abuse
  and Alcoholism, 298
National Long-Term Care
  Ombudsman Resource
  Center, 222
National Transitions of Care
  Coalition (NTOCC), 346
natural disasters. *See* disaster
neck assessment, 254–255
need for transparency, 4
neglect, 191, 215, 220*f*, 221*t*,
  244, 357
neighborhood conditions, 355
nervous system assessment,
  259–260
neurocognitive disorder, diagnostic
  criteria for, 187
neurologic disorders, 206*t*, 448
neuropathic pain, 272*t*
neuropsychological function, 193
New Ways for Better Days Tailored
  Activity Program, 374,
  379–380
New York City Human Rights Law
  for employees, 26
NHANES. *See* National Health and
  Nutrition Examination
  Survey (NHANES)
no personal control, 467
nociplastic pain, 271*t*
non-caregiver peers, 276
nonclinical care providers, 153
"normal" aging, 206
nose assessment, 253
NTOCC. *See* National Transitions of
  Care Coalition (NTOCC)
nurse-led management, meta-
  analysis of, 160
Nurses Improving Care for
  Healthsystem Elders
  (NICHE), 15, 168
nursing facilities, 383
nursing homes, 384
  geriatric assessments in, 385
nutritional assessment, 323–324
  health outcomes from under-nu-
    trition, 326–327
  tools, 327–328
  under-nutrition in older adults,
    324–326
nutritional deficiencies, 324
nutritional status, assessment
  of, 324

O

OAs. *See* older adults (OAs)
obesity, 324
  rate of, 450
older adult driver, 417–418
  Alzheimer's disease, 421–422
  assessing driving skills, 422–423
  behaviors and characteristics of,
    418–419
  crashes, 419
  crashes and older adults, 419
  dementia, 421–422
  driving retirement, 423
  ethical, legal, and policy issues, 424
  future trends in older adult
    mobility, 424–425
  mild cognitive impairment,
    421–422
  normal aging, 421–422
  older-driving safety behaviors, 419
  risk for motor vehicle crash,
    419–421
older adults (OAs), 197, 232,
    365, 402
  ability of, 373
  aging, 369
  AIP models for, 366
  aspect of care for, 74
  assessment of, 104
  challenging for, 373
  chronic conditions of, 9
  crashes and, 419
  with DD, 448
  dietary intakes of, 327
  as drivers, 424. *See also* older
    adult driver
  driving-related abilities in, 421
  examination of, 242
  functional status of, 232
  generation care planning for, 2
  health care for, 1
  healthcare regime for, 1
  illness severity, 403
  with impaired functional
    status, 403
  life expectancy improvements in
    the 20th century, 2*f*
  pain assessment and manage-
    ment in, 267
  pain experience in, 266
  personal goals, 2
  personal need for, 1
  postural hypotension in, 248
  psychosocial concerns for, 467

self-determination for, 451
sense of continuity for, 291
"sixth vital sign" for, 317
source of transportation for, 417
vulnerability in. *See* vulnerable
　populations
Older Americans Act, 118*t*, 119
older patients, initial impression
　of, 241
"one size fits all" solutions, 10
Open Notes, 60
　deployment of, 61
　documentation, 60
　medical records, 56
　patient portals with, 57
　policy, 61
　use of, 57
opioids, 291, 293
optimal care, 408
optimal team care outcomes
　changing healthcare system and
　　practice model, 128–129
　epidemiological challenges of
　　demographic changes,
　　126–127
　older adults benefit from,
　　129–130
　overview, 125–126
oral cavity assessment, 253–254
oral problems, 324
Osler maneuver, 247
osteoporosis, 449
Outcome and Assessment
　Information Set
　(OASIS-C2), 237
over-the-counter (OTC)
　medications, 306

P

8P Risk Assessment and
　General Assessment of
　Preparedness, 336
PACT. *See* Patient-Aligned Care
　Teams (PACT)
pain, 282, 408
　assessment. *See* pain assessment
　evaluation of, 269
　homeostenosis, 266
　management, 408, 409
pain assessment, 265–266, 452
　barriers and facilitators, 270–271
　demographics and prevalence
　　of, 266

effects on older adults' health,
　266–267
hierarchy of, 268*t*
importance of, 266–267
non-self-reporting individuals,
　269, 270*t*
practices, 267–270
self-reporting individuals,
　267, 268*t*
types of, 271–272*t*
Pain Assessment Checklist for
　Seniors with Limited
　Ability to Communicate
　(PACSLAC-II), 452
Palliative and Advanced Illness
　Research (PAIR) Center, 181
palliative care, 130, 286
Parkinson's disease, 317
partial or full capitation, 43
Patient Health Questionnaire
　(PHQ), 200, 201–202*f*, 237
patient needs, customization based
　on, 3
Patient Priorities Care, 70
Patient Self-Determination Act
　(PSDA), 180, 432
Patient-Aligned Care Teams
　(PACT), 52
"patient-centered" care over, 68
Patient-Reported Outcome
　Measurement Information
　System (PROMIS), 455
patient-reported outcome measures
　(PROMs), 58
patients. *See also* older adults (OAs)
　care, information technology
　　in, 332
　counseling, 335
　empowerment, 3
　needs and priorities of, 10
　vs. person-centered, 6–7
　self-assessment of, 359
　as source of control, 3
　voice, rules for ensuring, 3–4
Patient's Bill of Rights since 1979, 448
pay for performance, 43
payment bundling incentivizes,
　42, 42*f*
payment reform, 41–42
　bundling, 42–43, 42*f*
　joints, 43–47
PCP. *See* primary care provider (PCP)
PECs. *See* preexisting conditions
　(PECs)
Per capita Medicare, 6*f*
perceived clinical barriers, 71

performance testing, 319
performance-based assessment
　tools, 315–316*t*
performance-based outcomes, 319
performance-based road test, 421
peripheral nociceptive pain, 271*t*
persistent depressive disorder, 198
　diagnosis of, 198
persistent or chronic pain, 271*t*
person and family-centered, 3
personal health record (PHR), 56
person-centered care, 2, 68, 69, 81, 119
　approach, 66
　decision-making in healthcare,
　　3, 3*f*
　principles of, 7
person-centered, patient- *vs.*, 6–7
person-centeredness, 16
person-environment fit, 350
pet care, 466–467
Pew Charitable Trust, 150
pharmacies, 310–311
PHQ. *See* Patient Health
　Questionnaire (PHQ)
PHQ-9 depression screener, 207
PHR. *See* personal health record
　(PHR)
physical abuse, 215, 220*f*, 221*t*
physical assessment, 241–242,
　247–261
　of abdomen, 257–258
　approach to geriatric patient,
　　242–243
　of breasts, 258
　of ears, 252–253
　of eyes, 251–252
　of gait and balance, 260–261
　of genitourinary system and rec-
　　tal examination, 258–259
　of geriatric patient, 241
　of hair and nails, 250–251
　of head, 251
　of heart and lungs, 255–256
　of height, weight, and nutrition,
　　249–250
　history taking, 243–244
　of musculoskeletal system,
　　256–257
　of neck, 254–255
　of nervous system, 259–260
　of nose, 253
　of oral cavity, 253–254
　practice challenges of, 261
　sexual health assessment, 244–247
　of skin, 250
　of vital signs, 247–249

physical burden, 276
physical disability, 325
physical examination, 241
physical therapy, 410
physician orders for life-sustaining
        treatment (POLST), 180,
        432, 436
    forms, 183, 437–439
physician resistance, 59
physician-centric model, 143
plan of care, elements, 400*t*
policymakers, 15
POLST. *See* physician orders for
        life-sustaining treatment
polypharmacy, 306, 420
population, 67, 103
    based norms, 192
    health strategies, 166
    in United States, 165
post-acute care, 383, 384
    assessment in, 385
    vs. long-term care, 385*t*
post-hospitalization
        rehabilitation, 384
post-traumatic stress disorder
        (PTSD), 181, 469
potential abuse, 357
poverty, 368
    status among older adults,
        116, 116*f*
practice model, 128*f*
preexisting conditions (PECs), 411
preparedness, household
        disaster, 462
presbycusis, 57
prescription drug plans, 310
preventive health, 455
primary care
    internal medicine programs, 143
    lack of, 403
    multi-site study in, 292
primary care provider (PCP), 158,
        159, 161, 207, 345
prognosis, 182
Program of All-Inclusive Care for
        the Elderly (PACE), 15,
        33, 170
Project RED discharge, 336
Project Re-Engineered Discharge
        (Project RED), 335
PROMIS. *See* Patient-Reported
        Outcome Measurement
        Information System
        (PROMIS)
PROMs. *See* patient-reported
        outcome measures (PROMs)

PSDA. *See* Patient Self-
        Determination Act (PSDA)
psychiatric assessment schedule for
        adults with developmental
        disabilities (PAS-ADD), 454
psychiatric consultants, 211
psychological abuse, 215, 220*f*
psychosocial stressors, 206
PTSD. *See* post-traumatic stress
        disorder (PTSD)
public health, advances in, 127
public transportation, 93
PULSES Profile, 236

Q

Quadruple Aim, 147
quality improvement (QI)
        indicators, 408
quality of care for geriatric
        conditions, 158–159
quality of health and life, 7
quality of life, 15, 266, 350, 369,
        385, 419
quality pain care practice, 265
quality-based payment, 3–4

R

racism, 93
    negative health effects of, 94
Rand Corporation, 126
rapid assessment tool, disaster,
        465–466
Rapid Geriatric Assessment (RGA),
        388–389, 390–391*t*
readiness ruler, 299
real-time records, 129
Receiver Operator Characteristic
        curve (ROC), 109
red flags, 168
referrals, 424
    for treatment, 299
registered nurse (RN), 145–146, 174,
        350, 366, 367
Rehabilitation Act Amendments of
        1978, 447–448
reimbursement, 143
religion, 285
religious beliefs, 243
remote memory, 190
residential care communities, 368

respiration, 249
response registry, disaster, 467
"retail" approach, 42
RGA. *See* Rapid Geriatric
        Assessment (RGA)
risk, 217
    behavior, 292
Rita hurricane, 464
RN. *See* registered nurse (RN)
road performance tests, 422
Rogers' diffusion of innovation,
        35*f*, 36
"rolling" assessment, 193, 450
routine depression screening, 199

S

safety as system property, 4
Saint Louis University Mental Status
        Exam, 190
sarcopenia, 326
screening, 198
Screening, Brief Intervention, and
        Referral for Treatment
        (SBIRT), 294
    intervention, 298, 299
    interventions, 300
    model, 298, 299
Screening Tool of Older People's
        Prescriptions (STOPP)
        criteria, 307, 309
Screening Tool to Alert to Right
        Treatment (START) criteria,
        307, 309
SDOH. *See* social determinants of
        health (SDOH)
seizure disorders, 419, 448
self-care, 73–74
    best practices of, 75–76
    and older adults, 74–75
    practice challenges, 76
    problems, 354–355
self-efficacy, 3
self-management, 73–74, 126
    assessment of, 76–77
    "four pillars" of, 336
    interventions of, 74
self-report, 317, 452
    assessment tools, 315–316*t*
    measures of mobility, 319
    pain, 269
semi-structured diagnostic
        interview, 205
sensory problems, 354–355

sexual abuse, 215, 220*f*, 221*t*
sexual activity, patterns of, 246
sexual history, components of, 246
shared decision making, 3, 3*f*,
    10, 134
shared knowledge, 3
shared risk/shared savings, 43
shared savings, 43
Short Physical Performance Battery
    (SPPB), 315*t*
Short Portable Mental
    Status Questionnaire
    (SPMSQ), 109
short-term acute care, 150
short-term memory, 210
Sinclair Home Care, 367
situation, background, assessment,
    and recommendation
    (SBAR), 393–397*f*
6-Minute Walk Test, 316*t*
skill demonstration, 354
skilled nursing facilities (SNFs), 44,
    383, 410
skin
    assessment, 250
    problems, 326
    tags, 250
sleep disorders, 419
Snellen chart, 233
SNFs. *See* skilled nursing facilities
    (SNFs)
sniff test, 354
social determinants of health
    (SDOH), 89–90, 90, 91,
    117–118
    access to comprehensive health
        services, 90–91
    addressing, 94–96
    broader policy changes, 96
    discrimination based on race and
        ethnicity, 93–94
    food insecurity, 92
    housing and neighborhood
        settings, 92–93
    payment models, 96
    poverty and economic stability,
        91–92
    social isolation, 94
social differences, 104
social history information, 221
social movement theory, 37
Social Security, 326
social support, 121
social work assessment, 350
social workers, 90
social/social support assessment, 455

solar lentigenes, 250
soliciting, importance of, 3–4
specific care processes, 158
spiritual assessment, 281–282,
    282–283
    difficulties in performing, 286
    practice challenges in perform-
        ing, 285–286
    spirituality and health
        outcomes, 282
    tools, 283–285, 284*t*, 286
spiritual beliefs, 243
spiritual care, 282, 286
Spiritual Distress Assessment Tool
    (SDAT), 285
spiritual history, 283
spiritual needs, 285
spiritual suffering, 282
spiritual well-being, 282
spirituality, 243, 281
    comprehensive assessment
        of, 286
    definition of, 281–282
    exploration of, 283
standardized assessment tools, 336
standardized patient assessment
    data, 369
Stanford Chronic Disease Self-
    Management Program, 76
Stanford Medicine, 75
static visual acuity, 420
"Stop and Watch" early warning
    tool, 392, 392*f*
Stopping Elderly Accidents, Deaths,
    and Injuries (STEADI)
    toolkit, 369
stroke, 405
structured diagnostic interview, 205
subpar housing, 92
substance use assessment,
    291–294, 292
    alcohol screening instruments, 295
    brief discussion of brief
        intervention, 297–298
    decisional balance, 298–299
    drug screening instruments,
        295–296
    practice challenges, 299–300
    readiness ruler, 299
    referral for treatment, 299
    screening, brief intervention, and
        referral for treatment, 294
    team-based approaches to,
        299–300
subsyndromal depressive
    conditions, 210

suicide, 207–209
    assessment of, 207
    cases of, 207
    rate of, 109
    risk, 207–208
    screener, 208–209*f*
super-utilizers, 151
support, potential sources of, 71*f*
suppressed immune function, 327
swallowing, 324
systematic assessment, 231

T

Tailored Caregiver Assessment
    and Referral (TCARE)
    system, 278
team
    formation, phases of, 135
    maintenance, 136
    transformation, 142, 145
team building
    programs, 139
    resources for, 138*t*
team care on quality and
    outcomes, 158
    approaches to, 161
    best practices, 158–159
    co-management, 160–161
    Improving Mood-Promoting
        Access to Collaborative
        Treatment (IMPACT),
        159–160
    models, 160, 161
    overview, 157–158
    practice challenges, 161–162
team effectiveness, measuring, 139
team-based care, 135, 159
terminal illnesses, 282
tertiary referral centers, 421
therapeutic nihilism, 198
thriving in community, 373–374
    advancing better living for elders,
        376–379
    care of persons with dementia, 379
    community based services
        program, 374–375
    meals on wheels, 375–376
    models of aging, 374
    practice challenges of, 380–381
    tailoring activities for persons
        with dementia and
        caregivers, 379–380
    veteran-directed home, 374–375

TigerPlace, 367–368, 370
Timed Up and Go (TUG) test,
    236, 315*t*
TJR. *See* total joint replacement (TJR)
"top down" approach, 158
tornados, 465
total joint replacement (TJR), 43–47
    at Kaiser Permanente, 44, 45*f*
    today, 44–45
    tomorrow, 46–47
    yesterday, 44
toxins, detection of, 219
traditional nursing home, 370
tranquilizers, 291
transient ischemic attack, 405
transitional care model (TCM),
    170, 335
transitional care nurse, 336
transitions of care, 331–332,
    342–344*t*
    in era of value-based care,
        332–336
    key factors of, 332
    patient assessment in, 336,
        337–341*t*, 345
    resources for healthcare
        professionals, 346
transparency, need for, 4
transportation
    alternative means of, 418
    alternative modes of, 423
    modes of, 418
    older adults source of, 417
    options, 93
Trauma Quality Improvement
    Program (TQIP), 410
treatment, referral for, 299
treat-to-target approach, 211
Triple Aim, 31, 42

U

under-nutrition, 324, 326
    causes of, 324
    health consequences of, 326
    symptoms of, 324–325
understandable confusion, 32
unipolar depression, diagnosis
    of, 209
University of California, Los
    Angeles (UCLA) program,
    160, 172–173

U.S. healthcare system, 14
U.S. Preventive Services Task
    Force, 199

V

VA. *See* Veterans Affairs (VA)
VA Community Living Centers, 50
VA health system for older adults,
    49–52
    geriatric evaluation in, 52–54
value-based payment, 3–4
value-based (person-centered)
    care, 4
value-based purchasing (VBP),
    84–85
Values History, 432, 435–437,
    442–445
    clinical use of, 436–437
    preferences section, 435–436
    values section, 435
values, patient, 3
Vanderbilt Kennedy Center
    for Excellence in
    Developmental
    Disabilities, 454
VBP. *See* value-based purchasing
    (VBP)
Veteran-Directed Home and
    Community Based Services
    Program, 374–375
Veterans Administration
    system, 129
Veterans Administration (VA)
    hospital, 310
Veterans Affairs (VA), 49–52
Veterans Bureau, 49
Veterans Health Administration
    (VHA), 50
Veterans Millennium Benefits Act,
    Public Law 106-180, 51
VHA. *See* Veterans Health
    Administration (VHA)
vicarious traumatization, 470
VIEWS. *See* VitalPac Early Warning
    Score (VIEWS)
virtual team, 137
visual evaluation of house, 354
visual function, aspects of, 233
visual impairment, 419
VitalPac Early Warning Score
    (VIEWS), 411

VITALtalk, 184
vitamins, deficiencies of, 326
volume over value, 42
volunteerism, 22
vulnerability, 217
    to stressors in older
        population, 462
vulnerable older adults, 115
vulnerable populations
    clinical and functional
        characteristics, 117
    data for policymaking and pro-
        gram planning, 120–121
    definition of, 116
    economic characteristics, 116
    older adults, 118–120
    overview, 115–116
    programmatic issues and practice
        challenges, 121–122
    social determinants of health,
        117–118
    socioeconomic and health-related
        factors, 115

W

walking, 313
    difficulties of, 314
    epidemiology of, 314
warm handoff, 299, 356
Washington University Road Test
    (WURT), 422
water, lack of, 462
weight loss, 326
well-being
    of community residents, 96
    component of, 130
    functional, 232
    in older age, 20
    optimal, 98
    optimize function and, 53
    perceptions of, 20, 22
    sense of, 249
WURT. *See* Washington University
    Road Test (WURT)

Z

Zung Self-Rating Depression
    Scale, 205